注：本书彩图请登陆以下网址下载：Http://www.kbooks.cn/books/systems-biomedicine/

Systems Biomedicine
Concepts and Perspectives

系统生物医学
概念与展望

Edited by

Edison T. Liu and Douglas A. Lauffenburger

科学出版社
北京

图字:01-2010-4560 号

This is an annotated version of

Systems Biomedicine:Concepts and Perspectives
Edited by Edison T. Liu and Douglas A. Lauffenburger.

Copyright © 2010, Elsevier Inc.
ISBN 13: 978-0-12-372550-9

All rights reserved.
No part of this publication may be reproduced or transmitted in any form or by any means, electronic or mechanical, including photocopy, recording, or any information storage and retrieval system, without permission in writing from the publisher.

AUTHORIZED EDITION FOR SALE IN P. R. CHINA ONLY
本版本只限于在中华人民共和国境内销售

图书在版编目(CIP)数据

系统生物医学:概念与展望＝Systems Biomedicine:Concepts and Perspectives:英文/(新加坡)刘(Liu,E.T.)等编著. —北京:科学出版社,2010
  ISBN 978-7-03-028814-1

Ⅰ.①系… Ⅱ.①刘… Ⅲ.①生物医学工程-英文 Ⅳ.①R318

中国版本图书馆 CIP 数据核字(2010)第 168326 号

责任编辑:孙红梅　李小汀/责任印制:钱玉芬/封面设计:耕者设计工作室

斜 学 出 版 社 出版
北京东黄城根北街 16 号
邮政编码:100717
http://www.sciencep.com

北京佳信达欣艺术印刷有限公司 印刷
科学出版社发行　各地新华书店经销
*

2011 年 1 月第 一 版　开本:787×1092　1/16
2011 年 1 月第一次印刷　印张:28 1/2
印数:1—1 800　字数:675 000

定价:**108.00 元**
(如有印装质量问题,我社负责调换)

系统生物医学领域的一本切合时宜的好书

——评《系统生物医学：概念与展望》

陶生策

(上海交通大学系统生物医学研究院，上海，200240，E-mail：taosc@sjtu.edu.cn)

在过去的半个多世纪中，生命科学领域最为重要的发现莫过于 DNA 双螺旋结构的提出。在 DNA 双螺旋结构的基础上发展起来的分子生物学和其他相关实验手段则极大地加速了生命科学的进程，阐明了生命系统中的无数分子事件，生命科学也已从单基因、单蛋白质层面的研究转向了组学研究。这些组学研究包括基于大规模 DNA 测序的基因组分析、基于 DNA 芯片的表达谱分析、基于质谱的蛋白质组学研究，以及基于对代谢产物进行系统性分析的代谢组学研究等。组学研究的共同特点是可以在较短时间内产生海量数据，对这些数据的分析和深度发掘上的迫切需求促使包括生物学、计算机科学、化学甚至物理学等各个不同学科的专家坐到一起。对各类组学数据的整合，使得从系统层次来理解生物学问题成为可能，而且必要。在此基础上形成了一门迅速崛起的学科——系统生物学 (Systems Biology)。

系统生物学着眼于从系统角度认识和理解生命。试图从系统水平理解和阐明生命现象并非一个全新的理念，早在 20 世纪中叶以 Wiener 为代表的科学家就开始了最初的探索，但是由于缺乏有效的研究手段，他们不能从分子水平了解生命系统的细节，因此这些最初尝试的结果并不理想。由于生物学的进步，包括分子生物学在内的新技术手段的飞速发展，人们从来没有像今天这样对生命现象背后的分子机制有如此深刻的理解。因此，在试图从系统水平理解生命现象方面，虽然现代系统生物学并非首发，但的确是第一次试图将这种系统水平的理解建立在扎实、详尽、多层次的实验数据的坚实基础之上。那么，到底什么是现代意义上的系统生物学呢？一个比较公认的定义是由系统生物学创始人 Leory Hood 所给出的：在过去的 30 年中成功的生物学研究方式是一次只研究一个基因或者一个蛋白质，系统生物学与此不同，它所研究的是一个鲜活的生物系统中全部组分的行为和相互关系。系统生物学的终极目的是在系统性实验和分析的基础上，建立有效的数学模型，实现对生命系统的有效控制和设计。

在系统生物学的基础上，结合对中医药的深刻理解，陈竺院士最早在国内提出了系统生物医学 (Systems biomedicine) 的理念。其核心是以现代生物学研究手段为基础，以系统生物学的理论和方法，结合传统中医药的哲学思想和经验，研究临床医学实践中产生的重大科学问题，为实现预测、预防、参与和个体化医学做出实质性贡献。系统生物学和系统生物医学是新兴学科，尚在飞速的发展过程之中，目前国内的系统生物医学专门研究机构有陈竺院士领衔的上海交通大学系统生物医学研究院和程京院士领衔的清华大学医学系统生物学研究所，以及新近刚成立的北京大学系统生物医学研究所。

由新加坡基因组研究所 Edison T. Liu 和麻省理工学院的 Douglas A. Lauffenburger 主编的《系统生物医学：概念与展望》（*Systems Biomedicine: Concepts and Perspectives*）是系统生物医学领域的第一本专著，该书由数十位活跃在系统生物学领域的一流专家参与编写，内容精炼，囊括了系统生物医学的几个主要方面的最新进展。该书由三部分，共 18 章组成。第一部分为系统生物学的生物学基础，介绍了系统生物医学研究的概况以及系统生物学研究中的一些核心技术手段，具体包括基因组学技术，蛋白质组学技术等。同时还介绍了系统生物学研究的一些重要实例：细胞调节网络研究，microRNA 和转录因子调节网络，整合素调节的细胞附着中的蛋白质网络以及干细胞生物学研究等。第二部分为系统生物学中的计算和建模。重点介绍了系统生物学对计算和建模方面所带来的需求和挑战。作为案例，还介绍了虚拟细胞项目以及一些用于系统生物学数据处理的软件。第三部分介绍了系统生物学的应用。分别从生理组学（physiome）、发育、免疫、癌症研究、药物开发以及定量生物学等六个方面，以最新的研究为实例进行了介绍。

作者从系统生物医学的概念入手，将系统生物医学作为一个有机的整体，从生物学基础、计算和建模以及具体的应用三个方面进行了精炼的介绍。

本书切合时宜，适合作为研究生课程的教科书或参考书，对于从事基础医学和临床医学、高通量生物学、生物信息学以及生物系统集成的教学和科研人员均有重要的参考价值。

目 录

概论 ······ VII

I：系统生物学基础
1. 系统生物医学的基础：导言 ······ 3
2. 系统生物学中的基因组学技术 ······ 15
3. 蛋白质组学技术 ······ 45
4. 细胞调控网络 ······ 57
5. MicroRNA 与转录因子相互作用网络 ······ 109
6. 与整合素介导的黏附相关的蛋白质网络 ······ 139
7. 系统生物学和干细胞生物学 ······ 153

II：系统生物学中的计算建模
8. 系统生物学的发展对计算的挑战 ······ 177
9. 对生物系统的高层次建模 ······ 225
10. 系统生物学中的系统分析 ······ 249
11. 可视化细胞项目 ······ 273
12. 系统生物学中的软件工具 ······ 289

III：系统生物学的应用
13. 系统生物学中的生理组标记语言：模型的模块化和重复利用 ······ 317
14. 用于发育模式研究的系统化途径 ······ 329
15. 免疫建模在药物开发中的应用 ······ 351
16. 系统药学用于癌症研究 ······ 377
17. 药物开发中的系统生物学：利用预测生物医学来指导新型抗癌药物的研发 ······ 399
18. 定量生物学在临床实验中的地位和作用 ······ 415

索引 ······ 425

（陶生策　译）

概 论

Douglas Lauffenburger

对于什么是系统生物学，有多种不同的理解。Leory Hood 领导的系统生物学研究所的定义是："传统的生物学往往一次只研究一个特定的基因或者蛋白质，这一研究模式在过去的 30 年中取得了巨大的成功，而系统生物学则与此不同，系统生物学所试图研究的是有功能的生物系统中所有组分的行为和相互关系。"[Ideker et al.，2001]。美国国立卫生研究院国家通用医学研究中心的［NIH，2006］定义则是："系统生物学是一种新的多学科交叉研究模式，涉及到的学科包括生物学、数学、计算机科学、物理学以及工程学等。生物系统都非常复杂，即使采用当今最强的计算模型也不足以捕获生物系统的所有特性。一个有用的模型应该能够对所研究的系统进行准确的概念化并能进行可靠的预测。为了达到这一目的，我们必须进行简化，从而可以专注于我们所感兴趣的系统行为而忽略其他的细节。"以上两种定义非常清楚地认识到了生物系统复杂性的几个互补的侧面：前者强调需要同时研究的组分的数目，而后者则关注了定量预测能力，对系统组分、特性以及相互作用的概念性简化"。在我们看来，由于生物系统的复杂性和多维性，上述两种定义所强调的两个方面均很重要。为了能够预测性地理解分子组分的特性是如何决定细胞、组织、器官和机体的表型和行为，科学家和工程师必须将多个相互作用的组分以及与这些组分相关的定量信息整合到一起。此外，通过对生物系统组分和其相互作用的计算机建模能够使我们对生物系统的预测性理解达到一个更高的层次，而非靠单纯的直觉，并能够有助于假设的提出和检验。

由于这本书所关注的是系统生物学在医学方面的应用，我们需要考虑生物系统的第三维复杂性。这一维的复杂性代表的是需要将对分子过程的分析从简单的细胞培养实验系统上升到组织和器官层次，以及个体（患者）甚至群体层次。基因组学正在努力地将基因序列和表达信息同人的病理生理状态进行关联，毫无疑问的是，实现这一关联必须要通过建立计算机模型将基因组、蛋白质组与控制细胞功能的分子网络进行整合，然后将建立的模型推广到更大的空间尺度和时间尺度，并最终在分子水平上实现对机体的病理生理状态的预测。生物系统复杂性的三维概念如图所示（这一概念最初由 Peter Sorger 在 MIT 的计算与系统生物学讨论会上提出）。

在本书中，我们将对系统生物医学进行介绍和讨论，它是一种生物医学研究的全新手段。系统生物医学试图对生命系统中的分子和细胞过程的复杂的变量

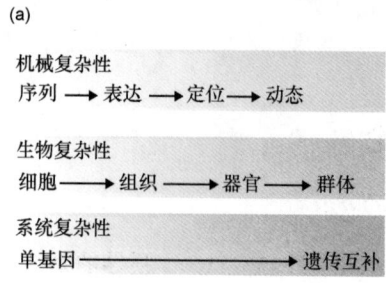
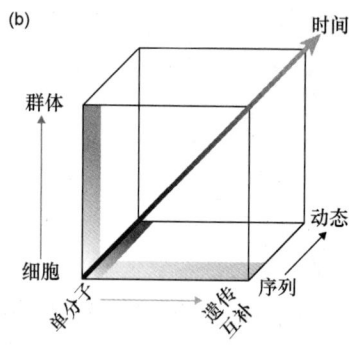

进行推断、标注和定量。系统生物医学的终极目的是针对生命系统建立模型，通过模型准确地预测系统对特定输入的反应。系统性的研究方式有如下几个特点：

1. 追求定量的和精确的数据；
2. 追求数据的完整性和全面性；
3. 关注系统各个组分之间的关联和网络；
4. 愿意定义、测量和操控生物系统的复杂性；
5. 有兴趣在计算（定量）的基础上去预测系统的反应。

　　当然，读者会说历史上所有的生物学研究都具有上述特点。任何以寻找隐藏的规律或模型为目的，对科学观察进行测量和系统化的努力，都将使得科学家能够对生物系统的结果进行预测。然而，正在发生的技术和实验手段的变革将会深刻地影响生物学研究的模式。全基因组序列使得我们能够了解一个物种的全部遗传信息。以表达谱芯片、多通道流式细胞技术以及高通量筛选为代表的多重分析能够提供精确和全面的数据。已有的和发展中的计算能足以应付基于计算模型的推论和预测，即便是系统的数量级（系统中的组分和相互作用关系的数目）和其相关的数据在持续增长。系统生物学与还原论生物学的区别在于我们能够分析复杂的数据以及由于数据的完整性所能达到的更高分析精度。

　　此外，系统生物学是一门快速发展的新学科，有非常快的更新速度。基于此，我们将本书组织成了一系列相关的章节，主要描述策略和过程。对于不同的主题，我们在不同的章节中会有深度的讨论并且鼓励争论。我们将主要澄清实事和强调概念，而非罗列过时知识。从这本备受期待的系统生物学著作将会衍生出许多东西，在本书中，我们讨论的范畴从模式系统，到人体生物学以及药学；我们将重点关注系统性研究手段在医学问题上的应用。读者也许会提出真正的系统性手段需要精确的数学模型，然而，由于在人体实验的复杂性，我们将讨论从系统生物学、系统定量到假设产生等更广泛的相关概念。

　　最后，我们将对系统生物医学进行进一步的讨论。通常，最合理的研究方式是针对简单并能被精确界定的模式系统进行研究，然后针对这些系统进行计算机建模，这些模式系统包括噬菌体、细菌以及酵母等。但现在的情况是，这样的系统性研究策略可用于更复杂的哺乳动物系统甚至是人类疾病，这类系统性研究必然与以原核生物为模型所进行的研究有所不同，并且可能不全面，其原因在于前者的解空间比后者的要大上几个数量级。尽管如此，研究者已经在包括药物开发在内的多个方面，进行了积极的尝试，并且取得了不错的效果。

我们在组织编写这本书时尽可能地体现实验生物学和医学研究的系统性策略的特点：全面（即使不能穷尽）地并定量地测量；针对所研究的系统采用定量的数据去建立模型；并且将复杂性作为一个实验依赖性变量。最终，我们将尝试将这些原则应用于生物医学问题研究。

我们是以记叙的方式来组织编写这本书的，而非简单地罗列一些没有相互关联的条目或章节。虽然无法预计读者将最终从这本书中学到什么，我们还是建议读者从第一章系统生物医学的概念性介绍开始，按照记叙文的方式按章节的排列顺序来阅读这本书。

这本书的第一部分介绍了实验基础。首先是基因组学技术（第二章）和蛋白质组学技术（第三章）的总结性介绍，这两项技术是所有观察和测量的基础，相关的计算模型源于此并且最终将被这两项技术所验证。第四章和第五章描述了调节细胞对外界输入作出何种反应的分子网络，这些分子网络是将要发展的多种模型的基础。紧随其后的是对两种不同的分子网络的介绍——细胞/基质黏附网络（第六章）以及调节干细胞行为的分子网络（第七章）。

本书的第二部分重点介绍用于对前述的分子网络和其后续的细胞行为进行建模的数学和计算机方法。第八章对分子网络建模中的挑战进行了概括，紧随其后的三章则描述了不同的建模方法。第九章关注"高层次"的方法，重点强调了分子和细胞过程中的关系性和逻辑性操作，而第十章和第十一章则关注于"低层次"的方法，在建模的过程中会引入生理和化学机制方面的细节。作为这一部分的结束，第十二章讨论了各种建模软件。

第三部分展示了系统生物学在特定的生物医学研究领域和制药业方面的初步尝试。在生理学方面，第十三章尝试对心血管疾病的病理生理进行系统建模，第十四章针对的则是发育调节，第十五章讨论了免疫系统的调节。本书的高潮在系统生物学/生物医学的重要实际应用上，第十六章讨论了疾病的药物治疗，第十七章描述了预测性系统分析在肿瘤药物发现中的应用，第十八章则讨论了系统性概念在临床试验中的应用。

本书的三个部分所涉及的系统生物医学研究领域均刚刚起步。实验技术的发展将会持续地加速，从而使得我们能够在对生物系统进行测量和操控的过程中，在接近全基因组水平上获取分子和细胞过程的更全、更准和更深层次的信息。这将会激发相关研究人员开发更加多样、复杂以及更有效的算法和模型，同时还将使研究者能够有较强的动力去对模型作出的预测进行测试和验证。更为重要的是，系统生物医学的成功研究实例必定会持续增加，虽然目前这一增加的速度可能比较慢,而且这些研究所针对的系统可能相对较小并且受到了约束,但我们仍然会从中得到不少新的认识和有用的预测。我们满怀信心地期待本书中所描述的系统生物医学的成功实例将会从学术界、生物技术业和制药业吸引来更多更好的资源,并最终使得系统生物学在更具前景的合理性治疗设计中发挥作用。

(陶生策 译)

Contents

Overview   VII

I
FOUNDATIONS OF SYSTEMS BIOLOGY

1. Foundations for Systems Biomedicine: An Introduction   3
2. Genomic Technologies for Systems Biology   15
3. Proteomics Technologies   45
4. Cellular Regulatory Networks   57
5. The Interface of MicroRNAs and Transcription Factor Networks   109
6. Protein Networks in Integrin-mediated Adhesions   139
7. Systems Biology and Stem Cell Biology   153

II
COMPUTATIONAL MODELING IN SYSTEMS BIOLOGY

8. Computational Challenges in Systems Biology   177
9. High-level Modeling of Biological Networks   225
10. Systems Analysis for Systems Biology   249
11. The Virtual Cell Project   273
12. Software Tools for Systems Biology   289

III
APPLICATIONS OF SYSTEMS BIOLOGY

13. Physiome Mark-up Languages for Systems Biology: Model Modularization and Re-use   317
14. Systems Approaches to Developmental Patterning   329
15. Applications of Immunologic Modeling to Drug Discovery and Development   351
16. Systems Pharmacology in Cancer   377
17. Systems Biology in Drug Discovery: Using Predictive Biomedicine to Guide Development Choices for Novel Agents in Cancer   399
18. Quantitative Biology and Clinical Trials: A Perspective   415

Index   425

Overview

Douglas Lauffenburger

Systems biology is different things to different people. One definition, from Lee Hood's Institute for Systems Biology [Ideker et al., 2001], is: *"Systems Biology does not investigate individual genes or proteins one at a time, as has been the highly successful mode of biology for the past 30 years. Rather, it investigates the behavior and relationships of all the elements in a particular biological system while it is functioning."* A second, from the US National Institute of General Medical Sciences [NIH, 2006], is: *"Systems biology is a new interdisciplinary science that derives from biology, mathematics, computer science, physics, engineering, and other disciplines... Most biological systems are too complex for even the most powerful computational models to capture all the system properties. A useful model, however, should be able to accurately conceptualize the system under study and provide reliable predictive values. To accomplish this, a certain level of abstraction may be required that focuses on the system behaviors of interest while neglecting some of the other details."* These two definitions clearly recognize complementary aspects of biological system complexity: the first emphasizes the number of components under consideration, while the second features the quantitative predictive capability and conceptual abstraction of system components, properties and interactions. From where we sit, both of these aspects are important, for biological system complexity is multi-dimensional. To gain predictive understanding of how phenotypic behavior of cells, tissues, organs, and organisms is dependent on molecular component characteristics, scientists and engineers must incorporate multiple interacting components and quantitative information concerning their properties into their studies. Moreover, this predictive understanding can most effectively be raised beyond the confines of mere intuition by constructing computational models of the components and interactions, both for hypothesis generation and hypothesis testing.

A third dimension of biological complexity must also be considered for purposes of this particular book, which is aimed at systems biology applications to human medical concerns. This dimension represents the need to move from analysis of molecular processes in simplified cell culture experimental systems, up to tissue and organ physiological contexts, to organisms (patients) and populations thereof. Although genomics by itself is currently striving to connect gene sequence and expression information directly to human pathophysiology, there is no question that the most powerful approach to this connection will be via computational models that move information from genome to proteome to molecular networks governing cell functions, then propagate these models to larger length-scales and time-scales for eventual prediction of organism pathophysiology in terms of molecular properties. The notion of these three dimensions of biological

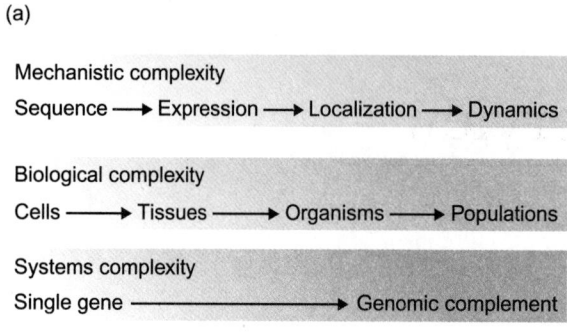
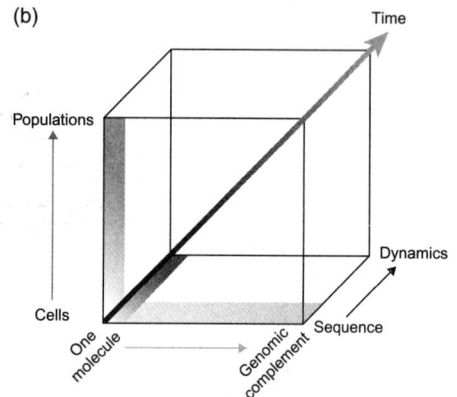

systems complexity is schematically illustrated in the figure (originally developed by Peter Sorger for the MIT Computational & Systems Biology Initiative).

In this book, then, systems biomedicine can be described as an emerging approach to biomedical science that seeks to integratively infer, annotate, and quantify multi-variate complexity of the molecular and cellular processes of living systems, with ultimate aim of constructing formal algorithmic models for prediction of process outcomes from component input. Systems approaches are characterized by several key attributes:

1. A pursuit of quantitative and precise data;
2. The comprehensiveness and completeness of the datasets used;
3. A focus on interconnectivity and networks of the component parts;
4. A willingness to define, measure, and manipulate biological complexity;
5. An interest to computationally (and therefore quantitatively) predict outcomes.

Certainly it can be said that all of biological research historically could be characterized by these descriptors. Any scientific endeavor seeks to measure and systematize observations (quantification) and, in finding underlying order (model), would allow scientists to predict outcome. However, there is an ongoing evolution of technologies and experimental approaches that is changing the conduct of biological research. The availability of whole genome sequences provides the complete catalog of genetic knowledge of an entire organism. Multiplex sensors such as expression arrays and multi-channel flow cytometry, and high throughput screening maneuvers generate precise and comprehensive data. Contemporary and developing computational capabilities are sufficiently powerful to envision capability for computing model-based inferences and/or predictions even as the magnitude of systems (in terms of number of components and their interactions) and associated data-sets continue increase. The difference between systems and reductionist biology is in the objectivity with which we can analyze complex data and the resolution afforded by the completeness of the datasets.

Furthermore, systems biology does not remain constant from year to year. Obsolescence occurs in a matter of months. For this reason, this book has been written and assembled as a series of linked essays that convey strategies and processes. The arguments are bolstered by commissioned chapters on specific topics discussed in depth. These should be considered as examples to clarify points and to stress concepts rather than as an encyclopedia of past knowledge. There will be more departures from an expected book on systems biology. Our discussion will extend from model systems to human biology and pharmacology. We will focus on applications of systems approaches to medical problems and thus the title Systems Biomedicine. Some would demand that true systems approaches require precise mathematical models; however, in this book, because of the experimental complexity in human systems, we wish to broaden the inclusion criteria for systems biology to qualitative systems and hypothesis generators.

Our attempt to describe systems medicine is our final experiment. Often, the most rational experimental strategy is to identify the simplest, most definable model system to study and then to construct a computational model around data output from such systems; ergo, the use of phage, microbial systems, and yeast. However, such systems strategies can now be applied to more complex mammalian systems and even to study human disease. The experimental systems approaches to studying a human problem will, by necessity, be different and potentially less complete than attacking a question using prokaryotes simply because the possible solution space is orders of magnitude greater. Nevertheless, productive strategies have been tried and the outcomes have proven useful even in drug development.

We are attempting to organize this book in a manner reflecting important distinguishing characteristics of systems strategies in experimental biology and medicine: comprehensive (even though not exhaustive) and quantitative measurement, using quantitative data to construct a model of the system, and defining complexity as an experimental dependent variable. Finally, we explore the applications of these principles to biomedical problems.

Rather than an assembly of independent entries or chapters, we have composed this book as a narrative. Whereas we cannot project how this book will ultimately benefit our readers, we suggest that it is best read in sequence as a narrative should be heard, starting with Chapter 1 (by Liu) which offers a conceptual introduction to systems biomedicine.

The first section of the book lays experimental groundwork. It begins with summaries of experimental technologies in genomics (Chapter 2, by Liu) and proteomics (Chapter 3, by Hanash), to set a foundation for the observations and measurements which motivate, populate, and test associated computational models. Chapters 4 (by Lauffenburger and Liu along with associated colleagues) and 5 (by Lim) describe molecular networks regulating cell functional responses to environmental inputs, which form a basis for a wide variety of envisioned models. These are followed by presentations of two particular manifestations of these networks – cell/matrix adhesion networks (Chapter 6, by Geiger and colleagues) and networks regulating stem cell behavior (Chapter 7, by Ng and colleagues).

The second section of the book focuses on mathematical and computational methods for modeling of these kinds of molecular networks and consequent cell behaviors. Chapter 8 (by Subramaniam and Maurya) starts by outlining fundamental challenges for network modeling, followed by three chapters describing different modeling approaches. Chapter 9 (by Janes, Woolf, and Peirce) focuses on "high level" approaches, which emphasize relational and logical operations of molecular and cellular processes, whereas Chapters 10 (by Doyle and Petzold and associates) and 11 (by Loew and associates) focus on "low level" approaches in which details of physico-chemical mechanism are incorporated. This section is rounded out by Chapter 12 (by Sauro and Bergmann) discussing modeling software.

Finally, the third section offers some early attempts at application of systems biology perspectives to particular biomedical science areas and pharmaceutical industry challenges. With respect to physiological areas, Chapter 13 (by Hunter and Cooling) directs systems modeling toward cardiac pathophysiology, Chapter 14 (by Asthagiri and Giurumescu) to developmental regulation, and Chapter 15 (by Young and colleagues) to immune system operation. Important practical focus provides a climax to this book, with Chapter 16 (by Liu and Qiang) on pharmacological treatment of disease, Chapter 17 (by Gaynor and associates at Eli Lilly) on predictive systems analysis for cancer drug discovery, and Chapter 18 (by Harrington and Hodgson) on the applications of systems concepts to clinical trials.

We close by noting that in each of these three sections the field is only in its infancy. There will be continuing acceleration of advance in experimental methods for gaining increasingly complete, accurate, and intensive information of molecular and cellular processes nearing genome-wide coverage in measurement and manipulation. This progress will motivate more diverse, sophisticated, and rigorous computational modeling algorithms, along with stronger insistence on dedicated test of model predictions. Most importantly, the number of "success stories" in which new insights and useful predictive understanding even of relatively small and constrained systems are demonstrated should at least slowly but surely increase. We confidently anticipate that these successes will motivate wider and stronger commitment of resources, in academia and in biotech/pharma industry, for applying the systems biology perspective to the larger promise of rationally informed therapeutics design.

Reference

Ideker, T., Galitski, T., Hood, L., 2001. A new approach to decoding life: systems biology. Annual Review of Genomics and Human Genetics 2, 343–372.

NIGMS Systems Biology Center RFA. (2006). http://grants.nih.gov/grants/guide/RFA-files/RFA-GM-07-004.html

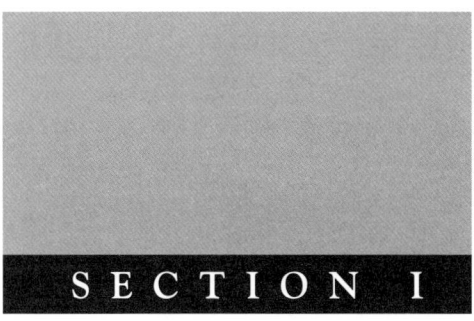

FOUNDATIONS OF SYSTEMS BIOLOGY

CHAPTER 1

Foundations for Systems Biomedicine: an Introduction

Edison T. Liu

Genome Institute of Singapore, Singapore

OUTLINE

Introduction	3	Circadian Cycles as a Relevant Model for Systems Biomedicine	9
Experimental Strategies in Systems Biology	6	Conclusion	11
Systems Biomedicine	7		

INTRODUCTION

Quantitative biology, mathematical biology and mathematical modeling have all been part of biological investigations in one form or another since the beginnings of investigative biology and medicine. Carl Linnaeus' creation of the binary nomenclature (*Systema Naturae*, Carolus Linnaeus, 1735) marked the origin of biologic taxonomy and provided the basis for phylogenic analysis. William Harvey (*An Anatomical Disquisition on the Motion of the Heart and Blood in Animals*, William Harvey, 1847) described the quantification of the amount of blood in the chambers of the heart, calculated the output of the heart by multiplying the volume by the number of heart beats per day, and noted that the output differed wildly from the volume of blood in an individual at any one time. With this information, he developed a model of circulating blood that could explain the blood volume discrepancies with supporting evidence from the anatomic presence of valves in veins. The mathematical tradition in biology therefore, runs long and deep.

However, systems biology, as we conceive of it, differs in scale and formalism from the earlier quantitative traditions. As with any new field, there are many opinions as to what systems biology is. For the purposes of this book, systems biology can be described as a discipline that seeks to quantify and annotate complexity in biological systems in order to construct algorithmic models with which to predict outcomes from component input. Systems biomedicine is an extension of these strategies into the study of biomedical problems. We believe that this demarcation is relevant, given the challenges of the complexity of the human organism and the human impact of the results of these investigations.

This definition of systems biomedicine highlights the difference between quantitative data acquisition and systems biology. The scale of data acquisition in biology today is unparalleled in history. Analog and descriptive data such as cellular images are now digitalized and converted to discrete data points. Genomic- and proteomic-scale information is registered in the gigabyte scale per experiment. This reality also demands formal mathematical and algorithmic conversion of experimental data in biology in order for them to be simply understood by the investigator. The interposition of computers and their algorithms as an essential part of biological research immediately places, at least a rudimentary, mathematical formalism around all experiments performed in this fashion.

Although measuring outcomes is standard in day-to-day biological experiments, these earlier quantitative approaches do not scale. While detailed biochemical kinetics can be calculated for a single biochemical reaction, most commonly, we have tended to resort to descriptive generalizations when we ascend to physiological scales. With current technologies that can acquire precise, comprehensive and quantitative data, biological complexity can now be quantitatively analyzed. The challenge, however, is to identify the optimal mathematical approaches most suited for this scale and complexity of analysis.

Physiologists and pharmacologists have always sought to quantify inputs and outputs in complex organisms, and the later generations of William Harveys had rendered pulmonary and cardiac physiology into equations. To a large extent, this approach has been remarkably successful, and has brought us many of the medical advances in cardiopulmonary medicine and surgery. The cardiac diagnostics from angiography, to echocardiography, to telemetry in which patient physiologic output is monitored and automated alerts generated, represent a culmination of such research in cardiac function. In a sense, physiology was the systems science in medicine. However, these organ-level models do not parse with molecular realities, because their unit of measure is in average blood flow, for example, and not in the flow dynamics of the red corpuscle. Therefore, in the past, quantitative physiologic models could not be unified with cellular models and, by scale, to molecular models. Moreover, the need that assumptions be greatly simplified in order to arrive at computationally tractable models also limited the relevance of many physiologic models.

Now, however, medicine is becoming amenable to complexity analysis. The understanding of the cell and molecular biology of human disease has dramatically advanced in the past 25 years. Whereas the pathophysiology of most human diseases was previously limited to the analysis of organ failure, most diseases now have a cellular and molecular explanation. It is precisely this reduction to common units of measure—to the cell and the molecules within the cell—that allows systems analyses to be applied across the entire human condition. Therefore, the pump dynamics of the heart after myocardial infarction can be resolved at the same level as pancreatic beta-cell function in diabetes mellitus. There is convergence.

The current systems biology now includes two important new characteristics that distinguish it from historical physiology and mathematical biology. First, there is a focus on complexity; secondly, the fundamental unit of study resides in the DNA (and, by association, protein) sequence.

That the unit of measure can be the nucleotide now provides the *lingua franca* that permits the direct translation of experimental results from biochemistry to cell biology, to physiology and to population genetics. Moreover, the ultra-high-throughput and multiplex genomic technologies allow for the digitalization of experimental data of such precision and comprehensiveness that the true complexity of a biological system can actually be measured and dissected. In all aspects—biological and mathematical—the greatest advance has been the availability of computational capabilities that can match the systems complexity. This reliance on these genomic and computational technologies and datasets that can be transmuted across species has broadened significantly the applicability of systems approaches to very complex systems such as human medicine.

Other thinkers have expounded on the new possibilities in integrating mathematics with biology. In an excellent essay, Joel E. Cohen (2004) noted that "mathematics is not only biology's next microscope, but in fact is better". He observed that, in biology, enormous complexity of up to 100 million species is built on just a few basic elements of carbon, nitrogen, hydrogen and oxygen. By contrast, the entire periodic table generates only several thousand kinds of minerals in the earth's crust. Thus the entire basis of biology is a complexity that produces ensemble or emergent properties of much greater function than the component parts. Cohen argued that mathematics can also benefit from attacking biological problems as it did in working through problems in physics. Calculus was developed in part to help solve the problems of celestial motion and of optics. Similarly, the multilayered complexity, interlocking control loops, distributed switch mechanisms and the differential use of the same components over developmental time challenges mathematical and computational solutions. It is likely that new mathematics will be required to deal with these ensemble properties and with the heterogeneity of the biological input that feeds into the organismic output.

Geneticists have already defined phenotypic interactions between genes or alleles as epistasis (Phillips, 2008). In many cases, new properties emerge: two white flowers that when crossed give a purple flower, or two genes that when individually mutated give no phenotype, but show a lethal outcome when both are mutated. The mathematical representation of epistasis can be:

$$W_{xy} = x + y + \delta \qquad (1.1)$$

where W is the observed phenotype, x and y are the individual effects of each allele at loci x and y, δ is the deviation that is due to epistasis. Systems biology, however, examines the sum of all epistatic relationships and hopes to uncover the hierarchy. This, indeed, has been the direction of this line of genetic research. Tong et al. (2004) crossed mutations in 132 "query" genes into a set of 4700 viable yeast gene deletion mutants to develop a genetic interaction map containing more than 4000 functional gene interactions. Classical genetics converges on systems biology.

Kitano (2007) noted the importance of control theory in describing biological systems, and described the primacy of "robustness" in the design of biological systems. He differentiated robustness from homeostasis, in that homeostasis seeks to return the system to the original state, whereas robustness will accommodate migration to another state to achieve survivability. One characteristic of evolvable systems described by the Highly Optimized Theory (HOT) states that such systems are robust against common perturbations, but are fragile against unusual ones (Carlson and Doyle, 2000). A common example is the World Wide Web, which, despite being robust because of its high interconnectivity, has been brought down by specific attacks at hubs of activity. Thus systems robustness is a matter of "trade-offs." Mathematical descriptions of robustness have been attempted.

Kitano (2007) provides a representation of robustness in the following equation, but also acknowledges that new mathematics may be necessary to accommodate these systems concepts in biology:

"Robustness (R) of the system (s) with regard to function (a) against a set of perturbations (P):

$$R_{a,P}^s = \int_P \psi(p) D_a^s(p) dp \quad (1.2)$$

The function ψ is the probability for perturbation 'p' to take place. P is the entire perturbation space, and D (p) is an evaluation function under perturbation (p)."

EXPERIMENTAL STRATEGIES IN SYSTEMS BIOLOGY

Systems approaches are characterized by several key attributes:

1. The measurement of quantitative and comprehensive data of an experimental system.
2. Assessment of the relationships between the component parts.
3. Perturbation of the system to detect response dynamics.
4. Intersection of orthogonal data to arrive at higher-order logic. (Orthogonal data are defined as datasets derived from different systems, perhaps addressing the same question in which the intersection of the two datasets can further resolve a problem: for example, the set of genes with binding sites of a transcription factor and the set of genes that are expressed with overexpression of the same transcription factor [see Chapter 4]).
5. Derivation of a model of the system that can be mathematical or qualitative.
6. Correct prediction of output based on the model.

The most complete analyses that engage all these attributes have been made in lower organisms. Bonneau and colleagues (2007) reported the construction of a complete functional biological network map for *Halobacterium salinarum*, an Archaea species that thrives in conditions of high salinity. The final network map describes the regulatory functional relationships among 80% of its genes. The predictive power of this model was evident in its ability to predict the transcriptional responses to challenge with novel environmental conditions or disruption of transcription factors. The predictive capability of this genome-wide, whole-organism predictive model was significant. In order to achieve this, Bonneau and colleagues accomplished the following in order to achieve their goal:

1. The 2.6 Mb *Halobacterium salinarum* genome was sequenced and functions were assigned to each gene using protein sequence and structural similarities (*know all the components*).
2. Cells were perturbed by varying concentrations of environmental factors and / or gene knockouts (*perturbation analysis*).
3. The transcriptional changes of all genes using microarrays were determined after each perturbation (*genomic readout for perturbation analysis*).
4. Diverse data (mRNA levels, evolutionary conservation in protein structure, metabolic pathways, and *cis*-regulatory motifs) were integrated to identify subsets of genes that are co-regulated in certain environment (*data integration*).
5. A dynamic network model was constructed for the of influence environmental and transcription factor changes on the expression of co-regulated genes (*model building*).
6. The resulting network was explored using software visualization tools within an integrator that enables software interoperability and database integration. This allowed for manual exploration and generation of hypotheses used to plan additional iterations of the systems analysis (*model testing*).

Similar strategies have been applied to the eukaryotic model system, yeast, with less predictive success (Luscombe, 2004; Tong, 2004; Yu, 2008). Nevertheless, the strategy still requires the integration of heterogeneous datasets, such as transcription factor binding sites, transcriptional profiles and protein–protein interactions (Fig. 1.1).

SYSTEMS BIOMEDICINE

Systems biomedicine is the analysis of medical problems using systems approaches; therefore pertinence to the human condition is a prerequisite. Given the complexity of mammalian systems, are we ready to study the ensemble properties of the human model, and are we sufficiently clever to use these approaches to understand and to treat human disease? Before 2001, perhaps, it would have been difficult to answer affirmatively. If access to the complete human genome is a prerequisite for a systems analysis, only after the sequencing of the human genome could this goal be conceived (Lander et al., 2001). Together with the advent of expression arrays in 1996 (Shalon, 1996) and their stable use by 2000, these technologies launched the next phase of growth for systems approaches to complex organisms like mammals. Network analyses have been conducted primarily where the system is cell-based, such as immunology (Kitano, 2006) or cancer (Segal et al., 2005), or where the tissue is homogeneous such as the heart (Olson, 2006) or liver (Schadt, 2008). Interestingly, computer scientists have looked to the natural immune system to develop analogous artificial immune systems for computer system security (Forrest and Beauchemin, 2007). There is much to be learned from biological systems that have had the benefit of more than a billion years of evolutionary history.

The experimental systems approaches to studying a human problem will, by necessity, be different and potentially less complete than those appropriate for attacking a question using prokaryotes. Such reconstruction of a regulatory network has been difficult in higher organisms, owing to the dramatically increased complexity of the contributing subsystems. Thus the possible solution space is orders of magnitude

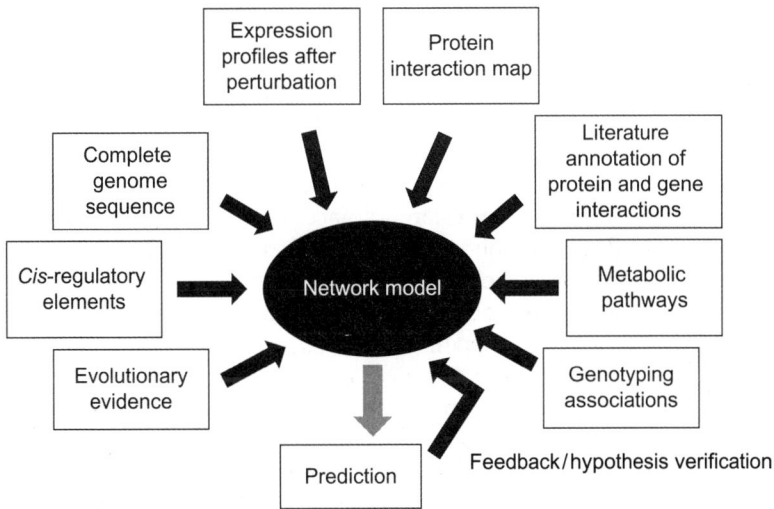

FIGURE 1.1 Input Information that can be Used to Construct a Network Model.

greater than that for lower organisms. Gene numbers increase in higher eukaryotes, but this is not the confounding factor: splice variants, transcription factors binding at great distances from the transcriptional start sites, gene duplication, post-transcriptional regulation by microRNAs and other non-coding RNA species, and complex post-translational modifications that change binding affinities all radically augment the complexity of the components.

Despite these challenges, network models of subsystems have been described, for example for the class of receptor tyrosine kinases (RTKs) (Amit et al., 2007a, 2007b; Katz, 2007). In these analyses, signaling hubs for the RTKs, such as RAF and the phosphoinositide 3' kinase PI3K–AKT nodes, are noted to be frequent points of attack by oncogenic viruses, in addition to being sites of *de-novo* mutations in primary cancers. Such hubs, independently identified by both viruses and cancer mutations, also are effective targets for anticancer therapeutics.

Exploiting kinase networks, Sachs et al. (2005) pursued an interesting alternative strategy. Using multicolor/multiparameter flow cytometry in which up to 11 different features can be determined when labeled with different fluorophores, they quantitatively assessed the combinatorial presence of specific phosphorproteins indicative of activated kinases. Because flow cytometry assesses the biochemical state of individual cells, a large number of observations can be accumulated that would otherwise be an average of the population. In this manner, Sachs and colleagues were able to construct a Bayesian network from these data. Bayesian network models disclose the dependent effect of each biomolecule on the others, and therefore can infer causal relationships. Examining signaling in T cells, they could construct a network map that faithfully portrayed known and experimentally validated kinase–substrate relationships. In a similar fashion, they mapped the signaling profiles of acute myeloid leukemia cells after cytokine challenge and found 36 node states, following 6 stimulation conditions assessing 6 signaling molecules. These states could separate acute myeloid leukemia cells into signaling classes that corresponded to cytogenetic and clinical parameters (Irish, 2004).

It has been said that biology asks six kinds of question (Cohen, 2004): How is it built? How does it work? How did it begin? What is it for? The remaining two questions are more in the domain of medicine: What goes wrong? How is it fixed? So, systems biomedicine focuses, not only on human biology, but also human disease. Efforts to examine perturbations in gene and protein networks for clues to disease etiology have been pursued and will be described in subsequent chapters in this book. Most efforts are in the bench-to-bedside direction, but one approach that starts commonly from the patient and is validated at the bench is in human and population genetics of disease genes.

Human variations in the form of single nucleotide polymorphisms (SNPs) are used to identify genetic loci statistically associated with disease when compared with control populations. When assessed on a genome-wide basis, this has been a powerful, unbiased means of uncovering disease-associated genes. When expression arrays are coupled with genetic markers, expression quantitative trait loci (eQTL) can be assigned. In eQTL analysis, each transcript on the array is considered to be a quantitative phenotype and is correlated with the SNP configuration at each locus in the genome (Cheung et al., 2005; Sieberts and Schadt, 2007). *cis*-eQTL represent those SNPs adjacent to the measured gene of which the configuration is correlated with transcript levels, whereas *trans*-eQTLs are those associated with SNPs that are distant from the transcribed gene. eQTLs in humans have been used as proof of the genetic basis of gene expression in humans (Cheung et al., 2008; Spielman et al., 2007). When viewed on a genome-wide basis, a transcriptional network of regulatory "influence" can be discerned by statistical association between individual SNPs and expression of genes anywhere in the genome. Schadt and his colleagues at Rosetta Pharmaceuticals have shown that combining genotypic data and expression data can increase precision of the discovery for disease-associated genes (Drake et al., 2005; Zhu et al., 2007).

CIRCADIAN CYCLES AS A RELEVANT MODEL FOR SYSTEMS BIOMEDICINE

An excellent example of a systems model that has medical importance is that of oscillators as regulators of the circadian rhythm. Oscillators are machines that cycle functions over time and are characterized by an automatic periodicity (see Chapter 4), and the best examples of biological oscillators are found in studies of circadian rhythm. The guiding motif for all living creatures is the ability to replicate, which imparts a cycling of functions. Over evolutionary time, there appeared to be an adaptive advantage to entrain such physiologic processes to an external clock defined by the day–night cycle. In order to do this, most organisms have found biochemical mechanisms to maintain this cycling, and mechanisms to sense the environment in order to modulate this periodicity.

The master circadian regulator in mammals is in the suprachiasmatic nucleus (SCN) in the brain. The molecular mechanism underpinning this oscillator has been elucidated. The basic helix–loop–helix containing transcription factor CLOCK interacts with BMAL1 to activate transcription of the *Per* and *Cry* genes. The Period (PER) and Cryptochrome (CRY) protein products heterodimerize and undergo negative feedback to inhibit their own transcription, and that of BMAL1. The PER–CRY repressor complex is degraded during the night, and *Clock-Bmal1* are de-repressed and can then induce transcription. There is a secondary feedback loop that involves the induction of a nuclear hormone receptor, REV-ERBα, by BMAL1/CLOCK. When REV-ERBα accumulates to threshold levels, it represses BMAL1/CLOCK. This secondary regulatory loop is not essential for the establishment of the circadian cycle, but it appears to be involved in stabilizing the regulatory framework. The oscillator function can be explained by a time delay in PER/CRY feedback inhibition of BMAL/CLOCK establishing a composite negative network motif with asymmetric timing. This oscillator is also affected by enzyme-families such as casein kinase 1 (CSNK1ε and CSNK1δ) that regulate the degradation of critical components like the PER protein (Fig. 1.2). (Takahashi et al., 2008).

Peripheral tissues also exhibit autonomous circadian rhythms but are subservient to and are entrained by the SCN. The SCN coordinates the peripheral clocks through humoral and neural signals that are not well understood, and by indirect means such as body temperature, wakefulness and food intake. Thus the entire circadian system is a hierarchy of subnetworks that extend from the molecular and biochemical level to the physiological level.

Components of the circadian clock are deeply involved in human physiology and disease. The most obvious association is with sleep disorders. Familial advanced sleep-phase syndrome (FASPS) is an autosomal dominant circadian rhythm disorder characterized by an abnormal phasing of the circadian cycle relative to the desired sleep–wake schedule. Here sleep onset and awakening times are 3–4 hours ahead of the desired times. Through linkage analysis, individuals with the syndrome were found to harbor a missense mutation, S662G, in the human *PER2* gene. This S662G mutation disrupts a phosphorylation site within a casein kinase 1 (CSNK1)-binding domain of *PER2*, resulting in the increased turnover of nuclear PER2. As evidence that FASPS has heterogeneous genetic origins, a mutation in a casein kinase isoform, CSNK1δ, was also found in FASPS.

Such sleep disorders are rare; however, there is the cumulative evidence that molecular

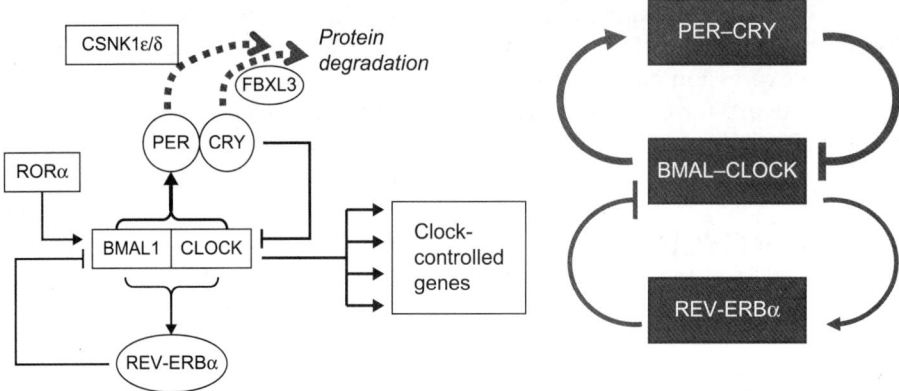

FIGURE 1.2 Schematic Representation of the Control Network for Circadian Cycling.
The core organization of the regulatory module is comprised of two interlocking negative-feedback network motifs with asymmetric timing. BMAL1, brain and muscle Arnt (aryl hydrocarbon receptor nuclear translocator)-like protein-1; CLOCK, Circadian Locomotor Output Cycles Kaput gene; CSNK1ε/δ, casein kinase 1 ε and δ; CRY, Cryptochrome; FBXL3, an E3 ubiquitin ligase; PER, Period; REV-ERBα: a retinoid-acid-related orphan nuclear hormone receptor; RORα, a retinoid-acid-related orphan nuclear hormone receptor.

components of the circadian oscillator may be involved in many common disorders. Gene profiling experiments demonstrated that up to 10% of the testable transcriptome shows circadian periodicity, and that the attributes of these clock-regulated genes are highly enriched for metabolic functions. Recall that the nuclear hormone receptors, RORα and REV-ERBα, are integral parts of the oscillator loop. Extending this analysis further, Yang and colleagues (2006) examined the detailed gene expression the 49 nuclear receptors in mice, and found that 28 display tissue-specific circadian rhythms. Given the function of nuclear receptors in metabolic regulation, their circadian control provides one explanation for the diurnal behavior of glucose and lipid metabolism.

Studies in animal models also continue to uncover associations between clock genes and metabolic phenotypes: homozygous *Clock*-mutant mice are hyperphagic, obese and exhibit a metabolic syndrome with hyperlipidemia, fatty liver, high circulating glucose concentrations and low circulating insulin concentrations (Turek et al., 2005). $Bmal1^{-/-}$ knockout mice not only have abnormal sleep patterns, but also show low body weight and sensitivity to insulin shock. Fibroblasts from these *Bmal1* knockout mice also cannot undergo adipocyte differentiation (Shimba et al., 2005). Clinically, a link between circadian cycles and metabolism has been observed. Epidemiologic studies in shift workers have shown an increase in body mass index, and in the rates of incidence of metabolic disorders and cardiovascular events (Ellingsen et al., 2007). It is also well understood that the specific sensitivity to exogenous insulin exhibited by diabetic patients changes over the time of day. Thus the circadian clock mechanisms are inextricably linked to metabolic functions, and may represent an adaptive evolutionary response to maximizing energy utilization that is dependent on a consistent environmental change—the planetary reality of the day/night cycle (Green et al., 2008).

An intriguing side observation that now has significant ramifications for cancer therapeutics is that liver detoxifying genes also show significant circadian oscillations and have been shown to be regulated by clock mechanisms. Doses of the chemotherapeutic agent, cyclophosphamide, given at different times of the circadian cycle can result in differences in mortality rates—from 20% to 100% (Gorbacheva et al., 2005). Exploring this phenomenon further, the investigators found that *Clock* and *Bmal1* knockout mice are sensitive to the toxic effects of cyclophosphamide, but *Cry1* and *Cry2* double-knockout mice are resistant. This resistance was not caused by pharmacokinetic differences, but appeared to be correlated with cellular insensitivity of B lymphocytes to the lymphotoxic effects of this drug. These experiments validate the clinical observations that timing of chemotherapeutic administration has an effect on drug toxicity and drug effectiveness (reviewed by Takahashi et al., 2008).

The growing body of knowledge of the mechanisms around circadian clocks and their impact on health has provided opportunities for the development of drugs targeting these molecules. Many of the clock-associated genes are amenable to the action of drugs or represent biochemical classes amenable to small-molecule modulation: the melatonin receptors are G-protein-coupled receptors; GSK3β is a kinase that modifies PER, and REV-ERBβ casein kinase 1 is another class of kinases; REV-ERB and ROR are nuclear hormone receptors (the ligand for REV-ERBα has been identified as heme). All these targets have candidate small-molecule modifiers. This has led companies to explore the use of cell-based screens to identify molecules that would disrupt or alter the circadian clock. Cell systems with luciferase reporter genes controlled by clock-dependent regulatory elements can be used to screen libraries of small molecules. The readout would be disruption of the periodicity (reviewed by Liu et al., 2007). Thus, starting from a simple oscillator, explanations of human physiology and identification of targets for therapy can be explored.

CONCLUSION

How is systems biomedicine different from other forms of systems studies? In my opinion, the differences are only ones of scale and experimental access. Clearly, the human genome and proteome is more complex than those of yeast and bacteria, and human genetic studies are more complex than those in mice. Moreover, the complexity of a multicellular and multi-organ system has yet to be configured into the equation. To date, the comparative extent of that complexity remains not quite known; therefore, how much more data and how much more computing will be necessary to achieve the same coverage as that described for *Halobacterium salinarum* is unclear, but will undoubtedly be more than the ratio of the size of our genome to that of this microbe. However, the approaches and the opportunities are the same.

Of course, in the final analysis, systems biomedicine, by directly benefiting human health, will be a significant endeavor. So any increment in improvement in prediction will help medicine and benefit society. The challenges, however, are logistical, computational and organizational. Logistical because first, for obvious ethical reasons, experimentation in human systems is slower and more ponderous; secondly, human variation will make initial estimates less generalizable; and thirdly, the further division into organ systems linked by circulation and endocrine factors will increase the number of studies needed in order to complete the human organism. The computational challenges have been alluded to, and are most critical: massive amounts of data requiring integration and iterative analysis of high computational complexity. The new technologies in sequencing, genotyping, proteomics and imaging are generating a hyper-exponential growth in data acquisition that is quickly outstripping the capabilities of most biological laboratories and departments. The physical sciences have pioneered the use of supercomputers with the capability of handling this challenge. However, the porting of the all biological, genetic and genomic algorithms to these new platforms and their continued development will be a prodigious task. Lastly, the simple fact is that our data standards do not routinely allow for cross-platform comparisons. Manual curation is still required for most high-level systems integration. There is a need for integration of heterogeneous data (e.g. protein–protein interaction, RNA expression information, biochemical pathways, genomic data and literature-based connections) and for visualization tools that will enable the presentation of large-scale data that are interpretable to bench biologists.

Finally, the organizational challenges, although man- made and therefore surmountable by man, are also daunting (Liu et al., 2005). These organizational challenges are rooted in the sometimes contradictory requirements of systems biology research and the operational intentions of our academic and funding institutions.

In systems research, scientists with very different skills (biology, mathematics, engineering, medicine) must be working closely together and have proximity with one another in what might almost be scientific collectives (Liu, 2009). Traditionally, bioinformatics resided in a computer science or biostatistics department, biology in a biochemistry department and a genomics center that was functionally dissociated from the previous two. However, the scale of this interaction requires coordinated resources from the funding agencies, much akin to the supercomputing program of the US National Science Foundation. This unfortunate disconnect would benefit from some conceptual realignment. Regarding data presentation, there is a need to provide more natural interfaces between humans and computers to service the non-expert user. There will be a demand for simplified interfaces specifically designed for biologists. This does not detract from the important need to train the next generation of biologists who are mathematically and computationally literate, and the next generation of mathematicians, computer scientists and engineers who are steeped in the nuances of biology.

Grants management is often at odds with collective efforts. Funding for critical technology platforms is too often bypassed as lacking scientific content. By discounting participation in collaborative projects and focusing exclusively on individual effort, University promotion processes historically encourage faculty insularity. Graduate student training, restrained by classical departmental boundaries and focused on individual faculty projects, is not responsive to the educational requirements for success in integrative and systems biology. Systems biology is deeply cross-disciplinary.

Daunting as these challenges are, the stakes are high. I believe that systems approaches in biology will become as common as molecular technologies are in current biological investigations. Molecular biology, which was a new creature in the 1970s and early 1980s and which spawned biotechnology companies and institutes and departments with "molecular biology" in their title, is now commonplace and integrated into the fabric of biological teachings. Current medical investigations are all molecular medicine. The same will be true of systems approaches.

Systems Biomedicine, indeed, is here to stay.

References

Amit, I., Citri, A., Shay, T., et al., 2007a. A module of negative feedback regulators defines growth factor signaling. Nat. Genet. 39, 503–512.

Amit, I., Wides, R., Yarden, Y., 2007b. Evolvable signaling networks of receptor tyrosine kinases: relevance of robustness to malignancy and to cancer therapy. Mol. Syst. Biol. 3, 151.

Bonneau, R., Facciotti, M.T., Reiss, D.J., et al., 2007. A predictive model for transcriptional control of physiology in a free living cell. Cell 131, 1354–1365.

Carlson, J.M., Doyle, J., 2000. Highly optimized tolerance: robustness and design in complex systems. Phys. Rev. Lett. 84, 2529–2532.

Cheung, V.G., Spielman, R.S., Ewens, K.G., Weber, T.M., Morley, M., Burdick, J.T., 2005. Mapping determinants of human gene expression by regional and genome-wide association. Nature 437, 1365–1369.

Cheung, V.G., Bruzel, A., Burdick, J.T., Morley, M., Devlin, J.L., Spielman, R.S., 2008. Monozygotic twins reveal

REFERENCES

germline contribution to allelic expression differences. Am. J. Hum. Genet. 82, 1357–1360.

Cohen, J.E., 2004. Mathematics is biology's next microscope, only better; biology is mathematics' next physics, only better. PLoS Biol. 2, e439.

Drake, T.A., Schadt, E.E., Davis, R.C., Lusis, A.J., 2005. Integrating genetic and gene expression data to study the metabolic syndrome and diabetes in mice. Am. J. Ther. 12, 503–511.

Ellingsen, T., Bener, A., Gehani, A.A., 2007. Study of shift work and risk of coronary events. J. R. Soc. Health 127, 265–267.

Forrest, S., Beauchemin, C., 2007. Computer immunology. Immunolog. Rev. 216, 176–197.

Green, C.B., Takahashi, J.S., Bass, J., 2008. The meter of metabolism. Cell 134, 728–742.

Gorbacheva, V.Y., Kondratov, R.V., Zhang, R., et al., 2005. Circadian sensitivity to the chemotherapeutic agent cyclophosphamide depends on the functional status of the CLOCK/BMAL1 transactivation complex. Proc. Natl. Acad. Sci. USA 102, 3407–3412.

Irish, J.M., Hovland, R., Krutzik, P.O., et al., 2004. Single cell profiling of potentiated phospho-protein networks in cancer cells. Cell 118, 217–228.

Katz, M., Amit, I., Citri, A., et al., 2007. A reciprocal tensin-3-cten switch mediates EGF-driven mammary cell migration. Nat. Cell Biol. 9, 961–969.

Kitano, H., 2006. The B-cell interactome. Available from http://amdec-bioinfo.cu-genome.org/html/BCellInteractome.html#Publication

Kitano, H., 2007. Towards a theory of biological robustness. Mol. Syst. Biol. 3, 137.

Kitano, H., Oda, K., 2006. Robustness trade-offs and host-microbial symbiosis in the immune system. Mol. Syst. Biol. 2, 2006–2022.

Lander, E.S., Linton, L.M., Birren, B., et al., 2001. For the international human genome sequencing consortium. Initial sequencing and analysis of the human genome. Nature 409, 860–921.

Liu, E.T., 2005. Systems biology, integrative biology, predictive biology. Cell 121, 505–506.

Liu, E.T., 2009. Integrative biology—a strategy for systems biomedicine. Nat. Rev. Genet. 10, 64–68.

Liu, A.C., Lewis, W.G., Kay, S.A., 2007. Mammalian circadian signaling networks and therapeutic targets. Nat. Chem. Biol. 3, 630–639.

Luscombe, N.M., Babu, M.M., Yu, H., Snyder, M., Teichmann, S.A., Gerstein, M., 2004. Genomic analysis of regulatory network dynamics reveals large topological changes. Nature 431, 308–312.

Olson, E.N., 2006. Gene regulatory networks in the evolution and development of the heart. Science 313, 1922–1927.

Phillips, P.C., 2008. Epistasis—the essential role of gene interactions in the structure and evolution of genetic systems. Nat. Rev. Genet. 9, 855–867.

Sachs, K., Perez, O., Pe'er, D., Lauffenburger, D.A., Nolan, G.P., 2005. Causal protein-signaling networks derived from multiparameter single-cell data. Science 308, 523–529.

Schadt, E.E., Molony, C., Chudin, E., et al., 2008. Mapping the genetic architecture of gene expression in human liver. PLoS Biol. 6, e107.

Segal, E., Friedman, N., Kaminski, N., Regev, A., Koller, D., 2005. From signatures to models: understanding cancer using microarrays. Nat. Genet. 37 (Suppl), S38–S45.

Shalon, D., Smith, S.J., Brown, P.O., 1996. A DNA microarray system for analyzing complex DNA samples using two-color fluorescent probe hybridization. Genome Res. 6, 639–645.

Shimba, S., Ishii, N., Ohta, Y., et al., 2005. Brain and muscle Arnt-like protein-1 (BMAL1), a component of the molecular clock, regulates adipogenesis. Proc. Natl. Acad. Sci. USA 102, 12071–12076.

Sieberts, S.K., Schadt, E.E., 2007. Moving toward a system genetics view of disease. Mamm. Genome 18, 389–401.

Spielman, R.S., Bastone, L.A., Burdick, J.T., Morley, M., Ewens, W.J., Cheung, V.G., 2007. Common genetic variants account for differences in gene expression among ethnic groups. Nat. Genet. 39, 226–231.

Takahashi, J.S., Hong, H.K., Ko, C.H., McDearmon, E.L., 2008. The genetics of mammalian circadian order and disorder: implications for physiology and disease. Nat. Rev. Genet. 9, 764–775.

Tong, A.H., Lesage, G., Bader, G.D., et al., 2004. Global mapping of the yeast genetic interaction network. Science 303, 808–813.

Turek, F.W., Joshu, C., Kohsaka, A., et al., 2005. Obesity and metabolic syndrome in circadian Clock mutant mice. Science 308, 1043–1045.

Yang, X., Downes, M., Yu, R.T., et al., 2006. Nuclear receptor expression links the circadian clock to metabolism. Cell 126, 801–810.

Yu, H., Braun, P., Yildirim, M.A., Lemmens, I., et al., 2008. High-quality binary protein interaction map of the yeast interactome network. Science 322, 104–110.

Zhu, J., Wiener, M.C., Zhang, C., et al., 2007. Increasing the power to detect causal associations by combining genotypic and expression data in segregating populations. PLoS Comput. Biol. 3, e69.

CHAPTER 2

Genomic Technologies for Systems Biology

Edison T. Liu[1], Sanket Goel[1], Kartiki Desai[1] and Mathijs Voorhoeve[2]

[1]Genome Institute of Singapore, Singapore
[2]Duke-National University of Singapore Graduate Medical School, Singapore

OUTLINE

Summary	16
Definitions	16
Introduction	16
DNA Sequencing: High-throughput Sequencing Technologies	17
Roche 454 Life Sciences: GS FLX Titanium	17
Illumina: Genome Analyzer	20
Applied Biosystems: SOLiD Sequencing	22
Applications of Sequencing in Systems Biology: The Transcriptome and Transcriptional Regulation	24
Expression Arrays	26
ChIP-on-chip Arrays	28
Interaction Analysis: Two-hybrid Screens	33
Gene-based Perturbation Studies: Transgenic Knockouts	34
Forward Genetics	34
Reverse Genetics	35
RNA Interference Approaches in Systems Biology	35

Summary

The term "genome-to-systems" used in systems biology is a reflection on how important genomic strategies are to the systems analysis of biological processes. The technical fundamentals of all genomic technologies are based on the principles of base-pair hybridization and DNA polymerization. From these basic steps comes the tool set of genome-to-systems work: quantitative polymerase chain reaction, expression and genomic arrays, DNA sequencing and nucleic-acid-based disruption of gene expression. Each tool provides one or more aspects of systems biological information: quantitative assessment, precise component determination and comprehensive coverage. We will describe each technology and explore their applications in systems biosciences.

Definitions

ChIP Chromatin immunoprecipitation
dsRNA Double-stranded RNA.
Hypomorph A genetic mutation that results in partial loss of function.
miRNA MicroRNA.
RISC RNA-induced silencing complex.
RNAi RNA interference.
RT-PCR Reverse transcriptase polymerase chain reaction.
SAGE Serial analysis of gene expression.
shRNA Short hairpin RNA.
siRNA Short interfering RNA.

INTRODUCTION

The sequencing of entire genomes and their annotation have been the critical enabling factors for all of systems biology. This information permitted the *in-silico* preparation of probes to assess both genomic and expression changes, enabled the use of short tags in genome re-sequencing and made possible the identification of peptide fragments from proteomic interrogations. The term "genome-to-systems" reflects the primary use of genomic information in systems analysis of biological processes. This is then coupled with characteristic systems approaches: the precise designation of each component under study, the comprehensive measurement of all components involved in a process, and the computation of complex information. Certainly, quantitative approaches have been used in the past, solely with protein or biochemical components, but the complexity of these systems was low, studying a limited number of components with the goal of rendering a mathematical model of a biochemical reaction. As such, early systems models were models of biochemical kinetics.

Knowledge of the genome and, in particular, the annotation of the transcriptome of model organisms including the human, has enabled the construction of genome-wide probes by *in-silico* (computationally-based) means, and precise gene assignment for genome-wide transcript analysis. The ability to assess the expression of all known gene transcripts in a quantitative fashion formed the basis for genome-wide systems analyses of biological processes. Thus transcriptional profiles were the first to be used in such a manner. This was followed by assessment of transcription factor binding and of the influence of epigenetic modifications on gene expression. The final call for precision in transcript ascertainment has led to the development of transcriptome re-sequencing and genome-scale mutational maps. Other gene-based technologies used for systems studies include two-hybrid screens for protein interaction mapping and gene silencing approaches (short interfering RNA [siRNA], short hairpin RNA [shRNA]) for perturbation analysis. Table 2.1 summarizes these technologies that contribute to the pursuit of genome-to-systems strategies.

TABLE 2.1 Technologies for Gene-to-Systems Strategies

---

1. DNA sequencing.
2. Comprehensive, precise and quantitative determination of transcripts expressed and their concentrations.
3. Transcription factor binding site analysis.
4. Interactions: two-hybrid screens.
5. Gene-based strategies for perturbation analysis:
   a. Transgenesis
   b. RNA interference.

DNA SEQUENCING: HIGH-THROUGHPUT SEQUENCING TECHNOLOGIES

The success of the Human Genome Project, completed in 2003, was primarily attributable to the development of high-throughput sequencing approaches and advanced computational capabilities. Earlier sequencing approaches relied on primer extension and fluorescent dye termination using DNA polymerase and specific nucleotide terminators (also called Sanger sequencing). The subsequent terminated fragments were then separated by capillary electrophoresis and the position of the specific nucleotide terminator deduced from the fragment sizes. The completed version of The Human Genome Project had fewer than 400 gaps and covered 99% of the genome, with an accuracy of more than 99.99% (Lander et al., 2001; Venter et al., 2001). It is apparent that in a human genome there were approximately 300 000 errors were found and 30 million bases remained elusive to sequence (Collins et al., 2004; Schmutz et al., 2004). Although an important technical advance that allowed for the sequencing of the human genome, this approach was sufficiently time-consuming and costly to limit the depth of sequencing and its use in time-course experiments. These limitations restricted the applicability of Sanger sequencing for systems biological experiments.

In the past few years, a dramatic change in sequencing technologies has allowed for improvements by orders of magnitude in speed and reduction in cost. These "second-generation" technologies have now superseded Sanger-based capillary electrophoresis sequencing and are the basis for the generation of data for genome-to-systems investigations. The fundamental shift that distinguishes this second-generation sequencing from Sanger sequencing is, first, the reliance on reading the DNA code by assessing the incorporation of each individual complementary nucleotide—sequencing-by-"synthesis" (as compared with sequencing by fragment length); alternatively, sequencing-by-hybridization is used, whereby precise sequences are deduced by specific hybridization of oligonucleotide probes. Secondly, this sequencing-by-synthesis is augmented in scale by arraying each sequencing reaction in a massively parallel fashion. The limiting factor is then the length of sequencing that can be achieved: until recently, sequencing lengths have been limited to 25–250 base pairs (bp). Now, however, computational algorithms for sequence assembly allow for the "stitching" of these fragmented sequences into contiguous sequences—called "contigs."

Second-generation sequencing has been championed by several technologies rooted in specific companies. We briefly review the commonly used platforms.

Roche 454 Life Sciences: GS FLX Titanium

In 2004, the Genome Sequencer 20 (GS 20) developed by the Roche company, 454 Life Sciences (Roche/454) was released as the first platform in the line of second-generation sequencers (Margulies et al., 2005). Subsequent improved versions of this platform were released: GS FLX and then GS Titanium. The Roche/454 sequencing platform relies upon a sequencing-by-synthesis strategy called "pyrosequencing"

(Ronaghi et al., 1996). Pyrosequencing is a biochemiluminescence-based assay in which pyrophosphate (PPi) is released during the DNA polymerase reaction during incorporation of a nucleotide (Fig. 2.1). This pyrophosphate is converted into visible light by two enzymatic reaction such that the light becomes measured as quanta of the number of nucleotides incorporated. The PPi is first converted to ATP by ATP sulfurylase, and is in turn used in the oxidation of luciferin by luciferase, which generates light. Knowledge of the order of the nucleotides incorporated reveals the sequence of the bases in the DNA template. The unreacted nucleotides and ATP are degraded by apyrase, allowing iterative addition of dNTP to the solution.

Library Preparation and Emulsion Polymerase Chain Reaction

Preparation of a universal DNA library from genomic DNA sample is the first and very important part in the Roche/454 sequencing strategy (Fig. 2.2). First, double-stranded (ds) DNA (3–5 μg) is fractioned into short double-stranded fragments (~300–1500 bp) by nebulization. This is

$$DNA_n + dNTP \xrightarrow{Polymerase} DNA_{n+1} + PPi$$

$$PPi + APS \xrightarrow{Sulfurylase} ATP$$

$$ATP + Luciferin \xrightarrow{Luciferase} AMP + PPi + CO_2 + Oxyluciferin + h\nu$$

$$ATP \xrightarrow{Apyrase} AMP + 2Pi$$

$$dXTP \xrightarrow{Apyrase} dXMP + 2Pi$$

FIGURE 2.1 Pyrosequencing.
Pyrosequencing is a four-enzyme processes in which four nucleotides (dXTP is any one nucleotide) are added stepwise to the template hybridized to a primer. The pyrophosphate (PPi) released in the DNA polymerase-catalyzed reaction is converted to light by the following two enzymatic reactions. A nucleotide-degrading enzyme, apyrase, continuously degrades the added nucleotides. The process of addition of the nucleotides is repeated, achieving longer stretches of the template. APS, adenosine-5′-phosphosulfate; hν, Energy of one photon with frequency ν (where h is the Planck constant); Pi, inorganic phosphate.

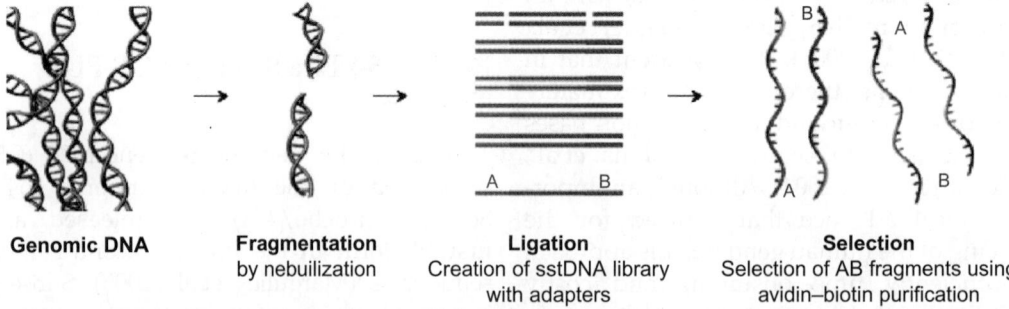

Genomic DNA | **Fragmentation** by nebulization | **Ligation** Creation of sstDNA library with adapters | **Selection** Selection of AB fragments using avidin–biotin purification

FIGURE 2.2 Process of DNA Library Preparation in the Roche/454 Sequencing System.
The genomic DNA is chopped into smaller fragments and short adapters are ligated onto the fragments. Finally, the sstDNA library undergoes size-selection and purification. Adapted from Roche literature, with permission (© Roche Diagnostics GmbH).

followed by the ligation of short adapters (A and B), providing the specific priming sequence required for both the amplification and sequencing steps. The adapters also provide the "sequencing key," a short sequence of four nucleotides used by the system software for base calling and to recognize legitimate library reads. Finally, the dsDNA fragments are separated into single strands and the quality of the library of single-stranded template DNA fragments (sstDNA library) is assessed. The library is quantified, to determine the amount of the library to use as input for emulsion-based clonal amplification.

After repair of any nicks in the double-stranded library, adapter B allows release of the unbound strand of each fragment (with 5'-adapter A). Adapter B also contains a biotin tag that allows for the immobilization of the library onto streptavidin beads. Fragments from the DNA library are immobilized onto the beads, with each bead carrying at most one amplifiable DNA molecule (Fig. 2.3) (Dressman et al., 2003). The bead-bound library is emulsified with the amplification reagents in water-in-oil mixture. Each bead is captured with the water-in-oil mixture and functions as its own microreactor in which polymerase chain reaction (PCR) amplification occurs. This results in bead-immobilized, clonal-amplified DNA fragments. Amplification is carried out in bulk, resulting in beads covered with tens of millions of copies of a single DNA fragment; while each bead contains a different fragment.

Sequencing

The unique feature of the sequencer is the flow cell, a custom-fabricated picotiter plate (PTP) with approximately 3.4 million wells to carry the 20μm amplified sstDNA library beads preincubated with DNA polymerase. The PTP is a fiberoptic faceplate with etched wells (each 29μm wide with 34μm pitch). Each PTP well holds a single DNA bead, providing a fixed location from which to monitor the sequencing reaction in real-time, using a closed-circuit digital (CCD) camera placed together with DTP. Smaller beads containing enzymes are centrifuged into the PTP to surround the DNA beads and fill the remaining space in the wells (Fig. 2.4).

The loaded PTP is placed into the instrument, where the fluidics subsystem causes sequencing reagents (containing buffers and nucleotides) to flow across the wells of the plate. Nucleotides are sequentially introduced across the PTP in a fixed order during a sequencing run. During the nucleotide flow, each of the million beads, each with millions of copies of DNA, is sequenced in parallel. If a nucleotide complementing the position on the template strand to be sequenced is captured in the well, the polymerase extends the existing DNA strand by adding nucleotide(s).

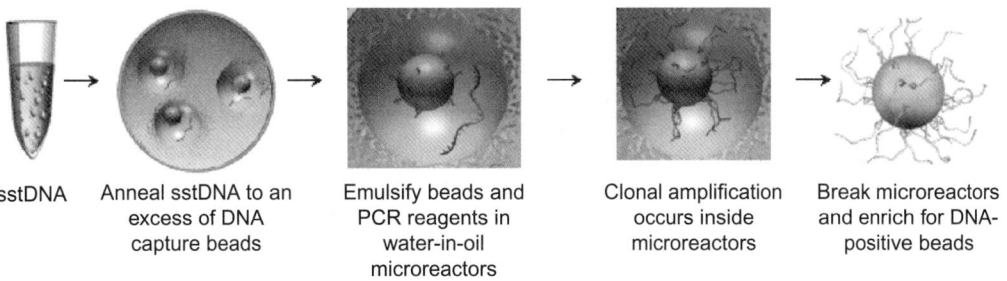

| sstDNA | Anneal sstDNA to an excess of DNA capture beads | Emulsify beads and PCR reagents in water-in-oil microreactors | Clonal amplification occurs inside microreactors | Break microreactors and enrich for DNA-positive beads |

FIGURE 2.3 The Emulsion Polymerase Chain Reaction Process.
The DNA fragments of the chosen size are immobilized onto the DNA capture beads. This follows the emulsification of the bead-bound library in a water-in-oil mixture, resulting in clonal-amplified DNA fragments immobilized on the beads. Adapted from Roche literature, with permission (© Roche Diagnostics GmbH).

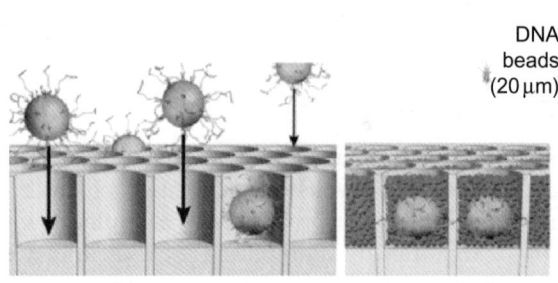
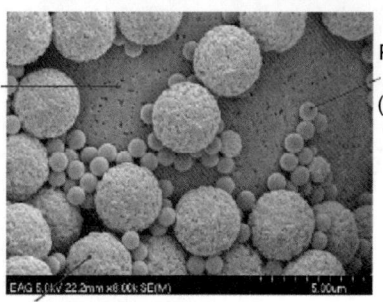

FIGURE 2.4 The Picotiter Plate.
DNA beads and enzyme beads are deposited into the wells of the picotiter plate. Packing beads fill the remaining gap in the wells. Adapted from Roche literature, with permission (© Roche Diagnostics GmbH).

Addition of one (or more) nucleotide(s) results in a reaction that generates a light signal, which is recorded by the CCD camera in the instrument. The signal strength is proportional to the number of nucleotides incorporated in a single nucleotide flow. Nucleotide incorporation is detected by the associated release of inorganic pyrophosphate and the generation of photons. Wells containing template-carrying beads are identified by detecting a known four-nucleotide "key" sequence embedded at the beginning of the read. This acts as an address for the sequencing run in each well.

The most recent version of the Roche/454 sequencing platform, Titanium, is able to produce more than 500 million bases in a single long run of 9 hours, with a read length of more than 400 bp. This platform has a unique advantage over other platforms in applications where longer read lengths are critical. To date, hundreds of articles have been published reporting the findings of research that was carried out using Roche/454 sequencers. After the completion of the human genome project, the first human genome (that of Nobel Laureate, James Watson, Wheeler, 2008) was completely sequenced on the Roche/454 sequencing platform, at a cost of approximately 2 million US dollars (roughly an order of magnitude less than it would have been using traditional machines) (Bentley et al., 2008).

Illumina: Genome Analyzer

Popularly known as Solexa, the Genome Analyzer from Illumina is another sequencing platform that is widely used these days. The unique feature of the sequencing scheme is the flow cell which, in contrast to the PTP flow cell in the Roche/454 platform, is a non-photolithographically fabricated chip and does not require physical positioning of the template. Here, the sequencing templates can be immobilized while the other sequencing reagents are accessed, and eight channels can be used to sequence the same or different libraries. The same flow cell can be used for both library amplification and sequencing processes. The Illumina Genome Analyzer uses reversible terminator-based sequencing chemistry (see below). This contrasts with the irreversible terminator-based sequencing chemistry of the classical Sanger sequencing approaches.

Library Preparation and Amplification

Figure 2.5 depicts the processes involved in preparing the DNA library and the amplification strategy used in the Illumina sequencing scheme. This relies on the attachment of randomly fragmented genomic DNA to a planar, optically transparent surface of the flow cell through specific adapters attached by ligation

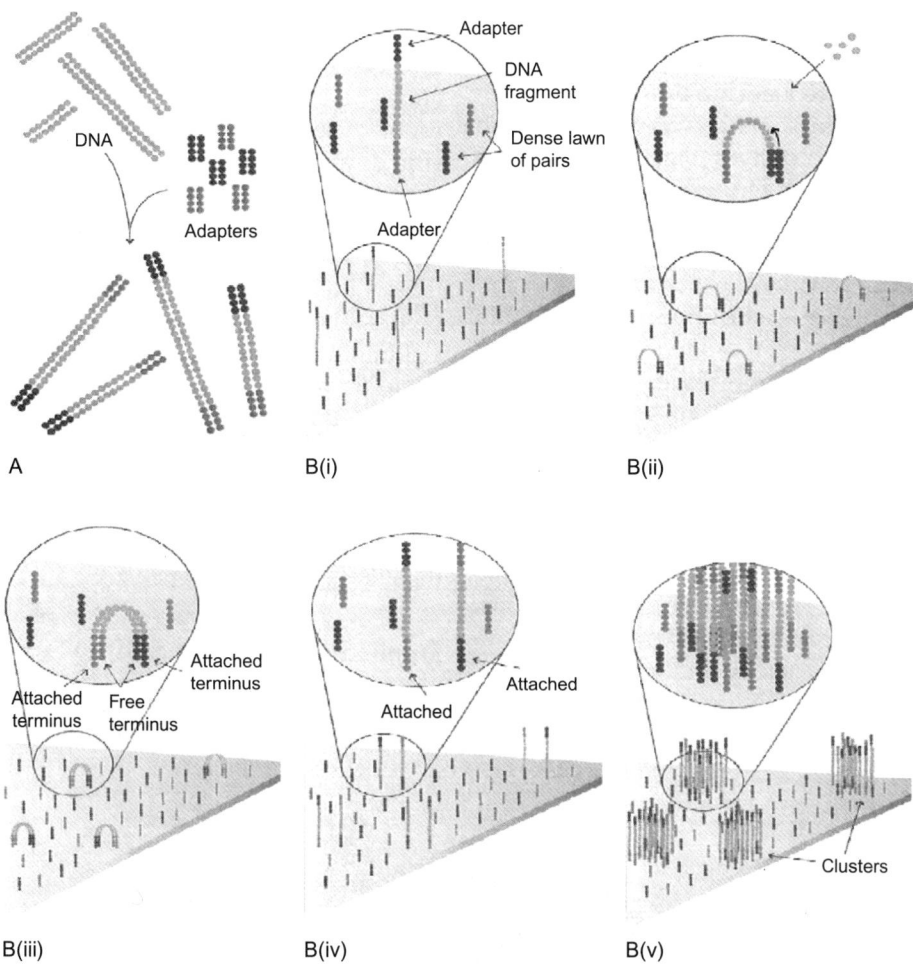

FIGURE 2.5 Upstream Process in the Illumina Genome Analyzer.
(A) Preparation of the genome library, in which the genomic DNA is randomly fragmented and adapters are ligated to both ends of the fragments. (B) Bridge amplification. B(i) The single-stranded fragments with adapters are bonded randomly to the inside surface of the flow-cell channels. B(ii) The solid-phase bridge amplification is started by the addition of unlabeled nucleotides and enzyme. B(iii) Double-stranded bridges are formed on the solid-phase substrate. B(iv) The single-stranded templates are left anchored to the surface as a result of denaturation. B(v) Completion of amplification of all clusters; the process is repeated to generate millions of dense clusters of double-stranded DNA. Adapted from Illumina literature, with permission.

(Adessi et al., 2000; Turcatti et al., 2008). Attached DNA fragments are extended and bridge amplified to create an ultra-high-density sequencing flow cell with 50 million clusters, each containing approximately 1000 copies of the same template (Adessi et al., 2000; Fedurco et al., 2006). The technical uniqueness is the use of bridge amplification, whereby an arc of DNA is anchored using the attached adaptors. The PCR amplification products are contained within the anchored sites (also called *in-situ* amplification). In this manner the signal can be augmented by PCR, and is kept at a specific site so that subsequent signals can be addressed.

Sequencing

The templates are sequenced using a robust four-color DNA sequencing-by-synthesis technology that uses reversible terminators with removable fluorescent dyes (Fig. 2.6). This novel approach ensures high accuracy and true base-by-base sequencing, eliminating sequence-context specific errors and thus enabling sequencing through homopolymers (e.g. A-A-A-A-A) and repetitive sequences, which are problematic in pyrosequencing.

High-sensitivity fluorescence detection is achieved using laser excitation and total internal reflection optics. Short sequence reads are aligned against a reference genome and genetic differences are called using specially developed data analysis pipeline software. Alternative methods of sample preparation allow the same system to be used for a range of applications, including gene expression, small RNA discovery and protein–nucleic acid interactions.

After completion of the first read, the templates can be regenerated *in situ* to enable a second read of more than 36 bp from the opposite end of the fragments. The Paired-End Module directs the regeneration and amplification operations to prepare the templates for the second round of sequencing. First, the newly sequenced strands are stripped off and the complementary strands are bridge amplified to form clusters. Once the original templates are cleaved and removed, the reverse strands undergo sequencing-by-synthesis. The second round of sequencing occurs at the opposite end of the templates.

Illumina Genome Analyzer is able to sequence up to 50 million clusters with a read length of approximately 35 bp and with a deliverable of more than 3 Gb per run. Recently, genomes of an Asian individual (Wang et al., 2008), an African male (Bentley et al., 2008) and a European woman (Ley et al., 2008) were sequenced using the Illumina Genome Analyzer.

Applied Biosystems: SOLiD Sequencing

Unlike other platforms, Sequencing by Oligonucleotide Ligation and Detection (SOLiD)

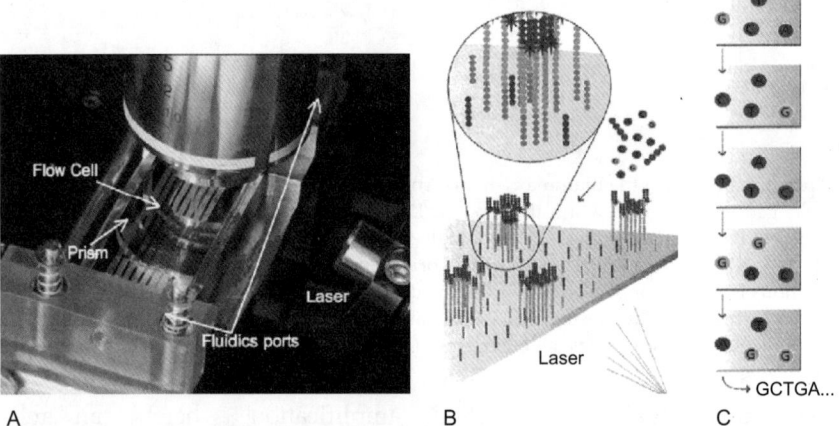

FIGURE 2.6 Sequencing Process in the Illumina Genome Analyzer.
(A) Flow-cell imaging by total internal reflection fluorescence. The imaging part of the machines: a typical flow cell with eight lanes. (B) Reversible terminator chemistry to determine a base. One sequencing cycle is initiated by the addition of all four reversible terminators, primers and DNA polymerase enzyme to the flow cell, followed by laser excitation. For each cluster, the emitted fluorescence image is captured and the identity of the first base is recorded. (C) The cycles are repeated for all clusters, the image is captured and the identification of the base is recorded. In this way the sequence of the bases in a given fragment is determined. Adapted from Illumina literature, with permission.

is based on sequential ligation with dye-labeled oligonucleotides (McKernan et al., 2006). The DNA fragments are immobilized on 1 mm magnetic beads and the sequencing function is performed by measurement of the serial ligation of oligonucleotides to the DNA by ligase.

Library Preparation and Emulsion Polymerase Chain Reaction

Similar to the Roche/454 sequencing platforms, the SOLiD platform uses an adapter-ligated library, and uses an emulsion PCR approach with magnetic beads to amplify the fragments for sequencing. There are two methods for creating the DNA library: fragment library and mate-paired library (Ng et al., 2005). The fragment library can be used for directed re-sequencing and the mate-paired (paired-end) library can be used for whole-genome sequencing (Fig. 2.7).

Clonal bead populations are prepared in microreactors containing template, PCR reaction components, 1 μm magnetic beads and primers. After PCR, the templates are denatured and bead enrichment is performed to separate beads with extended templates from undesired beads. The template on the selected beads undergoes a 3′ modification to allow covalent bonding to the slide. After the emulsion has been broken, beads bearing amplification products are selectively recovered (Fig. 2.8).

Sequencing

A custom-fabricated flow cell was used to immobilize the beads bearing amplification products to a solid planar substrate to generate a dense, disordered array. In this instrument, two flow cells can be loaded per run, each of which can be divided into one, four or eight chambers to contain different libraries or one single library.

The sequencing begins by hybridizing the universal primers complementary to the adapter sequence of each amplicon on each bead (Fig. 2.9).

The innovation in this strategy is the use of specific sequencing primers that interrogate dinucleotide sequences in a phased manner. One sequencing cycle involves the hybridization of octamers that have a specified dinucleotide sequence at the 5′ end (in Figure 2.9, it is AT), while the other bases are random, "wildcard" sequences, with one of four fluorescent colors linked to the 3′ end. This primer will hybridize if the template DNA to be sequenced has the complementary sequence (in Figure 2.9, it is TA) immediately after the universal primer. The provision of DNA ligase will covalently

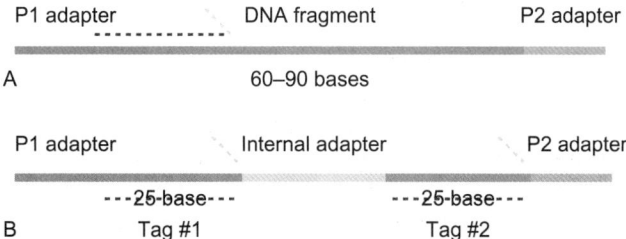

FIGURE 2.7 Two Types of Libraries Used in the SOLiD System.
(A) Creation of a fragment library. Any complex sample (genomic DNA, tag library or concatenated PCR products) is fragmented (60–90 bases) in either a random or a targeted fashion (mechanical sonication or enzymatic digestion). Subsequently, two adapters (P1 and P2) are ligated onto the fragmented samples. (B) Creation of a mate-paired library. After random fragmentation, the sample is selected in the size range from 0.6 Kb to 10 Kb. Thereafter, an internal adapter is ligated and the fragment with the internal adapter is circularized. The circularized molecule is cleaved such that two tags of known size are left attached to the two sides of the internal adapter, which follows the ligation of adapters P1 and P2. Adapted from Applied Biosystems literature, with permission.

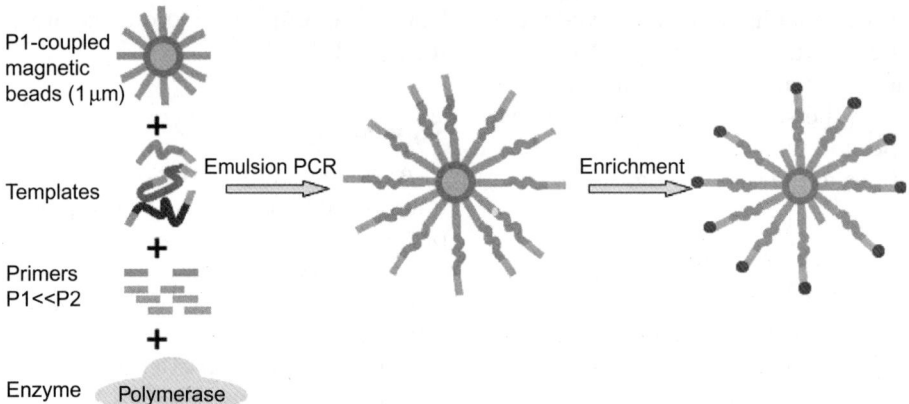

FIGURE 2.8 Emulsion Polymerase Chain Reaction.
P1-coupled beads, template, primers and DNA polymerase are mixed in microreactors containing oil-in-water emulsions. After emulsion PCR, the denaturization and enrichment steps are followed. Adapted from Applied Biosystems literature, with permission.

link the fluorescently labeled probe and will be registered after excitation. The image acquisition in four channels effectively collects data for the same base positions across all the beads. Subsequently, the fluorescence tag is removed by chemical cleavage of the octamer between positions 5 and 6. In the next round of hybridization, the second "universal" primer is offset by one base in the 5' direction (n − 1) and is prepared for another round of ligation, to enable sequencing and image acquisition of every 5th base. After the completion of one set of ligation, the new extended primer is denatured to reset the system, and ligation cycles are repeated sequentially five times. Different sets of interrogation positions can be selected by changing the position of the fluorescence label in the octamer or by using a different primer. With mate-paired sequencing, this process is repeated for the second 3' tag. Because synthesis is not required, the usual 5' to 3' directionality is not a limitation.

As each fluorescent tag on a ligated octamer correlates with two bases, the sequencing proceeds on a two-base encoding scheme that is offset by one base. This leads to the interrogation of each base position twice, making the system more prepared for miscalls and errors. Read lengths for SOLiD are user defined between 25 and 35 bp, and because of the massive parallel scale, each sequencing run yields 2–4 Gb of DNA sequence data. With improved chemistry and engineering, nowadays the platform can produce more than 10 Gb of sequence data.

APPLICATIONS OF SEQUENCING IN SYSTEMS BIOLOGY: THE TRANSCRIPTOME AND TRANSCRIPTIONAL REGULATION

The transcriptome is a collection of all transcripts in a cell. It can be assessed by expression arrays, or by direct sequencing approaches. Arrays have an advantage of speed and lower cost, but are limited to transcripts interrogated by the probes present on the array. Sequencing is accomplished by using reverse transcriptase to convert the messenger RNA (mRNA) code into complementary DNA (cDNA). A second round of polymerization renders this single-stranded cDNA into a double-stranded entity that can be inserted into appropriate vectors and cloned. cDNA libraries were the genomic

APPLICATIONS OF SEQUENCING IN SYSTEMS BIOLOGY: THE TRANSCRIPTOME 25

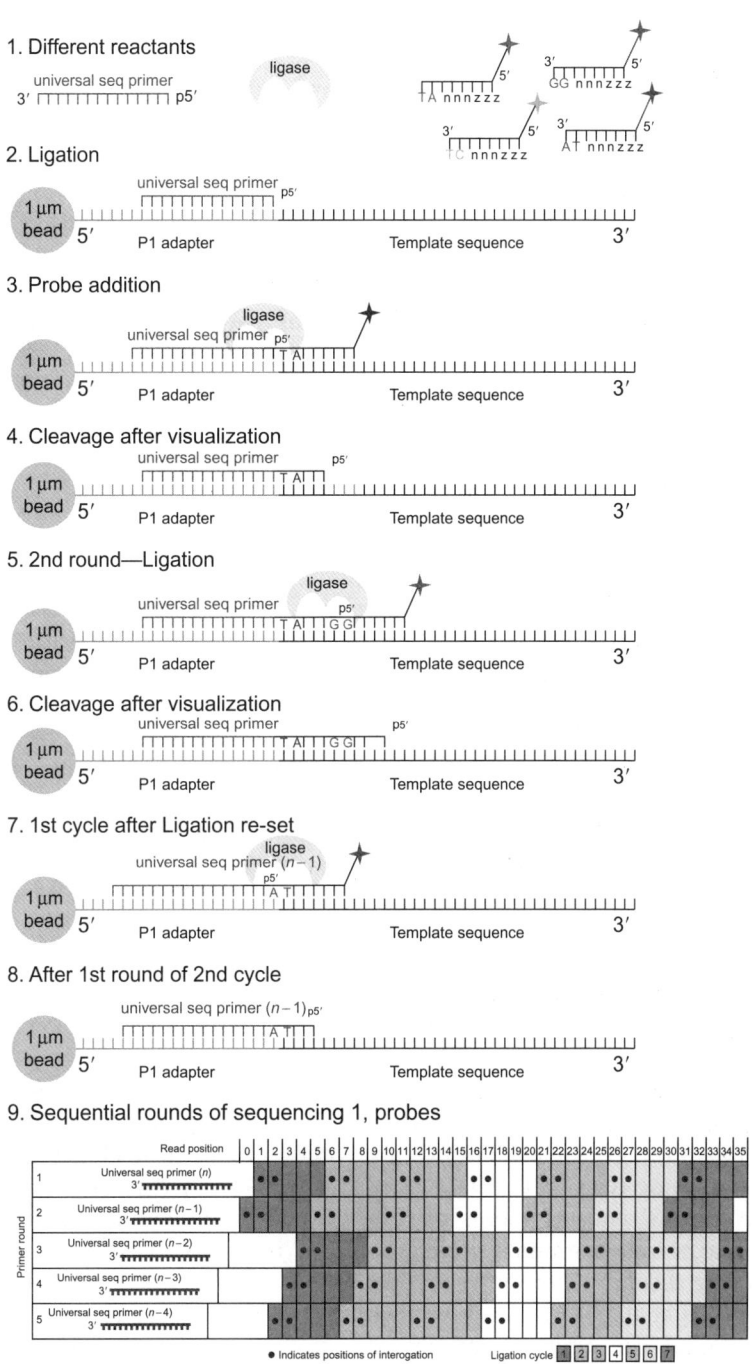

FIGURE 2.9 SOLiD Sequencing Chemistry. Adapted from Applied Biosystems literature, with permission.

I. FOUNDATIONS OF SYSTEMS BIOLOGY

representation of the transcriptome. However, cloning strategies add to the cost, and the massive abundance of some transcripts overwhelmed lower-abundance transcripts, leading to incomplete information. This has been overcome recently, by new cloning strategies and by the second-generation sequencing technologies.

Serial analysis of gene expression (SAGE) renders each cDNA into a representative short (14–21 bp) sequence fragment tag originating from the 3′ end of the cDNA, which can be concatenated to facilitate sequencing. In this approach, cDNA fragments first are 3′-labeled with biotin and bound to streptavidin-coated magnetic beads. These immobilized fragments are then digested with a 4 bp cleaving endonuclease and ligated with an adapter at the 3′ end that contains a recognition site for type II restriction endonucleases that cleave DNA distant from the recognition sequence. This allows for these restriction endonucleases to cleave the DNA 10 bp or 20 bp 5′ from its recognition sites, and permits the extraction of 14 bp SAGE tags or 21 bp LongSAGE tags from the 3′ end of each cDNA template. These short tags are then concatenated into longer DNA fragments, and then sequenced (Saha et al., 2002; Velculescu et al., 1995). The 14 or 21 bp tags can be mapped specifically to known and putative transcripts. Similarly, cap analysis gene expression (CAGE) isolates short (~20 nucleotide) sequence tags that originate from the 5′ end of full-length mRNAs (Kodzius et al., 2006). The major advance of this strategy is that the transcriptome could be assessed quantitatively in an unbiased manner.

Advancing this strategy, gene identification signature pair-end ditag (GIS-PET) cDNA cloning links the 5′ and 3′ end-fragments of full-length cDNAs into paired fragments, which can be sequenced using second-generation sequencing approaches (Wei et al., 2006). This approach has the same digital counting capabilities as SAGE, but is superior in that both the 5′ and 3′ ends are sequenced as a linked pair. This permits the annotation of the transcriptional start site of each transcriptional unit, which is important in assessing DNA regulatory regions. The disadvantage is that GIS-PET does not disclose the alternative spliced species and any sequences variations in the body of the cDNA. More recently, the complete transcriptome has been sequenced using a shotgun sequencing approach that fragments a cDNA library and computationally assembles all transcriptome sequences. This, in effect, provides the sequence of all cDNAs, including splice variants (Nagalakshmi et al., 2008; Wang et al., 2009).

Expression Arrays

Expression genomics is a strategy that examines gene expression in a comprehensive and massively parallel fashion. The simultaneous assessment of gene expression in this manner and across numerous cellular conditions uncovers higher-order organization in the gene transcriptional cassette of a cell. The ability to analyze this complexity is essential, because, often, the more genes and biological conditions studied, the more clear this underlying organization becomes. Thus the power of expression microarray data is not in viewing the technology as a collection of individual "northern" blots, but in generating a composite image of the expression profile of a cell. The core technology is found in expression *microarrays*, in which tens to hundreds of thousands of DNA *probes* are immobilized on a two-dimensional surface. The DNA probes are either double-stranded cDNAs specific to cloned genes, or gene-specific single-stranded sense oligonucleotides designed in a genome-wide manner. Spotted cDNAs are routinely used in custom arrays for specific queries, or for species for which the complete genome sequence is unavailable. The *oligo arrays* offer genome-wide transcription profiling and include known, unknown and predicted/annotated genes, and are a popular choice (Table 2.2). Affymetrix arrays (www.affymetrix.com)

TABLE 2.2 Expression Array Platforms

	Platform	Probe Sets	Coverage	Application
Affymetrix	GeneChip Exon 1.0 ST array	1.4 million, >5 500 000 features	4 probes along entire transcript	Alternate transcripts, different isoforms
	GeneChip Gene 1.0 ST array	764 885 probe sets, 28 869 genes	26 probes along the gene	Whole-transcript coverage
	GeneChip U133 Plus 2.0 array	>54 000 probe sets, 385 000 genes	11 pairs of probes per transcript	3′ Expression arrays
Agilent	Whole-genome oligo microarray	44 000 features representing all known genes	60-mer gene-specific oligomers	Whole-genome gene expression analysis
Illumina	Human HT-12, Human Ref-8 expression beadchips	48 000 probes, >25 000 annotated genes	50-mer gene-specific oligomers	Whole-genome expression array, in combination with DASL uses partially degraded RNA samples, FFPE samples

DASL, cDNA-mediated Annealing, Selection, extension and Ligation Assay; HT-12, high throughput 12: FFPE, formalin-fixed, paraffin-embedded; Ref-8, interrogates 8 samples at a time; ST, sense target.

have 25-mer oligos directly synthesized on the glass slide using photolithographic technology. Each probe set consists of matched and mismatched probes that are used to distinguish between specific and background signals. In contrast, Agilent (www.agilent.com) directly deposits 60-mer oligos using an inkjet printer. Illumina Beadarrays (www.illumina.com) use microbeads coated with 50-mer gene-specific oligonucleotides that are randomly distributed on a glass slide; detection of the hybridization signal is achieved by pseudo-sequencing of the bound signal. A comparative analysis of the performance of these platforms in terms of reproducibility, probe specificity and information content has been reported by de Reyniès et al. (2006).

All platforms use mRNA as the starting material, albeit in varying amounts, with Illumina Beadarrays requiring less than 100 ng of the sample, as opposed to 5 μg total RNA required for Affymetrix arrays. The mRNA is reverse transcribed using oligo-dT-T7 RNA polymerase primer and converted to dsDNA. T7 RNA polymerase is used to make antisense RNA using the dsDNA as template in the presence of fluorescent (cyanine 3)-labeled dUTP. The labeled cDNA or cRNA *target* is hybridized to the microarrays. The annealed target can be quantitatively assessed by various detection methods, including fluorescence- or luminescence-based approaches. The signal intensities for each probe are measured to approximate the actual levels of transcripts.

A key component is the analysis of microarray data to eliminate technical variation and random noise in order to quantify the biological variation amongst samples. Variation in array datasets occurs as a result of sampling errors, skewing introduced by poor quality of starting mRNA, biases introduced during the RNA amplification step, differential labeling of the cRNA and during probe-to-cRNA hybridization. The first level of analysis involves a statistical rendering of datasets: normalization of spot intensity, and a reproducibility check across biological replicates. The second level involves more sophisticated analysis to determine biological patterns embedded in the data. Most simple and intuitive is the analysis of differentially expressed genes across several samples by univariate analysis using *t*-tests, analysis of variance (ANOVA) or the Mann–Whitney test, depending upon the number of samples to be compared. To determine the effect of multiple gene expression patterns simultaneously, complex tests are required (Dupuy et al., 2007; Trevina et al., 2006). Commonly, in cancer datasets, group-specific gene expression signatures are used for class prediction, class discovery, response to chemotherapy, drug resistance and, more importantly, to determine prognostic signatures in cancer and their relationship to patient survival. The Affymetrix platform has been a popular choice in the clinical setting, and several diseases—including cancer, cardiovascular disease, inflammation, aging and stem cell differentiation—have been profiled.

A third level of complexity in microarray data analysis comes from studies that combine publicly available datasets or merge experimental data from several studies for meta-analysis. For these purposes, raw data need to be re-analyzed. In some meta-studies, the comparability of the different platforms appears to have been problematic (Severgnini et al., 2006). In contrast, exhaustive analysis by the multicenter Microarray Quality Control Consortium showed relatively high experimental reproducibility (Shi et al., 2006). It is thus important to adhere to a standard data exchange format, standard protocols and experimental design of array experiments. Another difficulty in merging datasets for analysis is the long list of genes that use different genome browsers and different nomenclature. The non-standard format of public data deposition makes it difficult to cross-compare datasets easily, especially across several species. Attempts to standardize this procedure have been made in the Minimum Information About a Microarray Experiment (MIAME) (Brazma et al., 2001).

ChIP-on-chip Arrays

Gene regulation consists of transcription factor binding to specific DNA sequence elements in gene regulatory regions. Microarray analysis and clustering of similarly regulated genes has prompted the need to develop tools for global patterning of DNA–protein interactions to investigate whether co-regulated genes are indeed controlled by the same transcription factor. Transcription factor binding sites are identified and validated by chromatin immunoprecipitation assay (ChIP) (Im et al., 2004). Samples/cells are cross linked with formaldehyde to covalently retain or "freeze" DNA–protein interactions. The complex is isolated and the DNA is sheared to 300–500 bp fragments using mechanical sonication. A small fraction of the complex is reserved as input DNA. Transcription-factor-specific antibodies are used to immunoprecipitate the protein-bound DNA fraction. DNA is then released from the DNA–protein–antibody complex by reverse cross linking, and is purified. If the transcription factor occupied the tested site, its corresponding DNA element would be enriched by ChIP. The occupancy and its strength are tested by using primers flanking the known or putative binding site DNA sequence and the input DNA, using real-time PCR analysis. Primer pairs located in the gene desert or a non-transcription factor binding region are used as an internal reference to normalize the PCR results. The real-time PCR cycles are a measure of the amount of enrichment at that site and the data are displayed as percentage of input.

Real-time PCR-based assays can allow only a finite number of binding sites to be investigated and, more importantly, require prior knowledge of the binding region/site of the transcription factor. However, there are more than 2000 known transcription factor–DNA binding proteins and combinations thereof that regulate gene transcription. Not all binding site sequences are known, and not all the regulatory regions have been characterized. To enable discovery and identification of existing and novel transcription factor binding sites in a genome wide manner, ChIP-on-chip technologies have emerged (Table 2.3). This platform combines

TABLE 2.3 ChIP-on-ChIP Array Platforms

	Platform	Probe Sets	Coverage		
Affymetrix	Chr 21/22 2.0R	25-mer probes, 16 bp tiling arrays with 2.3 million features	Whole-chromosome coverage		
Nimblegen	Whole-genome tiling array, HD2 format	50- to 75-mer probes, 100 bp probe interval, set of 10 arrays *or* > 200 bp probe interval, set of 4 arrays, 2.1 million probes	Whole-gene high-density coverage		
	Whole-genome 385 K	50-mer probes, 100 bp or less probe interval, across all unique regions	Whole-genome economy array		
				Distance from TSS (kb)	
				Upstream	Downstream
Affymetrix	Human promoter arrays 1R	25-mer probes, 35 bp tiling arrays with 4.6 million features, spanning 25 500 promoters		7.5	2.45
Nimblegen	2.1 M promoter array	50-mer probes, 100 bp probe interval or less, 2.1 million features, all promoters UCSC		7.25	3.25
	385 K set promoter array	50-mer probes, 100 bp probe interval or less, 385 000 features		3.5	0.75
	Refseq set promoter set	50-mer probes, 100 bp probe interval or less, all refseq genes		2.2	0.5

Chr, chromosome; HD2, high density 2 format; 1R, 2.0R; refseq, The reference sequence collection (http://www.ncbi.nlm.nih.gov/RefSeq/; TSS, transcription start site; UCSC, University of California, Santa Cruz.

ChIP assays with DNA microarrays. The DNA microarray was first generated using probes spanning promoter sequences up to 1 kb upstream of transcription start sites of 1500 genes (Ren and Dynlacht, 2004). The ChIP material obtained was labeled using fluorescent dyes in a manner similar to that in gene expression profiling arrays. The labeled probe was hybridized and the signal scanned after activation of the fluorophore to detect binding events. Subsequently, commercial platforms offering promoters up to 10 kb from known transcription start sites were designed (Table 2.3). The putative binding site of the transcription factor can be validated using ChIP and real-time PCR and gel-shift assays, and in promoter assays in heterologous systems. Although these arrays spanned a significant region upstream of the transcription start site, previous data indicate that, often, transcription factor binding sites were located in the gene body, downstream of the gene or several 100 kb away from the transcription start site. Therefore, the next generation arrays were developed using overlapping tiled probe sequences across chromosomes 21 and 22. The findings from initial experiments with nuclear hormone receptors, such as estrogen receptor ChIP-on-chip, suggested that distal binding sites could be detected using this technology. Recently, whole-genome tiled arrays are available for comprehensive mapping of the global binding site pattern of a transcription factor, irrespective of the location of the transcription start site.

ChIP-on-chip arrays, although expensive, offer several advantages, as they require small amounts of ChIP material, are biologically reproducible and can be used for perturbation or time-course experiments to study the dynamics of binding site utilization. However, ChIP-on-chip appears to be constrained by a low dynamic range of detection and by unique probe design challenges: for example, repeat DNA elements, structural complexities, regions of centromeres and GC-rich regions in the genome are often excluded from this array. Recently, we have shown the presence of important regulatory sites for the estrogen receptor in repetitive DNA and its importance in the evolution of binding sites across species. This calls for using a technology that is not dependent upon probe design or hybridization. With the advent of next-generation direct sequencing technologies, such as ChIP-sequencing discussed in later chapters, global mapping of binding sites has gained tremendously high throughput, and the intersection of several transcription factors and epigenetic modification datasets has revolutionized our understanding of gene expression. Combining both gene expression and ChIP-on-chip/ChIP-sequencing have provided complex and detailed information about transcriptional networks.

Reverse Transcriptase-Polymerase Chain Reaction

Early microarray data obtained from spotted arrays were validated with a gene-by-gene validation approach by simple qualitative changes in gene expression using a competitive primer strategy, or by limited multiplex PCR. Although useful, these techniques were time-consuming and laborious. With the sequencing of the human genome, the array platforms underwent rapid expansion and evolution to cover all known and predicted genes. Simultaneously, several tools for pathway analysis were generated, enabling grouping of genes in same biological process by anchoring functional biological data to observed changes. Used together on datasets, these overlapping tools showed that, often, genes in a pathway were simultaneously altered, which led to the emergence of a "gene signature" concept. Such signatures—defining class prediction, classification, disease states and therapeutic response to drugs—often comprised as few as five to as many as 78 genes. These data prompted the shift from gene-by-gene reverse transcriptase PCR (RT-PCR) to techniques of high-throughput PCR screening of several samples simultaneously that were fast, efficient and required small amounts of starting material for analysis and commonly used strategies are described in this section.

Radio-labeling of Polymerase Chain Reaction Products

This is the simplest, highly sensitive quantitative method available to determine levels of transcripts of various mRNAs across experimental samples. mRNA samples to be evaluated are reverse transcribed using standard procedures. Historically, equal amounts of cDNA were used in PCRs, with trace amounts of "spiked" $[^{32}P]dATP$ or $[^{32}P]dCTP$ nucleotides. An alternative strategy was to end-label the sense PCR primer. PCRs were carried out for varying number of cycles to allow the incorporation of the radionucleotide tracer, and the resultant product was analyzed on a gel. Densitometric scanning of the autoradiographs and images were quantified and compared, to determine fold changes in gene expression. These processes, although precise, are cumbersome and labor intensive. Importantly, a typical PCR reaction follows a geometric progression and tends to plateau over time as a result of depletion of nucleotides, exhaustion of the extension enzyme Taq polymerase, decreased template-to-primer ratio and increased competition between template–template vs. template–primer re-annealing. Such endpoint determinations that fall in the plateau region of the reaction often misrepresent actual amounts of starting cDNA template. Therefore quantification is performed by comparing the slopes of the linear portion of the amplification–cycle number curves.

Real-time Quantitative Polymerase Chain Reaction

To maintain the sensitivity of the radiolabel, but improve the scalability and accuracy of quantitative PCRs, several technologies have been developed that use fluorescence detectors but different chemistries to determine the outcome. Representative assays are described here (VanGuilder et al., 2008)

SyBR Green Incorporation

The first technology uses the incorporation of SyBr green dye during the PCR reaction, based on the linear relationship of SyBR green with DNA concentration. The dye intercalates in the minor groove of dsDNA, with little or no affinity to single-stranded DNA. The amount of fluorescence is recorded at each PCR cycle in real-time, unlike previous assays that only determined the concentrations of endpoint products. As the reaction progresses, the product remains undetected because of the low concentrations of DNA and SyBr green in the initial cycles. The first cycle in which the product is detected is called the threshold cycle (C_T). The C_T value is thus the most accurate determination of the starting amounts of cDNA in each reverse transcription product. Typically, a C_T value of 10 to 30 cycles is considered to be within the assay range. Above 30 cycles, often non-specific amplifications are evident. Using real-time PCR, several primer sets can be evaluated in a 96- or a 384-well format of PCR plates, thereby decreasing the time of reaction but allowing simultaneous detection of the gene signature and improving the scalability of the reaction to several samples. To determine the exact amounts of a gene-specific mRNA that is present, it would be necessary to run a dilution series using known amounts of an amplicon generated by the same set of primers as a positive control and plotting a standard curve using the C_T values. However, most validation PCRs that follow microarray analysis do not require exact quantification of mRNA, but a relative estimate of change across several samples.

To design this experimentally, a housekeeping gene that remains unchanged in expression is used for normalization as an internal reference, along with the test gene. Under ideal conditions, if equal amount of cDNA is taken from each test sample, the internal reference gene would have the same C_T value in all. Such a real-time PCR assay design typically generates two C_T values per sample, one specific for the test gene, the second specific for the reference gene; their difference gives the normalized amount of transcript in that sample (ΔC_T). Subtraction of ΔC_T values across various samples gives the relative fold change of gene-specific mRNA and is acquired by the formula

$$2^{-\Delta\Delta C_T} \qquad (2.1)$$

A potential drawback of the SyBr green system is that, along with desired products, non-specific amplifications and/or primer dimers may contribute and alter the C_T values, and cannot be distinguished from one another. However, the primer dimer issue is resolved to a large extent by plotting primer melting curves at each cycle: a single peak at the melting temperature of the primer suggests that the primers do not interact with each other. In addition, the non-specific products can be evaluated by conventional gel electrophoresis, to determine the size of the PCR product. Recent reports have shown that SyBr green PCRs have high accuracy and reproducibility, and are comparable to TaqMan assays for the validation of multiple-microarray platform data (Arikawa et al., 2008).

Laser Scanning Technology

TaqMan assays integrate PCR and laser scanning technology and, rather than quantifying the PCR product, tend to quantify the release of a fluorescent reporter dye (Applied Biosystems: https://products.appliedbiosystems.com/ab/

en/US/adirect/ab?cmd =catNavigate2&catID= 601267). In this assay, along with the conventional sense/forward and antisense/reverse primers, an additional primer is designed that spans the region between the gene-specific primers (Fig. 2.10). The middle probe primer is labeled with a VIC® reporter dye (R) at the 5' end and a quencher dye (Q) at its 3' end. The 3' end of the probe primer is blocked to prevent amplification from the middle probe primer. Upon annealing of the three primers, fluorescence of the VIC® reporter probe is prevented by its proximity to the quencher. As the reaction progresses, the 5' VIC® dye is cleaved by the 5' nuclease activity of AmpliTaq gold polymerase, thereby separating it from the quencher. The fluorescence of the released dye per cycle is a measure of the resultant products. This reaction is possible only if both the sense primer and the probe primer anneal on the same strand. Therefore, the use of the middle probe primer greatly improves the specificity of the primers and, to a large extent, prevents the detection of spurious and single-strand DNA amplifications. Furthermore, it improves the sensitivity of the PCR and allows for quantitative detection of relatively rare mRNAs.

Both these technologies improve the scalability of the assay without compromising accuracy, and serve most of the scientific community. However, both require ample starting material to assay several genes, whereas in the clinical setting the material available is especially limiting and sometimes processed as archival specimens. Moreover, plate-to-plate variations between primer sets in these assays can confound analysis across hundreds of samples. It is therefore desirable to have PCR assays that multiplex and assay several genes with several primer sets, using the same amount of starting material and in a single sample well.

The power of TaqMan PCRs is increased by 24 times using integrated microfluidics technology and nano valves to control the flow and mixing of PCR reagents (Warren et al., 2006). The Fluidigm Biomark (http://www.fluidigm.com/) assay is available in a 48 × 48 or 96 × 96 format, reading 2304 and 9216 samples, respectively. It is possible to test 96 samples simultaneously for 96 primer pairs in a single reaction. As opposed to the 10–20 μl reaction volume necessary in the previous platforms, this assay uses 5 μl of sample per reaction well, decreasing considerably the cost and the amount of starting material required. This assay covers six logs of magnitude, can detect single-copy mRNAs and has been successfully used to perform several gene PCRs on a single-cell mRNA with high reproducibility. This platform requires preamplification of the mRNA, which may lead to skewing of the PCR data; however, correct titration of starting mRNA quantities easily resolves this issue.

Branched DNA

Variations in the quality, efficiency of reverse transcription and amounts of purified RNA isolated from limited samples, together with the RNA amplification step required in the RT-PCR reactions previously described, all contribute to skewing of the data and imprecise PCR readouts.

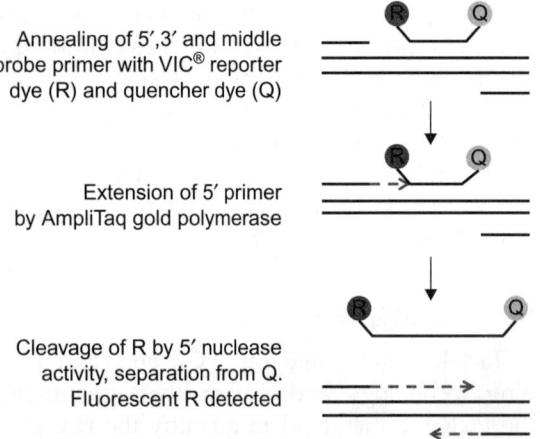

FIGURE 2.10 Schematic of the TaqMan Quantitative Polymerase Chain Reaction Assay.

Quantigene (Panomics: http://www.panomics.com/index.php?id=product_1) uses branched DNA technology that avoids all these steps. Gene-specific probe sets that contain 10 or more specific oligonucleotide primer pairs are hybridized to the sample mRNA. A preamplifier molecule that hybridizes to each oligonucleotide primer pair is added, followed by an amplifier molecule. Finally, several fluorescent-label probe oligonucleotides are added, thus allowing detection of the starting RNA using Luminex assays based on xMAP technology. Luminex color-codes 5.6μm beads using a mixture of two fluorophores that absorb in the infra-red to far-red region. The two dyes are mixed in different proportions to generate 100 types of microspheres with unique spectral signatures. Lasers excite the microspheres, identify each type of microsphere and detect the absorbed reporter dye. Together, the Quantigene assays can be plexed to 100; currently, 3–36 plex assays are available for gene expression analysis.

The cooperative hybridization steps ensure specificity of initial oligonucleotide primer pairs and the amplifiers circumvent the need for RNA amplification steps, thus increasing the overall specificity and sensitivity of this platform. A unique advantage of this technology is that it avoids purification of mRNA from DNA and cellular proteins, by using a specific buffer that allows direct detection of transcripts from cell/tissue extracts. It is one of the first methods compatible with and sensitive enough to multiplex *in-situ* PCR on archival formalin-fixed paraffin-embedded tissue sections and single-cell samples. This procedure makes Quantigene assays helpful in linking microarray technology to yet another high-content, high-throughput tissue microarray screening platform. The amplification signals for several genes are detected on the section, and their distribution encodes positional information of mRNA in tissue sections. Similarly in cell culture systems, the *in-situ* PCR technology enables temporal and spatial studies in the mRNA localization of several genes in a single cell after various perturbations. These applications of Quantigene not only serve to validate the microarray data, but also open up opportunities to discover novel mechanisms involved in transcription and mRNA biology.

INTERACTION ANALYSIS: TWO-HYBRID SCREENS

Two-hybrid screens were devised to identify candidates for protein–protein interactions on a genome-wide scale (Charbonnier et al., 2008; Suter et al., 2008). The molecular basis of this system is that the activating and binding domains of eukaryotic transcription factors are functionally separable modules, and can therefore act in close proximity to each other without being covalently linked. The fundamental strategy is to link the DNA binding portion (containing the DNA binding domain) of a yeast transcription factor with the protein of interest in an appropriate plasmid that is introduced into recipient yeast cells. This chimera is referred to as the "bait" of the two-hybrid system, and is focused on finding new binding partners of the protein of interest. A random primed cDNA library from a cell of interest is then constructed such that each cDNA is inserted into another plasmid engineered to produce a protein product in which the activation domain fragment is fused onto the protein product of the cDNA. The protein fused to the activation domain is the "prey" protein. The two-hybrid system utilizes a strain of mutant yeast that genetically lacks the ability to synthesize certain necessary amino acids or nucleic acids; these strains will not survive if grown in media that lack these nutrients. Once the library is transfected, if the bait and prey proteins interact by binding, the activation domain and binding domain of the transcription factor are physically brought together, bringing the activation domain in proximity to the transcription start site (Fig. 2.11). This initiates transcription of reporter gene(s)—commonly, a gene(s) that is missing in the biosynthetic pathway. In this way, a successful interaction between the bait and prey will allow the yeast clone to survive nutrient deprivation.

As with any screen, there will be false positives and false negatives. Therefore any results will need to be tested with more exacting assays, counter assays, to eliminate false data. However, the yeast two-hybrid screens have generated a number of important datasets of possible protein interactions. When integrated with other interactions datasets, the resultant interaction networks have been helpful in modeling cellular processes (de Chassey et al., 2008; Yu et al., 2008). Since the early descriptions, such two-hybrid systems have been structured in bacterial and in mammalian cells.

GENE-BASED PERTURBATION STUDIES: TRANSGENIC KNOCKOUTS

An important means of gaining understanding the biology of the candidate gene is through loss-of-function experiments. Sequencing of the human and mouse genomes established high gene-to-gene functional homology that displayed an organizational synteny along the chromosomes between the two species. Coupled with the advanced development of mouse transgenic and gene disruption strategies, large-scale mouse mutagenesis studies to develop models of human diseases were deemed plausible (Gondo, 2008). Two strategies that have been exploited for genome-wide mutagenesis are described here.

Forward Genetics

Random mutagenesis strategies involve treatment of the mouse sperm with *N*-ethyl-*N*-nitrosourea (ENU), an alkylating agent that results in single base-pair substitutions in the genome. Mutant sperm from mice treated with ENU is used for fertilization and the resultant progeny (G1) are screened for assayable phenotypes. Design of these phenotypic assays is crucial in identifying reliable and reproducible mutant lines. Although a potent mutagen, ENU induces mutants with partial function, rather than null alleles. Moreover, dominant mutations are represented by as few as 2–3% of the progeny, whereas recessive mutation rates are at least a 1000-fold higher. Phenotypic assays for recessive mutations require third-generation mice (G3) and these screens are often complicated by the number of mice that are needed to be handled per G1 type. A very low number of G3 mice resulting from recessive lethal mutations will be available for phenotype screens, limiting the use of this strategy. The screened mutant mice are then characterized by positional cloning and

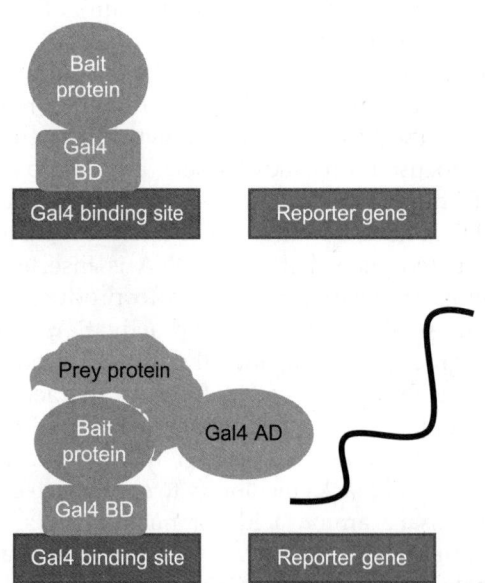

FIGURE 2.11 Schematic of the Molecular Components of a Yeast Two-hybrid Screen.
Gal4 is a yeast transcription factor. AD, activation domain; BD, binding domain; Gal4 AD, Gal4 transcription activation domain; Gal4 BD, Gal4 DNA binding domain.

gene trap experiments to identify the disrupted gene and its function. This process of phenotype-driven mutagenesis is termed "forward genetics." ENU mutagenesis appears to be labor intensive and costly, but initial screens led to dominant phenotypes and the identification of new genes (e.g. the *Clock* gene) (Vitaterna et al., 1994) and the development of ApcMin mice, the latter being an excellent model for human familial adenomatous polyposis (Su et al., 1992). This led to the establishment of large-scale mutagenesis programs using ENU, and cryopreservation of sperm representing approximately 40 000 G1 mouse lines. ENU mutagenesis has no "hot" or "cold" spots, and the G1 mouse lines are currently being characterized by next-generation sequencing.

Reverse Genetics

As opposed to random mutagenesis, gene-by-gene loss of function mutants can be achieved using homologous recombination strategies (Capecchi, 2005). In this genetic engineering application, gene disruption by homologous recombination is the process by which transfected DNA recombines with genomic segments in the recipient cell with homologous sequences. In this process, the target gene is first disrupted by site-specific recombination in mouse embryonic stem cells. The embryonic stem cells are injected into recipient mouse embryos and implanted into pseudopregnant mothers. The resultant progeny is analyzed for the mutation at the organismal level. Such a gene-to-phenotype approach is termed "reverse genetics." Knockout mice require sophisticated equipment and have a high cost, but they are indispensable to the study of recessive lethal mutations in genes. Embryonically lethal mice can be generated using genetically engineered inducible systems that allow for gene knockout in a manner specific to the tissue or the developmental stage (Sauer, 1998). In addition, knockout mice do not require the development of complex phenotype screens that are necessary for ENU mutagenesis or cumbersome downstream gene trap or positional cloning experiments. The mutations can be faithfully propagated over many generations. Moreover, genetic crosses of various knockout mice allow for the easy study of more complex phenotypes. These advantages form the basis of genome-side gene targeting efforts to determine gene function.

RNA Interference Approaches in Systems Biology

Loss-of-function assays for genes that can influence a given phenotype, such as genetic disruption by homologous recombination, are exact, but cumbersome and cannot scale. A relatively recent technical revolution, based on RNA interference (RNAi), is very promising. It greatly enhances the ease with which loss-of-function screens can be performed, shows a wider range of experimental models amenable to these interventions and can be applied on a genome-wide scale.

The recognition of RNAi as a biological mechanism was directly related to two phenomena of the 1990s: the advent of the Internet, and the whole-genome sequencing efforts that started to bear fruit (reviewed by Ruvkun, 2008). The increase in freely available genomic data and the possibility of searching this database on-line were some of the key factors that allowed the discovery that small RNAs can bind to 3'UTRs of genes and thereby inhibit their translation. These RNAs were dubbed "microRNAs" (miRNAs) and it was soon recognized by genomic comparison and cloning efforts that these small regulators were present in large numbers across the animal and plant kingdoms.

In plants and in *Caenorhabditis elegans* and *Drosophila melanogaster* there were also small endogenous RNAs that could inhibit gene expression through direct cleavage and subsequent degradation of mRNAs, provided they were completely complementary to their target. These silencing short interfering RNAs (siRNAs) share many of the features of miRNAs such as their size (19–22 nucleotides) and the protein machinery with which they associate to exert their actions (the RNA-induced silencing complex [RISC]). In animals, the largest difference between miRNAs and siRNAs is not so much their molecular identity, but their capacity for base pairing and the consequences: siRNAs will base pair with complete complementarity and result in degradation of the target mRNA, whereas the complementarity of base pairing by miRNAs to a target 3′UTR is generally restricted to the first eight nucleotides (the so-called seed), followed by incomplete base pairing for the rest of the miRNA–UTR duplex. These "bulged" small RNA–UTR duplexes are incapable of activating cleavage of the target RNA by RISC, but rather result in RISC-mediated translational inhibition in the absence of extensive mRNA degradation. However, by experimentally altering fully complementary target sites to bulged ones, or *vice versa*, siRNAs and miRNAs have been shown to be able to activate both the cleaving and translation-inhibiting activities of RISC toward target mRNAs, purely depending on the mode of binding to the target.

MicroRNAs have since been shown to be abundant and important endogenous genes in the genomes of all multicellular organisms; their production is regulated and, in their own turn, they have important and sometimes dramatic regulatory functions by fine tuning or suppressing many protein-coding genes. In contrast, siRNAs were initially found only to be expressed endogenously from repeats in *C. elegans* in a genomic defense mechanism against deleterious transposons and other mobile elements. However, as the cellular mechanisms used by miRNAs and siRNAs are largely overlapping, it was quickly recognized that exogenously introduced synthetic siRNAs could give rise to degradation of mRNA in a very sequence-specific manner (Elbashir et al., 2001). This opened up a tool box that has since very rapidly expanded and the impact of which is on par with the discovery of restriction enzymes and the polymerase chain reaction in previous decades (Fig. 2.12).

RNAi Tools

C. elegans and *D. melanogaster* use siRNA as a defense mechanism against repeats that generate dsRNA when they integrate sense and antisense to cellular promoters. They are therefore very efficient in converting long dsRNA into small RNAs of exactly the right size to trigger RNA interference. A crucial enzyme in this process is Dicer, which is an RNase that can bite off chunks of 19–22 nucleotides of a long dsRNA. Indeed, feeding *C. elegans* with bacteria that express two complementary RNAs (typically from a gene fragment that is placed in between two facing promoters [Fig. 2.12A]) is enough to ensure system-wide spread of siRNAs derived from this long RNA. This had already been realized, and was exploited to perform screens in *C. elegans* before RNAi was applied to mammalian cells (Fraser et al., 2000; Gönczy et al., 2000). Similarly, *Drosophila* cells can be soaked in dsRNA (generated by *in-vitro* transcription reactions of 150–700 bp amplicons of genomic DNA), which is taken up and expediently "Diced" into siRNAs (Lum et al., 2003). In both cases, care must be taken to avoid using regions of genes that are identical in two or more genes, as this will result in direct and specific cross-reactivity.

mRNAs are not fully accessible to the RISC complex, probably because of the secondary structure of RNA and shielding by RNA binding proteins; therefore, not all regions of the mRNA are susceptible to siRNA-mediated knockdown, and not all siRNAs will contribute equally to the knockdown efficiency. However, the efficiency of dsRNA-generated siRNAs in worms and flies is very high as, per construct, numerous independent siRNAs are generated that

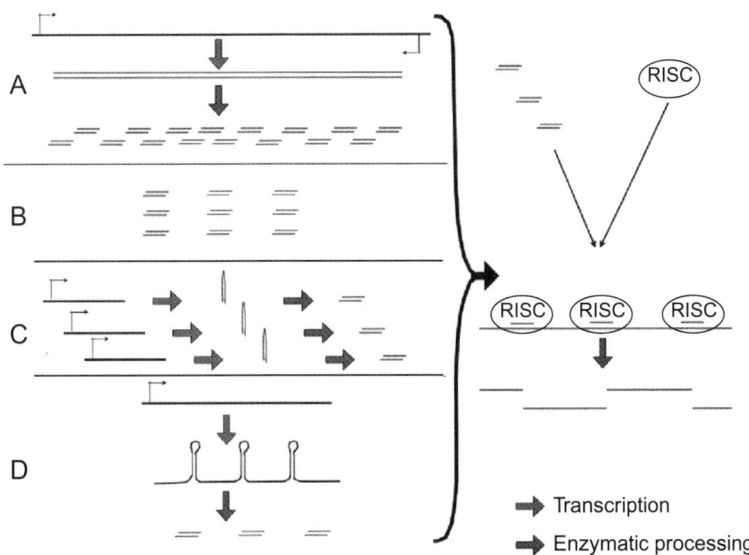

FIGURE 2.12 RNAi Delivery Methods.
The aim of all methods that use RNAi against a specific target is to generate small dsRNAs of approximately 19 nucleotides, which will be incorporated in the RISC and lead it to its target. The strategy of generating the dsRNAs differs from method to method. (A) In *C. elegans* and *Drosophila*, RNAi can be induced by introduction of two long complementary RNAs that are processed into a spectrum of small dsRNAs. (B) The simplest (but transient) method to introduce dsRNAs is to transfect annealed synthetic oligonucleotides into the cells (often as combinations of several siRNAs against one target). (C) For longer-term RNAi in mammalian cells, vectors are introduced that produce a precursor that is processed to dsRNAs. (D) Vectors based on miRNA precursors can be used for higher efficiency and simultaneous expression of multiple dsRNAs per construct.

are directed against various parts of the target gene. Furthermore, these organisms posses an RNA-dependent RNA polymerase that will use siRNA bound to an mRNA as a primer to generate a new dsRNA that generates new siRNAs, amplifying the amount of mRNA-specific siRNAs even further. Genome-wide collections of knockdown constructs are available for inhibition screens for both *C. elegans* and *Drosophila*.

RNAi in Mammalian Cells: Synthetic siRNAs

As a defense against exogenous (often virally derived) RNAs, vertebrates rely primarily on the interferon response that is triggered by dsRNA of more than 30 bp and leads to a general and a specific protein translation block, and to immune stimulation. This precludes the use of long dsRNA as source for siRNAs in vertebrate cell systems, which would be less efficient anyway, as these organisms lack the amplifying effect of an RNA-dependent RNA polymerase that *C. elegans* and *Drosophila* possess. However, the processing machinery is so conserved between the different species that synthetic dsRNAs, mimicking the dsRNA produced by Dicer-mediated cleavage of dsRNA, feed into the RISC machinery and can give rise to a fully functional siRNA response (Elbashir et al., 2001). This discovery brought RNA interference into the realm of mouse and human cell culture.

As mentioned above, not every siRNA can access the mRNA equally well, and therefore not every siRNA is equally efficient. To circumvent this problem, algorithms have been developed that are based on functional siRNAs, to preclude the use of siRNAs that are not processed very well, or those in which the wrong (sense) strand is incorporated into the RISC complex (Table 2.4). As the mRNA secondary structure is very difficult to predict, a large part of the siRNA selection process remains hit-and-miss. One common solution to this problem is to transfect pools of three or more independent siRNAs directed against the same mRNA, to achieve efficient knockdown. Because of the high number of these small molecules that can be transfected into cells, efficiencies of siRNA pools routinely reach around 90% protein reduction (Fig. 2.12B).

Vectors Encoding Short Hairpin RNAs

The duration of the knockdown response matches that of the presence of the siRNAs present in the cell, and in transient transfections the synthetic RNAs are not replenished when they are degraded or diluted during cell division. Chemical modifications can render these synthetic RNAs more stable, but eventually most experiments have a limit of 5–7 days during which the knockdown effect is significant. Therefore, an alternative approach was created using expression vectors that produce shRNAs feeding into the cellular miRNA processing machinery (Brummelkamp et al., 2002; Paddison et al., 2002). The vectors express a double-stranded stem-loop structure that is cut 19 nucleotides from the base of the stem. This leaves a dsRNA that is incorporated into the RISC complex, similar to double-stranded siRNAs or processed miRNAs precursors (Fig. 2.12C). These expression cassettes comprising a promoter and a hairpin-encoding piece of DNA can be incorporated into (retro) viral vectors and stably integrated into the genome, where they can generate a long-lasting knockdown effect.

The number of molecules produced by this system tends to be much lower than the number of siRNAs transfected into cells, as reported by, for example, Linsley et al. (2007). Therefore, the success rate per individual shRNA tested is lower, as there is less excess of small RNA than of mRNA to compensate for lower efficiency. There are also additional restrictions on the sequence of the shRNA precursor, resulting from requirements for efficient processing of the precursor hairpin, which do not apply to the "preprocessed" siRNAs (Table 2.4).

A next generation of shRNA vectors is directly based on miRNA precursors in which the mature miRNA sequence (and its complementary sequence that helps to form the miRNA precursor hairpin) is replaced by a custom shRNA sequence. This is the most direct mimic of endogenous small RNA production, and seems to give a high yield of effective shRNAs (although the success rate is still less than 50%)(Fig. 2.12D).

Libraries of vectors encoding shRNAs against human and mouse genes are available. The libraries vary in their set-up, in their specificity and in their cost: pools of shRNAs against all genes, families of genes, single-well pools of several shRNAs targeting one gene and single-well shRNAs, sometimes validated to target that gene efficiently. One advantage of shRNA vectors over siRNA oligonucleotides is that the vectors can be tracked using a barcode, approach once they have integrated into the host genome. This allows the identification of RNAi species that confer both positive and negative selection. In tracking negative selection, a library should be transferred into recipient cells such that the efficiency of gene transfer is one shRNA to one cell. The cells are then subjected to a particular screen such as growth under specific conditions. Over time, shRNAs that inhibit genes necessary for growth will disappear from the cellular population. At steady state, the shRNAs that become underrepresented in the cellular population are those against genes essential for growth. Detecting this loss from the population puts extra demands on the system, such as low levels of noise in the barcode detection and the absence of non-functional, point-mutated shRNA variants that share a barcode with a functional shRNA construct.

TABLE 2.4 Intelligent Design of RNAi

	Website	Features
siRNA Algorithm		
BIOPREDsi	www.biopredsi.org; www.qiagen.com	Artificial neural network design; validated siRNA or custom design
Deqor	http://cluster-1.mpi-cbg.de/Deqor/deqor.html	Design of siRNA or esiRNA
RFR-siRNA	www.bioinf.seu.edu.cn/siRNA/index.htm	Random forest regression for siRNA design
siDirect	http://genomics.jp/sidirect/	Target-specific siRNA design
SMARTselection	www.dharmacon.com	Predesigned or custom siRNA design
Wadsworth Center Sfold	http://sfold.wadsworth.org	Software for statistical folding and siRNA design
Whitehead siRNA Selection	http://jura.wi.mit.edu.libproxy1.nus.edu.sg/bioc/siRNA	siRNA selection
shRNA Algorithm		
The RNAi Consortium	http://www.broad.mit.edu/genome_bio/trc/rules.html	Vector-based shRNA design rules
Genelink	http://www.genelink.com/sirna/shRNAi.asp	On-line form based on simple rules
iRNAi	http://www.mekentosj.com/irnai	Desktop program based on simple rules

esiRNA, endoribonuclease-prepared siRNAs short interfering RNA; iRNAi, name of Mac OSX program to design shRNA RNA interference; RFR-siRNA, Design of siRNA with Random Forest Regression Model Coupled with Database Searching (Name of method) short interfering RNA; RNAi, RNA interference; shRNA, short hairpin RNA.

Scientific Art Copies Nature

A special class of RNAi libraries is one in which the "design" of the interfering RNA also is derived from nature: miRNA libraries. By cloning the precursor for all known miRNA genes into a series of retroviral expression vectors, it is possible to create libraries that express the majority of known miRNAs. These small RNAs have been selected during evolution to exert strong biological effects on regulatory networks, as is also reflected in their—sometimes striking—conservation between species. Although their biological potency is very high, the information they give in screens is limited. This is due to the diffuse nature of their predicted targets. As miRNAs have a very limited requirement for consecutive homologous base-pairing to achieve their effect, a major obstacle in deciphering their mode of action is the identification of the true and relevant targets from amongst the hundreds of potential target genes that contain a sequence complementary to the 7- or 8-mer seed sequence of the miRNA. These may be many (*see* Chapter 5). Although using these genes in RNAi high-throughput screens can identify them as important regulators in themselves, unless there is a consistent and reliable way to pinpoint their mRNA targets, the information gained about biological networks is limited.

RNAi in Systems Biology

An obvious use of RNAi in any of its forms (dsRNA, siRNA, shRNA vectors) is the rapid and efficient reduction of expression of the genes under investigation, which allows researchers to quickly test hypotheses generated from model signaling networks. This has sped up the validation process, as previous gold standards for testing the function of a gene were time consuming and were at risk of organismal adaptations (in mouse knockout studies) or artifacts (in studies using overexpressed proteins or dominant negative constructs). However, from the viewpoint of systems biology, RNAi has much more to offer than just its convenience to validate the presumed function of a gene. Provided the weaknesses and strengths of RNAi are accounted for, the use of RNAi can offer answers that are both quantitatively and qualitatively different than those obtained with previous techniques. We will therefore describe the major differences of RNAi with other systems, and highlight some of the weak points that need to be addressed during the design of large scale investigations of gene networks or in the interpretation of their results.

Traditionally, loss-of-function genetic screens were confined to model organisms such as yeast, *C. elegans* and *Drosophila*, in which the gene inactivation was achieved by random chemical mutagenesis or random insertion of mobile genetic elements. In general, these conventional approaches have been characterized by long delays between characterization of the phenotype and identification of the responsible gene, and truly genome-wide screens using these approaches are very costly and time consuming. RNAi approaches, however, take full advantage of the available genomic information and the results are believed to be gene targeted. However, RNAi screens have some limitations that are inherent to the method. Mutagenesis studies can result in very informative correlations between the type of mutation (point mutations or partial deletions of genes) and variations in phenotype. One striking example is the loss of the 3′UTR of the heterochronic gene, lin-14 (which controls the timing of developmental events in diverse cell types), leading to its resistance to *lin-4*-mediated repression. This mutation ultimately led to the discovery of miRNAs. Another difference between RNAi and mutagenesis or gene-targeting approaches is that RNAi leaves a residual amount of protein product, which is not present in genetic knockouts. This means that some functions of genes may be overlooked. For instance, using classical genetic means, it was shown that a low (10%) level of expression of the mismatch repair gene MutS homolog 2 (*Msh2*) from a hypomorph allele was enough to reconstitute its mismatch repair function, but not other functions of the gene (Claij and Te Riele, 2002). However, as every disadvantage has its advantage, the residual expression of some genes may allow the identification of interesting functions that would be masked by lethality resulting from the total loss of expression of that gene.

Factors Influencing Experimental Design

When RNAi screening approaches are being used, there are several factors that are important in the design of genome-wide screens. The first consideration is the experimental system to be used, including deciding the best approach to scoring the phenotype. The other considerations are technical: the possible routes of RNAi administration for this system, and the desired duration of inhibition needed to achieve a reliable readout.

In mammalian cell lines, knockdown of gene expression for short-term experiments (up to 1 week) is generally achieved by transfection of siRNAs. These are commercially available as pools of synthetic dsRNA, designed for optimum efficiency and minimal knockdown of unrelated targets. For screens that require a long-term effect, such as rescue of the ability for anchorage-independent growth, vector-encoded shRNAs is the method of choice. Permanent inhibition of a gene can be achieved using RNA interference through an integrating retrovirus. Moreover, for screens using pools of vectors that incorporate a separate barcode, PCR of the barcode from genomic DNA before and after selection, followed by differential hybridization to custom microarrays, or direct high-throughput sequencing, allows detection of enriched or depleted RNAi encoding constructs (Silva et al., 2008).

The lower efficiency of shRNAs compared with that of siRNAs requires that more shRNA vectors per gene need to be used to achieve full genome coverage. Therefore, many screens use three shRNA vectors per gene, expecting that the penetrance of the screen is suboptimal. In addition, efforts are under way to generate libraries that contain more than nine shRNA vectors per gene. To reduce the costs of such screens, many laboratories opt to use subcategories of the whole genome. Favorites are the kinome, phosphatome, druggable enzymes in general, or custom sets of genes selected for their likelihood to be involved in the phenotype under scrutiny (Moffat and Sabatini, 2006). There is clearly a trade-off here between breadth of search and cost of doing the screen. Another reason to opt for smaller libraries is to decrease the number of false positives resulting from a phenomenon that plagues every RNAi screen: off-target effects.

Off-target effects of any specific probe can affect other unintended pathways, often as a result of extended shared sequence homology between the intended target and bystander genes (Fig. 2.13). Typical siRNAs are 19 nucleotides long, and siRNA or shRNA sequences should be avoided that have fewer than three mismatches to other sequences in the transcriptome. Another, and more difficult to avoid, effect is caused by the similarity between the siRNA and miRNA pathways that are targeted by RNAi tools in mammalian cells. Not only are short dsRNAs processed and incorporated into the RISC where they can cleave their target mRNAs, they will also act as surrogate miRNAs, which have more diffuse effects across a larger number of genes. The sequence specificity of miRNA–target interactions is dependent on a 7–8 nucleotide seed. This means that any short RNA can, in principle, also exert biological functions through a miRNA-like action that is unrelated to the primary target against which it was designed. Indeed, in several screens using large shRNA collections, constructs were isolated that gave a reproducible and strong effect on the phenotype in question. However, when tested, these constructs failed to downregulate their

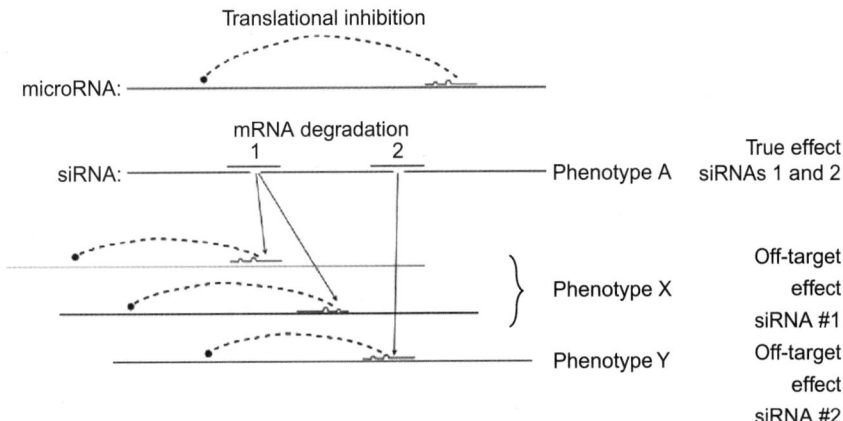

FIGURE 2.13 Off-target Effects.
Two siRNAs (1 and 2) are depicted that inhibit the same gene through mRNA degradation, and therefore both induce the same phenotype (A). However, both siRNAs could also bind to one or more other mRNAs in a miRNA-like fashion, inhibit their expression through translational inhibition (dashed lines) and thus elicit additional phenotypes (X and Y). As independent siRNAs are unlikely to share the same seed sequence required for the miRNA-like action, use of two active siRNAs should allow distinction between direct (A) and off-target (X or Y) effects.

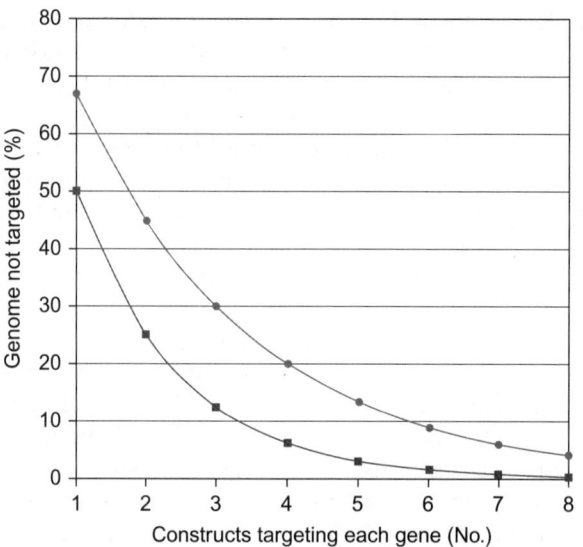

FIGURE 2.14 The Numbers Game.
With an average success rate of 1 in 3 for each shRNA (–♦–), eight constructs per gene are needed to inactivate more than 95% of the genome. For a genome of 20 000 genes, that means 160 000 constructs are necessary to target the majority (missing 544 genes). Even if the algorithm and expression vectors are optimized so that 1 in 2 shRNAs gives sufficient knockdown (–■–), 100 000 vectors are needed to target more than 95% of the genes. MicroRNAs are in large part directed to their targets by their seed sequence of seven nucleotides at the 5′ end. There are (4^7) or 16 384 possible 7-mers, which means that any genome-wide library has an approximately six- to 10-fold representation of each possible miRNA seed. When both sense and anti-sense RNA, produced by transfecting in dsRNA or made from shRNA stem-loops, are taken into account, this doubles to 12- to 20-fold. The Figure shows the percentage of the genome that is not functionally targeted when an increasing number of constructs is used. The asymptote is approached by the 7th or 8th construct.

intended target, and, conversely, constructs that indeed downregulated the intended target did not reproduce the phenotype. As it is already difficult to identify the targets of true miRNAs, finding the precise targets for these spurious miRNA-like effects has been very difficult, and not productive.

Correction for off-target false positives can be made in several ways (Echeverri et al., 2006). The amount of target mRNA reduction can be tested and correlated with the activity of the shRNA. The effect of the shRNA can be abrogated by expression of the target mRNA containing "silent" mutations that make it insensitive to the shRNA but will not affect gene function. This is a reasonable approach when validating a relatively small number of positive hits from an initial screen; however, such validation strategies do not scale in genome-wide screens. In reducing false discovery in large-scale shRNA screens, one solution is to expand the libraries so that every gene is targeted at least twice by a functional shRNA (Fig. 2.14). Another approach is to generate a library containing only shRNAs that have been validated for their activity, by quantitative PCR. This reduces the number of shRNA constructs in the library, with less chance of an off-target effect and increased chance of finding two shRNAs per target gene that result in the same phenotype.

When all factors are taken into account, RNAi strategies are among the most precise approaches to gene-targeted screening that are available.

References

Adessi, C., Matton, G., Ayala, G., et al., 2000. Solid phase DNA amplification: characterization of primer attachment and amplification mechanisms. Nucleic Acids Res. 28, e87.

Arikawa, E., Sun, Y., Wang, J., et al., 2008. Cross-platform comparison of SYBR Green real-time PCR with TaqMan PCR, microarrays and other gene expression measurement technologies evaluated in the MicroArray Quality Control (MAQC) study. BMC Genomics 9, 328.

Bentley, D.R., Balasubramanian, S., Swerdlow, H.P., et al., 2008. Accurate whole human genome sequencing using reversible terminator chemistry. Nature 456, 53–59.

Brazma, A., Hingamp, P., Quackenbush, J., et al., 2001. Minimum information about a microarray experiment (MIAME)-toward standards for microarray data. Nat. Genet. 29, 365–371.

Brummelkamp, T.R., Bernards, R., Agami, R., 2002. A system for stable expression of short interfering RNAs in mammalian cells. Science 296, 550–553.

Capecchi, M.R., 2005. Gene targeting in mice: functional analysis of the mammalian genome for the twenty-first century. Nat. Rev. Genet. 6, 507–512.

Charbonnier, S., Gallego, O., Gavin, A.C., 2008. The social network of a cell: recent advances in interactome mapping. Biotechnol. Annu. Rev. 14, 1–28.

Claij, N., Te Riele, H., 2002. Methylation tolerance in mismatch repair proficient cells with low MSH2 protein level. Oncogene 21, 2873–2879.

Collins, F.S., Lander, E.S., Rogers, J., Waterston, R.H., et al., 2004 for the International Human Genome Sequencing Consortium. Finishing the euchromatic sequence of the human genome. Nature 431, 931–945.

de Chassey, B., Navratil, V., Tafforeau, L., et al., 2008. Hepatitis C virus infection protein network. Mol. Syst. Biol. 4, 230.

de Reyniès, A., Geromin, D., Cayuela, J.M., et al., 2006. Comparison of the latest commercial short and long oligonucleotide microarray technologies. BMC Genomics 7, 51.

Dressman, D., Yan, H., Traverso, G., Kinzler, K.W., Vogelstein, B., 2003. Transforming single DNA molecules into fluorescent magnetic particles for detection and enumeration of genetic variations. Proc. Natl. Acad. Sci. USA 100, 8817–8822.

Dupuy, A., Simon, R.M., 2007. Critical review of published microarray studies for cancer outcome and guidelines on statistical analysis and reporting. J. Natl. Cancer Inst. 99, 147–157.

Echeverri, C.J., Beachy, P.A., Baum, B., et al., 2006. Minimizing the risk of reporting false positives in large-scale RNAi screens. Nat. Methods 3, 777–779.

Elbashir, S.M., Harborth, J., Lendeckel, W., Yalcin, A., Weber, K., Tuschl, T., 2001. Duplexes of 21-nucleotide RNAs mediate RNA interference in cultured mammalian cells. Nature 411, 494–498.

Fedurco, M., Romieu, A., Williams, S., Lawrence, I., Turcatti, G., 2006. BTA, a novel reagent for DNA attachment on glass and efficient generation of solid-phase amplified DNA colonies. Nucleic Acids Res. 34, e22.

Fraser, A.G., Kamath, R.S., Zipperlen, P., Martinez-Campos, M., Sohrmann, M., Ahringer, J., 2000. Functional genomic analysis of C. elegans chromosome I by systematic RNA interference. Nature 408, 325–330.

Gönczy, P., Echeverri, C., Oegema, K., et al., 2000. Functional genomic analysis of cell division in C. elegans using RNAi of genes on chromosome III. Nature 408, 331–336.

Gondo, Y., 2008. Trends in large-scale mouse mutagenesis: from genetics to functional genomics. Nat. Rev. Genet. 9, 803–810.

Im, H., Grass, J.A., Johnson, K.D., Boyer, M.E., Wu, J., Bresnick, E.H., 2004. Measurement of protein-DNA interactions in vivo by chromatin immunoprecipitation. Methods Mol. Biol. 284, 129–146.

Kodzius, R., Kojima, M., Nishiyori, H., et al., 2006. CAGE: cap analysis of gene expression. Nat. Methods 3, 211–222.

Lander, E.S, Linton, L.M., Birren, B., et al., for the International Human Genome Sequencing Consortium. Finishing the euchromatic sequence of the human genome. Nature 431:931–945.

Ley, T.J., Mardis, E.R., Ding, L., et al., 2008. DNA sequencing of a cytogenetically normal acute myeloid leukaemia genome. Nature 456, 66–72.

Linsley, P.S., Schelter, J., Burchard, J., et al., 2007. Transcripts targeted by the microRNA-16 family cooperatively regulate cell cycle progression. Mol. Cell Biol. 27, 2240–2252.

Lum, L., Yao, S., Mozer, B., et al., 2003. Identification of Hedgehog pathway components by RNAi in Drosophila cultured cells. Science 299, 2039–2045.

Margulies, M., Egholm, M., Altman, W.E., et al., 2005. Genome sequencing in microfabricated high-density picolitre reactors. Nature 437, 376–380.

McKernan, K., Blanchard, A., Kotler, L., Costa, G., 2006. Reagents, methods, and libraries for bead-based sequencing. US patent application 20080003571.

Moffat, J., Sabatini, D.M., 2006. A lentiviral RNAi library for human and mouse genes applied to an arrayed viral high-content screen. Cell, vol. 124 (6), 1283–1298.

Nagalakshmi, U., Wang, Z., Waern, K., et al., 2008. The transcriptional landscape of the yeast genome defined by RNA sequencing. Science 320, 1344–1349.

Ng, P., Wei, C.L., Sung, W.K., et al., 2005. Gene identification signature (GIS) analysis for transcriptome characterization and genome annotation. Nat. Methods 2, 105–111.

Paddison, P.J., Caudy, A.A., Hannon, G.J., 2002. Stable suppression of gene expression by RNAi in mammalian cells. Proc. Natl. Acad. Sci. USA 99, 1443–1448.

Ren, B., Dynlacht, B.D., 2004. Use of chromatin immunoprecipitation assays in genome-wide location analysis of mammalian transcription factors. Methods Enzymol. 376, 304–315.

Ronaghi, M., Karamohamed, S., Pettersson, B., Uhlén, M., Nyrén, P., 1996. Real-time DNA sequencing using detection of pyrophosphate release. Anal. Biochem. 242, 84–88.

Ruvkun, G., 2008. The perfect storm of tiny RNAs. Nat. Med. 14, 1041–1045.

Saha, S., Sparks, A.B., Rago, C., et al., 2002. Using the transcriptome to annotate the genome. Nat. Biotechnol. 20, 508–512.

Sauer, B., 1998. Inducible gene targeting in mice using the Cre/lox system. Methods 14, 381–392.

Schmutz, J., Wheeler, J., Grimwood, J., et al., 2004. Quality assessment of the human genome sequence. Nature 429, 365–368.

Severgnini, M., Bicciato, S., Mangano, E., et al., 2006. Strategies for comparing gene expression profiles from different microarray platforms: application to a case-control experiment. Anal. Biochem. 353, 43–56.

Shi, L., Reid, L.H., Jones, W.D. For the MAQC Consortium, et al., 2006. The MicroArray Quality Control (MAQC) project shows inter- and intraplatform reproducibility of gene expression measurements. Nat. Biotechnol. 24, 1151–1161.

Silva, J.M., Marran, K., Parker, J.S., et al., 2008. Profiling essential genes in human mammary cells by multiplex RNAi screening. Science 319, 617–620.

Su, L.K., Kinzler, K.W., Vogelstein, B., et al., 1992. Multiple intestinal neoplasia caused by a mutation in the murine homolog of the APC gene. Science 256, 668–670.

Suter, B., Kittanakom, S., Stagljar, I., 2008. Two-hybrid technologies in proteomics research. Curr. Opin. Biotechnol. 19, 316–323.

Turcatti, G., Romieu, A., Fedurco, M., Tairi, A.P., 2008. A new class of cleavable fluorescent nucleotides: synthesis and optimization as reversible terminators for DNA sequencing by synthesis. Nucleic. Acids Res. 36, e25.

VanGuilder, H.D., Vrana, K.E., Freeman, W.M., 2008. Twenty-five years of quantitative PCR for gene expression analysis. Biotechniques 44, 619–626.

Velculescu, V.E., Zhang, L., Vogelstein, B., Kinzler, K.W., 1995. Serial analysis of gene expression. Science 270, 484–487.

Venter, J.C., Adams, M.D., Myers, E.W., et al., 2001. The sequence of the human genome. Science 291, 1304–1351.

Vitaterna, M.H., King, D.P., Chang, A.M., et al., 1994. Mutagenesis and mapping of a mouse gene, Clock, essential for circadian behavior. Science 264, 719–725.

Wang, J., Wang, W., Li, R., et al., 2008. The diploid genome sequence of an Asian individual. Nature 456, 60–65.

Wang, Z., Gerstein, M., Snyder, M., 2009. RNA-Seq: a revolutionary tool for transcriptomics. Nat. Rev. Genet. 10, 57–63.

Warren, L., Bryder, D., Weissman, I.L., Quake, S.R., 2006. Transcription factor profiling in individual hematopoietic progenitors by digital RT-PCR. Proc. Natl. Acad. Sci. USA 103, 17807–17812.

Wei, C.L., Wu, Q., Vega, V.B., et al., 2006. A global map of p53 transcription-factor binding sites in the human genome. Cell 13, 207–219.

Wheeler, D.A., Srinivasan, M., Egholm, M., et al, 2008. The complete genome of an individual by massively parallel DNA sequencing. Nature 452, 872–876.

Yu, H., Braun, P., Yildirim, M.A., et al., 2008. High-quality binary protein interaction map of the yeast interactome network. Science 322, 104–110.

CHAPTER 3

Proteomics Technologies

Sam Hanash
Fred Hutchinson Cancer Research Center, Seattle

OUTLINE

Summary	45	Microarray-based Approaches	50
Introduction	45	Computational Aspects of Proteomics	52
Cell-based Proteomics	46	Conclusion	53
Proteomics of Biological Fluids	48		

Summary

The proteome represents the most functional component encoded for in the genome. A system approach to biology and disease benefits substantially from integration of proteome- and genome-level studies. Current approaches for profiling cell populations and biological fluids and related computational aspects of proteomics are reviewed, with emphasis on addressing issues of quantification and depth of analysis.

INTRODUCTION

The current interest in proteomics is due in part to its power to interrogate the functional component encoded for in the genome, namely the proteins. Much progress has been made in developing strategies for mining complex proteomes using technologies that are suitable for analyzing particular aspects of proteins that encompass quantifying their overall concentrations, determining their occurrence in various cellular compartments, their activity and their post-translational modifications and structure, their binding properties and their occurrence as part of complexes (Mann and Kelleher, 2008). With the advent of mass spectrometry, proteomics is increasingly relied upon for understanding basic cellular and physiologic processes in an unbiased systems-wide fashion (Cravatt et al., 2007) and in a disease context, for identifying critical pathways and biomarkers relevant to risk assessment and early disease detection, and for molecular classification and monitoring of disease progression or regression (Hanash et al., 2008). This chapter will address in-depth quantitative proteomics approaches currently in use that are applicable to cell populations and to biological fluids. Discovery technologies that allow comprehensive unbiased proteomics investigations will be considered, in contrast to assays that target a relatively small set of proteins.

CELL-BASED PROTEOMICS

A multitude of approaches for cell protein analysis have yielded quantitative information with respect to cellular protein composition and responses to environmental changes and to gene manipulations (analysis of single cells by means of affinity reagents is covered in Chapter 4). Label-free methods have been utilized to derive quantitative data from mass spectrometry, with some success (Haqqani et al., 2008). Alternatively, *in-vitro* stable isotope labeling of proteins or of amino acids in cell culture (SILAC) (Elia et al., 2002) has become widely used to study the proteomes of various cell types and of organisms from microbes to mice and how they change in response to various conditions (Ong and Mann, 2006). For cell isotopic labeling, cells are grown in culture in the presence of one amino acid such as lysine for which all the ^{12}C are substituted by ^{13}C. Incorporation of the isotopically labeled amino acid occurs in the process of cell growth, protein synthesis and turnover. Isotopic labeling allows "light" and "heavy" proteomes to be distinguished by mass spectrometry. In one study using SILAC to label differentiated brown adipocytes (Kruger et al., 2008), seven phosphoproteins not previously described in insulin signaling were identified using high resolution mass spectrometry in combination with phosphotyrosine immunoprecipitation. The combination of quantitative phosphoproteomics with SILAC made it possible to decipher insulin signaling pathways in intact cells. In another study (Guha et al., 2008), SILAC-based quantitative mass spectrometry was relied upon to identify tyrosine phosphorylated proteins in isogenic human bronchial epithelial cells and human lung adenocarcinoma cell lines, expressing mutant epidermal growth factor receptor (EGFR) or a mutant KRAS (KRAS) allele. Tyrosine phosphorylation of signaling molecules was found to be greater in cells expressing mutant EGFR compared with those expressing mutant wild-type EGFR or mutant KRAS. Signaling molecules not previously implicated in oncogene ErbB (EGFR) receptor signaling were also found to be differentially phosphorylated.

As part of a search for potential diagnostic markers for lung cancer, apical surface fluids from aberrantly differentiated squamous metaplastic human tracheobronchial epithelial cells in culture and from normal counterparts were compared (Kim et al., 2007), yielding identification of 22 proteins associated with metaplasia. In another illustrative study of breast cancer cell lines, proteomic analysis of conditioned media provided a rich dataset of secreted proteins with established roles in breast cancer development and identification of additional potential candidate biomarkers (Kulasingam and Diamandis, 2007).

A broader de-complexing of cellular processes using proteomics encompasses in-depth analysis of whole-cell lysates, of proteins localized to various compartments—notably the cell surface, which mediates cell–cell interactions—and of responses to changes in the microenvironment and proteins released into the extracellular compartment through secretion or other processes (Fig. 3.1).

In one such study, the repertoire of proteins expressed both in ovarian adenocarcinoma cell lines and in ovarian cancer cells enriched from ascites fluid was substantially elucidated (Faca et al., 2008b). Separate analyses of proteins released into culture media and of cell surface proteins, using total cell lysates as a reference,

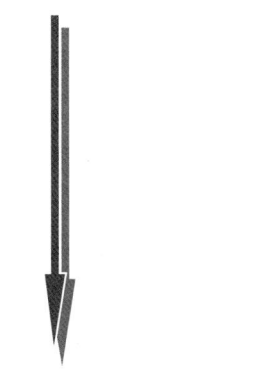

FIGURE 3.1   Cell-based Proteomics Discovery Workflow.

were subjected to fractionation and high resolution mass spectrometry. Some 6400 proteins were identified, with high confidence. Estimation of the abundance of identified proteins on the basis of spectral counts (Liu et al., 2004) allowed assessment of their enrichment in the subproteome compartments investigated. Substantial concordance was observed between subcellular location and predictions made from database searches and sequence analysis. An interesting finding that emerged was the close similarity of the proteomic profiles of freshly isolated cancer and those of ovarian cancer cell lines of the same subtype. Analysis of ovarian cancer cell derived proteins in culture media provided evidence for shedding of several hundred proteins annotated as membrane proteins. Related peptides identified were found to be largely derived from extracellular domains of cell surface proteins, suggestive of a generalized process of cleavage and release of ectodomains. A large proportion of the shed proteins were found to be related to processes of cell adhesion and cell movement. Several integrins, cadherins and ADAM protein family members were identified.

Glycoproteins represent a subset of proteins that play important functions such as cell–cell interaction and exhibit alterations in disease states. Several technologies are available to capture and analyze cell and tissue glycoproteins (Pilobello and Mahal, 2007; Zhao et al., 2008). An illustrative study focused on the effects of cell–cell interactions on N-linked glycans in epithelial cells (Iijima et al., 2006). N-Glycans were purified from whole-cell lysates and then detected by high performance liquid chromatography and mass spectrometry. N-Acetylglucosamine (GlcNAc)-containing N-glycans, which are dependent on N-acetylglucosaminyltransferase III (GnT-III), were found to be substantially increased in cells cultured under dense conditions compared with those cultured under low-density conditions. Concordant increases in levels of expression and activities of GnT-III, but not other glycosyltransferases, were also found. Disruption of E-cadherin-mediated adhesion by treatment with ethylenediamine tetra-acetic acid (EDTA) or a neutralizing anti-E-cadherin antibody abolished the upregulation of expression of GnT-III. The data suggested that an E-cadherin-dependent pathway regulated GnT-III expression. The findings of this study emphasize the interplay of glycosylation enzymes with other regulatory systems and their impact on glycoproteins.

Besides phosphorylation and glycosylation, there are numerous post-translational modifications that play important roles in regulating cellular activities. However, few have been systematically explored in the same way as phosphorylation and, for the most part, the extent of such modifications and their relevance to biological processes remain largely unknown.

Aside from studies of protein concentrations and modification, other approaches that are focused on function include activity-based protein profiling, which relies on active site-directed probes to interrogate, for example, the functional state of enzyme families (Cravatt et al., 2008). The delineation of enzyme activities selectively associated with disease processes has the potential to yield a rich source of targets for diagnosis and treatment. In one study (Salisbury and Cravatt, 2007), an active site-directed chemical probe for profiling histone deacetylases in native proteomes and live cells was used to profile both the activity state of histone deacetylases and the binding proteins that regulate their function. The probe was applied to assess differences in acetylase content and complex assembly in human disease models.

PROTEOMICS OF BIOLOGICAL FLUIDS

Proteomics is particularly promising for the analysis of biological fluids and biomarker identification. Biomarkers are indicators of specific physiologic and pathologic states. Disease biomarkers can aid in diagnosis and/or patient management by defining subtypes and predicting or monitoring response to treatment and disease progression or regression (Hanash 2003; Hanash et al., 2008; Ludwig and Weinstein, 2005). The search for biomarkers that can be assayed in biological fluids—notably serum and plasma—has relied on various strategies, each with its own advantages and disadvantages related in part to depth of analysis and throughput. By and large, high throughput strategies tend to lack depth of analysis or depend on a preselected set of proteins, whereas in-depth, comprehensive approaches tend to be labor intensive and have low throughput.

Serum and plasma from which serum is derived are among the most accessible biological materials and have been relied upon for screening and diagnosis perhaps more than any other type of specimens. However, the plasma proteome is particularly challenging because of its complexity, its within- and between-subject variability and because of its vast dynamic range. Plasma contains several thousand proteins that, in their abundance, span from as high as 20–50 mg/ml for serum albumin to femtomolar concentrations for some known biomarkers (States et al., 2006). Most plasma proteins occur in multiple forms as a result of alternative splicing, cleavage or other post-translational modifications that occur in the tissues from which they are derived or after proteins leave the cells and enter the circulation (Misek et al., 2005; Nedelkov et al., 2005). This plethora of protein forms, combined with the vast dynamic range of concentrations, presents the greatest challenge to serum and plasma profiling and biomarker discovery. Mass spectrometry has evolved sufficiently to detect and identify femtomoles of peptides, but the dynamic range of detection is still a limiting factor and currently does not exceed 3 to 4 orders of magnitude for complex mixtures such as plasma (Aebersold and Mann, 2003; Mann and Kelleher, 2008; Wang and Hanash, 2005).

There are three basic strategies to achieve depth of analysis of biological fluids: (i) removal of high-abundance proteins, such as albumin and immunoglobulins that interfere with the detection of less abundant proteins, by means such as immunodepletion (Liu et al., 2006); (ii) fractionation of samples by chromatographic or other means of separation, resulting in individual fractions with a reduced complexity that is better suited for mass spectrometry (Wang and Hanash, 2005) and (iii) isolation of targeted protein or peptide subsets of interest such as glycoproteins or phosphoproteins (Zhou et al., 2007). Using a combination of depletion of abundant proteins and extensive fractionation, together with isotopic labeling (Fig. 3.2), our group was able to identify several cancer biomarkers in plasma other than non-specific inflammatory and acute phase protein markers.

In one study that illustrated integration of proteome-level and genome-level data, a pancreatic cancer mouse model was investigated for the discovery of blood-based pancreatic cancer biomarkers applicable to humans (Faca et al., 2008a). Refined genetically engineered mouse models of human cancer have been shown to recapitulate faithfully the molecular, biological and clinical features of human disease. Plasma was sampled from mice at early and advanced stages of pancreatic cancer development and from matched controls. Some 1442

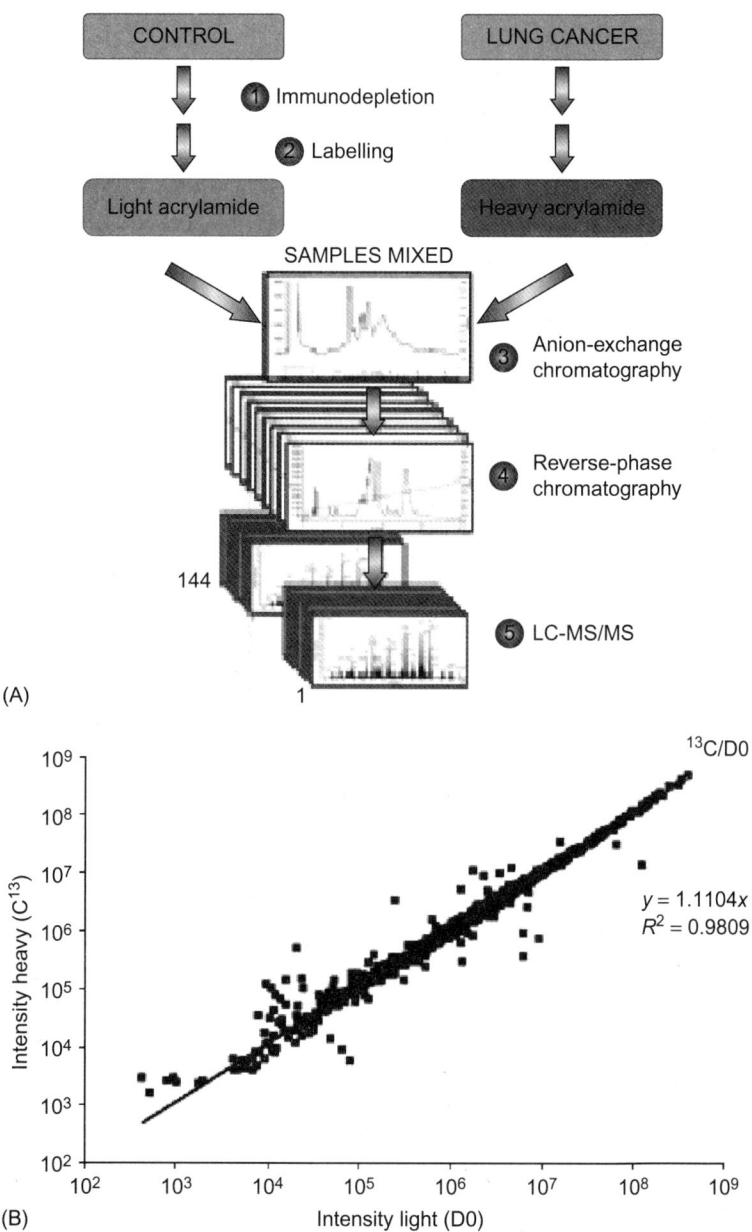

FIGURE 3.2 Five-step Analysis of Plasma Proteins for Disease-related Changes.
(A) Plasmas (e.g. from lung cancer cases and from controls), are separately subjected to immunodepletion for the removal of high-abundance proteins and separately labeled with acrylamide isotopes (Faca et al., 2006). After mixing, samples are fractionated at the intact protein level into a large number of fractions that are separately analyzed by LC-MS/MS after protein digestion with trypsin. (B) Analysis of self–self aliquots of plasma by LC-MS/MS as with the above proteomics workflow, showing distribution of identified proteins over five orders of magnitude based on ion intensities, indicating a dynamic range of detection and reliable quantitation suitable for biomarker identification.

proteins were confidently identified. Analysis of proteins chosen on the basis of increased concentrations in plasma from tumor-bearing mice and corroborating tissue protein or RNA analysis, demeonstrated concordance in the blood from humans with pancreatic cancer relative to control specimens. A panel of five proteins selected on the basis of their increased concentration at an early stage of tumor development in the mouse was tested in a blinded study of serum and was demonstrated to discriminate pancreatic cancer cases from matched controls in specimens obtained between 7 and 13 months before the development of symptoms and clinical diagnosis of pancreatic cancer.

While the above strategy provides in-depth quantitative analysis of biological fluids, it is limited in its ability for multiplexing. Important aspects with regard to biomarker discovery and validation in biological fluids are throughput and relative quantification. An approach that allows multiplexing is the isobaric tag labeling method, iTRAQ, developed at Applied Biosystems, which allows multiplexing up to eight samples (Wiese et al., 2007). The chemistry of this system leads to a labeling of all resulting tryptic peptides without affecting their ionization. The tags utilized have the same total mass and consist of a peptide reactive group, a balance group and a reporter group. Each peptide from each of up to eight different samples is labeled with a different tag, but generates the identical mass in a mass spectrometry scan. After labeling, the samples are mixed together as in the case of intact protein labeling with the Intact Protein Analysis System (IPAS), and the peptides are analyzed by LC-MS/MS (LC-MS/MS). The MS/MS spectrum is used for both quantification and identification of the proteins in a single data-dependent LC-MS/MS experiment. The feasibility of this strategy for successfully profiling several hundred proteins has been demonstrated. In a study of hepatocellular carcinoma using iTRAQ, some 600 proteins were quantified and 59 proteins and 92 proteins were over- and under-expressed, respectively,

in cancerous tissue as compared with adjacent normal tissue (Chaerkady et al., 2008). A subset of proteins was further validated using immunoblotting and immunohistochemical labeling. The study revealed that all the enzymes of urea metabolic pathway were altered in tumor tissue. Although multiplexing strategies, notably iTRAQ, have worked well with cell and tissue specimens within a limited dynamic range, exceedingly complex samples such as serum and plasma represent something of a challenge. Other labeling methods in use include $^{16}O/^{18}O$ labeling of peptide mixtures resulting from tryptic digestion. Labeling is achieved using $[^{18}O]$ water by means of post-digestion ^{16}O-to-^{18}O exchange (Qian et al., 2005). Comparison of differentially labeled peptides provides information on relative abundance. With the addition of labeled reference peptides from a mixture to samples to be compared, each identified peptide in the different samples will have abundance information relative to the standard based on the isotopic $^{16}O/^{18}O$ ratios.

MICROARRAY-BASED APPROACHES

With the development and success of DNA microarrays, protein microarrays have emerged as a promising approach to meet the pressing need for systematic analysis of thousands of proteins in parallel. Protein microarrays provide a high-throughput and low-volume sample consumption platform for various assays, including determining the interactions between proteins and other molecules of interest, such as other proteins, antibodies, drugs and other ligands (Kingsmore, 2006). Such assays have utility for investigations in physiologic or pathologic processes and for the identification of biomarkers and therapeutic targets.

From a conceptual point of view, a protein microarray is an array of protein spots on solid supports—typically, modified glass slides. A need for optimizing the surface chemistries specifically for protein microarrays has been recognized to improve binding capacity, increase signal-to-noise ratio, prevent immobilized proteins from denaturing, and orient proteins properly. Various surfaces using specialized immobilization chemistries have been reported, including the use of nitrocellulose-coated slides to immobilize proteins with reliance on hydrophobic interactions (Stillman and Tonkinson, 2000), immobilization of biotinylated proteins onto a streptavidin-coated surface (Lesaicherre et al., 2002) and immobilization of His-tagged proteins onto Ni^{2+} chelating surfaces (Zhu et al., 2001).

There are generally two major classes of protein microarray. One is intended for protein profiling, in which several protein capture agents (usually antibodies) are spotted to assay the abundance of corresponding antigens or epitopes in a biological sample such as cell or tissue lysate or biological fluid. Alternatively, several biological samples are spotted to assay for proteins that interact with a specific analyte in the biological samples applied to the array. Another class is intended for functional protein analysis, in which large numbers of purified proteins are spotted to study their biochemical properties.

The detection of binding in protein microarrays can be based on a sandwich immunoassay in which an immobilized antibody or any other type of capture agent is utilized to capture proteins of interest in a biological sample and a second labeled antibody or capture agent is used to detect and determine the abundance of the protein. Such an approach therefore requires two capture agents that recognize different epitopes on proteins of interest. This dual-capture agent requirement creates constraints for interrogating the abundance of large numbers of proteins simultaneously in a biological sample because it is difficult to have access to high-quality matched antibody pairs.

An alternative to sandwich assays is to label the biological samples before they are hybridized to the arrays. The biological samples can be labeled with either a fluorophore for the direct detection method or a hapten tag such as biotin for the indirect detection method. In the latter case, the arrays are further incubated with fluorophore-conjugated streptavidin.

The success of protein microarrays relies on sensitive detection methods, as only nanoliter volumes of protein samples are printed for each spot. Substantial efforts have been made to improve detection sensitivity without loss of resolution or increase in background. Isothermal rolling-circle amplification (RCA) has been applied to protein microarrays to increase sensitivity (Zhou et al., 2004). An alternative is the "Tyramide Signal Amplification System" developed by Perkin Elmer, which amplifies both fluorescent and chromogenic signals (http://www.perkinelmer.com).

One concern with the labeling of biological samples is that the labeled biotin or fluorophore might interfere with protein interactions. Methodologies have been developed to detect binding of proteins to the arrays without any pretreatment of the biological samples, using mass spectrometry, surface plasmon resonance (SPR) (Rich et al., 2002), or atomic force microscopy (ATM) (Lynch et al., 2004). These label-free approaches provide more flexibility for experimental design and preserve protein conformation in the biological samples that may be disrupted by labeling. However, these approaches are still at the proof-of-concept stage.

Array-based approaches also have been implemented for glycomic analysis. Lectin arrays have been developed as tools for the elucidation of carbohydrate structures (Chen et al., 2007b). Such arrays have been used for the characterization of differences in carbohydrate expression patterns on normal and tumorigenic human breast cell lines, and lines that differ in their metastatic homing capacity. An alternative strategy for the study of glycans relies on antibody microarray capture of multiple proteins, followed by detection with lectins or glycan-binding antibodies. Chemical derivatization of the glycans on the spotted antibodies prevents lectin binding to glycans. A lectin-binding profile of captured proteins is developed, with the use of multiple lectins as detection probes. Glycan alterations in MUC1 (MUC1) and carcinoembryonic antigen (CEA), associated with pancreatic cancer, have been found by profiling both protein and glycan variation using parallel sandwich and glycan-detection assays (Chen et al., 2007a).

COMPUTATIONAL ASPECTS OF PROTEOMICS

An expanding menu of commercial and open-source software is currently available to process and analyze proteomics data. Some are highly specialized and others address proteomics needs more broadly, particularly as they relate to mass spectrometry. One such suite is the Computational Proteomics Analysis System (CPAS), which is an open-source LC-MS/MS analysis pipeline specifically developed to integrate data standards and open algorithms to foster data exchange and integration (Rauch et al., 2006). CPAS documents the experimental protocols used to generate data and process all data in a uniform manner and allows a flexible means of using criteria for various applications, notably protein identification.

The need to mine mass spectrometry data beyond protein identification becomes more pressing as instrument resolution and mass accuracy improve. Proteomic analysis would therefore be substantially enriched if it were possible to identify, more fully than has been the case, protein variation caused by polymorphism or mutation or resulting from post-translational modification or cleavage. In fact, such variation is likely to represent an important source of biomarkers. For example, cleavage products of tumor-derived proteins have been proposed as potential cancer biomarkers. Increased concentrations of calreticulin and PDIA3 fragments have been found in serum of patients with hepatocellular carcinoma (Chignard et al., 2006). Tools to mine protein variation include embedding single-nucleotide polymorphisms into mass spectrometry search engines for their identification (Schandorff et al., 2007), and the development, by UniProt, of UniMod as an ontology for protein post-translational modification based on the RESID Database of Protein Modifications (Garavelli, 2004).

A large number of databases have been developed for depositing and retrieving proteomic datasets, including PRIDE (Jones et al., 2006), PeptideAtlas (Deutsch et al., 2005), UniPep (Zhang et al., 2006), the Global Proteome Machine (Craig et al., 2004), Proteopedia (Mathivanan et al., 2008) and Proteome Commons and its Tranche file-sharing system (www.tranche.proteomecommons.org).

Initial analysis of proteomics data focuses on identifying individual proteins of interest, but computational tools have led to the ability to discern relevant networks and pathways from the data. There are currently no standard approaches for this purpose. However, approaches being applied to transcriptomic data also have utility for proteomic data; these include Gene Ontology (http://www.geneontology.org), Kyoto Encyclopedia of Genes and Genomes (KEGG; http://www.genome.jp/kegg), Ingenuity (http://www.ingenuity.com), Metacore (http://www.metacore.com) and gene set enrichment (Mootha et al., 2003; Tian et al., 2005). From such analyses, over-representation of particular pathways may be discerned, which has the added advantage of increasing confidence in identification. Therefore the approach of integrative genomics, assimilating data and information from several sources, also has relevance to proteomics.

Integration of several datasets is valuable for deriving hypotheses, developing a list of candidate markers to guide subsequent studies (Fig. 3.3). A recent effort to facilitate mining

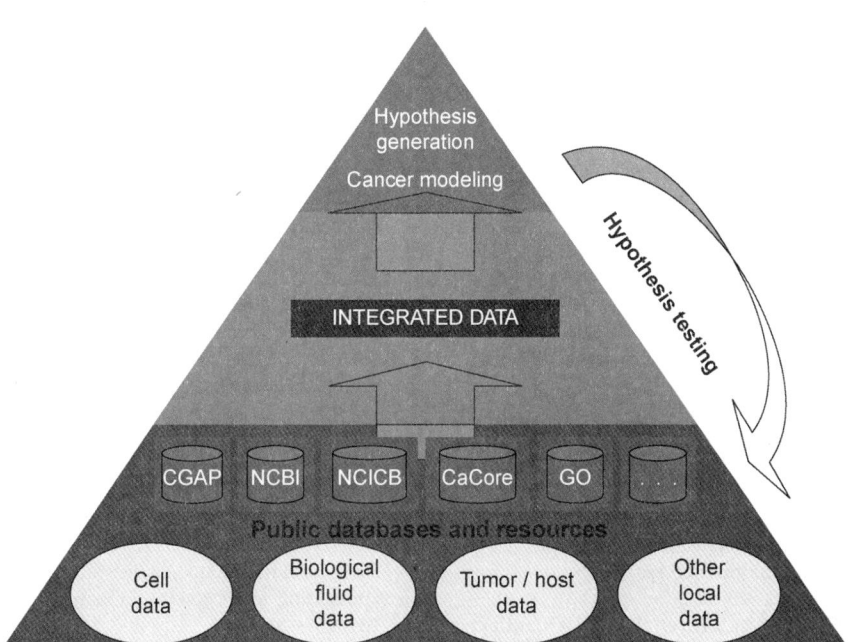

FIGURE 3.3 Integration of Proteomic Data with Other Datasets. For discovery studies and hypothesis generation, leading to hypothesis testing.

of proteomics data for biomarker discovery is BiomarkerDigger (http://biomarkerdigger.org), with its automated data analysis, searching. Its metadata-gathering function searches available proteome databases for protein–protein interaction, Gene Ontology, protein domain and tissue expression profile information and integrates it into protein dataset profiles accessible by search functions in BiomarkerDigger.

CONCLUSION

The field of proteomics is experiencing rapid growth, with technologies achieving ever increasing accuracy, sensitivity and throughput, and computational tools to address particular applications. A near exhaustive analysis of the protein content of cells is currently possible, and analysis of biological fluids spanning seven logs of protein abundance is feasible with the utilization of fractionation technologies. In the near future, top-down mass spectrometry will gradually complement current strategies based on analysis of protein digests. Microarrays with expanded content reaching the entire genome complement in recombinant proteins and a large repertoire of affinity-capture agents are likely to emerge, thus further empowering a system-wide approach to mining proteomes in health and in disease.

References

Aebersold, R., Mann, M., 2003. Mass spectrometry-based proteomics. Nature 422, 198–207.

Chaerkady, R., Harsha, H.C., Nalli, A., et al., 2008. A quantitative proteomic approach for identification of potential biomarkers in hepatocellular carcinoma. J. Proteome Res. 7, 4289–4298.

Chen, S., LaRoche, T., Hamelinck, D., et al., 2007a. Multiplexed analysis of glycan variation on native proteins captured by antibody microarrays. Nat. Methods. 4, 437–444.

Chen, S., Zheng, T., Shortreed, M.R., Alexander, C., Smith, L.M., 2007b. Analysis of cell surface carbohydrate expression patterns in normal and tumorigenic human breast cell lines using lectin arrays. Anal. Chem. 79, 5698–5702.

Chignard, N., Shang, S., Wang, H., et al., 2006. Cleavage of endoplasmic reticulum proteins in hepatocellular carcinoma: detection of generated fragments in patient sera. Gastroenterology 130, 2010–2022.

Craig, R., Cortens, J.P., Beavis, R.C., 2004. Open source system for analyzing, validating, and storing protein identification data. J. Proteome Res. 3, 1234–1242.

Cravatt 3rd, B.F., Simon, G.M., Yates, J.R., 2007. The biological impact of mass-spectrometry-based proteomics. Nature 450, 991–1000.

Cravatt, B.F., Wright, A.T., Kozarich, J.W., 2008. Activity-based protein profiling: from enzyme chemistry to proteomic chemistry. Annu. Rev. Biochem. 77, 383–414.

Deutsch, E.W., Eng, J.K., Zhang, H., et al., 2005. Human plasma peptide atlas. Proteomics 5, 3497–3500.

Elia, G., Silacci, M., Scheurer, S., Scheuermann, J., Neri, D., 2002. Affinity-capture reagents for protein arrays. Trends Biotechnol. 20, S19–S22.

Faca, V., Coram, M., Phanstiel, D., et al., 2006. Quantitative analysis of acrylamide labeled serum proteins by LC-MS/MS. J. Proteome Res. 5, 2009–2018.

Faca, V.M., Song, K.S., Wang, H., et al., 2008a. A mouse to human search for plasma proteome changes associated with pancreatic tumor development. PLoS Med. 5, e123.

Faca, V.M., Ventura, A.P., Fitzgibbon, M.P., et al., 2008b. Proteomic analysis of ovarian cancer cells reveals dynamic processes of protein secretion and shedding of extra-cellular domains. PLoS ONE 3, e2425.

Garavelli, J.S., 2004. The RESID Database of Protein Modifications as a resource and annotation tool. Proteomics 4, 1527–1533.

Guha, U., Chaerkady, R., Marimuthu, A., et al., 2008. Comparisons of tyrosine phosphorylated proteins in cells expressing lung cancer-specific alleles of EGFR and KRAS. Proc. Natl. Acad. Sci. USA 105, 14112–14117.

Hanash, S., 2003. Disease proteomics. Nature 422, 226–232.

Hanash, S.M., Pitteri, S.J., Faca, V.M., 2008. Mining the plasma proteome for cancer biomarkers. Nature 452, 571–579.

Haqqani, A.S., Kelly, J.F., Stanimirovic, D.B., 2008. Quantitative protein profiling by mass spectrometry using label-free proteomics. Methods Mol. Biol. 439, 241–256.

Iijima, J., Zhao, Y., Isaji, T., et al., 2006. Cell-cell interaction-dependent regulation of N-acetylglucosaminyltransferase III and the bisected N-glycans in GE11 epithelial cells. Involvement of E-cadherin-mediated cell adhesion. J. Biol. Chem. 281, 13038–13046.

Jones, P., Cote, R.G., Martens, L., et al., 2006. PRIDE: a public repository of protein and peptide identifications for the proteomics community. Nucleic Acids Res. 34, D659–D663.

Kim, S.W., Cheon, K., Kim, C.H., et al., 2007. Proteomics-based identification of proteins secreted in apical surface fluid of squamous metaplastic human tracheobronchial epithelial cells cultured by three-dimensional organotypic air-liquid interface method. Cancer Res. 67, 6565–6573.

Kingsmore, S.F., 2006. Multiplexed protein measurement: technologies and applications of protein and antibody arrays. Nat. Rev. Drug Discov. 5, 310–320.

Kruger, M., Kratchmarova, I., Blagoev, B., Tseng, Y.H., Kahn, C.R., Mann, M., 2008. Dissection of the insulin signaling pathway via quantitative phosphoproteomics. Proc. Natl. Acad. Sci. USA 105, 2451–2456.

Kulasingam, V., Diamandis, E.P., 2007. Proteomic analysis of conditioned media from three breast cancer cell lines: a mine for biomarkers and therapeutic targets. Mol. Cell. Proteomics 6, 1997–2011.

Lesaicherre, M.L., Lue, R.Y., Chen, G.Y., Zhu, Q., Yao, S.Q., 2002. Intein-mediated biotinylation of proteins and its application in a protein microarray. J. Am. Chem. Soc. 124, 8768–8769.

Liu 3rd, H., Sadygov, R.G., Yates, J.R., 2004. A model for random sampling and estimation of relative protein abundance in shotgun proteomics. Anal. Chem. 76, 4193–4201.

Liu, T., Qian, W.J., Mottaz, H.M., et al., 2006. Evaluation of multiprotein immunoaffinity subtraction for plasma proteomics and candidate biomarker discovery using mass spectrometry. Mol. Cell Proteomics 5, 2167–2174.

Ludwig, J.A., Weinstein, J.N., 2005. Biomarkers in cancer staging, prognosis and treatment selection. Nat. Rev. Cancer. 5, 845–856.

Lynch, M., Mosher, C., Huff, J., Nettikadan, S., Johnson, J., Henderson, E., 2004. Functional protein nanoarrays for biomarker profiling. Proteomics 4, 1695–1702.

Mann, M., Kelleher, N.L., 2008. Precision proteomics: the case for high resolution and high mass accuracy. Proc. Natl. Acad. Sci. USA 105, 18132–18138.

Mathivanan, S., Ahmed, M., Ahn, N.G., et al., 2008. Human Proteinpedia enables sharing of human protein data. Nat. Biotechnol. 26, 164–167.

Misek, D.E., Kuick, R., Wang, H., et al., 2005. A wide range of protein isoforms in serum and plasma uncovered by a quantitative Intact Protein Analysis System (IPAS). Proteomics 5, 3343–3352.

Mootha, V.K., Lindgren, C.M., Eriksson, K.F., et al., 2003. PGC-1alpha-responsive genes involved in oxidative phosphorylation are coordinately downregulated in human diabetes. Nat. Genet. 34, 267–273.

Nedelkov, D., Kiernan, U.A., Niederkofler, E.E., Tubbs, K.A., Nelson, R.W., 2005. Investigating diversity in human plasma proteins. Proc. Natl. Acad. Sci. USA 102, 10852–10857.

Ong, S.E., Mann, M., 2006. A practical recipe for stable isotope labeling by amino acids in cell culture (SILAC). Nat. Protoc. 1, 2650–2660.

Pilobello, K.T., Mahal, L.K., 2007. Deciphering the glycocode: the complexity and analytical challenge of glycomics. Curr. Opin. Chem. Biol. 11, 300–305.

Qian, W.J., Monroe, M.E., Liu, T., et al., 2005. Quantitative proteome analysis of human plasma following in vivo lipopolysaccharide administration using 16O/18O labeling and the accurate mass and time tag approach. Mol. Cell. Proteomics 4, 700–709.

Rauch, A., Bellew, M., Eng, J., et al., 2006. Computational Proteomics Analysis System (CPAS): an extensible, open-source analytic system for evaluating and publishing proteomic data and high throughput biological experiments. J. Proteome Res. 5, 112–121.

Rich, R.L., Hoth, L.R., Geoghegan, K.F., et al., 2002. Kinetic analysis of estrogen receptor/ligand interactions. Proc. Natl. Acad. Sci. USA 99, 8562–8567.

Salisbury, C.M., Cravatt, B.F., 2007. Activity-based probes for proteomic profiling of histone deacetylase complexes. Proc. Natl. Acad. Sci. USA 104, 1171–1176.

Schandorff, S., Olsen, J.V., Bunkenborg, J., et al., 2007. A mass spectrometry-friendly database for cSNP identification. Nat. Methods. 4, 465–466.

States, D.J., Omenn, G.S., Blackwell, T.W., et al., 2006. Challenges in deriving high-confidence protein identifications from data gathered by a HUPO plasma proteome collaborative study. Nat. Biotechnol. 24, 333–338.

Stillman, B.A., Tonkinson, J.L., 2000. FAST slides: a novel surface for microarrays. Biotechniques 29, 630–635.

Tian, L., Greenberg, S.A., Kong, S.W., Altschuler, J., Kohane, I.S., Park, P.J., 2005. Discovering statistically significant pathways in expression profiling studies. Proc. Natl. Acad. Sci. USA 102, 13544–13549.

Wang, H., Hanash, S., 2005. Intact-protein based sample preparation strategies for proteome analysis in combination with mass spectrometry. Mass Spectrom. Rev. 24, 413–426.

Wiese, S., Reidegeld, K.A., Meye, H.E., Warscheid, B., 2007. Protein labeling by iTRAQ: a new tool for quantitative mass spectrometry in proteome research. Proteomics 7, 340–350.

Zhang, H., Loriaux, P., Eng, J., et al., 2006. UniPep—a database for human N-linked glycosites: a resource for biomarker discovery. Genome Biol. 7, R73.

Zhao, Y.Y., Takahashi, M., Gu, J.G., et al., 2008. Functional roles of N-glycans in cell signaling and cell adhesion in cancer. Cancer Sci. 99, 1304–1310.

Zhou, H., Bouwman, K., Schotanus, M., et al., 2004. Two-color, rolling-circle amplification on antibody microarrays for sensitive, multiplexed serum-protein measurements. Genome Biol. 5, R28.

Zhou, Y., Aebersold, R., Zhang, H., 2007. Isolation of N-linked glycopeptides from plasma. Anal. Chem. 79, 5826–5837.

Zhu, H., Bilgin, M., Bangham, R., et al., 2001. Global analysis of protein activities using proteome chips. Science 293, 2101–2105.

CHAPTER 4

Cellular Regulatory Networks

Brian A. Joughin[1], Edwin Cheung[3], R. Krishna Murthy Karuturi[3], Julio Saez-Rodriguez[2], Douglas A. Lauffenburger and Edison T. Liu[3]

[1]The David H. Koch Institute for Integrative Cancer Research at MIT,
Massachusetts Institute of Technology, Cambridge
[2]Department of Systems Biology, Harvard Medical School,
Boston and Biological Engineering Department,
Massachusetts Institute of Technology, Cambridge
[3]Genome Institute of Singapore, Agency for Science Technology and Research,
Singapore

OUTLINE

Introduction	58	Part II. Protein Phosphorylation Networks	84
Part I. Transcriptional Networks	58	Phosphopeptide Databases	85
Transcriptional Machinery	59	Kinase–Substrate Connections	86
Transcriptional Regulatory Elements	61	In-vivo Functions of Protein Phosphorylation	89
Epigenetic Control of Transcription	63	Protein Networks	92
Post-transcriptional Control: MicroRNAs	64	Analysis of Protein Interaction and Signaling Networks	93
Complexity of the Transcriptome	65	Epidermal Growth Factor Receptor as a Model for Protein Signaling Networks	97
Transcriptional Regulation on a Genomic Scale in Medicine	65		
Principles of Transcriptional Network Analysis	72		
Estrogen Receptor as a Model for Transcriptional Complexity	82	Acknowledgements	99

INTRODUCTION

For many decades, cell signaling has been a focus of study as the key to understanding the fate decisions of a cell. Earlier investigations, which focused on binary enzyme–substrate interactions with dichotomized (on–off) outputs, have been superseded by studies of signaling networks associated with complex and diffuse processes often resulting in subtle biological consequences. In building such network maps for higher mammalian systems pertinent to medicine, protein–protein interactions and generalized enzyme–substrate databases have formed one foundation, and transcriptional regulatory networks have formed the second foundation. The challenges in making use of these of these datasets lie in uncovering hierarchy of effect, integration of heterogeneous data and the incorporation of dynamical, time-dependent data in order to improve the predictive value of the models. Herein, we will discuss the strategies and approaches used to develop understanding of complex signaling networks, with focus on two layers as templates: transcriptional regulatory processes as an ultimate controller of cell function, and protein kinase pathways as a crucial upstream "information processing" governor located downstream of environmental stimuli.

PART I. TRANSCRIPTIONAL NETWORKS

The basis of mapping transcriptional regulatory networks began with the development of expression arrays (for a review of these technologies, *see* Chapter 2). Earlier efforts in using expressed tag sites to assess the transcriptome were deficient because of the cost of sequencing, which limited the depth of data extracted. Thus sampling error and confounding by abundant RNA species, which overwhelmed the signals, dampened the utility of this strategy. Expression arrays now use oligonucleotide probes targeting the 3' end of known transcripts and, although not lacking in bias, are sufficiently representative of most transcripts that expression patterns and profiles can be discerned. It is the coordinate expression of specific gene sets that is of greatest interest in systems analyses of transcription. The assumption in this framework is that the gene expression profile of a cell, when in a specific cellular state or when challenged, is a measurable readout of a functional response.

Although network mapping for protein and transcriptional systems are similar, they differ in one organizational aspect: proteins fundamentally have a radiating network of interactions that usually operate as a tandem series of branching reactions; transcription is controlled by a direct and specific interaction between a transcription factor and many discrete locations within the genome, guided by a DNA sequence recognition motif. Thus proteins form branching networks often emanating from different subcellular locations, whereas transcriptional networks are, in the first instance, a large collection of parallel interactions that are registered as a coordinate transcriptional response. That transcriptome analyses can be performed with relative quantitative precision, on a complete-genome scale and aided by the ability to amplify the signal using polymerase chain reaction, makes transcriptional systems simpler to interrogate than protein networks. To understand the whole system, we must first examine the components.

A primary control point in the regulation of differential gene expression is transcription. This is one of the major mechanisms the cell utilizes to modulate gene activities involved in numerous important biological processes, including DNA synthesis and cell cycle progression. Consequently, deregulation of transcription can frequently lead to disease. In general, transcription of a gene involves several steps and the recruitment of numerous proteins and protein complexes to the promoter, in concert with changes to the structure of the local chromatin environment, including nucleosome remodeling and histone modification. These processes are tightly regulated, directly or indirectly, by protein factors with discrete *cis*-acting DNA sequence elements upstream or downstream of the transcription start site (TSS). Below, we review the different types of transcriptional regulatory elements (e.g. promoter, enhancer, silencer, locus control region) and the associated protein factors (e.g. general transcription factors, activators, repressors, enhanceosomes) that interact with the regulatory elements to control the precise level of gene expression.

Transcriptional Machinery

The transcriptional machinery that is responsible for the precise temporal and spatial regulation of RNA synthesis in eukaryotic cells consists of many protein factors and protein complexes. These can be broadly categorized into three classes (Figs. 4.1 and 4.2): (i) general transcription factors (GTFs), (ii) sequence-specific DNA binding transcription factors/activators and (iii) co-regulatory proteins.

General Transcription Factors

T7 and other bacteriophage RNA polymerases can recognize a specific promoter, transcribe the corresponding gene and terminate transcription,

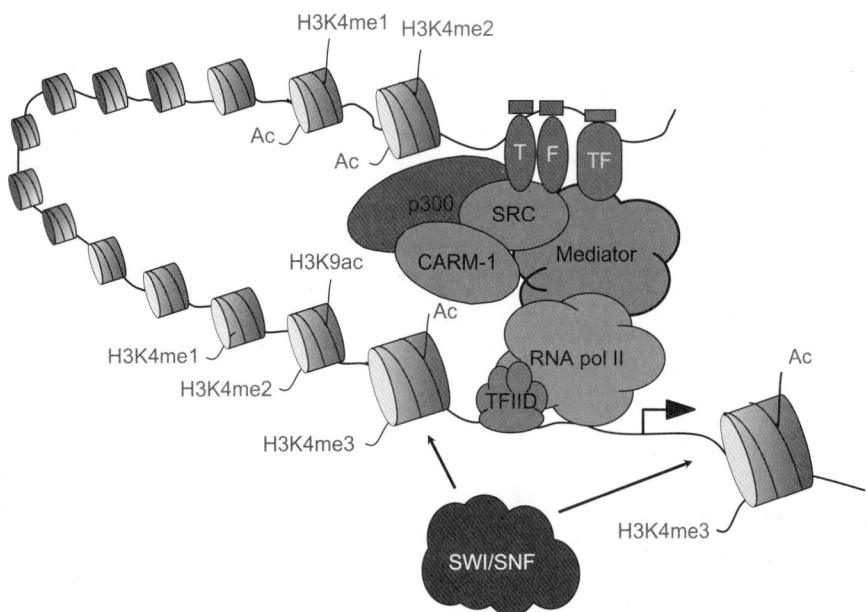

FIGURE 4.1 The Transcription Apparatus.
Schematic diagram showing the components of the transcription machinery required for correct activation of transcription. To overcome the general repressive effects of chromatin (nucleosomes denoted as cylinders), activators, which are sequence-specific DNA binding transcription factors (TF), recruit a host of factors to the promoter of genes, including co-activators (e.g. p300, SRC, CARM-1), chromatin remodeling complexes (SWI/SNF) and the Mediator complex. Together, these factors cooperate to bring the general transcription factors (e.g. TFIID and RNA pol II) to the promoter to initiate transcription. Ac, acetylation of histone tails; H3K9ac, N-terminal lysine-9-acetylated histone H3; H3K4me1-3, N-terminal lysine-4-methylated, dimethylated or trimethylated histone H3.

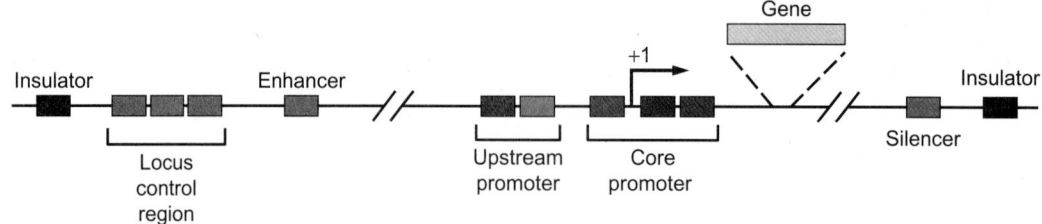

FIGURE 4.2 The Transcriptional Regulatory Region of a Gene.
Schematic diagram showing the various transcriptional regulatory elements and their location relative to the promoter.

with a single polypeptide. In eukaryotes, however, the transcription process is much more complex because RNA polymerase II (RNA pol II) (Fig. 4.1) cannot specifically recognize TSSs on its own (Matsui et al., 1980). Instead, for accurate initiation of transcription, RNA pol II needs to be recruited to the promoter by a complex of basal transcription factors or GTFs (Matsui et al., 1980). GTFs consist of TFIIA, TFIIB, TFIID, TFIIE, TFIIF, TFIIH and RNA pol II. These factors are recruited onto the promoter of genes in an ordered stepwise fashion, forming the preinitiation complex (Buratowski et al., 1989; Van Dyke et al., 1988). The initial step of this process is the binding of TFIID (a multiprotein complex consisting of TATA-binding protein (TBP) and TBP-associated factors (TAFs) to the TATA box, which is then followed by the subsequent recruitment of TFIIs A, B, E, F and H (Thomas and Chiang, 2006). Finally, RNA pol II is brought to the promoter to initiate transcription at the TSS (Thomas and Chiang, 2006).

Sequence-specific DNA Binding Transcription Factors/Activators

The recruitment and assembly of the preinitiation complex at the promoter leads to only a low or basal level of transcription. To control the rate and specificity of transcriptional activation, another factor, namely an activator, is required. Generally, activators are sequence-specific DNA binding transcription factors the binding sites of which can be located either upstream or downstream of the TSSs (Kadonaga, 2004). There are thousands of different activators in eukaryotes, and they can be grouped into different families on the basis of their DNA binding domain properties (e.g. zinc finger, homeobox, helix–loop–helix) (Kadonaga, 2004). Besides having a DNA binding domain, activators also contain one or more activation domains that are necessary for the stimulation of transcription. The binding sites for activators are called transcription factor binding sites, which are typically short DNA sequences with lengths varying from 6 to 12 bp. Activators can enhance transcription by several means, including directly contacting GTFs, or indirectly by recruiting co-regulatory proteins. In addition, they can recruit co-regulatory proteins containing enzymatic activities. All these actions ultimately lead to an increase in preinitiation complex formation.

Co-regulators

The activity of transcription factors can be modulated by co-regulatory proteins (Fig. 4.1) (Glass and Rosenfeld, 2000; Robyr et al., 2000). Co-regulatory proteins comprise two major groups, co-activators and co-repressors. Co-activators enhance, whereas co-repressors inhibit transcription. One group of co-activators possesses acetyltransferase activity capable of acetylating histones and other proteins, including p300/CBP, PCAF (p300/CBP-associated factor) and the SRC/p160 group of proteins (steroid receptor co-activators, including SRC1, SRC2 and SRC3) (Glass and Rosenfeld, 2000; Robyr et al., 2000). A second group of co-activators include DRIP and TRAP complexes, which are human homologs of the yeast mediator complex (Glass and Rosenfeld, 2000; Robyr et al., 2000). Co-activators are thought to enhance transcription by simultaneously contacting the activators and basal transcription machinery, and by helping to remodel the chromatin at the promoter through acetylation of histones. Co-repressors include nuclear receptor co-repressor (N-CoR) and silencing mediator for retinoid and thyroid receptors (SMRT), which act to repress basal transcription (Glass and Rosenfeld, 2000). N-CoR and SMRT function by recruiting Sin3 and histone deacetylases (HDACs) to repress transcription through targeted histone deacetylation (Glass and Rosenfeld, 2000).

Enhanceosomes

The precise transcription of a gene is often controlled by more than one specific activator. Several activators can bind together in close proximity, forming an "enhanceosome" at the enhancer binding sites of genes, to stimulate transcription (Thanos and Maniatis, 1995). The activators in this cluster act cooperatively, integrate multiple stimuli and operate as a single discrete functional module. The best characterized enhanceosome is found in the promoter of the human interferon-beta (*IFN-β*) gene. Upon virus infection, several activators, including nuclear factor κB (NF-κB), the interferon activator IRF-3/IRF-7 and the ATF-2/c-Jun complex, all bind to a compact 55 bp stretch of the upstream enhancer of *IFN-β*. Another protein, HMGA1, which is important for stabilization of the enhanceosome, is also recruited as part of the complex (Merika et al., 1998; Thanos and Maniatis, 1995). The findings of recent molecular and X-ray crystallographic studies suggest that the enhanceosome does not activate transcription as a result of synergistic binding of the activators to the enhancer, because there was a lack of physical interaction detected between them; rather, activation is a result of the activators working together to simultaneously contact the co-activator CBP/p300 (Merika et al., 1998; Panne et al., 2007). In that study, recruitment of the co-activator was most optimal when all of the activators in the enhanceosome had their activation domains present together.

Transcriptional Regulatory Elements

Core Promoter

RNA pol II promoters are characterized by core-promoter sequence elements that reside within a 100 bp region of the TSS that specifies the binding of GTFs (Juven-Gershon et al., 2008; Smale and Kadonaga, 2003) (Fig. 4.2). Located in this region, approximately 30 bp upstream of the start site in mammalian promoters is a conserved AT-rich sequence known as the TATA box, that the GTF, TFIID occupies (Buratowski et al., 1989; Van Dyke et al., 1988). However, not all promoters contain TATA boxes. Instead promoters can contain other core promoter sequence element near the TSS, such as an initiator element (Inr), TFIIB-recognition element (BRE), motif ten element (MTE), downstream promoter element (DPE) or downstream core element (DCE), in which TFIID or TFIIB can bind (Burke and Kadonaga, 1996; Juven-Gershon et al., 2008; Lagrange et al., 1998; Lewis et al., 2000; Lim et al., 2004; Smale and Kadonaga, 2003). Thus there is sequence heterogeneity at the DNA recognition site for the basal transcriptional machinery.

Upstream Promoter Elements

Binding of GTFs to the core promoter ensures accurate initiation from the start site, but produces only a low rate or basal level of transcription. Enhanced or activated transcription is mediated by the binding of regulatory factors to gene-specific *cis*-acting elements in regions either proximal to or distal from the core promoter. *Cis*-elements located in the proximal promoter region are known as upstream promoter elements (UPE) (Kadonaga, 2004). A typical UPE consists of a consensus sequence of 6–12 bp. Examples of UPEs include GC (or Sp1) and CCAAT boxes, which are common to many pol II genes (Courey and Tjian, 1988; Kadonaga et al., 1988; Santoro et al., 1988). There are other less common elements, and they are usually found in promoters that are subject to specialized transcriptional regulation, such as response to hormonal stimulation, growth factors and heat shock.

Enhancers

Distal promoter elements are known as en-hancers, and are capable of activating transcrip-tion in an orientation- and distance-independent manner relative to the promoter (Banerji et al., 1981). In general, enhancers are clusters of transcription factor binding sites that are closely grouped together and function cooperatively as a single cohesive unit to stimulate transcription (Szutorisz et al., 2005; West and Fraser, 2005). Enhancers have properties similar to those of UPEs, such that the same activators can bind to both types of site. Therefore, what constitutes an enhancer or UPE can sometimes be unclear. Furthermore, the actual boundary between the upstream promoter region and the enhancer region remains an arbitrary cut-off that is determined by the investigator. However, we know that enhancers are often located very far from the core promoter, residing as far as several hundred kilobases away, and can activate transcription whether it is located in the 5′ or the 3′ of the promoter, in the intron or even downstream of the gene (Szutorisz et al., 2005; West and Fraser, 2005).

Silencers

Silencers are DNA elements that have a net negative/repressive effect on transcription (Gaston and Jayaraman, 2003; Thiel et al., 2004). They share properties very similar to those of enhancers, in that they function in a manner that is independent of the promoter in both orientation and distance (Gaston and Jayaraman, 2003; Thiel et al., 2004). Therefore, like enhancers, silencers can be found at very far distances from the promoter of their target gene, and can be located anywhere relative to the promoter and gene. Silencers are binding sites for repressors, which have been shown to inhibit transcription by several potential mechanisms, including (i) preventing the binding of an activator to a proximal adjacent site, (ii) directly competing for the same binding site, (iii) forming a repressive chromatin environment through the recruitment of co-repressors containing histone-modifying activities (e.g. HDACs), thus preventing activators or GTFs from being recruited to the promoter, or (iv) directly inhibiting preinitiation complex formation at the promoter (Gaston and Jayaraman, 2003; Thiel et al., 2004). It is noteworthy that, under certain conditions or stimuli, an activator can function as a repressor by switching co-regulatory factor recruitment from a co-activator to a co-repressor.

Locus Control Regions

Locus control regions (LCRs) are groups of transcription regulatory elements that regulate clusters of genes often involved in cellular differentiation and development (Dean, 2006; West and Fraser, 2005). An LCR typically contains a complex collection of enhancer and silencer elements distributed along a large genomic region and marked by DNAse I hypersensitive sites (DHS) (Dean, 2006; West and Fraser, 2005). Each individual component of the LCRs is bound by activators or repressors that in turn recruit co-activators, repressors, and co-regulatory factors to regulate the expression of the genes in the cluster in a precise temporal and spatial manner (Dean, 2006; West and Fraser, 2005). Similar to enhancers and silencers, LCRs typically act from a large distance from their target gene. They can also function in a position-independent manner, in which they can sometimes be located in the introns of neighboring genes. Numerous LCRs have been identified; the best characterized include the loci of β-globin, major histocompatibility complex (MHC) class II HLA-DRA, T_H2 cytokine and human growth hormone (Fields et al., 2004; Ho et al., 2004; Masternak et al., 2003; Tolhuis et al., 2002).

Insulators/Boundary Elements

Insulators are DNA elements that block the transcriptional effects of neighboring genes (Bushey et al., 2008). These elements are necessary because of the ability of enhancers and silencers to regulate genes that can be located hundreds of kilobases away and in an orientation-independent manner. Thus insulators are an important means for (i) preventing the inappropriate regulation of adjacent genes by the transcriptional activities of another and (ii) segregating the genome into individual functional and non-functional transcription units (Bushey et al., 2008). Insulators generally regulate transcription in a position-dependent (usually between the enhancer and promoter or silencer and promoter of the adjacent gene) and orientation-independent (Bushey et al., 2008) fashion. It remains unclear exactly how insulators achieve their blocking abilities; however, evidence suggests that they most probably function by interacting with the activator or repressor to disrupt enhancer/silencer–promoter interactions, and by recruiting histone-modifying co-regulators that in turn create barriers against the spreading of condensed chromatin (heterochromatin) onto active chromatin (euchromatin) (Bushey et al., 2008). To date, the only protein factor identified in vertebrates that binds to insulators is CCCTC-binding factor (CTCF) (Bell and Felsenfeld, 2000; Bell et al., 1999). CTCF has been shown to regulate numerous loci, including T cell receptor for antigen (TCR) and insulin-like growth factor-2 (IGF-II) (Bell and Felsenfeld, 2000; Bell et al., 1999). In addition, recent ChIP-on-chip analysis revealed that there are approximately 15,000 CTCF insulator sites in the human genome, suggesting an important role for insulators in regulating gene expression (Kim et al., 2007).

Epigenetic Control of Transcription

Eukaryotic genomes are packaged into chromatin, the physiological template for cellular processes, including transcription. Epigenetic mechanisms that control transcription include alterations in the chromatin structure such as DNA methylation and covalent modification of histone tails (e.g. methylation, acetylation, phosphorylation, ubiquitination, sumoylation and ADP-ribosylation). DNA methylation is generally associated with transcriptional silencing (Klose and Bird, 2006). For example, a majority of the promoters in the human genome are located near CpG islands, genomic regions containing high GC content and CpG dinucleotides. CpG dinucleotides are normally unmethylated, but methylation of CpG dinucleotide is believed to block transcriptional activators from binding to their recognition sites, resulting in silencing of the gene (Klose and Bird, 2006). DNA methylation also occurs in other regulatory regions of the genome such as insulators, the methylation of which inhibits insulator activity by preventing CTCF from binding (Bell and Felsenfeld, 2000; Bushey et al., 2008; Hark et al., 2000). In addition to DNA methylation, modification of specific residues on the N-terminal tails of histone is also believed to be a major epigenetic mechanism in gene regulation. For example, acetylation of lysine-9 (K9) and lysine-14 (K14), di- or trimethylation of K4 and phosphorylation of S10 at the N-terminal tail of histone H3 are generally associated with gene activation, whereas di- or trimethylation of K9 and trimethylation of K27 at histone H3 is associated with repressed genes (Kouzarides, 2007; Lennartsson and Ekwall, 2009). There is a close interplay between DNA methylation and histone modification in gene regulation: the modification of one can affect the modification of the other. For example, methylation of CpG dinucleotides has been shown to stimulate the recruitment MeCP2, which in turn recruits histone-modifying co-regulators such as HDACs to the deacetylated histones, resulting in a repressive chromatin environment (Jones et al., 1998; Nan et al., 1998).

Many of the regulatory elements described above, such as enhancers, silencers, insulators and LCRs, are typically located far away from the promoter and, in certain cases, can be found downstream of the gene. So how do these elements relay their transcriptional effects over great physical distances from their target genes? Several mechanisms have been proposed, but recent technical advances have provided a strong support for a model based on "looping." Results from fluorescent *in-situ* hybridization (FISH) and the newly developed molecular techniques, chromosome conformation capture (3C) and RNA tagging and recovery of associated proteins (RNA-TRAP), demonstrated for the first time that the LCR of β-globin was positioned in close physical proximity to the *β-globin* genes (Carter et al., 2002; Dekker et al., 2002; Tolhuis et al., 2002). Subsequent studies showed this long-range interaction to be dependent on the insulator protein, CTCF (Splinter et al., 2006). CTCF has also been shown to be involved in long-range loop formation at the mouse imprinted *H19/Igf2* locus (Kurukuti et al., 2006; Murrell et al., 2004). At this locus, CTCF regulates expression of the allele-specific gene by binding specifically to the unmethylated maternal imprinting control region (ICR) and forming a loop with another region called the DMR1, which results in the sheltering of the promoter of the *Igf* gene from the enhancer (Bell and Felsenfeld, 2000; Murrell et al., 2004). CTCF has also been implicated in regulating gene expression via long-range interaction in other systems, including the major histocompatibility gene cluster and X-chromosome inactivation (Donohoe et al., 2007; Filippova et al., 2005; Majumder et al., 2006, 2008).

In addition to the above studies, similar long-range interactions have been reported in other systems, including immune response, hormonal signaling and maintenance of pluripotency in stem cells (Carroll et al., 2005; Levasseur et al., 2008; Spilianakis and Flavell, 2004; Tsytsykova et al., 2007). From these studies, long-range chromosomal looping is well accepted as a basic mechanism of transcriptional regulation. However, one major question currently eluding the field is, how widespread is the use of this mechanism for transcription regulation in the cell? Numerous genome-wide analyses of transcription binding sites have revealed that many transcription factors are preferentially located at regions distal to the promoter, suggesting that there is a strong possibility that long-range chromosomal interaction may be a general mode of transcriptional regulation by transcription factors (Bolton et al., 2007; Carroll et al., 2006; Lin et al., 2007; So et al., 2007). However, to identify all these interactions using 3C would be a tedious and time-consuming task. Newer techniques have been developed, such as 4C and 5C, but are these are biased and are not genome-wide approaches (Dostie et al., 2006; Simonis et al., 2006; Zhao et al., 2006). Thus the current goal in the field is to develop new methods that will be able to map all the long-range interactions in the genome in an unbiased manner.

Post-transcriptional Control: MicroRNAs

Mature microRNAs (miRNAs) are short (~22 nucleotides), non-coding RNAs that post-transcriptionally repress gene expression by two mechanisms. First, miRNAs that engage in perfect pairing to target mRNAs induce mRNA cleavage and destruction. Secondly, miRNAs that bind by imperfect pairing to target mRNAs can inhibit translation although preserving mRNA structure (*see* Chapter 5). In animals, miRNA-mediated repression is often relatively weak compared with transcription-factor-mediated repression, which appears to be stronger. MicroRNAs therefore have a unique repressor function that broadly inhibits a large number of transcripts, but most commonly does so only partially. MicroRNAs are transcribed as a primary miRNA (pri-mRNA) transcript by the enzyme Drosha, and converted to precursor miRNAs (pre-mRNAs) that are hairpin structures of ~70 nucleotides. These then are further processed to mature miRNAs by the enzyme, Dicer.

Taken together, the RNA pol II/basal transcriptional machinery can be viewed as the engine of the system. The enhancers function as accelerators; silencers and microRNAs as brakes. Insulators function as borders; the epigenetic marks and DNA topology act as both the roads and the road signs that guide transcription. The challenge now is to manage the traffic.

Complexity of the Transcriptome

The universe of all RNA species is called the "transcriptome." Previously, the focus had been on the <2% of the protein-encoding genome that generates polyadenylated and processed transcripts; thus it had been assumed that only a small percentage of the genome was ever transcribed. However, genomic interrogation of the transcriptome, first with whole-genome-tiling arrays and then with RNA (complementary DNA [cDNA]) sequencing, revealed that the transcriptome is very much larger. It has been estimated that from 60% to 90% of the genome can be transcribed, that most of the transcripts in the transcriptome are therefore non-coding (ncRNA) and that these ncRNAs range from very short segments to long and mature RNA species. Originally, the majority of these transcripts were believed to be the detritus of normal transcription. However, this is no longer the thinking.

There are specific subclasses of ncRNAs that have specific functions, such as the miRNAs mentioned above, and ncRNAs with specific developmental functions, such as H19 and XIST, as a class. Moreover, ncRNAs can form DNA–DNA–RNA triple helices inhibiting promoter activity; they can be involved in sense–antisense pairing with, and thus modulating, the function of coding transcripts, and they can also act in *trans* by binding to chromatin and mediating epigenetic control. The larger body of ncRNAs, however, is highly diverse and is generated from a very large number of genomic templates. It is therefore possible that this widespread transcription is a necessary concomitant to transcription itself. Recently, collective behavior of genome-wide transcription was described. Ebisuya and colleagues (2008) demonstrated that immediate early gene transcription after growth factor induction is followed by waves of transcription in nearby genomic regions even in intergenic segments. This generates a ripple effect that may organize coordinated expression of nearby genes. Separately, Core et al. (2008) showed that promoters of genes (55% of all genes and 77% of active genes) engage polymerases that embark on transcription in divergent directions. Bidirectional or divergent promoters appear to be the norm for active promoters, rather than the exception.

The act of transcription, when viewed from the whole-cell perspective, is far ranging—from very controlled and purposeful mechanisms to stochastic and "messy" processes the purpose of which we are still divining. It is, however, in examining populations of transcripts and their regulatory units that meaning emerges.

Transcriptional Regulation on a Genomic Scale in Medicine

Transcriptional regulation on a genomic scale is based on an organizational structure in which a single transcription factor controls the expression of many genes (including other transcription factors) and many transcription factors conjointly regulate individual genes. The overlay of these two organizational principles provides the necessary flexibility for an organism to respond to a wide range of conditions. Similarly, this creates complexity in inferring regulatory relationships from gene expression information. This has been assessed in a detailed genome-wide scale using a simplified model of gene regulation found in yeast. Here, transcription factors usually bind, upstream to the TSSs of genes, to specified DNA sequence motifs, which then leads to differential expression of gene cassettes. These simplifications allow for computational rendering of expression and motif data so that functional inferences can be made.

Classification

Segal et al. (2003a, 2003b) examined 2355 genes and 173 expression arrays from the yeast *Saccharomyces cerevisiae*, across a large number of stress conditions (Box 4.1). Using probabilistic graphical strategies associating the presence of transcription factor recognition motifs with gene expression, they inferred the presence of 50 module networks with 46 of the 50 organized as a functionally coherent set of genes (e.g. assigned to functions such as glycolysis, oxidative stress or protein folding). Thirty of the 50 modules included genes previously known to be regulated by the module's predicted regulators, and 15 of the 50 had a match between a predicted regulator and its known *cis*-regulatory motif. A *cis*-regulatory motif is a short (~6–20 bp long) nucleotide sequence pattern in the genome to which a specific transcription factor binds in order to regulate the expression of an associated gene. In this experimental system, predicted regulatory modules could be validated by gene disruption approaches easily accomplished in yeast.

The basis of this analysis is the identification of context rules that can describe the behavior of regulator genes controlling the expression of genes in a specific expression module. These sets of rules are then organized as a regression tree in which the response in each context is modeled as a normal distribution. This procedure is repeated and, in each iteration, genes are reassigned to modules having programs that best predict their behavior.

Although the transcriptional consequences of altering the expression of a single transcription factor had been described previously in the biological literature, the characteristic of this systems strategy is the integration of the combinatorial genetic influences on the expression of a regulatory program specifying a gene cassette. The importance of this work using a simpler model system in yeast is that it confirmed experimentally that such complex regulatory modules exist and can be inferred computationally. This is a case in which a system trains the analytical process.

Extrapolating from this work, transcriptional signatures in human conditions may therefore be reasonable representations of transcriptional regulatory programs associated with important physiologic functions (Box 4.2). The disease for which there has been the greatest translational impact is perhaps breast cancer. The examination of transcriptional signatures was responsible for a change in the classification of breast cancers that has had an impact on the selection of treatment strategies.

BOX 4.1

CIS-REGULATORY MOTIFS

Regulatory sequences can be placed either close to the gene they regulate (*cis*-) or distant from that gene (*trans*-). Therefore, a *cis*-regulatory motif is a sequence motif that is positioned close to the gene that it regulates.

> **BOX 4.2**
>
> **BIOLOGICAL HETEROGENEITY OF BREAST CANCER**
>
> The mammary gland that makes up the breast is a complex tissue comprising lobules that produce the milk, ducts that conduct and add to the characteristics of the milk, basal cells that are believed to hold the committed mammary stem cells, and stroma that not only form the scaffold for the lobules and ducts, but also support their growth and biology. Each of these components or cellular lineages can give rise to different types of breast cancer.

In a seminal study, Perou et al. (2000) showed that the biological heterogeneity of breast cancer could be largely explained by information embedded in the ordered transcriptional architecture represented by the transcriptional signature of a tumor. Using hierarchical analysis, numerous clusters of genes with recurrent coordinate expression patterns could be recognized as biologically distinct networks of individual tumors. These molecular portraits led to the discovery of an "intrinsic" gene signature that could distinguish new cancer subtypes, which, we now believe, are based on the cell type of origin (see Box 4.2). In breast cancer, these subtypes derived from the coordinate expression of specific gene cassettes were first termed luminal A, luminal B (tumor types that are estrogen receptor [ER] positive and together are the most frequent subclass of breast cancer), ErbB2+, and basal-like (collectively called Perou–Sørlie subtypes). Subsequent studies showed these to be stable and reproducible subclasses observable in different patient populations, and significantly correlated with tumor recurrence and patient survival (Sørlie et al., 2001, 2003). Before this classification, breast tumors were first defined on the basis of their histologic appearance (inflammatory, low or high grade, medullary, intraductal or lobular), which also inferred the cell type of origin (e.g. intraductal vs. lobular). Subsequently, subclassification was based on the specific molecular marker (ER positive or negative, and HER2/ErbB2 positive or negative). The latter molecular markers had significance, not only because of prognosis, but because they were also the direct targets for specific therapeutic agents. The discovery of these biomarkers led to the belief that specific subsets of breast cancers could be discerned by the combinatorial presence or absence of individual markers (add to this p53 and epidermal growth factor receptor [EGFR]). Since their first description, the genomic-based classifications of luminal A and B and basal (also called triple-negative because of their association with ER negative, progesterone receptor [PR] and HER2 negative tumors) have now taken hold as clinically meaningful assignments. For example, it is now believed that luminal A tumors are all ER positive, hormonally sensitive and associated with good prognosis. By contrast, luminal B tumors, although ER positive, have a worse prognosis. HER2 overexpressing/amplified breast cancers appear to be sensitive to a specific class of chemotherapy called anthracyclines, and susceptible to treatment with anti-HER2 antibodies such as Herceptin. The triple-negative (basal-like) tumors are aggressive cancers and, if untreated, are associated with very poor prognosis, but appear to be specifically sensitive to non-anthracycline and alkylator-based chemotherapy.

In the studies linking luminal and basal cellular phenotypes and breast cancer transcriptional signatures, it was surmised that the transcriptional signature was a mark of the specific cellular lineage (i.e., which cell type of origin) of a cancer, rather than a signature of an end-stage of a progression pathway. This would suggest that the molecular "point of origin" of a cancer (which can also be considered a tumor regulatory module) would define the transcriptional signature of the final tumor. Desai et al. (2002) profiled breast tumors arising from transgenic mice bearing different mammary-gland-specific onco transgenes (MMTV-*Ha-ras*, MMTV-*neu*, MMTV-*myc*, MMTV-polyoma middle T antigen, C3T-SV40 Large T antigen and WAP-SV40 Large T antigen). They identified expression cassettes unique to the different transgenes, indicating that transcriptional footprints of the earliest initiating oncogenic events could be found within the end-stage tumors. Bild and colleagues (Bild et al., 2006) found that specific oncogene transcriptional configurations (e.g. *HRAS*, *MYC*, *E2F* and *SRC*) could be detected as modules in primary tumors bearing the same genetic lesions. Moreover, these signatures could be used to enrich for tumors sensitive to targeted therapeutic agents. Miller et al. (2005) exploited the association between p53 mutations and gene expression in primary breast cancers and identified a 32-gene signature capable of distinguish p53-mutant and p53-wild-type breast tumors with good accuracy (85%). Survival analysis of patients with breast cancer showed that those with the mutant-like signature had a significantly shorter disease-free survival than those with the wild-type-like profile. Furthermore, these studies suggest that the p53 expression signature, as an endpoint measure of the entire p53 pathway, may be more predictive of p53 function than even the mutational status as ascertained by direct sequencing of the p53 locus.

Application to Cancer Patient Prognosis

An important translational goal is to develop molecular markers that can predict clinical outcome. van't Veer et al. (2002) and Wang et al.(2005) both focused on the identification of gene expression "signatures" (rather than tumor subtypes) that could predict outcome in patients with early-stage breast cancer (specifically, those breast cancers that have not metastasized to the local and regional lymph nodes). The signature identified by van't Veer et al. (also known as the Amsterdam signature) was comprised of 70 genes, whereas the predictor identified by Wang et al. (also known as the Rotterdam signature) used 76 genes. A description of how the expression signatures were extracted in these early studies is informative. van't Veer and her colleagues followed a combination of unsupervised and supervised learning strategies to select the 70-gene signature. In the first unsupervised selection step, 5000 genes were selected in which the expression differed twofold from a reference. In the second supervised learning step, the 5000 genes were tested for their correlation with the disease outcome; 231 genes were identified. The 231-gene signature was reduced to a 70-gene signature that maintained accuracy but minimized complexity. Wang's group, however, followed a strict supervised learning strategy to select their 76-gene signature and used the Cox Proportional Hazards model to test the relevance of gene expression to the disease outcome. They measured the performance of the 76-gene classifier using receiver operator characteristic (ROC) analysis instead of other measures of accuracy.

In both the above studies, the prognostic power of the signature was independent of, and even superior to, conventional risk factors (e.g. tumor size, histologic grade, patient age). Importantly, these signatures were better at predicting which patients should not receive adjuvant therapy than were the existing consensus guidelines for patient selection for adjuvant chemotherapy, potentially sparing a significant proportion of patients from over-treatment. Whereas many of the prognostic transcriptional signatures were identified by supervised clustering of genes associated with clinical outcome, others have pursued a different strategy of uncovering gene expression modules associated with specific pathways pertinent in cancer. Termed "mechanism-derived biomarker discovery," this approach focuses on the identification of regulatory modules in human cancers specified by a physiologic or molecular process (Liu, 2005). It then takes the signature of such a regulatory module and assesses its clinical translational potential. If such molecular or physiologic processes are selected to be ones with prior associations with tumor virulence, there would be a high likelihood that such transcriptional signatures would have clinical prognostic utility.

Early microarray studies on breast cancer cell lines uncovered a large cluster of coordinately expressed genes associated with cell proliferation (Chang et al., 2004; Ross et al., 2000; Whitfield et al., 2002). Later called the "proliferation signature," these genes appear to be associated with various aspects of cancer biology in breast and other cancer types, including neoplastic transformation (Rhodes et al., 2004), histologic grade (Ivshina et al., 2006; Ma et al., 2003; Sotiriou et al., 2006) and poor patient survival (Dai et al., 2005; Rosenwald et al., 2002). Furthermore, these signature genes were expressed in specific phases of the cell cycle in cell synchronization experiments involving HeLa cells (cervical carcinoma) (Whitfield et al., 2002).

Clinically, the pathologist's microscopy reading of tumor proliferation is the histologic grade of the cancer. Although histologic grade (measured from I to III) is regarded as a strong indicator of disease recurrence, its utility as a prognostic marker has been limited by the subjective nature of the grading process with its inter-observer variability. Several groups used the expression profiles of grade I and III tumors as a training set to uncover minimal transcriptional signature of grade, and then tested the prognostic value of this signature by assessing outcome in grade II patients. These efforts resulted in a five-gene genetic grade signature (Ivshina et al., 2006) and a 97-gene genomic grade index (Sotiriou et al., 2006), both capable of discriminating grade I (G1) and grade III (G3) tumors with high accuracy, but both partitioning intermediate grade II (G2) tumors into G1-like and G3-like classes. Patients with G2 disease classified as G1-like and G3-like showed significantly different 10-year survival curves—similar to those of patients with histologic G1 and G3 tumors, respectively. Thus there is surprising precision in these multigene predictors that capture the prognostic essence of histologic grade and cellular proliferation, particularly for patients with G2 disease. Moreover, such studies may redefine pathology practice by suggesting that there is no grade II, only low- and high-grade tumors with confounding histologic appearance. From a biological perspective, these findings suggest that tumors of low and high grade/proliferation may reflect discrete biological entities, rather than a continuum through which cancer progresses.

Chang and colleagues (Adler et al., 2006; Chang et al., 2004, 2005) exploited the similarity of the behavior of cells involved in wound healing and of those involved in cancer progression that were used in extracting a clinically useful transcriptional signature. They defined an expression signature of serum response in fibroblasts (after proliferation genes had been subtracted) that was expressed in breast and other epithelial cancer datasets (Chang et al., 2004). As wound healing is a composite physiologic process that includes cell motility, angiogenesis and growth factor release, in addition to cell proliferation, it is believed that this serum response might reflect these other cell biological modules. Intriguingly, this wound response signature was subsequently found to be prognostic of survival for patients with breast, lung and gastric cancers. In this approach, the transcriptional signature of a physiologic process associated with cancer was derived using an "orthogonal" source—primary human fibroblasts. This strategy of "orthogonality," by using data generated from a biologically related process but from different and distinct experimental systems, is a powerful approach that can uncover hidden physiologic processes and simultaneously generate clinically useful expression cassettes (Fig. 4.3).

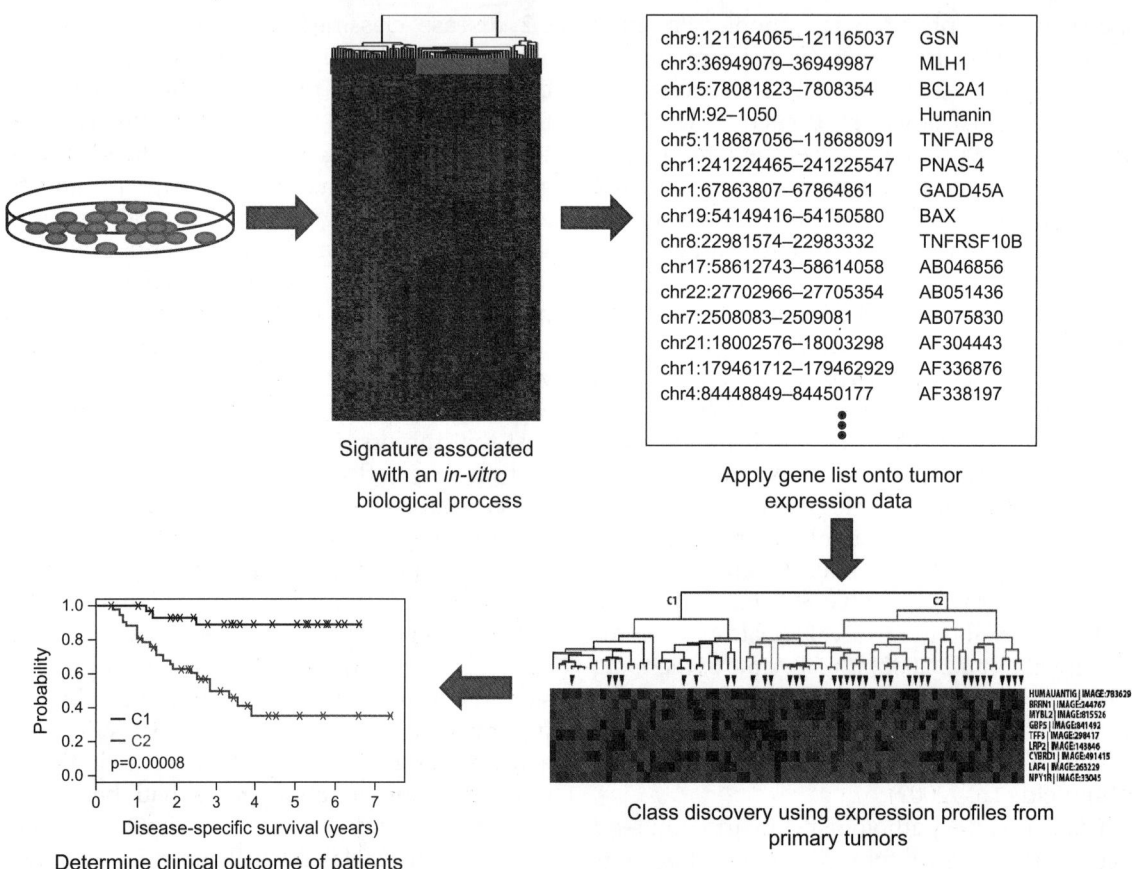

FIGURE 4.3 Use of Orthogonal Data to Derive Clinical Significance of a Biological Process.
By intersecting the higher-level data generated from studying a specific biological process, but from different and distinct experimental systems, hidden order can be uncovered. In this case, the first dataset are genes that are responsive to an *in-vitro* stimulus, and the second dataset are genes that are differentially expressed in primary tumors, with clinical outcome information. These genes that intersect are putatively representative of that physiological process operative in primary cancers, and can be assessed for their prognostic potential.

Cleverly exploiting intersection of orthogonal data, Wong and colleagues (2008) addressed the question of the importance of a stem cell phenotype on cancer behavior. To this end, using publicly available datasets, they first identified an embryonic stem cell (ESC) expression module. When applied to a range of expression data from primary cancers, this ESC-like module was able, not only to distinguish normal from cancer tissues, but also to divide breast cancers into defined prognostic groups. Wong's group extended their findings by mining the 335 genes that determine the ESC-like module for *cis*-acting transcription factor binding sites and found that the binding motif for Myc was highly enriched. Their work concluded by experimentally showing that exogenously introduced *myc* can induce an ESC-like expression in primary epithelial cells that is associated with enhanced cancer-initiating cell characteristics: the fraction of tumor initiating cells could be increased 150-fold in primary keratinocytes transduced with exogenous *c-myc*. Intriguingly, others working in the stem cell field had determined that Myc is an important transcriptional initiator for the reprogramming of differentiated cells into stem cells (Hanna et al., 2008; Lowry et al., 2008).

This strategy of intersecting *cis*-regulatory motifs with gene expression profiles is therefore used as an unbiased approach to enrich for genes involved in expression modules. It should be noted that such regulatory motifs can be represented in different ways. A *cis*-regulatory motif may be described as a simple sequence which is a lower-order representation. This is often inadequate, because of the many permissive representations of the binding motifs. Position × weight matrix (PWM) is a higher-order representation of motifs that takes into account the variability of a consensus recognition sequence. A PWM is a matrix of $4 \times L$ dimension, with L being the length of the motif and the 4 rows representing A, C, G and T nucleotides. PWM_{ij} is the probability of the *i*th base being at the *j*th position of the motif. PWM for a transcription factor is inferred from a set of short *cis*-regulatory sequences experimentally determined to bind the transcription factor of interest. A motif is rated by its over-representation in the given *cis*-regulatory sequences compared with the background (Tompa et al., 2005).

In one example, Rhodes and colleagues (2005) extracted specific cancer-associated signatures from 6348 arrays archived in Oncomine and explored any enrichment of known transcription factor binding site motifs in the immediate region of the TSSs. They observed that, across all cancers, the presence of E2F binding motifs predominated, suggesting a mechanistic role for E2F transcription factors in the genesis or maintenance of human cancers. Other transcription factors such as Rel and Myc were found, but associated with more restricted forms of cancer: Myc with small-cell lung cancers and Rel with diffuse large B-cell lymphomas. In truth, the realities of transcription factor–DNA interactions limit the utility of this approach in higher organisms. Regulatory transcription factors commonly bind far away from the TSS. Moreover, binding site motifs are degenerate and often are short segments that are almost ubiquitous in the genome; thus any assumptions of significance simply by scoring their presence should be made with great care.

On occasion, the comprehensive analysis of DNA binding sites may also reveal network associations. Chen et al. (2008) conducted a genome-wide sequence analysis of chromatin-immunoprecipitated fragments for binding of 13 transcription factors operative in mouse ESC biology. What was noteworthy was the observation that the co-occupancy of ESC-specific binding of several transcription factors within 100 bp of each other was much greater than by chance alone. Moreover, there were specific clusters of transcription factors that aggregated on DNA regions in enhanceosomes associated with coordinate regulation of downstream genes. For example, Nanog–Oct4–Sox2 co-clustered in many multiple-transcription-factor binding loci, whereas the Myc-associated clusters were found in different regions. This suggested co-evolution of transcription factor binding to sites that attract structurally diverse sets of transcription factors that recognize different sequence motifs. On the basis of these convergent binding site and gene expression data, Chen and colleagues drew a network map that was more richly populated than previously understood. Through a map of this complexity, they were able to discern higher-order regulatory architecture that had ramifications on the coordinated expression of developmental genes. This higher-order structure was mediated by the co-clustering of transcription factors into distinct classes based on transcription factor co-occupancy.

Parsing Pathways for Targeted Therapy

An example of how mechanism-based approaches may uncover molecular pathways predisposing sensitivity to specific therapeutic interventions has been found also in diffuse large B-cell lymphomas (DLBCLs). Alizadeh et al. (2000) used expression microarrays and discerned transcriptional patterns that could separate DLBCLs into at least two classes associated with different characteristics of normal B-cell physiology. One class showed expression of genes commonly induced in germinal center B cells, whereas the other was characterized by expression of genes associated with growth-stimulated B cells (termed the activated B cell [ABC]-like class). Importantly, these two classes showed distinct clinical responses to chemotherapy: patients with germinal center B-cell-like disease had twice the 5-year survival rate of those with ABC-like class disease (Alizadeh et al., 2000; Rosenwald et al., 2002; Wright et al., 2003). These expression microarray data also revealed that NF-κB target genes were more highly expressed in the ABC-like class (Davis et al., 2001). On the basis of this array information, it was subsequently shown that constitutive NF-κB activity was required for the survival of the ABC-like class, but not that of the germinal center B-cell-like class, therefore NF-κB may protect cells from death induced by certain chemotherapeutic agents and may be responsible for the poor survival outcomes found in the ABC-like subclass of DLBCLs. This suggests that patients of the poor-outcome ABC-like class, as defined by gene expression profiling, may benefit from treatment with NF-κB inhibitors that are known to work in synergy with chemotherapy to enhance cell death. Such expression-derived hypotheses are currently being tested in clinical trials.

Principles of Transcriptional Network Analysis

The overriding assumption in the study of cancer is that there are unifying molecular principles of transformation that are true for all forms of cancer of different cellular origin. A further assumption that drives the clinical translational work is that the output of these principles could explain clinical behavior of the cancers. Therefore the earlier work in transcription profiling in cancer assumed that the prognostic expression cassettes from different studies on the same cancer would have significant overlap. This was not to be the case. Although the gene lists from the two major studies providing the best breast cancer prognostic signatures were driven by the same basic scientific question and used similar patient cohorts, only three genes were found in common to both signatures (Wang et al., 2005). Moreover, as more mechanism-based prognostic signatures emerged, there was very little overlap between these (p53, wound healing, etc.), with each other and with the original clinical studies. This was also true when fundamental cellular processes were assessed using expression modules. Wong et al. (2008) noted that the 184-gene signature that defined the profiles of enriched breast cancer cell "stem cells" (relative to normal breast tissues) overlapped by only four genes with their 335-gene core ESC-like gene module. Various technical differences have been proposed to account for this discrepancy, but others have noted that many pathways contribute to prognosis, thus converging on the same underlying clinical biology (Wang et al., 2005). In addition, with the intricate interactions between these pathways, it is not likely that clear demarcations of a stem-cell-like module and a wound-healing module, for example, will be feasible. Therefore, these prognostic signatures are likely to be gene cassettes derived from sampling from a much larger list of genes associated with the fundamental biology of the tumor that affects clinical outcome. Alternatively stated, these findings show that prognostic transcriptional signatures are a summation of a number of expression cassettes representing different physiologic processes. This concept of summation of transcriptional signatures is the rationale for many of the biological and medical applications of transcriptional profiling. The challenge which remains unsolved is how to measure the relative contribution of these expression cassettes to the overall transcriptional picture.

Statistical Approaches

In the analysis of clinically relevant array data, the goal is to assess statistical associations between genes and clinical attributes of the samples, or cassettes of genes and clinical outcome. The first order of business often is to ascertain if there is an ordered architecture to the expression profiles of the tumors. To establish gene clusters and sample/tumor classes, clustering strategies have been used. Clustering is an unsupervised analysis strategy that arranges the genes/samples into distinct groups on the basis of a predefined notion of similarity. Genes grouped together are essentially co-regulated in a population of samples; samples grouped together exhibit similar gene expression, and therefore may have similar clinical attributes. Two common types of conceptually different clustering strategies are hierarchical clustering and K-means clustering.

Hierarchical clustering elicits a gradient of similarity between different genes/samples in the form of dendrogram or a tree. The change of gradient is used to identify different subpopulations of distinctly co-regulated genes (on one axis) and subgroups of samples (on the other axis). In contrast, K-means clustering partitions genes into K distinct groups of co-regulated gene sets (with K being defined by the investigator) and biologically homogeneous samples. Genes in each group are more closely co-regulated, whereas the regulation of each group is measurably dissimilar from the genes in the other groups. Samples in each cluster have similar patterns of expression and may share similar biological behavior.

The major advantage of hierarchical clustering is in visualizing gradients of similarity of co-regulation and thereby giving visual flexibility of choice in defining major clusters. However, the choice-of-similarity threshold may leave out many singletons—that is, genes not assigned to any major clusters. Moreover, the tree structure may not be robust, especially if the number of genes/samples clustered is not large enough. Conversely, K-means clustering conveniently partitions all genes into K number of groups, with an explicit objective of high within-group similarity and low between-group similarity. A disadvantage of K-means clustering is its inability to handle outliers, and the inadequate statistical approaches to define the choice of a meaningful K (i.e., the number of groups).

Both strategies have been used logically to assemble groups of elements (genes or tumors) into distinct groups or classes so that associations with specific outputs such as cellular phenotype or survival can be discerned. The next step is to assess the association of such clusters with clinically relevant parameters. Assessing the clinical associations from a compact expression dataset can be carried out using statistical tests such as Fisher's exact test or the chi-square test. The association with disease outcome can be effectively tested by the Cox Proportional Hazards model. Central to the statistical association testing are the *P value* and the *false discovery rate* (FDR). The *P* value is the probability that the observed relative change is possible purely by chance as a result of sampling variation; in other words, the *P* value is the probability that the observed effect is not different from the reference. The FDR is the expected proportion of false predictions in the set of predictions. For example, an FDR of 0.2 in an analysis that identifies 1000 genes means that 800 are likely to be correct. The FDR accounts for errors arising from multiple testing carried out in gene expression studies in which tens of thousands of probes are studied.

A potential advantage of genomic medical approaches is that the genomic dataset for each patient is sufficiently comprehensive that, potentially, further re-testing will not be necessary: all pertinent information will have been acquired. As the fundamental unit is the nucleotide sequence, the information should be highly flexible, and can be used by many scientists for many different purposes and exchanged freely. Despite this goal, there are common experimental challenges that limit the desired exchangeability of the data, such as batch and operator effects and differences between the experimental platforms (e.g. Affymetrix vs. Illumina expression arrays). For datasets from different sources to be useful in meta-analyses, normalization or data equalization is required. For datasets generated by the same technology platform (e.g. Affymetrix U133A, U133B, U133+), this is commonly accomplished by quantile normalization, which equalizes the distributions of the measurements of all arrays and batches—that is, every quantile from all arrays is made to be the same.

Besides normalization, more sophisticated approaches may also have to be used to eliminate or reduce the batch effects. In their molecular characterization of soft tissue tumors, Nielsen et al. (2002) used the batch correction method based on singular value decomposition that was proposed by Alter et al. (2000). Later, Garman et al. (2008) used the distance weighted discrimination method proposed by Benito and colleagues (2004) to correct for batch-dependent bias in a hierarchical fashion—that is, normalizing two batches at a time if the number of batches is greater than two. In contrast to batch-wide analysis, Li and Wong (2003) proposed a location/scale procedure that estimates the batch-dependent location and scale parameters of the expression of each gene and makes corrections using a linear regression model. This accounts for both additive batch effects and multiplicative batch effects, which have been recently augmented by Johnson et al. (2007) in their COMBAT algorithm by estimating the batch-associated location and scale parameters using an empirical Bayes approach. COMBAT was successfully deployed by Acharya et al. (2008) in their recent study to identify gene expression signatures by combining expression data of early-stage breast cancer patients from different Affymetrix gene chip platforms. If the array platforms are not of the same type, the batch-effect elimination procedures have to be preceded by probe mapping as used by Acharya's group (2008). Recently, Shabalin et al. (2008) have proposed a more direct method of integrating data from different platforms such as Affymetrix and Illumina using a block linear model and K-means clustering.

In contrast to data equalization procedures, meta-analysis procedures compute the association of a gene with a clinical attribute by combining results from several studies using non-parametric or parametric analysis procedures. The non-parametric procedures combine the P values or the statistical significance using methods such as Fisher's inverse chi-square method. They are based on an important property of the P value distribution: the P values in multiple testing are distributed uniformly in the interval $[0, 1]$. The final P value is derived by combining the P values, which follows a certain distribution depending on the combination procedure under a no-change hypothesis. For example, in Fisher's inverse chi-square method, $-2\log$ (product of P values) is computed, which follows a chi-square distribution of degrees of freedom, double that of the number of P values used. An important drawback of the non-parametric procedures is that they give equal weight to all studies, irrespective of the number of samples and their quality.

Clinically relevant genes as chosen by the above procedure may be reduced to a compact signature that can best predict the clinical outcome or attribute. To achieve such an objective, a classifier will be built using the selected clinically relevant genes. A classifier can typically be a one of diagonal linear discriminant analysis (DLDA), support vector machine (SVM), K nearest neighbor (KNN) and decision tree analysis. The strategy frequently used to identify a compact set of genes for classification is the gene-wrapper strategy. In this strategy, a series of classifiers are built using series of gene lists of increasing size. The difference in the size of any consecutive gene list may vary from one to five genes. The analysis of size of gene list used and the performance measured give a saturating point of maximum attainable performance. The size of the gene list that achieves the saturation point is delivered as a compact gene set predictive of the clinical outcome. If the complexity of the classifier exceeds the size of the training data, which is the case in a typical genomics study, the estimate of the performance of the classifier using the training data alone could be far greater than that of its true performance. This problem is called "overfitting."

To circumvent the problem of overfitting, an N-fold cross-validation procedure is used to estimate the performance or generalization in which a series of N classifiers is built using the same set of genes and training parameters for N different training sets derived from the same set of samples by reserving the Nth number of the samples only for testing, and the performance is measured on the reserved samples. Another approach to account for overfitting is bootstrapping, in which a series of training sets is derived by sampling with replacement, so that classifier stability is estimated. Miller et al. (2005) used DLDA in conjunction with leave-one-out cross-validation (onefold cross-validation) to find their 32-gene list that achieved least error to predict p53 functional status. van't Veer et al. (2002) used a similar strategy to identify their 70-gene signature. In contrast, Wang et al. (2005) used bootstrapping to obtain relapse scores by maximizing the area under the ROC curve and identified a 76-gene signature.

Network Motifs and Modules

Most network maps for disease states primarily describe gene relationships and clusters, and are static representations. Certainly, the goal of these efforts is to use this understanding to model dynamic processes in order to predict cellular output, given component input. This can be accomplished by knowing the following components: the transcription factors involved, the complete inventory of true binding sites, the relationship of the binding sites to the gene regulated (induced, repressed or irrelevant), the intensity of the response and the effect of the protein induced or repressed. This approach has been most successful in prokaryotic systems, not only because of the smaller genomes and therefore fewer transcription factors, but also because the organization of the transcriptional regulatory system is simpler and more uniform. The structure of the regulatory mechanism in prokaryotes is a binding site, followed by a short distance to the TSS of the regulated gene. This organizational module can therefore be used in a general model of transcriptional regulation of the whole microbe. Eukaryotic systems are significantly more complex, and mammalian systems pertinent to biomedicine are among the most complicated. The added layers of transcriptional regulators such as miRNAs, and distant locus control regions, confound simple models. These complexities will be discussed further later in this chapter.

Much has been learned from work on simpler organisms in constructing transcriptional network models. From these lessons, integrated with understanding of more complex network systems, several organizing frameworks emerge. First, networks can be devolved into networks of subnetworks composed of many simple network motifs, which are unit control elements that describe basic regulatory relationships. The output of the entire system is therefore a dynamic integration of all the control functions within each subunit. Secondly, dynamical networks evolve into scale-free networks that are no longer a random collection of interactions, but are characterized by a limited number of hubs with many connections, and many nodes with few connections. It is hoped that knowledge of such subnetworks, network motifs and network hubs will be helpful in cell biology, in the study of human diseases and in developing

4. CELLULAR REGULATORY NETWORKS

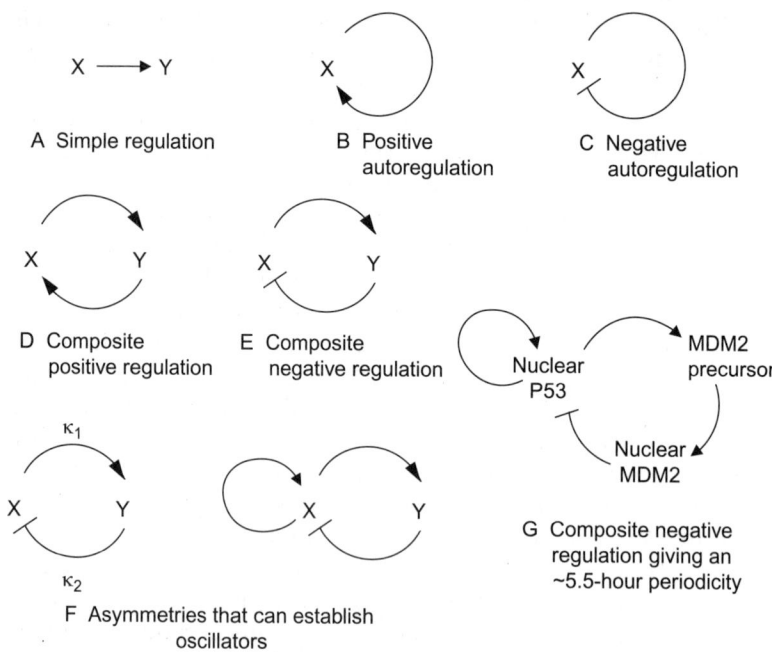

FIGURE 4.4 Examples of Network Motifs.

new therapeutic agents: destruction of a hub leads to disease or maybe an efficient target for therapeutics, whereas finessing a subnetwork and the mechanics of a network motif can give selective advantage of one drug over another.

The simplest network motifs are single-edge reactions in which X induces or represses Y. There are also autoregulatory functions in which X inhibits its own transcription (negative autoregulation) or augments its own transcription (positive autoregulation) (Alon, 2007) (Fig. 4.4). When more nodes are added to the network motif, the possibilities of composite directions of control (induction in one and repression in the other edge), branch-points at the nodes and different reaction velocities for each edge provide nuanced and complex responses for the organism. Extending the negative regulation motif, composite network motifs involve more than one element involved in divergent controls. The proteins P53 and MDM2 provide an example of a two-member loop involved in negative feedback control: P53 transcriptionally induces the expression of MDM2, which then biochemically reduces P53 function. Depending on the kinetic relationship linking the two nodes, the output can be a self-delimited induction, or can create oscillations. In the case of P53 and MDM2, using a cancer cell line system transfected with P53 marked with cyan-fluorescent protein and MDM2 marked with yellow fluorescent protein, Lahav and colleagues (Geva-Zatorsky et al., 2006; Lahav, 2008; Lahav et al., 2004) found that the two proteins exhibited oscillations that were slightly out of phase, with an average periodicity of approximately 5.5 hours, after induction by gamma irradiation. The number of cells exhibiting these oscillations, but not the amplitude or frequency, increased with the dose of radiation given, suggesting that the irradiation functioned to initiate the oscillations, but that the characteristics of the oscillations were cell dependent. This also appears to be the case in the delayed negative-feedback relationship between inhibitor

I. FOUNDATIONS OF SYSTEMS BIOLOGY

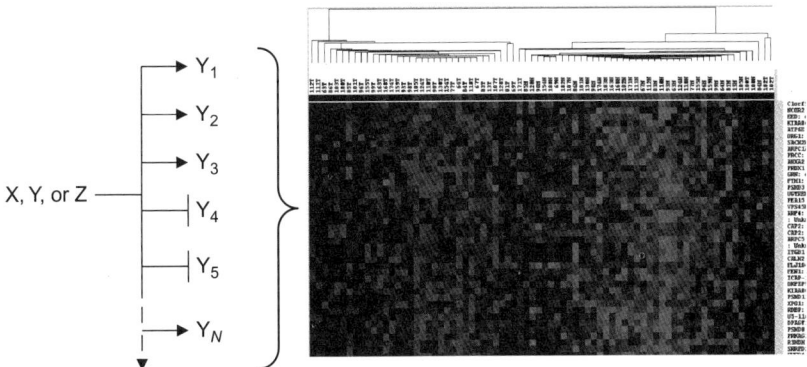

FIGURE 4.5 Single-input Modules in Parallel, Generating Tumor Signatures.
A single transcription factor regulates a number of downstream genes as a mechanism to generate specific tumor signatures.

IκB and its cytosolic target, NF-κB, on the nuclear localization of NF-κB. From single-cell time-lapse images, oscillations of NF-κB localization were found in the nucleus after a cellular stimulus (Nelson et al., 2004). These oscillations decreased in frequency with increased IκB transcription, and appeared to be correlated with transcription of NF-κB downstream target genes.

More complex modules have branch-points at the origin. The single-input module denotes a model in which a single transcription factor regulates many downstream genes (Fig. 4.5). This model is the theoretical basis for generating the cancer-associated transcriptional signatures discussed previously: cancer-associated transcriptional signatures of coordinately up- and downregulated genes linked to a disease phenotype. This has been a useful simplification of transcriptional regulation with which to infer the involvement of specific oncogenic transcription factors. By adjusting specific parameters, the single-input module network can also allow for ordered expression of downstream genes (Y) if the threshold for activation by the inducer (X) also is ordered (Fig. 4.6). Such regulatory strategies can be seen in development and in response to external signals.

Another important family of more complex network motifs are the feed-forward loops (FFLs), consisting of three components, X that

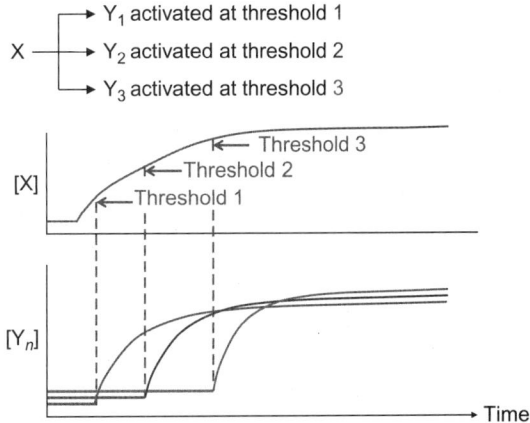

FIGURE 4.6 Single-input Module, One Transcription Factor Regulating Three Genes.
The three genes have different thresholds of activation: $3 > 2 > 1$. This arrangement generates a temporally ordered gene induction of a transcriptional cassette.

regulates Z, but also regulates Y, that itself regulates Z (Fig. 4.7A). A coherent feed-forward loop is present when the output of the branching controls from X are in the same direction (i.e., both inducing or both repressing), whereas incoherent FFLs are those in which the output of the two controls on Z are in the opposite direction (i.e., both outputs from X result in either induction or repression). The kinetics of the induction or repression can be tuned to generate

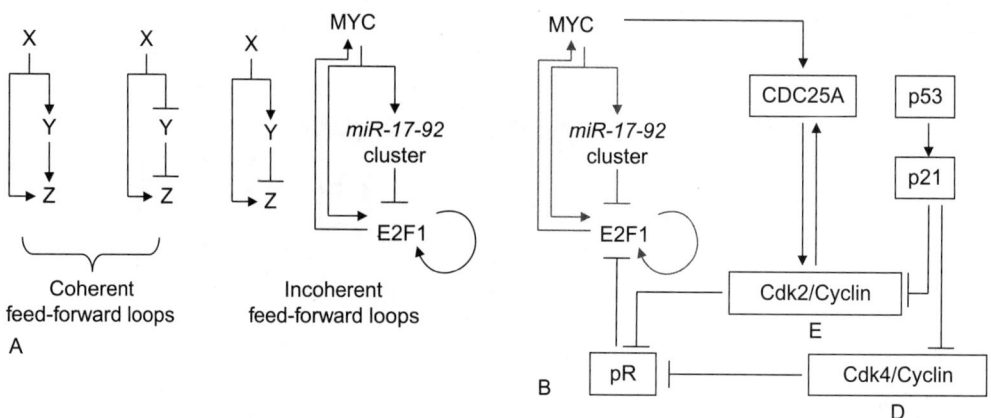

FIGURE 4.7 Complex Network Motifs in the Form of Coherent and Incoherent Feed-forward Loops. (A) Coherent feed-forward loops (FFLs) generate branching output in the same direction, whereas incoherent FFLs have branch outputs in the opposite direction. An example of a relevant incoherent FFL is MYC and E2F1. (B) Diagram of the MYC/E2F1 FFL in the context of the larger cell cycle regulatory network. Adapted from Aguda et al. (2008), with permission.

a desired pattern for Z as the outcome. An example of an incoherent FFL pertinent to cancer biology involves MYC as activator X, the miRNA *miR-17-92* cluster as repressor Y, and E2F1 as the target gene, Z. Such incoherent feed-forward loops can be modeled to induce a pulse of activity by accelerating the induction. Thus *miR-17-92*-mediated inhibition of translation could induce a pulse of E2F activity. Equally important, because Myc and E2F1 reciprocally induce each other, phased induction of *miR-17-92* may act to dampen Myc and E2F1 to prevent "runaway" activation (Coller et al., 2007). Aguda et al. (2008) computationally analyzed this *miR-17-92*–E2F–Myc interaction and created a model that correctly predicted that steady levels of *miR-17-92*, E2F and Myc will change in the same direction. Their model also suggested that *miR-17-92* is likely to play an important part in positioning of the on–off switch for the system by determining the "on" levels for these proteins (Fig. 4.7A,B). Thus the versatility of such a FFL is that slight modulations of individual parameters around the component genes can give different patterns of behavior for the entire system. Given the central position of E2F and Myc in many oncogenic processes, this threshold-setting function may be critical in determining susceptibility to cancer. The importance of this pathway has led others to construct a refined interaction map specifically of the pRB/E2F pathway that encompasses 78 proteins, 176 genes and 165 chemical reactions that revealed a modular organization of network. When applied to a bladder cancer expression dataset, the analysis predicted the downregulation of Wee1, APC, E2F4-5 and E2F608 modules in invasive cancers (Calzone et al., 2008).

Gene transcripts, when organized at a higher level, allow for transcriptional modules to emerge. Transcription modules are sets of co-regulated genes exhibiting coordinate responses to different conditions, and an associated set of conditions that can perturb the expression of the genes in that module (Segal et al., 2003b). Conceptually, transcription modules have greater information content than either individual gene expression behavior or a collection of clusters of co-expressed genes, because transcription modules comprise both genes and conditions joined by common functions. They have been called "self-consistent regulatory units," in which all conditions of a module affect all genes within the module.

Transcriptional modules were initially discovered purely from massive gene expression data using bi-clustering or co-clustering techniques (Ihmels et al., 2004; Kluger et al., 2003). The transcriptional modules were further refined by integrating heterogeneous data. Segal et al. (2003a) integrated promoter motifs data with the expression data to identify transcription modules by requiring genes in a transcriptional module to have the same common motif profile. Stuart et al. (2003) integrated expression data and ortholog gene sets data from humans, flies, worms and yeast to discover evolutionarily conserved transcriptional modules. They developed a network that links metagenes across the four model organisms and is operative in at least two, and organizes them according to the degree of correlation. Using this approach, they showed that predictions of individual gene function made by using the annotation label of neighboring genes in this multispecies network outperformed predictions using the networks of individual species. Ihmels et al. (2005) examined the co-expression of genes within two yeast species and noted a discordance in the co-expression of several major classes. Expression of *S. cerevisiae* genes encoding mitochondrial functions, notably the mitochondrial ribosomal proteins (MRPs), was not correlated with genes encoding ribosomal RNA (rRNA) processing genes and cytoplasmic ribosomal proteins, whereas, in *Candida albicans*, the expression of MRP genes was strongly correlated with the expression of ribosomal protein genes and rRNA processing genes. In examining the *cis*-regulatory elements associated with these genes in the two species, Ihmels and colleagues discovered that a specific regulatory element, AATTTT, was missing upstream of *S. cerevisiae* MRP genes, although it was present in *C. albicans*. This wholesale rewiring of the *cis*-regulatory framework of MRP genes appeared to coincide with the evolutionary genome duplication event that then allowed for phenotypic differentiation: *C. albicans* requires oxygen for growth, whereas *S. cerevisiae* can grow rapidly in anaerobic conditions. In all cases, transcriptional module networks were uncovered by integrating/intersecting heterogeneous sources of information: literature-derived associations, evolutionary conservation, response after environmental challenge or association with *cis*-regulatory motifs. The reasoning is that the higher-order relationships can be uncovered when orthogonal sources of data correlate.

This approach has been applied to biomedical questions with some limited success. Segal et al. (2004) integrated the expression data from 1975 microarrays obtained from 22 tumor types, from which 2849 biologically meaningful gene sets (co-expressed genes, tissue-type-specific genes and genes belonging to the same functional pathway) and 456 gene modules could be extracted. The analysis then assessed the relationship between clinical conditions (such as tumor type, molecular markers, prognostic information) and the gene modules as a representation of biological function. Some observations were not surprising. That some brain tumors and liver cancers lacked neural- and liver-associated modules, respectively, was consistent with the de-differentiation of the cancer relative to the tissues of origin. Several observations, however, shed light on the mechanisms of maintenance of the cancer. A growth-inhibitory module appeared to be repressed in a subset of acute leukemias. Some of these genes are repressors of extracellular-signal-regulated kinase 1 (ERK1), which is an activator of cell proliferation also found to be constitutively active in acute leukemias. Moreover, the signature suggested that the apoptosis repressor, p38, would be activated. Thus the coordinated downregulation of these growth suppressors might induce tumor growth. In another example, the induction of a bone osteoblastic module was seen in a subset of breast cancer tumors that is known to metastasize to bone and, unusually, can induce bone formation (osteoblastic metastases).

Mani, et al. (2008) used an interesting different approach in analyzing B-cell lymphomas. They posited that molecular interactions in normal B cells would be disrupted in the malignant state, and sought to uncover those interaction modules. To this end, they used an annotated B-Cell Interactome (BCI) database for their comparison base. The BCI is an interaction network representing key molecular interaction types in the human B cell. These include transcriptional expression, protein–DNA and protein–protein interactions. Mani's group first assembled a collection of microarray expression profiles from normal, tumor and experimentally manipulated B cells, to identify those BCI interactions that exhibited either a gain of correlation or a loss of correlation with the phenotype of interest as compared with background. These dysregulated interactions are pooled and genes having a statistically high number of these aberrant interactions were identified and ranked. Not surprisingly, they found *MYC* as a major gene potentially driving B-cell lymphomas, along with other genes involved in translocations, such as *MLL* and *PRDM2*. However, they also uncovered a number of novel candidate genes such as *POU6F1* and the ER gene, *ESR1*, which deserve further exploration.

Taken together, these observations lead to the underlying message that the higher-order expression architecture of a cell is a source of gene discovery in human diseases. These observations also raise the question of how such networks of regulatory hubs and linking edges determine the characteristics of the whole system.

Topological Analysis

If molecules in a cell simply contacted one another randomly, their number of interactions would follow a normal, bell-shaped, distribution. However, biological interactions that form networks follow a power-law distribution. Power laws describe a relationship characterized by the equation: $f(x) = C(1/x)^\alpha$ which

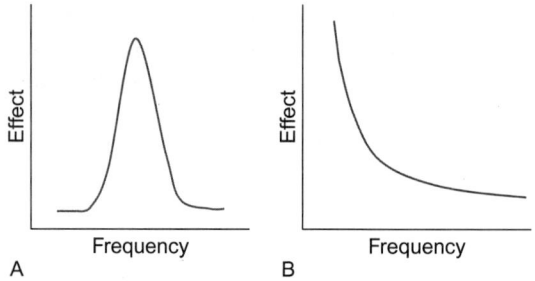

FIGURE 4.8 Graphical Representation of the Relationship Between the Frequency of an Event and the Effect or Impact of That Event.
(A) As a Poisson distribution; (B) as a power-law distribution. Biological interactions that form networks follow a power-law distribution. For these networks, the Y-axis would represent the number of linkages of a node with other nodes, and the X-axis would represent frequency of nodes with a specific number of linkages.

may represent the relationship between biological connectivity and their component parts surprisingly well. Simply stated, most nodes have just a few connections, whereas only a few nodes will have large numbers of connections (Fig. 4.8). Such networks are called "scale free," in that there is no normal distribution of the number of linkages that any node has with other nodes; that is, there is no natural upper limit to the number of connections. The power law describes the relationship of many other systems, such as the number of links experienced by websites in the World Wide Web, or how many citations scientists have for their publications (a few scientists account for most of the literature cited by others). Such power-law distributions are a consequence of an evolutionary process that requires that, as nodes are added to the system, the better nodes become more connected over time. It should be noted that all power-law relationships are context specific; therefore, a member that is highly connected in one context (most-cited scientist) may not be the most linked in another context (richest person). Moreover, such a relationship also suggests that, although all nodes contribute to the final outcome, most nodes are dispensable.

In gene networks, the same power-law relationship is found. Although there might be many genes involved in the entire network, only a few genes act as connectivity hubs. In transcription networks, this is evident in how mature somatic cells such as fibroblasts can be reprogrammed into induced pluripotent stem cells by the transfection of four master transcription factors, Oct4, Sox2, Myc and Klf4 (Takahashi and Yamanaka, 2006). As a reflection of how transcription factor hubs are context specific, three different transcription factors are capable of inducing lineage reprogramming from a pancreatic exocrine cell to an insulin-secreting beta cell: Pdx1, Ngn3 and MafA (Zhou et al., 2008; also reviewed by Gurdon and Melton, 2008). At a different level, most transcription factors bind to many sites in the genome, but only a smaller number of these sites, including those far away from the TSS, are actually important in regulating gene expression. These observations have several theoretical ramifications.

Systems characterized by scale-free networks are characterized by robustness to external perturbations. These systems are robust because the great majority of nodes are only marginally connected, and can be removed without compromising the whole. This characteristic makes these systems fault tolerant, in that chance challenges to the system probably will not perturb its function. In this manner, the dynamics resemble a phase shift in which little is changed until a threshold has been surpassed and the system shifts to a new position. Such added stability in biological systems functions will be favored in evolution. The trade-off, however, is that an attack on the network hubs might severely affect the entire system. This is often described as the Achilles' heel of power-law systems. Nevertheless, the relative stability to frequent insults still confers an advantage.

Because of their resemblance to buffer systems, genetic networks have been referred to as genetic buffers. Such buffering capacity is necessary, because transcription is a "noisy" process.

Single-cell measurements in prokaryotic and eukaryotic systems show random bursts of expression that, when averaged over the entire cell population, often will escape detection (Blake et al., 2003; Chubb et al., 2006; Elowitz et al., 2002). In development, dampening of such transcriptional noise may prevent premature or inappropriate induction of morphogenetic pathways, and can be accomplished by decoupling rates of protein synthesis and/or maturation (slow) from transcriptional bursts (fast).

A case in point is the effect of mutations in the heat-shock protein 90 gene (*hsp90*) on the variability of phenotypic expression. HSP90 is a chaperone the function of which is to facilitate the correct folding and maturation of a range of client proteins. Under environmental stress such as temperature challenges, HSP90 has a critical role that can be limiting, depending on the degree of stress. Under these conditions, there emerge phenotypically cryptic mutations in the genome that have accumulated under neutral selection. Hypomorphs of HSP90 in which function is partially attenuated in both *Drosophila* and Zebrafish are viable, but permit the penetrance of these cryptic genetic variants (Rutherford and Lindquist, 1998; Yeyati et al., 2007). If such a variant is beneficial to the stressed organism, then positive selection will enhance the expansion of that variant. Conversely, under normal conditions, HSP90 functions as a "buffer" for genetic variations that might otherwise adversely affect organismal robustness, and in this manner, permits the storage of a wider range of functional genetic variants to meet unknown environmental challenges.

Transcriptional control networks appear to also act as buffers for naturally occurring transcriptional spikes or bursts. In the case of *miR-17-92*, it has been speculated that the translational attenuation by this microRNA helps minimize noise in the concentrations of the E2F1 protein. As logical as it may seem for the control of E2F1, the presence of a complex and imperfect system such as miRNAs (e.g. many overlapping targets with partial inhibition) raises the question of its overarching function to enhance evolutionary robustness. In the worm, *Caenorhabditis elegans*, the genetic elimination of 95 miRNAs revealed a small minority with essential survival functions for the individual miRNAs (Miska et al., 2007). This suggests that individual miRNAs act as modulators of processes, rather than imparting critical survival functions. Mice with mutations in miRNAs involved in hematopoiesis (*miR-155*, *miR-150* or *miR-223*) exhibit abnormalities in immune cell numbers that can affect survival following immune challenge, but are viable and fertile. Similarly, mice with mutations in miRNAs such as *miR-1-2* or *miR-208* exhibit defects in cardiac function upon stress (reviewed by Flynt and Lai, 2008). These findings suggest that miRNAs have evolved to provide survivability after environmental challenges.

Stochasticity

For biologists, stochastic and random processes are often considered noise, and are believed to be usually detrimental to biological systems, especially for essential genes and those involved in multicomponent complexes in which the activity of the complex is determined by the weakest component (Fraser et al., 2004). However, Kussell and Leibler (2005) provided an intriguing theoretical argument for the importance of stochasticity in cellular systems. As described above, organisms adapt to consistently varying environments such as circadian cycles by evolving internal circadian clocks. When severe environmental fluctuations that challenge survival are irregular, organisms have responsive mechanisms to adjust to the changes. There is, however, an energetic cost, because active sensory processes must be maintained. This responsive switching strategy is associated, therefore, with a specific sensory cost. An alternative strategy is stochastic switching, in which the phenotype of the population is randomized by some stochastic process, generating limited diversity in the population. This process does not require environmental sensing, but does have a specific diversity cost that is extracted by harboring less-adapted individuals in the population. This recognized strategy of phenotype randomization to provide adaptive advantage in fluctuating environments is known as "bet-hedging." On the basis of their calculations, Kussell and Leibler concluded that a stochastic switching mechanism is the better solution if the environmental changes are unpredictable and infrequent. This strategy ensures that up to 50% of the elements in a population are poised to withstand such environmental challenges. Stochasticity in populations can confer robustness. Kitano (2007) noted that instability in a systems component can confer robustness to an entire system.

This concept is similar to that of neutral drift in population genetics, advanced by Motoo Kimura in the 1960s, which states that most of the sequence changes in individual genomes are the result of "genetic drift"—random changes that are not undergoing selection. This concept was modified by Ohta (2002), who advanced the idea of "near neutrality." This concept suggests that variants that are near neutral will survive, and may provide selective advantage to the population when challenged. The sense from these discussions is that the randomness may not be just noise, but may be a strategy to achieve greater systems robustness.

Estrogen Receptor as a Model for Transcriptional Complexity

The ER belongs to the large superfamily of nuclear hormone receptor proteins that are ligand-regulated DNA-binding transcription factors (Green and Carroll, 2007; Heldring et al., 2007). Since its discovery more than 50 years ago, a large body of biochemical, molecular and structural information on this transcription factor has accumulated, thus making it an excellent candidate for systems studies. ER is activated upon the binding of estrogen (17β-estradiol). This induces a conformational change in the structure of the ligand binding domain that promotes the dissociation of heat-shock proteins, the dimerization of ER and subsequent binding of the dimerized receptor to its cognate DNA binding sites, the estrogen response element (ERE) (Green and Carroll, 2007; Heldring et al., 2007). Once the receptor has bound to DNA, it alters the expression of target genes by recruiting a host of co-regulatory proteins (to promote local changes in histone modifications and chromatin structure) and the basal transcription machinery to the promoter, resulting in activated transcription. *In-vivo* studies have shown that ER has key roles in growth, differentiation and cell-specific gene regulation in a variety of tissues, including those of the male and female reproductive tracts, central nervous system and skeleton (Heldring et al., 2007). Moreover, from clinical studies, ER has been demonstrated to have important functions in hormone-dependent diseases such as breast cancer and osteoporosis, and over the years numerous therapeutic drugs (e.g. tamoxifen and raloxifene) have been successfully developed to target the receptor (Heldring et al., 2007).

Until recently, most of the literature on ER was from single-gene studies using classical molecular and biochemical approaches. However, the emergence and application of genomic approaches has provided us with a new way of understanding how ER functions as a transcription factor. Several studies in which chromatin immunoprecipitation (ChIP)-on-chip and ChIP-sequencing were used have revealed that ER is bound to thousands of sites across the breast cancer genome, perhaps in the range of 10 000 in the MCF7 cell line (Carroll et al., 2006; Hua et al., 2008; Lin et al., 2007). More importantly, these studies provided several novel mechanistic findings that would not have been possible using single-gene studies alone. For example, these studies revealed that the sequence of most binding sites, EREs, are highly variable, with only a minor fraction containing the historical consensus ERE motif, which suggests there is a high degree of degeneracy in the ERE motif (Carroll et al., 2006; Hua et al., 2008; Lin et al., 2007). The canonical ERE is an inverted repeat—AGGTCA-NNN-TGACCT—with the half site, AGGTCA, also sufficient to confer ER binding. However, the presence of the ERE motif does not determine ER binding. In fact, it is estimated that there are nearly a million ERE-like sequences in the genome, but only several thousand are used by the cell in any tissue. This implies that ER binding requires factors in addition to the ERE motif. Furthermore, a large portion of ER binding sites were found to be enriched for binding sites for many transcription factors, including AP-1, Sp1, C/EBP and Oct, suggesting that ER binds and regulate genes by co-operating with other DNA binding transcription factors (Carroll et al., 2006; Hua et al., 2008; Lin et al., 2007). One of the more interesting transcription factors that was enriched was FoxA1, which was shown to function as a pioneer factor for ER in regulating a subset of estrogen-regulated genes (Carroll et al., 2006). Such a pioneer factor is believed to engage potential ER binding sites, and is released upon ER binding. Other modulators of transcriptional regulation appear also to interact with ER and have been mapped, for example co-activators, RNA pol II and histone modifications (Carroll et al., 2006; Cheng et al., 2006; Kininis et al., 2007; Kwon et al., 2007; Lupien et al., 2008).

Unlike the transcriptional regulatory systems of lower eukaryotes, most of the ER binding sites identified were located at large distances away from the TSS of genes. It was observed that 95% of experimentally determined ER binding sites identified in genome-wide studies are more than 5 kb distal to the TSSs. This suggests that ER can regulate transcription from afar, extending up to several hundred kilobases via DNA looping; this has been experimentally proven. Very often, a regulated gene will have a number of ER binding sites, with the sites distal to the TSS being the more important regulators. Intriguingly, several studies have now demonstrated ER binding in proximity to the TSS to be associated with upregulation of genes, whereas no preferential positioning is seen for binding sites associated with repressed genes.

The genome-wide positioning and characteristics of these ER binding sites challenged the standard molecular biology deterministic construct of binding and gene regulation. The variability of the ER binding motif, the multiplicity of binding sites around a regulated gene, the irregular positioning of the ER binding sites and their distance from the TSSs are not consonant with any exact mechanism. This raises the question of whether most of the ER binding sites represent evolutionary noise and are irrelevant to gene regulation. However, other genome-wide transcription factor binding studies show similar results in terms of indistinctness of position, sequence and intensity of binding (Wei et al., 2006). This suggests that this strategy might confer adaptive robustness to transcriptional regulatory systems.

These results were further confounded by the observation that the majority of the binding sites (about 50–70%) for any human transcription factor are not conserved in evolution. Bourque et al. (2008) examined this question in detail and found that many (about 20–50%) of these non-conserved binding sites across six transcription factors are carried by specific repetitive elements with origins from endogenous retroviruses and transposable elements. These repeat-associated binding sites are functional in that they bind their cognate transcription factor and appear to regulate adjacent genes. It is known that these transposable elements have populated genomes throughout evolution. This work suggests that one evolutionary advantage that these transposable elements provide is to generate binding-site heterogeneity. Consistent with this, it was observed that more ancient repeat families have a greater proportion of response element motifs that are functional in transcription factor binding. This means that after, a wave of transpositional dispersal, there is subsequent evolutionary selection of those sites for functional binding, which may take millions of years to reach a population equilibrium.

For the organism to tolerate this rate and range of binding site generation (which by this mechanisms of transposable elements is mostly random), a compensatory mechanism needed to be adopted to minimize disruption. It is therefore fortuitous that the regulatory mechanism for transcription factors has loose constraints: these sites can regulate across long distances, 3' and 5' to the target gene, and often work in concert with other sites. That genetic diversity confers population robustness is akin to the advantage of the high genetic mutational rate of the human immunodeficiency virus noted by Kitano (2007). In higher organisms, genetic diversity allowing for a range of phenotypic responses to environmental challenges at the adult stage of the animal is also likely to be highly beneficial. However, the process of early development does not tolerate mutational loads. The compromise might have been provided by the generation of diversity in transcriptional regulation. It is possible that this diversity imparted by the repeat-associated binding sites generated through evolution confers that benefit without perturbing the transcriptional cassette required during the critical stages in development.

PART II. PROTEIN PHOSPHORYLATION NETWORKS

Phosphoproteins are of tremendous importance in eukaryotic cellular signaling and regulation. Protein kinases—proteins that catalyze the phosphorylation of other proteins—are the third most common family of proteins in the human genome, with 518 members (Manning et al., 2002). It has been estimated that 30% of human proteins are substrates for these kinases (Cohen, 2002), with resulting effects in nearly every aspect of biology. Protein kinases catalyze the transfer of a phosphate moiety from a molecule of ATP to a protein. Although other residues can be phosphorylated, the vast majority of stable protein phosphorylations in eukaryotes occur on the hydroxyl moiety of serine, threonine and tyrosine amino acid side chains. An analysis of several eukaryotic genomes suggested that 75% of eukaryotic kinases phosphorylate serine and threonine residues, while the remaining 25% are tyrosine-specific (Rubin et al., 2000).

Phosphorylation of proteins by protein kinases is regulated at several levels. First, the kinase and potential ligand must be co-localized in the cell. Secondly, the kinase activity is generally increased when the kinase is in an active structural conformation. The catalytic domains of most protein kinases share a similar active state conformation, but are often activated by a conformational change from a less similar inactive state, driven by a variety of mechanisms (Huse and Kuriyan, 2002). These mechanisms include phosphorylation of the kinase itself on a flexible "activation" loop (Johnson and Lewis, 2001), inter- or intramolecular allostery (Gonfloni et al., 2000) and release of an intramolecular substrate-competitive inhibitor sequence (Lei et al., 2000). It has been noted (Huse and Kuriyan, 2002) that the diversity among kinase domain inactive state conformations lends itself to the design of kinase inhibitors that function specifically by stabilization of the kinase-specific inactive states, as the anticancer drug, imatinib mesylate (Gleevec), does in the case of the Abl kinase (Zimmermann et al., 1997), rather than less specifically by obstructing the ATP binding site, which is relatively well conserved among kinases. Finally, kinase activity on a substrate is also influenced by recognition of the substrate amino acid sequence surrounding the phosphate receptor side chain (Kennelly and Krebs, 1991).

Phosphopeptide Databases

A number of general databases of protein information include information on phosphorylation as one component among many. UniProtKB/Swiss-Prot (Boutet et al., 2007) (http://www.uniprot.org/) is a manually curated knowledge base for proteins across a variety of species, concentrating on common model systems. Among the types of data catalogued are protein sequence, domain structure, known function, tissue and developmental expression data, interaction data and data on post-translational modifications, including phosphorylation. All data are referenced back to the literature from which they were drawn. Bulk download of proteins in particular categories, or those that match search criteria, is facilitated, simplifying novel analyses.

The Human Protein Reference Database (HPRD; Keshava Prasad et al., 2009) (http://www.hprd.org/) contains literature-curated information on human proteins, specific, when possible, at the level of individual isoforms. HPRD focuses on protein–protein interactions and post-translational modifications. Unlike UniProt, HPRD accepts direct input by users of new information, through an interface at the Human Proteinpedia (http://www.humanproteinpedia.org/). This information must be experimentally derived, and is presented to users of HPRD on the same webpage as, but distinctly from, data curated by HPRD itself, along with attribution to the scientist who added the data.

Other databases exist specifically to catalog known instances of protein phosphorylation. Phospho.ELM (Diella et al., 2008) (http://phospho.elm.eu.org) is a manually curated database of known phosphorylation sites on eukaryotic proteins. Each phosphorylated site in a phosphoprotein is tied to the original literature.

When known, the site is associated with the kinase or kinases that phosphorylate it, and with phosphopeptide binding domains that interact with it. A notation indicates whether the site has been identified in a low- or high-throughput experiment, or both. Data are accepted from all metazoan species, but largely consist of mouse and human phosphoproteins. The entire Phospho.ELM dataset is available for download, making it extremely useful for novel batch analyses.

PhosphoSitePlus (http://www.phosphosite.org/), like Phospho.ELM, is a curated database of phosphorylation sites. PhosphoSitePlus explicitly tracks homology among phosphorylated proteins in different species, showing sites phosphorylated in each species for any given query. Nonetheless, the focus of PhosphoSitePlus is on mouse and human phosphorylations. PhosphoSitePlus is maintained by Cell Signaling Technologies, a private company. When known, the cellular functions of individual phosphorylations are noted, and links are provided to information on antibodies that recognize phosphorylation sites. The full dataset underlying PhosphoSitePlus is not freely available, although academic users can gain access to the portion of the data that is derived from the literature.

PHOSIDA (Gnad et al., 2007) (http://www.phosida.com/) contains data from UniProtKB/Swiss-Prot, in addition to data derived in the research group of Matthias Mann, where PHOSIDA is maintained. In addition, data from other selected publications are sometimes included in PHOSIDA. Because the data in PHOSIDA are maintained in large part by the researchers who generated the data, PHOSIDA includes specialized information specific to the studies in which the phosphorylated sites were identified. In human phosphoproteins, this information includes time dynamics downstream of epidermal growth factor (EGF) stimulation (Olsen et al., 2006) and cell-cycle dynamics (Daub et al., 2008). PHOSIDA also includes a

TABLE 4.1 URLs for Selected On-line Protein Phosphorylation Resources

UniProtKB/Swiss-Prot	http://www.uniprot.org/
Human Protein Reference Database (HPRD)	http://www.hprd.org/
Human Proteinpedia	http://www.humanproteinpedia.org/
Phospho.ELM	http://phospho.elm.eu.org/
PhosphoSitePlus	http://www.phosphosite.org/
PHOSIDA	http://www.phosida.com/
ELM	http://elm.eu.org/
PROSITE	http://ca.expasy.org/prosite/
Scansite	http://scansite.mit.edu/
NetworKIN	http://networkin.info/
NetPhorest	http://netphorest.info/
KinasePhos 2.0	http://kinasephos2.mbc.nctu.edu.tw/
PredPhospho	http://pred.ngri.re.kr/PredPhospho.htm/
NetPhosK	http://www.cbs.dtu.dk/services/NetPhosK/
PPSP	http://bioinformatics.lcd-ustc.org/PPSP/
MetaPredPS	http://metapred.umn.edu/MetaPredPS/

tool to predict sites of protein phosphorylation on the basis of conservation of serine, threonine and tyrosine sites across species.

Table 4.1 lists Internet resources related to protein phosphorylation and kinase–substrate connections.

Kinase–Substrate Connections

In general, the experimental demonstration that a particular protein kinase phosphorylates a particular protein substrate is onerous. There are three generally accepted requirements (Cohen, 1997). First, the kinase must be capable of phosphorylating the putative substrate *in vitro* with physiologically relevant K_m and V_{max}. Secondly, the substrate must be phosphorylated *in vivo* at the same amino acid side chain in response to a signal that activates the protein kinase. Finally, as there are kinases that share both activating signal and substrate specificity, the substrate should be shown not to be phosphorylated when the kinase of interest is specifically inactivated, whether chemically, genetically or at the transcriptional or translational level. Because of the difficulty of such a characterization, experimental and theoretical tools have been developed for generating hypotheses connecting phosphoproteins and kinases.

There are two families of techniques for identifying potential downstream products of an individual kinase. The first is direct: individual proteins are identified that are phosphorylated, generally *in vitro*, as a response to the activity of a kinase of interest. The laboratory of Kevan Shokat has made notable advances in this area, designing variant kinases that accept as a phosphate donor a radiolabeled analog of ATP that does not interact with wild-type kinases (Liu et al., 1998). The analog is added to cell lysates, and radiolabeled proteins, putatively phosphorylated by the variant kinase, are subsequently identified. Other "direct" approaches include affinity reagents such as phosphomotif antibodies that can be used, in some cases, to purify phosphorylated peptides and proteins (Rush et al., 2005; Ting et al., 2001) for identification. A number of other techniques exist for querying the phosphorylation state of the proteome more globally that can be used to generate hypothetical kinase–substrate relationships (de Graauw et al., 2006) for further testing, including 2-dimensional gel electrophoresis and mass spectroscopy. Conversely, however, to date there is no direct method of identifying the kinase responsible for a phosphorylation of interest from the entire kinome without some prior hypothesis. Such a hypothesis can be generated on the basis of knowledge of which kinases are active under specific conditions and in the cellular compartment in which the site of interest is phosphorylated, and of knowledge of which kinases have motif specificity compatible with the phosphorylated sequence and which antagonists inhibit the phosphorylation of interest (Obenauer et al., 2003; Yaffe et al., 2001).

The second set of techniques is more indirect. Characterizations of the substrate specificities of the kinases are generated on the basis of the amino acid sequence, and those characterizations are used to search a protein sequence database to generate hypotheses connecting substrates and kinases of interest. Phosphorylation motifs have been determined by peptide library screening (Songyang and Cantley, 1998; Yaffe et al., 2001), in which a pool of degenerate peptides containing a fixed—or "oriented"—serine, threonine or tyrosine is exposed to a kinase, and the phosphorylated subset of the pool is purified by chromatography and batch sequenced to provide a consensus sequence. In a modification of this technique, libraries of degenerate phosphopeptides have been spotted on membranes, and exposed to a kinase of interest and radiolabeled ATP (Hutti et al., 2004). The spotting allows for parallelization; libraries can be searched with every amino acid fixed at every position relative to the fixed phosphate acceptor residue in a high-throughput manner. In an alternative approach, peptide libraries have been immobilized on beads, exposed to a kinase and then sorted by fluorescence-activated cell sorting (FACS) after incubation with a phosphospecific fluorophore (Gast et al., 1999). Libraries containing fusions of peptides to the mRNAs that encode them have also been screened by immunoprecipitation with a phosphospecific antibody, followed by analysis on a cDNA microarray (Cujec et al., 2002). Once the phosphorylation motif for a particular kinase is determined, database techniques can be applied to scan the set of known protein sequences for matches, which can all be considered for further testing as putative kinase targets. It is possible to discover a great number of leads for experimental validation quickly in this manner, although the identification of motif sequences by a database search provides no direct experimental evidence for the phosphorylation of target proteins. Moreover, it is important to note that the majority of eukaryotic kinases do not have a known substrate amino acid sequence motif.

One class of database tools for connecting kinases to putative substrates consists of maintained lists of fairly simple expressions of linear amino acid sequence motifs. HPRD, for example, compiles a list of literature-reported motifs, sometimes many per kinase, which themselves come from library screens or from expert annotation for the most part (Keshava Prasad et al., 2009). It is important to note that such specific motifs may be neither necessary nor sufficient for kinase–substrate interaction. Likewise, ELM (http://elm.eu.org/), which stands for Eukaryotic Linear Motif, catalogs a list of linear motifs in biology, not limited to phosphorylation (Puntervoll et al., 2003). These motifs are maintained as regular expressions, a type of representation of character strings common in computer science. This makes it trivial to copy a motif directly from ELM in a computer- and human-readable format. Motifs in ELM are also associated with filters on cellular localization, protein domain structure and taxonomy with which they are compatible. These serve to reduce the number of false-positive results associated with amino acid sequence motifs. PROSITE (http://ca.expasy.org/prosite/) is a third site that maintains sets rules and patterns for short amino acid sequence motifs indicative of the existence of protein domains, families and functional sites (Hulo et al., 2006). Phosphorylation motifs make up a very small fraction of the available patterns.

A second class of tools for identifying putative substrates of kinases relies on more complicated models of kinase–substrate preference. One of the earliest of these, Scansite (Yaffe et al., 2001) (http://scansite.mit.edu/) converts the results of kinase-specific peptide library screens to position-specific scoring matrices. These matrices mathematically encode the fitness of any given peptide sequence for phosphorylation by a kinase *in vitro*, subject to an assumption of interpositional independence within the putative substrate. This fitness measure can be converted to a statistical significance value by ranking it among all potential sites in the human proteome.

NetworKIN (Linding et al., 2007, 2008) (http://networkin.info/) uses Scansite to suggest which families of kinase would be most likely to phosphorylate a given substrate. Because kinases in the same family frequently phosphorylate similar amino acid sequences, the selection of which kinase within a family is most likely to phosphorylate the substrate in question is further informed by the context of the protein interaction network of the substrate. The protein–protein interaction database STRING (Jensen et al., 2009) is used to build a probabilistic Bayesian framework for selecting the kinase within a family nearest to the substrate of interest. The authors found that over 60% of the capability to identify a kinase–substrate relationship comes from network context, rather than information on sequence motifs.

NetPhorest (Miller et al., 2008) (http://netphorest.info) uses both position-specific scoring matrices and more complicated sequence models trained using artificial neural networks on known kinase substrates. All models are simultaneously examined at various levels of the phylogeny of known kinases, and a set of models are chosen which globally do an optimal job of connecting kinases and substrates together. The resulting atlas contains substrate sequence models for 179 protein kinases.

Prediction of kinase–substrate interactions is a rich field of research, and many other online resources exist that use a wide variety of machine learning and computational classification techniques. KinasePhos 2.0 (Wong et al., 2007) (http://kinasephos2.mbc.nctu.edu.tw/)

and PredPhospho (Kim et al., 2004) (http://pred.ngri.re.kr/PredPhospho.htm) use support vector machines to classify likely substrates of individual kinases. NetPhosK (Blom et al., 2004) (http://www.cbs.dtu.dk/services/NetPhosK/) utilizes neural networks; PPSP (Xue et al., 2006) (http://bioinformatics.lcd-ustc.org/PPSP/) instead uses Bayesian decision theory. More recently, MetaPredPS (Wan et al., 2008) (http://metapred.umn.edu/MetaPredPS/) has been devised to accumulate the data from a number of previously existing kinase–substrate prediction resources and perform a weighted voting meta-analysis which outperforms all of the input predictors.

In-vivo Functions of Protein Phosphorylation

There are a number of mechanisms by which the phosphorylation of a protein can serve to propagate a signal to further biological effect.

Induction of Conformational Change

The steric bulk and strong anionic charge of the phosphate ion can prompt a conformational change in a peptide upon phosphorylation. The first known example of conformational change as the effect mechanism of phosphorylation was in the protein, glycogen phosphorylase (Johnson, 1992). Phosphorylation of glycogen phosphorylase at residue serine 14 prompts a local conformational rearrangement that leads to large-scale allosteric shift of both the monomeric and multimeric protein structure, resulting in the activation of the enzyme. The activities of many protein kinases, including insulin receptor kinase (IRK) (Hubbard et al., 1994) and the mitogen-activated protein kinases (MAPKs) ERK2 (Canagarajah et al., 1997) and p38 (Derijard et al., 1995) are also regulated by a phosphorylation-dependent conformational change in the kinase activation loop, again resulting in a conformational change that results in enzyme activation.

Generation of a Docking Site for a Phosphopeptide Binding Domain

Rather than a conformational change, it is possible for protein phosphorylation to affect protein function by the creation of a binding site for a phosphopeptide binding domain (Yaffe, 2002; Yaffe and Elia, 2001). Generally,

TABLE 4.2 Phosphopeptide Binding Domains and Their Specificities

Domain	Example Protein	Specificity	References
SH2	Src	**pY**-E-E-I	Songyang et al. (1993)
PTB	SHC	N-P-x-**pY**	Songyang et al. (1995)
14-3-3	14-3-3 ζ	R-(S/F/W/Y)-X-(**pS/pT**)-X-P or R-X-(S/F/W/Y)-X-(**pS/pT**)-X-P	Yaffe et al. (1997)
Group IV WW	Pin1	(**pS/pT**)-P	Lu et al. (1999)
FHA	Rad53 FHA1	**pT**-X-X-D	Durocher et al. (2000)
WD40	β-TrCP	D-**pS**-G-X-X-**pS**	Winston et al. (1999)
MH2	Smad2	S-**pS**-M-**pS**-COOH	Wu et al. (2001)
Polo-box	Plk1	S-(**pS/pT**)-P	Elia et al. (2003b)
BRCT	BRCA1	(**pS/pT**)-X-X-(F/Y)	Manke et al. (2003)

phosphopeptide binding domains have specificity for a phosphorylated amino acid, in addition to at least partial specificity for some amino acids in a short sequence motif surrounding the phosphorylated residue (Table 4.2). Although the various known phosphopeptide binding domains do not share much structural similarity, there are a number of physicochemical properties general to phosphopeptide binding sites (Joughin et al., 2005).

A number of roles have been discovered for phosphopeptide-binding domains in a range of important biological processes, from apoptosis to cell-cycle control and differentiation. Some of the isoforms of the phosphopeptide binding protein 14-3-3 exert a tumor-suppressing function in the DNA damage pathway by isolating the pro-mitotic phosphatase, Cdc25, in the cytosol when Cdc25 has been phosphorylated by the DNA damage kinase, Chk1 (Kumagai and Dunphy, 1999). The S. cerevisiae protein, Ess1, the budding yeast homologue of Pin1, contains a WW domain that exerts regulatory effects in transcription by phosphodependently binding the C-terminal domain of RNA pol II. A second, catalytic, proline isomerase domain of Ess1 then isomerizes the bound peptide (Morris et al., 1999). The Polo-box domain of the Plk family of kinases, which regulate aspects of mitosis and cytokinesis, is required for protein localization, and probably for substrate targeting also, by binding to peptides containing the motif "S-(pS/pT)-P" (Elia et al., 2003b). A defect in the wild-type ability of the BRCA1 BRCT domain to bind phosphopeptides predisposes women to breast and ovarian cancer (Yu et al., 2003). BRCA1 mutations linked to inherited cancer-related phenotypes are enriched in the BRCT domains of the protein.

In conjunction with kinases and phosphatases with which they have fully or partially overlapping ligand specificities, phosphopeptide binding domains are capable of exerting combinatorial control over cell signaling by temporally and spatially controlling the assembly and disassembly of signaling complexes. Phosphopeptide binding domains that bind some, but not all, of the substrates of particular kinases allow for branching within signaling pathways.

Identification of the Substrates of a Phosphopeptide Binding Domain

The process of identifying the ligands of a phosphopeptide binding domain is quite similar to the identification of kinase substrates. Targets can be identified directly, by affinity purification using as bait the domain of interest (Pozuelo Rubio et al., 2004). Oriented peptide library screening has been used extremely successfully as a more indirect technique, first to identify in batch all peptides from a random library that bind to a domain of interest (Yaffe and Cantley, 2000), and then to use the consensus profile to predict in-vivo ligands (Yaffe et al., 2001). Recent work in the laboratory of Gavin MacBeath has focused on printing large numbers of phosphopeptide binding domains on protein arrays and analyzing binding with phosphopeptides of interest in a large-scale, multiplexed way (Gordus et al., 2009; Jones et al., 2006; Kaushansky et al., 2008).

Identifying Phosphopeptide Binding Domains Specific for a Site of Interest

Two of the most recently described phosphopeptide binding domains, the Polo-box domain and the BRCT domain, were identified using a proteomic screen for proteins that bind to a target peptide library phosphospecifically (Elia et al., 2003a; Manke et al., 2003). Proteins were translated in vitro in pools, and pools were tested for binding to phosphorylated and non-phosphorylated peptide libraries. Members of pools that showed specificity were then searched for specific clones responsible for the activity. The Plk1 Polo-box was identified in a search for proteins specific to the motif "pS/pT-P" generated by mitotic kinases. The WW domain of Pin1, known to share that specificity, was also re-identified. The BRCT domains of BRCA1 and PTIP were identified in an equivalent screen for domains that bound the motif "pS/pT-Q," generated by the DNA damage kinases. Interestingly, although in the optimal motif for the BRCT domain, a phenylalanine at the pS/pT + 3 position seems to be much more important than a pS/pT + 1 glutamine. In both cases, the experimental design was driven by a desire to understand the downstream regulation prompted by the activity of a particular kinase family; however, neither domain had specificity identical to that of the targeted kinase. Kinases and phosphopeptide binding domains, having incompletely overlapping specificity, are able to exert a combinatorial control in signaling.

Software Tools Connecting Phosphopeptide Binding Domains and Substrates

Because phosphopeptide binding domains, like kinases, are somewhat specific for amino acid sequence motifs on their substrate peptides, many of the tools for developing hypotheses connecting kinases and their substrates have also been used here. HPRD and ELM maintain curated annotations of phosphopeptide binding domain substrate motifs. Scansite and NetPhorest both predict binding domain–substrate interactions alongside those of kinases.

Phosphorylation-mediated Disruption of Sequence-specific Effects

In some cases, the effect of phosphorylation is to disrupt some other sequence-mediated function. It has been shown, for example, that phosphorylation of 14-3-3 ζ by MAPK-activated protein kinase 2 impairs the ability of 14-3-3 ζ to dimerize (Powell et al., 2003). Phosphorylation of Cdc25C at serine-214 prevents phosphorylation at serine-216, in turn preventing the binding and cytosolic sequestration of Cdc25C by 14-3-3 (Bulavin et al., 2003). Phosphorylation of the Forkhead transcription factor AFX at serine-193 in the middle of a nuclear localization sequence motif results in an increase in cytosolic AFX, and a decrease in AFX transcriptional activity (Brownawell et al., 2001). Because phosphorylation results in a significant change in the steric and electrostatic properties of any local peptide sequence, it is quite easy to imagine the direct disruption of nearly any non-phosphorylated sequence-motif-mediated effect by phosphorylation. Function can also be altered indirectly, through binding a phosphopeptide binding domain. 14-3-3 binds to the transcription factor FKHRL1, and in so doing exposes on FKHRL1 a nuclear export sequence, prompting it to leave the nucleus (Brunet et al., 2002).

Protein Phosphatases

Protein phosphorylations are removed by the action of protein phosphatases, providing the aspect of reversibility to phosphoregulation. Protein phosphatases are fewer in number than protein kinases, and demonstrate a much broader specificity *in vitro* (Rubin et al., 2000). *In vivo*, regulation and targeting of phosphatases is handled, in at least some cases (including the protein phosphatase 1 family of serine/threonine phosphatase), by the complexing of phosphatase with other proteins to form a number of separate holoenzymes (Bollen, 2001; Cohen, 2002). In contrast, many protein tyrosine phosphatases are found in tandem with other protein domains that seem to have the capacity for generating target specificity through localization or direct binding through SH2 and PTB domains (Alonso et al., 2004). Interestingly, this modular multidomain structure is similar to that found in protein tyrosine kinases. Unlike serine/threonine phosphatases, there are similar numbers of tyrosine kinases and phosphatases (Manning et al., 2002), indicating that perhaps, in the case of phosphotyrosine regulation, there is more mechanism shared between kinases and phosphatases.

Protein Networks

Individual protein–protein interactions, whether structural or enzymatic, combine together to form signaling networks. Signaling networks are the mechanisms by which stimuli are converted to a cellular or systemic response. In this section, we will focus on networks comprised only of proteins; in a later section, we will discuss protein–genetic interactions, which represent the interface between signaling and genetic networks.

Protein interaction networks are topologically described as undirected node-edge graphs in which nodes represent proteins and undirected edges represent the occurrence of binding between proteins (Pieroni et al., 2008). Signal transfer, however, requires not only interaction among proteins, but also that an actual transfer of information between the proteins takes place, prompting a functional change in the state of the protein. Such a state change might take the form of a post-translational modification such as phosphorylation, or a protein translocation into a different cellular compartment. This causal information leads to a second type of network, protein signaling networks, that are represented as directed node-edge graphs wherein the nodes represent proteins in a specific or partially specified signaling state, and the edges represent the causal effects that lead to these modifications and state changes.

Protein Interaction Networks

While the most trustworthy protein–protein interactions are discovered through targeted, low-throughput study, there are three major classes of high-throughput experiment that reveal large numbers of protein–protein interactions. In the first, tandem affinity purification-mass spectroscopy, a protein of interest is labeled with an affinity tag and purified from a cell lysate. Putative interactors may remain associated with the labeled protein, and can then be identified by mass spectroscopy (Ewing et al., 2007; Kocher and Superti-Furga, 2007). In the second approach, the two-hybrid assay, pairs of proteins are analyzed in a strain of yeast engineered to demonstrate a genetic regulatory response if the two proteins are capable of interacting (Ito et al., 2002; Parrish et al., 2006). While the two-hybrid approach is best suited to identifying binary interactions, the affinity purification approach identifies stably associated groups of proteins without providing definitive evidence of direct interactions. An additional relevant approach relies on protein arrays (MacBeath and Schreiber, 2000; Zhu et al., 2001). Individual proteins of interest are densely spotted on slides, and incubated with a labeled potential interactor. Quantification of the label reflects the level of interaction between the two binding partners.

An alternative approach to the construction of protein interaction networks is by curation of existing data from the available literature. The number of databases that do so is quite large, with many commonalities, but also different strengths and weaknesses. A detailed review of the databases available is beyond the scope of this review, but we can recommend Pathguide (Bader et al., 2006) (http://www.pathguide.org), a compendium of web-accessible protein network databases, as a starting point for beginners in the area. Although providing an invaluable resource, the quality of literature-curated protein interaction networks is lower than might be expected, perhaps because of the error-prone process of the curation of literature (Cusick et al., 2009). An additional resource worth special mention is the database, STRING (Jensen et al., 2009) (http://string.embl.de/). STRING contains, in addition to curated interactions, other interactions inferred from a combination of genomic, co-expression and literature data, among other types. The probability of interaction between pairs of individual proteins is evaluated in a Bayesian framework, from the presence or absence of supporting data of all types.

Protein Signaling Networks

The amount of data on protein signaling networks is far less extensive than that on interaction networks, but has been increasing rapidly, thanks to novel technical developments that allow researchers to generate large proteomic and phosphoproteomic datasets. These methods rely on different technologies such on quantitative mass spectrometry (Kumar, Wolf-Yadlin, et al., 2005, 2007), protein arrays (Jones et al., 2006), bead-based sandwich enzyme-linked immunosorbent assay methods (Pelech, 2004) and flow cytometry (Hale and Nolan, 2006). The data are used to reverse-engineer the underlying signaling network using tools such as differential equations (Nelander et al., 2008) and Bayesian networks (Sachs et al., 2005). As with protein interaction networks, the myriad available web databases of protein signaling interactions are well reviewed by Pathguide (http://www.pathguide.org/).

Knowledge Integration for Protein Networks

As described above, the number of databases with information on protein interaction and signaling networks is enormous. As of February 2009, Pathguide contained about 300 web-accessible biological pathway and network databases. There are databases that aim to provide the same type of information (e.g. hand-curated human protein interaction information), but the content varies in quality and completeness, as well as in format and level of interaction with the user (Adriaens et al., 2008). Therefore, creating a high-quality network pertinent to a biological process of interest still requires a time-consuming, manual curation work flow to combine difference sources. Several efforts are under way to help automate this process. Biological Pathway Exchange (BioPAX; http://www.biopax.org/) is a standard exchange format for biological pathways (Luciano and Stevens, 2007). It has a dedicated ontology, and provides a common format, vocabulary and conceptual framework for pathway information, allowing integration and query of data from several sources. In addition, databases supporting BioPAX format can be integrated into a common repository, Pathway Commons (http://www.pathwaycommons.org). Pathway Commons allows users to query information across these databases, and also to filter the information depending on the nature of the source (for example, if one is interested only in hand-curated data). Currently, Pathway Commons integrates information from databases describing both protein interaction networks and protein signaling networks.

Obviously, protein interaction networks and protein signaling networks are closely related. In a way, the former represent the skeleton on which the latter operate. A kinase, for example, must bind transiently to its substrate, and possibly to other proteins required to regulate the process, in order to phosphorylate it. Furthermore, the same event may be present in both interaction and signaling networks: binding of one protein to another might enhance or inhibit the activity of one of the proteins. Therefore, a simple binding event can be a signaling-relevant edge in a protein signaling network. One effort to bridge these two worlds is provided by CellCircuits (Mak et al., 2007) (http://www.cellcircuits.org), an explicit attempt to build a repository of signaling pathway models derived from protein interaction data.

Table 4.3 lists some of the available databases giving information on protein interaction and signaling networks.

Analysis of Protein Interaction and Signaling Networks

There exist several tools to analyze both protein interaction and protein signaling networks. Arguably, the most popular software is Cytoscape (Cline et al., 2007). The focus of Cytoscape is to visualize networks and to integrate

TABLE 4.3 URLs for Selected On-line Protein Interaction and Signaling Network Resources

Pathguide	http://www.pathguide.org/
STRING	http://string.embl.de/
BioPAX	http://www.biopax.org/
Pathway Commons	http://www.pathwaycommons.org/
CellCircuits	http://www.cellcircuits.org/
Cytoscape	http://www.cytoscape.org/
NeAT	http://rsat.ulb.ac.be/rsat/index_neat.html/
Ingenuity Pathway Analysis	http://www.ingenuity.com/
Pathway Studio	http://www.ariadnegenomics.com/products/pathway-studio/
VisANT	http://visant.bu.edu/
Pajek	http://vlado.fmf.uni-lj.si/pub/networks/pajek/
SNAVI	http://code.google.com/p/snavi/
CellNetAnalyzer	http://www.mpi-magdeburg.mpg.de/projects/cna/cna.html
GinSim	http://gin.univ-mrs.fr/
Pathway Logic	http://pl.csl.sri.com/

them with external data such as gene expression profiles. In this manner, the pathway visualization provides context, acting as a skeleton for the added external data. In addition, there are about 50 plug-ins for Cytoscape, generated by an active community of developers, which allow users to perform many analyses such as graph-based studies, network inference, functional enrichment studies and more.

Another toolkit, Network Analysis Tools (NeAT), provides web-based access to a collection of modular tools for the analysis of networks. The tools comprising NeAT have less sophisticated visualization routines than Cytoscape, but provide powerful clustering methods, are designed to cope with large datasets and are able to analyze networks that are either stored in various databases (protein interactions, regulation and metabolism) or obtained from high-throughput experiments (two-hybrid, mass-spectrometry and microarrays). They also provide predefined analysis work flows that facilitate the study of networks. NeAT tools can be used independently as a web service, or easily integrated with other available resources (Brohee et al., 2008).

One popular commercial tools-suite is Ingenuity Pathways Analysis (IPA; http://www.ingenuity.com/), which combines both hand-curated protein signaling pathways and protein interactions automatically mined from the literature with the ability to analyze high-throughput experimental data. Another commercial suite is Pathway Studio (Nikitin et al., 2003) (http://www.ariadnegenomics.com/products/pathway-studio/) from Ariadne Genomics, that also allows the user to mine literature and perform gene expression analysis.

Other tools for analyzing protein networks include VisANT (Hu et al., 2008) (http://visant.bu.edu/), Pajek (Batagelj and Mrvar, 2002) (http://vlado.fmf.uni-lj.si/pub/networks/pajek/) and SNAVI (Ma'ayan et al., 2009) (http://code.google.com/p/snavi/), to name but a few.

Topological Analysis

Many analyses of protein interaction networks study different graph-based properties such as scale-free features (Barabasi and Oltvai, 2004), identification of modules (Rives and Galitski, 2003) and identification of recurrent motifs (Alon, 2007). Many of the methods applicable to topological analysis of genetic networks (see Principles of Transcriptional Network Analysis: Topological Analysis, in Part I) also apply to protein interaction network topology. Recently, with the advent of human interactomes (Rual et al., 2005), applications to human disease have begun to appear (Ideker and Sharan, 2008; Russell and Aloy, 2008). One clearly important application is the study of the network properties of disease-related genes: for example, oncogenes seem to be highly connected nodes in protein interaction networks (Jonsson and Bates, 2006). Other studies are attempts to identify novel genes related to a disease of interest on the basis of the hypothesis that proteins that are neighbors in interaction networks may be related to the same diseases. For example, new disease genes were predicted from genetically mapped disease loci without identified disease genes, on the basis of their proximity, in protein interaction networks, to genes known to be related to a certain disease (Oti et al., 2006).

Protein interaction data can also be combined with other information to construct a disease-relevant subnetwork. For example, Pujana and colleagues (2007) constructed a network around four oncogenes known to be associated with breast cancer (*BRCA1*, *BRCA2*, *ATM* and *CHEK2*), using co-expression data with genetic and protein interactions, in addition to phenotypic profiling. Looking at network neighbors of these four genes, they were able to identify a gene, *HMMR*, as being strongly functionally associated with the oncogene, *BRCA1*. The *HMMR* locus was then found to be associated with a greater risk of breast cancer. An additional application is the development of improved means to classify cancers according to their transcriptional signatures, by using as markers the combined transcriptional signature of genes present in disease-relevant subnetworks of protein interaction networks as markers (Chuang et al., 2007; Mani et al., 2008), as described in Transcriptional Regulation on a Genomic Scale in Medicine: Application to Cancer Patient Prognosis, in Part I. A final interesting and novel application is the use of protein–protein interaction data to help determine the structure of macromolecular assemblies. The research group of Andrej Sali developed a method to integrate a number of biophysical and bioinformatic data types, including interaction data based on affinity purification, to constrain and approximate the structure of large macromolecular assemblies (Alber et al., 2007).

Protein signaling networks allow researchers to analyze certain properties of signal transfer, as exemplified by the findings of Ma'ayan and colleagues (2005), who studied ligand-induced signal flow through a large, hand-curated signaling network in neurons. However, even protein signaling networks do not completely capture the logic of cellular biochemistry, and are thus not suited to perform functional studies. They are useful as descriptive means, but not detailed enough to construct predictive models; the existence of a structural or enzymatic interaction between proteins does not contain information on kinetics or on conditions necessary and sufficient for the interaction to occur.

Computational Modeling

Other chapters in this volume will provide extensive depth and detail on computational modeling of cell signaling networks, so we will offer only a superficial sketch here to end our chapter. Figure 4.9 illustrates the spectrum of computational modeling approaches that have been brought to bear on protein signaling network problems (Ideker and Lauffenburger, 2003). This spectrum ranges from highly abstracted approaches for problems in which little prior knowledge concerning the network topology—or even the key components—exists, to highly specified approaches for problems in which there is substantial prior knowledge concerning the network topology and perhaps even interaction mechanisms among key components. The approach likely to be most productive for a given problem depends heavily on the biological question being asked and the kind of data available for modeling.

The most commonly employed approach relies on differential equations describing the underlying biochemical and biophysical interactions among components believed to be important in the network operation (Aldridge et al., 2006). An important application of differential equation models is to study the emergence of dynamic and signal-transfer properties not present when studying individual proteins

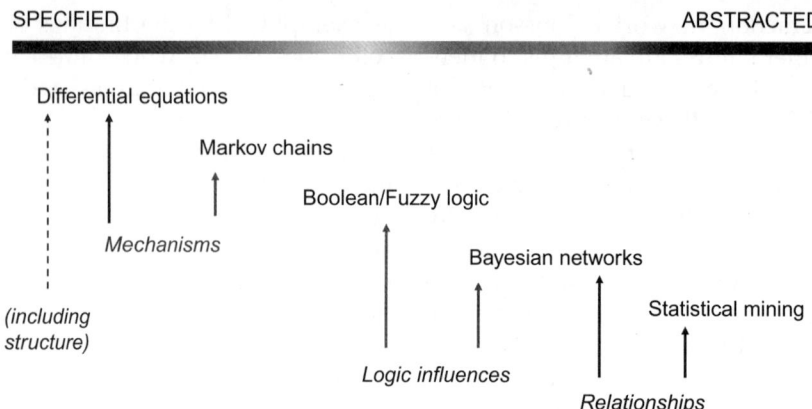

FIGURE 4.9 The Spectrum of Computational Modeling Approaches Applied to Signaling Networks.
This spectrum ranges from strategies that deal with concrete output data for systems with substantial prior knowledge of the connections, to highly abstracted approaches in systems in which little prior knowledge of the connections or even the key components exists.

and local interactions alone (Bhalla and Iyengar, 1999). One of the largest models of this sort was recently published by Chen and colleagues (2009). They constructed a model comprised of 28 proteins, describing the family of ErbB receptors and their downstream pathways leading to the activation of the phosphatidyl inositol 3-kinase (PI3K)/AKT and the Raf/MAPK kinase (MEK)/extracellular-signal-regulated kinase (ERK) MAPK cascades. The model extends a previous model by Schoeberl et al. (2002) describing the activation of ERK triggered by the ErbB ligand, EGF. The model uncovered emergent high-level properties of the system, such as an extreme sensitivity of the receptors to ligand concentration as a result of the ability of both MAPK and PI3K cascades to amplify signals in a non-linear manner. Remarkably, the behavior of each cascade is very different when considered in isolation, underscoring the importance of studying signal transfer in the correct cellular context and from a system-wide perspective.

These differential equation models are powerful tools of analysis, but are not feasible for networks of more than a few dozen proteins—far from the hundreds that a protein signaling network can comprise. For modeling of large protein signaling networks, simpler formalism can be used. A next step in the spectrum represents the logic of influences among components in the network. One relatively simple formalism within this category is a Boolean logic description, wherein proteins are either active (ON) or inactive (OFF), and are connected by logic gates describing their causality. This approach has proven feasible and useful for large signaling networks (Saez-Rodriguez et al., 2007). Recently, a Fuzzy logic extension of this approach has been provided, allowing continuous characterization of network states, rather than the discretized characterization of the Boolean approach, without adding a substantial degree of interpretation or computational cost (Aldridge et al., 2009). A significantly more complex formalism, with respect to both interpretation and computational effort, is represented by Bayesian networks, which permit inference of highly non-intuitive dependencies of "child" nodes on "parent" nodes. This kind of algorithm works best for large numbers of replicates or conditions for which measurement of the network node activities are made, and has been applied to a small number of cell signaling network problems in recent years (Sachs et al.,

2005, 2009; Woolf et al., 2005). At the extreme of abstracted methods, principal components analysis (PCA) and partial least-squares regression (PLSR) algorithms yield statistical relationships, among signals and between signals and cell behavioral responses, respectively, across diverse conditions. These methods have been applied productively toward elucidation of key signal combinations associated with cell treatment conditions and phenotypic behaviors (Janes et al., 2005; Kemp et al., 2007; Miller-Jensen et al., 2007).

Formal software tools exist for computational modeling of cell signaling (and gene regulatory) networks. For Boolean logic models, there are CellNetAnalyzer (Klamt et al., 2007) (http://www.mpi-magdeburg.mpg.de/projects/cna/cna.html) and GinSim (Gonzalez et al., 2006) (http://gin.univ-mrs.fr/). Other tools, such as Pathway Logic (Talcott et al., 2004) (http://pl.csl.sri.com/), rely on more general and abstract languages inspired in computer science, such as pi-calculus, rewriting logic, Petri nets and others. There also can be found a number of software packages for biophysical/biochemical differential equation modeling (Alves et al., 2006).

Epidermal Growth Factor Receptor as a Model for Protein Signaling Networks

The family of EGFRs and associated ligands, known as the ErbB family, represents an excellent example for our general discussion; the summary following is largely derived from a recent review (Lazzara and Lauffenburger, 2009). The ErbB family is appreciated as a highly appropriate application for the systems biology paradigm (Wiley et al., 2003). Oda and co-workers (2005) have delineated a "comprehensive pathway map," derived from 242 earlier publications. This map comprises 322 entities involved in 211 interactions among 122 particular protein components. These proteins include the four Erb family receptors: ErbB1 (EGFR), ErbB2, ErbB3 and ErbB4; they also include the contemporaneously identified 14 ErbB family ligands, which bind, with various selectivities and affinities, to the receptors (with the exception of ErbB2, which does not bind ligand). Downstream of ligand–receptor couplings and upstream of their ultimately regulated processes (transcriptional, metabolic and cytoskeletal), 32 kinases, 3 ion channels, 22 adapters and 6 G-protein subunits were configured into what the authors termed a "bow-tie" structure.

The earliest set of publications offering mathematical models representing generation of specific downstream pathway signals resulting from ErbB receptor–ligand interactions were by Kholodenko et al. (1999), Haugh et al. (2000) and Schoeberl et al. (2002). Each of these used mass-action kinetic ordinary differential equation (ODE) models, comprising a relatively small number of molecular species. Kholodenko's group addressed activation of the Shc/Grb2 and the phospholipase C (PLC)γ pathways during the initial 2 minutes following stimulation with EGF at low and high concentrations; Haugh and colleagues analyzed PLCγ-mediated hydrolysis of phosphatidylinositol bisphosphate during a 30-minute period following stimulation with either EGF or transforming growth factor-α (TGFα) across a range of dose concentrations; Schoeberl and co-workers focused on activation of ERK during a 1-hour period following EGF stimulation at low and high concentrations. In all these models, attention was restricted to signals generated by EGFR–EGFR homodimers. In each of these efforts, the most notable features were the highly transient nature of downstream pathway activities and the non-linear relationships between the degree of EGFR activation (characterized by level of phosphorylation) and the degree of downstream pathway activation.

Major advances beyond this early body of literature have come from three aspects of expansion of this kind of ODE modeling approach. One aspect is inclusion of other ErbB receptor family members, especially ErbB2 and ErbB3 (relatively little is still known about ErbB4), and

EGF family ligands that induce homodimeric and heterodimeric interactions among them. A second aspect is simultaneous incorporation of several downstream pathways within a given model. Birtwistle et al. (2007) demonstrated both of these aspects, building on the original Kholodenko framework by including the Ras/Raf/MEK/ERK and PI3K/AKT pathways as extensions of the receptor-proximal Shc/Grb2 activation events. As noted above, the most recent and largest model of this kind was recently published by Chen et al. (2009). They constructed a model comprised of 28 proteins, describing the family of ErbB receptors and their downstream pathways leading to the activation of the PI3K/AKT and the Raf/MEK/ERK MAPK cascades. A third aspect of advance has been more explicit investigation of the effects of receptor–ligand trafficking processes on downstream signaling dynamics. The importance of this facet has become clear as investigators have broadened their attention to longer time-periods of signaling network activity. Resat et al. (2003) developed a novel Monte Carlo stochastic simulation of EGFR homodimer activity and induction of downstream signals, with emphasis on the effects of endocytic internalization and pH-sensitive endosomal ligand–receptor complex dissociation. They spliced Kholodenko and colleagues' (1999) original model for Shc/Grb2 into their receptor/ligand dynamics simulation, and found significant differences for EGF-elicited signaling in comparison with TGFα-elicited signaling. Most notably, pathways activated primarily by receptor–ligand complexes associated with the plasma membrane were found to be increased for EGF stimulation relative to TGFα stimulation. These differences arose from the enhanced dissociation of TGFα–EGFR complexes relative to EGF–EGFR complexes, as a result of the greater pH sensitivity of the former. Hendriks et al. (2005) considered how overexpression of HER2 alters the activity of ERK downstream of EGF stimulation over a 2-hour period, during which the modulation of EGFR–EGFR homodimers and EGFR–HER2 heterodimers by endocytic trafficking processes has significant effects. It had been previously observed that ERK signaling is increased in HER2-overexpressing cells, such as are found in many breast cancers, but the mechanism for this increase was unclear; for instance, speculation had been raised in various quarters that HER2 possesses an unusually strong capability to activate the ERK pathway. Hendriks and colleagues used a combination of quantitative experimental measurement and mathematical modeling to ascertain that this was not the case, but that, rather, EGFR–EGFR homodimers and EGFR–HER2 heterodimers each lead, on a *per capita* basis, to essentially identical levels of ERK activity. Moreover, they showed that HER2 heterodimerizes to EGFR with an essentially identical association equilibrium constant as EGFR homodimerizes with itself, rather than having an especially high proclivity for interactions with other ErbB members. Finally, they determined that the ratios of ERK activity to EGFR–EGFR homodimer or EGFR–HER2 heterodimer numbers depends on stimulating concentration of EGF, with lower ratios for higher EGF concentrations; this result was consistent with the nonlinear, asymptotically saturating dependence of downstream signaling on receptor activity previously found for EGFR–EGFR homodimers.

A challenge in systems biology is understanding of how signals generated by environmental stimuli connect to phenotypic cell behavioral responses. Developing effective models for ligand–receptor interactions and for generation of signals downstream of such interactions is certainly difficult, but it is fairly straightforward because the biochemistry can, in principle, be followed experimentally. In contrast, the roads from signals to phenotypic responses are at present darkly shrouded, for many reasons. Not surprisingly, then, there exist to date only a few publications successfully describing predictive models for the mechanisms by which phenotypic responses are related to signaling network activities. Moreover, these models fall into the more "abstracted" realm, compared with the more "specified" realm of the computational modeling spectrum (Janes and Lauffenburger, 2006).

Kumar et al. (2007) applied PLSR modeling to ascertain the principal components, representing quantitatively weighted combinations of signals, most strongly correlated with (or against) the phenotypic cell behaviors (proliferation, migration) measured concomitantly with the tyrosine phosphopeptide sites assessed by mass spectrometry. From the 62 phospho sites on 45 proteins quantified across six conditions (two cell types: parental and HER2-overexpressing human mammary epithelial cells; three ligand treatments: EGF, heregulin (HRG) and autocrine stimulation), this analysis led to the construction of a model comprising two principal components containing nine phospho sites on six key proteins. Training the weighting coefficients on the associated data from the parental cells across the three ligand treatments yielded a model that could successfully predict the behavior of the HER2-overexpressing cells, on the basis of the corresponding set of signal measurements. This quantitative combination of nine phospho sites was proffered to provide a "network gauge," such that its calculation from direct measurement indicates the state of the EGFR/HER2 regulatory system governing proliferation and migration of these human mammary epithelial cells across the landscape of ligand treatment conditions and HER2 expression level. This perspective was tested directly by Kumar et al. (2008), who used an analogous partial least-squares modeling approach to predict how modulation of key kinase pathways by pharmacological inhibitors alters the migration behavior of HER2-overexpressing mammary epithelial cells in response to EGF and HRG. The signal measurements were limited to western blot assays for phosphorylation states of ERK, AKT and p38, along with that of EGFR (two phosphorylation sites), to demonstrate utility for commonly accessible experimental datasets. The most important insight gained from this contribution was that, whereas a quantitative combination of these five phospho sites on four key proteins could successfully comprehend the effects of kinase inhibitors on cell phenotypic behavior across several treatment conditions, no individual signal alone was able to. This finding emphasizes that signal-to-response relationships will, in general, require several signaling pathways to be included in the model, and that attempts to predict how cells will behave on the basis of a single pathway are most likely to be in vain.

With this particular example manifesting the general perspective described in this section, it is clear that a vast and rapidly growing amount of information is available on protein interaction and signaling networks. The development in recent years of methods to obtain large amounts of network information in human cells opens fascinating areas of study and research, particularly in understanding the functioning of signaling in health and disease, with huge potential implications for drug discovery and development. Advances in this area will strongly depend on the success of efforts to integrate the heterogeneous emergent data types and sources, and to provide powerful and user-friendly tools.

ACKNOWLEDGEMENTS

The authors (MIT) thank Joel Wagner, Bruce Tidor and Michael B. Yaffe for critical reading of this work in an early form. Funding was provided by NIH grants CA112967 to the MIT Integrative Cancer Biology Program and GM68762 to the MIT Cell Decision Processes Center and by Pfizer.

The authors (GIS) thank Chaylan Long for editorial support. Funding is provided by the Agency for Science Technology and Research (A*STAR) from the Ministry of Trade and Industry, Singapore.

References

Acharya, C.R., Hsu, D.S., Anders, C.K., et al., 2008. Gene expression signatures, clinicopathological features, and individualized therapy in breast cancer. JAMA 299, 1574–1587.

Adler, A.S., Lin, M., Horlings, H., Nuyten, D.S., van de Vijver, M.J., Chang, H.Y., 2006. Genetic regulators of large-scale transcriptional signatures in cancer. Nat. Genet. 38, 421–430.

Adriaens, M.E., Jaillard, M., Waagmeester, A., Coort, S.L., Pico, A.R., Evelo, C.T., 2008. The public road to high-quality curated biological pathways. Drug Discov. Today 13, 856–862.

Aguda, B.D., Kim, Y., Piper-Hunter, M.G., Friedman, A., Marsh, C.B., 2008. MicroRNA regulation of a cancer network: consequences of the feedback loops involving miR-17-92, E2F and Myc. Proc. Natl. Acad. Sci. USA 105, 19678–19683.

Alber, F., Dokudovskaya, S., Veenhoff, L.M., et al., 2007. Determining the architectures of macromolecular assemblies. Nature 450, 683–694.

Aldridge, B.B., Burke, J.M., Lauffenburger, D.A., Sorger, P.K., 2006. Physicochemical modelling of cell signalling pathways. Nat. Cell Biol. 8, 1195–1203.

Aldridge, B.B., Saez-Rodriguez, J., Mulich, J., Sorger, P.K., Lauffenburger, D.A., 2009. Fuzzy logic analysis of kinase pathway crosstalk in TNF/EGF/insulin-induced signaling. PLoS Comput. Biol. 5, e1000340.

Alizadeh, A.A., Eisen, M.B., Davis, R.E., et al., 2000. Distinct types of diffuse large B-cell lymphoma identified by gene expression profiling. Nature 403, 503–511.

Alon, U., 2007. Network motifs: theory and experimental approaches. Nat. Rev. Genet. 8, 450–461.

Alonso, A., Sasin, J., Bottini, N., et al., 2004. Protein tyrosine phosphatases in the human genome. Cell 117, 699–711.

Alter, O., Brown, P.O., Botstein, D., 2000. Singular value decomposition for genome-wide expression data processing and modeling. Proc. Natl. Acad. Sci. USA 97, 10101–10106.

Altschul, S.F., Gish, W., Miller, W., Myers, E.W., Lipman, D.J., 1990. Basic local alignment search tool. J. Mol. Biol. 215, 403–410.

Alves, R., Antunes, F., Salvador, A., 2006. Tools for kinetic modeling of biochemical networks. Nat. Biotechnol. 24, 667–672.

Bader, G.D., Cary, M.P., Sander, C., 2006. Pathguide: a pathway resource list. Nucleic. Acids Res. 34, D504–D506.

Banerji, J., Rusconi, S., Schaffner, W., 1981. Expression of a beta-globin gene is enhanced by remote SV40 DNA sequences. Cell 27, 299–308.

Barabasi, A.L., Oltvai, Z.N., 2004. Network biology: understanding the cell's functional organization. Nat. Rev. Genet. 5, 101–113.

Batagelj, V., Mrvar, A., 2002. Pajek—analysis and visualization of large networks. Lect. Notes Comput. Sci. 2265, 477–478.

Bell, A.C., Felsenfeld, G., 2000. Methylation of a CTCF-dependent boundary controls imprinted expression of the Igf2 gene. Nature 405, 482–485.

Bell, A.C., West, A.G., Felsenfeld, G., 1999. The protein CTCF is required for the enhancer blocking activity of vertebrate insulators. Cell 98, 387–396.

Benito, M., Parker, J., Du, Q., et al., 2004. Adjustment of systematic microarray data biases. Bioinformatics 20, 105–114.

Bhalla, U.S., Iyengar, R., 1999. Emergent properties of networks of biological signaling pathways. Science 283, 381–387.

Bild, A.H., Yao, G., Chang, J.T., et al., 2006. Oncogenic pathway signatures in human cancers as a guide to targeted therapies. Nature 439, 353–357.

Birtwistle, M.R., Hatakeyama, M., Yumoto, N., Ogunnaike, B.A., Hoek, J.B., Kholodenko, B.N., 2007. Ligand-dependent responses of the ErbB signaling network: experimental and modeling analyses. Mol. Syst. Biol. 3, 144.

Blake, W.J., Kaern, M., Cantor, C.R., Collins, J.J., 2003. Noise in eukaryotic gene expression. Nature 422, 633–637.

Blom, N., Sicheritz-Ponten, T., Gupta, R., Gammeltoft, S., Brunak, S., 2004. Prediction of post-translational glycosylation and phosphorylation of proteins from the amino acid sequence. Proteomics 4, 1633–1649.

Bollen, M., 2001. Combinatorial control of protein phosphatase-1. Trends Biochem. Sci. 26, 426–431.

Bolton, E.C., So, A.Y., Chaivorapol, C., Haqq, C.M., Li, H., Yamamoto, K.R., 2007. Cell- and gene-specific regulation of primary target genes by the androgen receptor. Genes Dev. 21, 2005–2017.

Bourque, G., Leong, B., Vega, V.B., et al., 2008. Evolution of the mammalian transcription factor binding repertoire via transposable elements. Genome Res. 18, 1752–1762.

Boutet, E., Lieberherr, D., Tognolli, M., Schneider, M., Bairoch, A., 2007. UniProtKB/Swiss-Prot: the manually annotated section of the UniProt KnowledgeBase. Methods Mol. Biol. 406, 89–112.

Brohee, S., Faust, K., Lima-Mendez, G., Vanderstocken, G., van Helden, J., 2008. Network Analysis Tools: from biological networks to clusters and pathways. Nat. Protoc. 3, 1616–1629.

Brownawell, A.M., Kops, G.J., Macara, I.G., Burgering, B.M., 2001. Inhibition of nuclear import by protein kinase B (Akt) regulates the subcellular distribution and activity of the forkhead transcription factor AFX. Mol. Cell Biol. 21, 3534–3546.

Brunet, A., Kanai, F., Stehn, J., et al., 2002. 14-3-3 transits to the nucleus and participates in dynamic nucleocytoplasmic transport. J. Cell Biol. 156, 817–828.

Bulavin, D.V., Higashimoto, Y., Demidenko, Z.N., et al., 2003. Dual phosphorylation controls Cdc25 phosphatases and mitotic entry. Nat. Cell Biol. 5, 545–551.

REFERENCES

Buratowski, S., Hahn, S., Guarente, L., Sharp, P.A., 1989. Five intermediate complexes in transcription initiation by RNA polymerase II. Cell 56, 549–561.

Burke, T.W., Kadonaga, J.T., 1996. Drosophila TFIID binds to a conserved downstream basal promoter element that is present in many TATA-box-deficient promoters. Genes Dev. 10, 711–724.

Bushey, A.M., Dorman, E.R., Corces, V.G., 2008. Chromatin insulators: regulatory mechanisms and epigenetic inheritance. Mol. Cell. 32, 1–9.

Calzone, L., Gelay, A., Zinovyev, A., Radvanyi, F., Barillot, E., 2008. A comprehensive modular map of molecular interactions in RB/E2F pathway. Mol. Syst. Biol. 4, 173.

Canagarajah, B.J., Khokhlatchev, A., Cobb, M.H., Goldsmith, E.J., 1997. Activation mechanism of the MAP kinase ERK2 by dual phosphorylation. Cell 90, 859–869.

Carroll, J.S., Liu, X.S., Brodsky, A.S., et al., 2005. Chromosome-wide mapping of estrogen receptor binding reveals long-range regulation requiring the forkhead protein FoxA1. Cell 122, 33–43.

Carroll, J.S., Meyer, C.A., Song, J., et al., 2006. Genome-wide analysis of estrogen receptor binding sites. Nat. Genet. 38, 1289–1297.

Carter, D., Chakalova, L., Osborne, C.S., Dai, Y.F., Fraser, P., 2002. Long-range chromatin regulatory interactions in vivo. Nat. Genet. 32, 623–626.

Chang, H.Y., Sneddon, J.B., Alizadeh, A.A., et al., 2004. Gene expression signature of fibroblast serum response predicts human cancer progression: similarities between tumors and wounds. PLoS Biol. 2, E7.

Chang, H.Y., Nuyten, D.S., Sneddon, J.B., et al., 2005. Robustness, scalability and integration of a wound-response gene expression signature in predicting breast cancer survival. Proc. Natl. Acad. Sci. USA 102, 3738–3743.

Chen, X., Xu, H., Yuan, P., et al., 2008. Integration of external signaling pathways with the core transcriptional network in embryonic stem cells. Cell 133, 1106–1117.

Chen, W.W., Schoeberl, B., Jasper, P.J., et al., 2009. Input-output behavior of ErbB signaling pathways as revealed by a mass action model trained against dynamic data. Mol. Syst. Biol. 5, 239.

Cheng, A.S., Jin, V.X., Fan, M., et al., 2006. Combinatorial analysis of transcription factor partners reveals recruitment of c-MYC to estrogen receptor-alpha responsive promoters. Mol. Cell 21, 393–404.

Chuang, H.Y., Lee, E., Liu, Y.T., Lee, D., Ideker, T., 2007. Network-based classification of breast cancer metastasis. Mol. Syst. Biol. 3, 140.

Chubb, J.R., Trcek, T., Shenoy, S.M., Singer, R.H., 2006. Transcriptional pulsing of a developmental gene. Curr. Biol. 16, 1018–1025.

Cline, M.S., Smoot, M., Cerami, E., et al., 2007. Integration of biological networks and gene expression data using Cytoscape. Nat. Protoc. 2, 2366–2382.

Cohen, P., 1997. The search for physiological substrates of MAP and SAP kinases in mammalian cells. Trends Cell Biol. 7, 353–361.

Cohen, P.T., 2002. Protein phosphatase 1—targeted in many directions. J. Cell Sci. 115, 241–256.

Coller, H.A., Forman, J.J., Legesse-Miller, A., 2007. "Myc'ed messages": myc induces transcription of E2F1 while inhibiting its translation via a microRNA polycistron. PLoS Genet. 3, e146.

Core, L.J., Waterfall, J.J., Lis, J.T., 2008. Nascent RNA sequencing reveals widespread pausing and divergent initiation at human promoters. Science 322, 1845–1848.

Courey, A.J., Tjian, R., 1988. Analysis of Sp1 in vivo reveals multiple transcriptional domains, including a novel glutamine-rich activation motif. Cell 55, 887–898.

Cujec, T.P., Medeiros, P.F., Hammond, P., Rise, C., Kreider, B.L., 2002. Selection of v-abl tyrosine kinase substrate sequences from randomized peptide and cellular proteomic libraries using mRNA display. Chem. Biol. 9, 253–264.

Cusick, M.E., Yu, H., Smolyar, A., et al., 2009. Literature-curated protein interaction datasets. Nat. Methods 6, 39–46.

Dai, H., van't Veer, L., Lamb, J., et al., 2005. A cell proliferation signature is a marker of extremely poor outcome in a subpopulation of breast cancer patients. Cancer Res. 65, 4059–4066.

Daub, H., Olsen, J.V., Bairlein, M., et al., 2008. Kinase-selective enrichment enables quantitative phosphoproteomics of the kinome across the cell cycle. Mol. Cell 31, 438–448.

Davis, R.E., Brown, K.D., Siebenlist, U., Staudt, L.M., 2001. Constitutive nuclear factor kappaB activity is required for survival of activated B cell-like diffuse large B cell lymphoma cells. J. Exp. Med. 194, 1861–1874.

de Graauw, M., Hensbergen, P., van de Water, B., 2006. Phospho-proteomic analysis of cellular signaling. Electrophoresis 27, 2676–2686.

Dean, A., 2006. On a chromosome far, far away: LCRs and gene expression. Trends Genet. 22, 38–45.

Dekker, J., Rippe, K., Dekker, M., Kleckner, N., 2002. Capturing chromosome conformation. Science 295, 1306–1311.

Derijard, B., Raingeaud, J., Barrett, T., et al., 1995. Independent human MAP-kinase signal transduction pathways defined by MEK and MKK isoforms. Science 267, 682–685.

Desai, K.V., Xiao, N., Wang, W., et al., 2002. Initiating oncogenic event determines gene-expression patterns of human breast cancer models. Proc. Natl. Acad. Sci. USA 99, 6967–6972.

Diella, F., Gould, C.M., Chica, C., Via, A., Gibson, T.J., 2008. Phospho.ELM: a database of phosphorylation sites--update 2008. Nucleic. Acids Res. 36, D240–D244.

Donohoe, M.E., Zhang, L.F., Xu, N., Shi, Y., Lee, J.T., 2007. Identification of a Ctcf cofactor, Yy1, for the X chromosome binary switch. Mol. Cell 25, 43–56.

Dostie, J., Richmond, T.A., Arnaout, R.A., et al., 2006. Chromosome Conformation Capture Carbon Copy (5C): a massively parallel solution for mapping interactions between genomic elements. Genome Res. 16, 1299–1309.

Durocher, D., Taylor, I.A., Sarbassova, D., et al., 2000. The molecular basis of FHA domain:phosphopeptide binding specificity and implications for phospho-dependent signaling mechanisms. Mol. Cell 6, 1169–1182.

Ebisuya, M., Yamamoto, T., Nakajima, M., Nishida, E., 2008. Ripples from neighbouring transcription. Nat. Cell Biol. 10, 1106–1113.

Elia, A.E., Cantley, L.C., Yaffe, M.B., 2003a. Proteomic screen finds pSer/pThr-binding domain localizing Plk1 to mitotic substrates. Science 299, 1228–1231.

Elia, A.E., Rellos, P., Haire, L.F., et al., 2003b. The molecular basis for phosphodependent substrate targeting and regulation of Plks by the Polo-box domain. Cell 115, 83–95.

Elowitz, M.B., Levine, A.J., Siggia, E.D., Swain, P.S., 2002. Stochastic gene expression in a single cell. Science 297, 1183–1186.

Ewing, R.M., Chu, P., Elisma, F., et al., 2007. Large-scale mapping of human protein-protein interactions by mass spectrometry. Mol. Syst. Biol. 3, 89.

Fields, P.E., Lee, G.R., Kim, S.T., Bartsevich, V.V., Flavell, R.A., 2004. Th2-specific chromatin remodeling and enhancer activity in the Th2 cytokine locus control region. Immunity 21, 865–876.

Filippova, G.N., Cheng, M.K., Moore, J.M., et al., 2005. Boundaries between chromosomal domains of X inactivation and escape bind CTCF and lack CpG methylation during early development. Dev. Cell 8, 31–42.

Flynt, A.S., Lai, E.C., 2008. Biological principles of microRNA-mediated regulation: shared themes amid diversity. Nat. Rev. Genet. 9, 831–842.

Fraser, H.B., Hirsh, A.E., Giaever, G., Kumm, J., and Eisen, M.B., 2004. Noise minimization in eukaryotic gene expression. PLoS Biol. 2, e137.

Garman, K.S., Acharya, C.R., Edelman, E., et al., 2008. A genomic approach to colon cancer risk stratification yields biologic insights into therapeutic opportunities. Proc. Natl. Acad. Sci. USA 105, 19432–19437.

Gast, R., Glokler, J., Hoxter, M., Kiess, M., Frank, R., Tegge, W., 1999. Method for determining protein kinase substrate specificities by the phosphorylation of peptide libraries on beads, phosphate-specific staining, automated sorting and sequencing. Anal. Biochem. 276, 227–241.

Gaston, K., Jayaraman, P.S., 2003. Transcriptional repression in eukaryotes: repressors and repression mechanisms. Cell Mol. Life Sci. 60, 721–741.

Geva-Zatorsky, N., Rosenfeld, N., Itzkovitz, S., et al., 2006. Oscillations and variability in the p53 system. Mol. Syst. Biol. 2, 0033.

Glass, C.K., Rosenfeld, M.G., 2000. The coregulator exchange in transcriptional functions of nuclear receptors. Genes Dev. 14, 121–141.

Gnad, F., Ren, S., Cox, J., et al., 2007. PHOSIDA (phosphorylation site database): management, structural and evolutionary investigation and prediction of phosphosites. Genome Biol. 8, R250.

Gonfloni, S., Weijland, A., Kretzschmar, J., Superti-Furga, G., 2000. Crosstalk between the catalytic and regulatory domains allows bidirectional regulation of Src. Nat. Struct. Biol. 7, 281–286.

Gonzalez, A.G., Naldi, A., Sanchez, L., Thieffry, D., Chaouiya, C., 2006. GINsim: a software suite for the qualitative modelling, simulation and analysis of regulatory networks. Biosystems 84, 91–100.

Gordus, A., Krall, J.A., Beyer, E.M., et al., 2009. Linear combinations of docking affinities explain quantitative differences in RTK signaling. Mol. Syst. Biol. 5, 235.

Green, K.A., Carroll, J.S., 2007. Oestrogen-receptor-mediated transcription and the influence of co-factors and chromatin state. Nat. Rev. Cancer 7, 713–722.

Gurdon, J.B., Melton, D.A., 2008. Nuclear reprogramming in cells. Science 322, 1811–1815.

Hale, M.B., Nolan, G.P., 2006. Phospho-specific flow cytometry: intersection of immunology and biochemistry at the single-cell level. Curr. Opin. Mol. Ther. 8, 215–224.

Hanna, J., Markoulaki, S., Schorderet, P., et al., 2008. Direct reprogramming of terminally differentiated mature B lymphocytes to pluripotency. Cell 133, 250–264.

Hark, A.T., Schoenherr, C.J., Katz, D.J., Ingram, R.S., Levorse, J.M., Tilghman, S.M., 2000. CTCF mediates methylation-sensitive enhancer-blocking activity at the H19/Igf2 locus. Nature 405, 486–489.

Haugh, J.M., Wells, A., Lauffenburger, D.A., 2000. Mathematical modeling of epidermal growth factor receptor signaling through the phospholipase C pathway: mechanistic insights and predictions for molecular interventions. Biotechnol. Bioeng. 70, 225–238.

Heldring, N., Pike, A., Andersson, S., et al., 2007. Estrogen receptors: how do they signal and what are their targets. Physiol. Rev. 87, 905–931.

Hendriks, B.S., Orr, G., Wells, A., Wiley, H.S., Lauffenburger, D.A., 2005. Parsing ERK activation reveals quantitatively equivalent contributions from epidermal growth factor receptor and HER2 in human mammary epithelial cells. J. Biol. Chem. 280, 6157–6169.

Ho, Y., Liebhaber, S.A., Cooke, N.E., 2004. Activation of the human GH gene cluster: roles for targeted chromatin modification. Trends Endocrinol. Metab. 15, 40–45.

Hu, Z., Snitkin, E.S., DeLisi, C., 2008. VisANT: an integrative framework for networks in systems biology. Brief Bioinform. 9, 317–325.

Hua, S., Kallen, C.B., Dhar, R., et al., 2008. Genomic analysis of estrogen cascade reveals histone variant

H2A.Z associated with breast cancer progression. Mol. Syst. Biol. 4, 188.

Hubbard, S.R., Wei, L., Ellis, L., Hendrickson, W.A., 1994. Crystal structure of the tyrosine kinase domain of the human insulin receptor. Nature 372, 746–754.

Hulo, N., Bairoch, A., Bulliard, V., et al., 2006. The PROSITE database. Nucleic. Acids Res. 34, D227–D230.

Huse, M., Kuriyan, J., 2002. The conformational plasticity of protein kinases. Cell 109, 275–282.

Hutti, J.E., Jarrell, E.T., Chang, J.D., et al., 2004. A rapid method for determining protein kinase phosphorylation specificity. Nat. Methods 1, 27–29.

Ideker, T., Lauffenburger, D., 2003. Building with a scaffold: emerging strategies for high- to low-level cellular modeling. Trends Biotechnol. 21, 255–262.

Ideker, T., Sharan, R., 2008. Protein networks in disease. Genome Res. 18, 644–652.

Ihmels, J., Bergmann, S., Barkai, N., 2004. Defining transcription modules using large-scale gene expression data. Bioinformatics 20, 1993–2003.

Ihmels, J., Bergmann, S., Gerami-Nejad, M., et al., 2005. Rewiring of the yeast transcriptional network through the evolution of motif usage. Science 309, 938–940.

Ito, T., Ota, K., Kubota, H., et al., 2002. Roles for the two-hybrid system in exploration of the yeast protein interactome. Mol. Cell Proteomics 1, 561–566.

Ivshina, A.V., George, J., Senko, O., et al., 2006. Genetic reclassification of histologic grade delineates new clinical subtypes of breast cancer. Cancer Res. 66, 10292–10301.

Janes, K.A., Lauffenburger, D.A., 2006. A biological approach to computational models of proteomic networks. Curr. Opin. Chem. Biol. 10, 73–80.

Janes, K.A., Albeck, J.G., Gaudet, S., Sorger, P.K., Lauffenburger, D.A., Yaffe, M.B., 2005. A systems model of signaling identifies a molecular basis set for cytokine-induced apoptosis. Science 310, 1646–1653.

Jensen, L.J., Kuhn, M., Stark, M., et al., 2009. STRING 8—a global view on proteins and their functional interactions in 630 organisms. Nucleic. Acids Res. 37, D412–D416.

Johnson, L.N., 1992. Glycogen phosphorylase: control by phosphorylation and allosteric effectors. FASEB J. 6, 2274–2282.

Johnson, L.N., Lewis, R.J., 2001. Structural basis for control by phosphorylation. Chem. Rev. 101, 2209–2242.

Johnson, W.E., Li, C., Rabinovic, A., 2007. Adjusting batch effects in microarray expression data using empirical Bayes methods. Biostatistics 8, 118–127.

Jones, P.L., Veenstra, G.J., Wade, P.A., et al., 1998. Methylated DNA and MeCP2 recruit histone deacetylase to repress transcription. Nat. Genet. 19, 187–191.

Jones, R.B., Gordus, A., Krall, J.A., MacBeath, G., 2006. A quantitative protein interaction network for the ErbB receptors using protein microarrays. Nature 439, 168–174.

Jonsson, P.F., Bates, P.A., 2006. Global topological features of cancer proteins in the human interactome. Bioinformatics 22, 2291–2297.

Joughin, B.A., Tidor, B., Yaffe, M.B., 2005. A computational method for the analysis and prediction of protein:phosphopeptide-binding sites. Protein Sci. 14, 131–139.

Juven-Gershon, T., Hsu, J.Y., Theisen, J.W., Kadonaga, J.T., 2008. The RNA polymerase II core promoter-the gateway to transcription. Curr. Opin. Cell Biol. 20, 253–259.

Kadonaga, J.T., 2004. Regulation of RNA polymerase II transcription by sequence-specific DNA binding factors. Cell 116, 247–257.

Kadonaga, J.T., Courey, A.J., Ladika, J., Tjian, R., 1988. Distinct regions of Sp1 modulate DNA binding and transcriptional activation. Science 242, 1566–1570.

Kaushansky, A., Gordus, A., Chang, B., Rush, J., MacBeath, G., 2008. A quantitative study of the recruitment potential of all intracellular tyrosine residues on EGFR, FGFR1 and IGF1R. Mol. Biosyst. 4, 643–653.

Kemp, M.L., Wille, L., Lewis, C.L., Nicholson, L.B., Lauffenburger, D.A., 2007. Quantitative network signal combinations downstream of TCR activation can predict IL-2 production response. J. Immunol. 178, 4984–4992.

Kennelly, P.J., Krebs, E.G., 1991. Consensus sequences as substrate specificity determinants for protein kinases and protein phosphatases. J. Biol. Chem. 266, 15555–15558.

Keshava Prasad, T.S., Goel, R., Kandasamy, K., et al., 2009. Human Protein Reference Database—2009 update. Nucleic. Acids Res. 37, D767–D772.

Kholodenko, B.N., Demin, O.V., Moehren, G., Hoek, J.B., 1999. Quantification of short term signaling by the epidermal growth factor receptor. J. Biol. Chem. 274, 30169–30181.

Kim, J.H., Lee, J., Oh, B., Kimm, K., Koh, I., 2004. Prediction of phosphorylation sites using SVMs. Bioinformatics 20, 3179–3184.

Kim, T.H., Abdullaev, Z.K., Smith, A.D., et al., 2007. Analysis of the vertebrate insulator protein CTCF-binding sites in the human genome. Cell 128, 1231–1245.

Kimura M., 1968. Evolutionary rate at the molecular level. Nature 217, 624–626.

Kininis, M., Chen, B.S., Diehl, A.G., et al., 2007. Genomic analyses of transcription factor binding, histone acetylation and gene expression reveal mechanistically distinct classes of estrogen-regulated promoters. Mol. Cell Biol. 27, 5090–5104.

Kitano, H., 2007. Towards a theory of biological robustness. Mol. Syst. Biol. 3, 137.

Klamt, S., Saez-Rodriguez, J., Gilles, E.D., 2007. Structural and functional analysis of cellular networks with CellNetAnalyzer. BMC Syst. Biol. 1, 2.

Klose, R.J., Bird, A.P., 2006. Genomic DNA methylation: the mark and its mediators. Trends Biochem. Sci. 31, 89–97.

Kluger, Y., Basri, R., Chang, J.T., Gerstein, M., 2003. Spectral biclustering of microarray data: coclustering genes and conditions. Genome Res. 13, 703–716.

Kocher, T., Superti-Furga, G., 2007. Mass spectrometry-based functional proteomics: from molecular machines to protein networks. Nat. Methods 4, 807–815.

Kouzarides, T., 2007. Chromatin modifications and their function. Cell 128, 693–705.

Kumagai, A., Dunphy, W.G., 1999. Binding of 14-3-3 proteins and nuclear export control the intracellular localization of the mitotic inducer Cdc25. Genes Dev. 13, 1067–1072.

Kumar, N., Wolf-Yadlin, A., White, F.M., Lauffenburger, D.A., 2007. Modeling HER2 effects on cell behavior from mass spectrometry phosphotyrosine data. PLoS Comput. Biol. 3, e4.

Kumar, N., Afeyan, R., Kim, H.D., Lauffenburger, D.A., 2008. Multipathway model enables prediction of kinase inhibitor cross-talk effects on migration of Her2-overexpressing mammary epithelial cells. Mol. Pharmacol. 73, 1668–1678.

Kurukuti, S., Tiwari, V.K., Tavoosidana, G., et al., 2006. CTCF binding at the H19 imprinting control region mediates maternally inherited higher-order chromatin conformation to restrict enhancer access to Igf2. Proc. Natl. Acad. Sci. USA 103, 10684–10689.

Kussell, E., Leibler, S., 2005. Phenotypic diversity, population growth, and information in fluctuating environments. Science. Sep 23;309(5743): 2075–2078.

Kwon, Y.S., Garcia-Bassets, I., Hutt, K.R., et al., 2007. Sensitive ChIP-DSL technology reveals an extensive estrogen receptor alpha-binding program on human gene promoters. Proc. Natl. Acad. Sci. USA 104, 4852–4857.

Lagrange, T., Kapanidis, A.N., Tang, H., Reinberg, D., Ebright, R.H., 1998. New core promoter element in RNA polymerase II-dependent transcription: sequence-specific DNA binding by transcription factor IIB. Genes Dev. 12, 34–44.

Lahav, G., 2008. Oscillations by the p53-Mdm2 feedback loop. Adv. Exp. Med. Biol. 641, 28–38.

Lahav, G., Rosenfeld, N., Sigal, A., et al., 2004. Dynamics of the p53-Mdm2 feedback loop in individual cells. Nat. Genet. 36, 147–150.

Lazzara, M.J., Lauffenburger, D.A., 2009. Quantitative modeling perspectives on the ErbB system of cell regulatory processes. Exp. Cell Res. 315, 717–725.

Lei, M., Lu, W., Meng, W., et al., 2000. Structure of PAK1 in an autoinhibited conformation reveals a multistage activation switch. Cell 102, 387–397.

Lennartsson, A., Ekwall, K., 2009. Histone modification patterns and epigenetic codes. Biochim. Biophys. Acta Jan 8 [Epub ahead of print].

Levasseur, D.N., Wang, J., Dorschner, M.O., Stamatoyannopoulos, J.A., Orkin, S.H., 2008. Oct4 dependence of chromatin structure within the extended Nanog locus in ES cells. Genes Dev. 22, 575–580.

Lewis, B.A., Kim, T.K., Orkin, S.H., 2000. A downstream element in the human beta-globin promoter: evidence of extended sequence-specific transcription factor IID contacts. Proc. Natl. Acad. Sci. USA 97, 7172–7177.

Li, C., Wong, W.H., 2003. DNA-Chip analyzer (dChip). In: Parmagianai, G., Garett, E.S., Irizarry, R.A., Zeger, S.L. (Eds.) The Analysis of Gene Expression Data: Methods and Software. Springer, New York, pp. 120–141.

Lim, C.Y., Santoso, B., Boulay, T., Dong, E., Ohler, U., Kadonaga, J.T., 2004. The MTE, a new core promoter element for transcription by RNA polymerase II. Genes Dev. 18, 1606–1617.

Lin, C.Y., Vega, V.B., Thomsen, J.S., et al., 2007. Whole-genome cartography of estrogen receptor alpha binding sites. PLoS Genet. 3, e87.

Linding, R., Jensen, L.J., Ostheimer, G.J., et al., 2007. Systematic discovery of in vivo phosphorylation networks. Cell 129, 1415–1426.

Linding, R., Jensen, L.J., Pasculescu, A., et al., 2008. NetworKIN: a resource for exploring cellular phosphorylation networks. Nucleic. Acids Res. 36, D695–D699.

Liu, E.T., 2005. Mechanism-derived gene expression signatures and predictive biomarkers in clinical oncology. Proc. Natl. Acad. Sci. USA 102, 3531–3532.

Liu, Y., Shah, K., Yang, F., Witucki, L., Shokat, K.M., 1998. Engineering Src family protein kinases with unnatural nucleotide specificity. Chem. Biol. 5, 91–101.

Lowry, W.E., Richter, L., Yachechko, R., et al., 2008. Generation of human induced pluripotent stem cells from dermal fibroblasts. Proc. Natl. Acad. Sci. USA 105, 2883–2888.

Lu, P.J., Zhou, X.Z., Shen, M., Lu, K.P., 1999. Function of WW domains as phosphoserine- or phosphothreonine-binding modules. Science 283, 1325–1328.

Luciano, J.S., Stevens, R.D., 2007. e-Science and biological pathway semantics. BMC Bioinformatics 8 (suppl 3), S3.

Lupien, M., Eeckhoute, J., Meyer, C.A., et al., 2008. FoxA1 translates epigenetic signatures into enhancer-driven lineage-specific transcription. Cell 132, 958–970.

Ma, X.J., Salunga, R., Tuggle, J.T., et al., 2003. Gene expression profiles of human breast cancer progression. Proc. Natl. Acad. Sci. USA 100, 5974–5979.

Ma'ayan, A., Jenkins, S.L., Neves, S., et al., 2005. Formation of regulatory patterns during signal propagation in a mammalian cellular network. Science 309, 1078–1083.

Ma'ayan, A., Jenkins, S.L., Webb, R.L., et al., 2009. SNAVI: desktop application for analysis and visualization of large-scale signaling networks. BMC Syst. Biol. 3, 10.

MacBeath, G., Schreiber, S.L., 2000. Printing proteins as microarrays for high-throughput function determination. Science 289, 1760–1763.

Majumder, P., Gomez, J.A., Boss, J.M., 2006. The human major histocompatibility complex class II HLA-DRB1 and HLA-DQA1 genes are separated by a CTCF-binding enhancer-blocking element. J. Biol. Chem. 281, 18435–18443.

Majumder, P., Gomez, J.A., Chadwick, B.P., Boss, J.M., 2008. The insulator factor CTCF controls MHC class II gene expression and is required for the formation of long-distance chromatin interactions. J. Exp. Med. 205, 785–798.

Mak, H.C., Daly, M., Gruebel, B., Ideker, T., 2007. CellCircuits: a database of protein network models. Nucleic. Acids Res. 35, D538–D545.

Mani, K.M., Lefebvre, C., Wang, K., et al., 2008. A systems biology approach to prediction of oncogenes and molecular perturbation targets in B-cell lymphomas. Mol. Syst. Biol. 4, 169.

Manke, I.A., Lowery, D.M., Nguyen, A., Yaffe, M.B., 2003. BRCT repeats as phosphopeptide-binding modules involved in protein targeting. Science 302, 636–639.

Manning, G., Whyte, D.B., Martinez, R., Hunter, T., Sudarsanam, S., 2002. The protein kinase complement of the human genome. Science 298, 1912–1934.

Masternak, K., Peyraud, N., Krawczyk, M., Barras, E., Reith, W., 2003. Chromatin remodeling and extragenic transcription at the MHC class II locus control region. Nat. Immunol. 4, 132–137.

Matsui, T., Segall, J., Weil, P.A., Roeder, R.G., 1980. Multiple factors required for accurate initiation of transcription by purified RNA polymerase II. J. Biol. Chem. 255, 11992–11996.

Merika, M., Williams, A.J., Chen, G., Collins, T., Thanos, D., 1998. Recruitment of CBP/p300 by the IFN beta enhanceosome is required for synergistic activation of transcription. Mol. Cell 1, 277–287.

Miller, L.D., Smeds, J., George, J., et al., 2005. An expression signature for p53 status in human breast cancer predicts mutation status, transcriptional effects, and patient survival. Proc. Natl. Acad. Sci. USA 102, 13550–13555.

Miller, M.L., Jensen, L.J., Diella, F., et al., 2008. Linear motif atlas for phosphorylation-dependent signaling. Sci. Signal 1, ra2.

Miller-Jensen, K., Janes, K.A., Brugge, J.S., Lauffenburger, D.A., 2007. Common effector processing mediates cell-specific responses to stimuli. Nature 448, 604–608.

Mishra, G.R., Suresh, M., Kumaran, K., et al., 2006. Human protein reference database—2006 update. Nucleic. Acids Res. 34, D411–D414.

Miska, E.A., Alvarez-Saavedra, E., Abbott, A.L., et al., 2007. Most *Caenorhabditis elegans* microRNAs are individually not essential for development or viability. PLoS Genet. 3, e215.

Morris, D.P., Phatnani, H.P., Greenleaf, A.L., 1999. Phosphocarboxyl-terminal domain binding and the role of a prolyl isomerase in pre-mRNA 3'-end formation. J. Biol. Chem. 274, 31583–31587.

Murrell, A., Heeson, S., Reik, W., 2004. Interaction between differentially methylated regions partitions the imprinted genes Igf2 and H19 into parent-specific chromatin loops. Nat. Genet. 36, 889–893.

Nan, X., Ng, H.H., Johnson, C.A., et al., 1998. Transcriptional repression by the methyl-CpG-binding protein MeCP2 involves a histone deacetylase complex. Nature 393, 386–389.

Nelander, S., Wang, W., Nilsson, B., et al., 2008. Models from experiments: combinatorial drug perturbations of cancer cells. Mol. Syst. Biol. 4, 216.

Nelson, D.E., Ihekwaba, A.E., Elliott, M., et al., 2004. Oscillations in NF-kappaB signaling control the dynamics of gene expression. Science 306, 704–708.

Nielsen, T.O., West, R.B., Linn, S.C., et al., 2002. Molecular characterisation of soft tissue tumours: a gene expression study. Lancet 359, 1301–1307.

Nikitin, A., Egorov, S., Daraselia, N., Mazo, I., 2003. Pathway studio—the analysis and navigation of molecular networks. Bioinformatics 19, 2155–2157.

Obenauer, J.C., Cantley, L.C., Yaffe, M.B., 2003. Scansite 2.0: proteome-wide prediction of cell signaling interactions using short sequence motifs. Nucleic. Acids Res. 31, 3635–3641.

Oda, K., Matsuoka, Y., Funahashi, A., Kitano, H., 2005. A comprehensive pathway map of epidermal growth factor receptor signaling. Mol. Syst. Biol. 1, 0010.

Ohta, T., 2002. Near-neutrality in evolution of genes and gene regulation. Proc. Natl. Acad. Sci. USA 99, 16134–16137.

Olsen, J.V., Blagoev, B., Gnad, F., et al., 2006. Global, in vivo, and site-specific phosphorylation dynamics in signaling networks. Cell 127, 635–648.

Oti, M., Snel, B., Huynen, M.A., Brunner, H.G., 2006. Predicting disease genes using protein-protein interactions. J. Med. Genet. 43, 691–698.

Panne, D., Maniatis, T., Harrison, S.C., 2007. An atomic model of the interferon-beta enhanceosome. Cell 129, 1111–1123.

Parrish Jr., J.R., Gulyas, K.D., Finley, R.L., 2006. Yeast two-hybrid contributions to interactome mapping. Curr. Opin. Biotechnol. 17, 387–393.

Pelech, S., 2004. Tracking cell signaling protein expression and phosphorylation by innovative proteomic solutions. Curr. Pharm. Biotechnol. 5, 69–77.

Perou, C.M., Sørlie, T., Eisen, M.B., et al., 2000. Molecular portraits of human breast tumours. Nature 406, 747–752.

Pieroni, E., de la Fuente van Bentem, S., Mancosu, G., Capobianco, E., Hirt, H., de la Fuente, A., 2008. Protein networking: insights into global functional organization of proteomes. Proteomics 8, 799–816.

Powell, D.W., Rane, M.J., Joughin, B.A., et al., 2003. Proteomic identification of 14-3-3zeta as a mitogen-activated protein kinase-activated protein kinase 2 substrate: role in dimer formation and ligand binding. Mol. Cell Biol. 23, 5376–5387.

Pozuelo Rubio, M., Geraghty, K.M., Wong, B.H., et al., 2004. 14-3-3-Affinity purification of over 200 human phosphoproteins reveals new links to regulation of cellular metabolism, proliferation and trafficking. Biochem. J. 379, 395–408.

Pujana, M.A., Han, J.D., Starita, L.M., et al., 2007. Network modeling links breast cancer susceptibility and centrosome dysfunction. Nat. Genet. 39, 1338–1349.

Puntervoll, P., Linding, R., Gemund, C., et al., 2003. ELM server: a new resource for investigating short functional sites in modular eukaryotic proteins. Nucleic. Acids Res. 31, 3625–3630.

Resat, H., Ewald, J.A., Dixon, D.A., Wiley, H.S., 2003. An integrated model of epidermal growth factor receptor trafficking and signal transduction. Biophys. J. 85, 730–743.

Rhodes, D.R., Yu, J., Shanker, K., et al., 2004. Large-scale meta-analysis of cancer microarray data identifies common transcriptional profiles of neoplastic transformation and progression. Proc. Natl. Acad. Sci. USA 101, 9309–9314.

Rhodes, D.R., Kalyana-Sundaram, S., Mahavisno, V., Barrette, T.R., Ghosh, D., Chinnaiyan, A.M., 2005. Mining for regulatory programs in the cancer transcriptome. Nat. Genet. 37, 579–583.

Rives, A.W., Galitski, T., 2003. Modular organization of cellular networks. Proc. Natl. Acad. Sci. USA 100, 1128–1133.

Robyr, D., Wolffe, A.P., Wahli, W., 2000. Nuclear hormone receptor coregulators in action: diversity for shared tasks. Mol. Endocrinol. 14, 329–347.

Rosenwald, A., Wright, G., Chan, W.C., et al., 2002. The use of molecular profiling to predict survival after chemotherapy for diffuse large-B-cell lymphoma. N. Engl. J. Med. 346, 1937–1947.

Rosenwald, A., Wright, G., Leroy, K., Yu, X., Gaulard, P., et al., 2003. Molecular diagnosis of primary mediastinal B cell lymphoma identifies a clinically favorable subgroup of diffuse large B cell lymphoma related to Hodgkin lymphoma. J. Exp. Med. 15 198(6),851–862.

Ross, D.T., Scherf, U., Eisen, M.B., et al., 2000. Systematic variation in gene expression patterns in human cancer cell lines. Nat. Genet. 24, 227–235.

Rual, J.F., Venkatesan, K., Hao, T., et al., 2005. Towards a proteome-scale map of the human protein-protein interaction network. Nature 437, 1173–1178.

Rubin, G.M., Yandell, M.D., Wortman, J.R., et al., 2000. Comparative genomics of the eukaryotes. Science 287, 2204–2215.

Rush, J., Moritz, A., Lee, K.A., et al., 2005. Immunoaffinity profiling of tyrosine phosphorylation in cancer cells. Nat. Biotechnol. 23, 94–101.

Russell, R.B., Aloy, P., 2008. Targeting and tinkering with interaction networks. Nat. Chem. Biol. 4, 666–673.

Rutherford, S.L., Lindquist, S., 1998. Hsp90 as a capacitor for morphological evolution. Nature 396, 336–342.

Sachs, K., Perez, O., Pe'er, D., Lauffenburger, D.A., Nolan, G.P., 2005. Causal protein-signaling networks derived from multiparameter single-cell data. Science 308, 523–529.

Sachs, K., Itani, S., Carlisle, J., Nolan, G.P., Pe'er, D., Lauffenburger, D.A., 2009. Learning signaling network structures with sparsely distributed data. J. Comput. Biol. 16, 201–212.

Saez-Rodriguez, J., Simeoni, L., Lindquist, J.A., et al., 2007. A logical model provides insights into T cell receptor signaling. PLoS Comput. Biol. 3, e163.

Santoro, C., Mermod, N., Andrews, P.C., Tjian, R., 1988. A family of human CCAAT-box-binding proteins active in transcription and DNA replication: cloning and expression of multiple cDNAs. Nature 334, 218–224.

Schoeberl, B., Eichler-Jonsson, C., Gilles, E.D., Muller, G., 2002. Computational modeling of the dynamics of the MAP kinase cascade activated by surface and internalized EGF receptors. Nat. Biotechnol. 20, 370–375.

Segal, E., Shapira, M., Regev, A., et al., 2003a. Module networks: identifying regulatory modules and their condition-specific regulators from gene expression data. Nat. Genet. 34, 166–176.

Segal, E., Yelensky, R., Koller, D., 2003b. Genome-wide discovery of transcriptional modules from DNA sequence and gene expression. Bioinformatics 19 (Suppl 1), i273–i282.

Segal, E., Friedman, N., Koller, D., Regev, A., 2004. A module map showing conditional activity of expression modules in cancer. Nat. Genet. 36, 1090–1098.

Shabalin, A.A., Tjelmeland, H., Fan, C., Perou, C.M., Nobel, A.B., 2008. Merging two gene-expression studies via cross-platform normalization. Bioinformatics 24, 1154–1160.

Simonis, M., Klous, P., Splinter, E., et al., 2006. Nuclear organization of active and inactive chromatin domains uncovered by chromosome conformation capture-on-chip (4C). Nat. Genet. 38, 1348–1354.

Smale, S.T., Kadonaga, J.T., 2003. The RNA polymerase II core promoter. Annu. Rev. Biochem. 72, 449–479.

So, A.Y., Chaivorapol, C., Bolton, E.C., Li, H., Yamamoto, K.R., 2007. Determinants of cell- and gene-specific transcriptional regulation by the glucocorticoid receptor. PLoS Genet. 3, e94.

Songyang, Z., Cantley, L.C., 1998. The use of peptide library for the determination of kinase peptide substrates. Methods Mol. Biol. 87, 87–98.

Songyang, Z., Shoelson, S.E., Chaudhuri, M., et al., 1993. SH2 domains recognize specific phosphopeptide sequences. Cell 72, 767–778.

Songyang, Z., Margolis, B., Chaudhuri, M., Shoelson, S.E., Cantley, L.C., 1995. The phosphotyrosine interaction domain of SHC recognizes tyrosine-phosphorylated NPXY motif. J. Biol. Chem. 270, 14863–14866.

Sørlie, T., Perou, C.M., Tibshirani, R., et al., 2001. Gene expression patterns of breast carcinomas distinguish tumor subclasses with clinical implications. Proc. Natl. Acad. Sci. USA 98, 10869–10874.

Sørlie, T., Tibshirani, R., Parker, J., et al., 2003. Repeated observation of breast tumor subtypes in independent gene expression data sets. Proc. Natl. Acad. Sci. USA 100, 8418–8423.

Sotiriou, C., Wirapati, P., Loi, S., et al., 2006. Gene expression profiling in breast cancer: understanding the molecular basis of histologic grade to improve prognosis. J. Natl. Cancer Inst. 98, 262–272.

Spilianakis, C.G., Flavell, R.A., 2004. Long-range intrachromosomal interactions in the T helper type 2 cytokine locus. Nat. Immunol. 5, 1017–1027.

Splinter, E., Heath, H., Kooren, J., et al., 2006. CTCF mediates long-range chromatin looping and local histone modification in the beta-globin locus. Genes Dev. 20, 2349–2354.

Stuart, J.M., Segal, E., Koller, D., Kim, S.K., 2003. A gene-coexpression network for global discovery of conserved genetic modules. Science 302, 249–255.

Szutorisz, H., Dillon, N., Tora, L., 2005. The role of enhancers as centres for general transcription factor recruitment. Trends Biochem. Sci. 30, 593–599.

Takahashi, K., Yamanaka, S., 2006. Induction of pluripotent stem cells from mouse embryonic and adult fibroblast cultures by defined factors. Cell 126, 663–676.

Talcott, C., Eker, S., Knapp, M., Lincoln, P., Laderoute, K., 2004. Pathway logic modeling of protein functional domains in signal transduction. *Pac. Symp. Biocomput.* 568–580.

Thanos, D., Maniatis, T., 1995. Virus induction of human IFN beta gene expression requires the assembly of an enhanceosome. Cell 83, 1091–1100.

Thiel, G., Lietz, M., Hohl, M., 2004. How mammalian transcriptional repressors work. Eur. J. Biochem. 271, 2855–2862.

Thomas, M.C., Chiang, C.M., 2006. The general transcription machinery and general cofactors. Crit. Rev. Biochem. Mol. Biol. 41, 105–178.

Ting, A.Y., Witte, K., Shah, K., et al., 2001. Phage-display evolution of tyrosine kinases with altered nucleotide specificity. Biopolymers 60, 220–228.

Tolhuis, B., Palstra, R.J., Splinter, E., Grosveld, F., de Laat, W., 2002. Looping and interaction between hypersensitive sites in the active beta-globin locus. Mol. Cell 10, 1453–1465.

Tompa, M., Li, N., Bailey, T.L., et al., 2005. Assessing computational tools for the discovery of transcription factor binding sites. Nat. Biotechnol. 23, 137–144.

Tsytsykova, A.V., Rajsbaum, R., Falvo, J.V., Ligeiro, F., Neely, S.R., Goldfeld, A.E., 2007. Activation-dependent intrachromosomal interactions formed by the TNF gene promoter and two distal enhancers. Proc. Natl. Acad. Sci. USA 104, 16850–16855.

Van Dyke, M.W., Roeder, R.G., Sawadogo, M., 1988. Physical analysis of transcription preinitiation complex assembly on a class II gene promoter. Science 241, 1335–1338.

van't Veer, L.J., Dai, H., van de Vijver, M.J., et al., 2002. Gene expression profiling predicts clinical outcome of breast cancer. Nature 415, 530–536.

Wan, J., Kang, S., Tang, C., et al., 2008. Meta-prediction of phosphorylation sites with weighted voting and restricted grid search parameter selection. Nucleic. Acids Res. 36, e22.

Wang, Y., Klijn, J.G., Zhang, Y., et al., 2005. Gene-expression profiles to predict distant metastasis of lymph-node-negative primary breast cancer. Lancet 365, 671–679.

Wei, C.L., Wu, Q., Vega, V.B., et al., 2006. A global map of p53 transcription-factor binding sites in the human genome. Cell 124, 207–219.

West, A.G., Fraser, P., 2005. Remote control of gene transcription. Hum. Mol. Genet. 14 (Spec. No. 1), R101–R111.

Whitfield, M.L., Sherlock, G., Saldanha, A.J., et al., 2002. Identification of genes periodically expressed in the human cell cycle and their expression in tumors. Mol. Biol. Cell 13, 1977–2000.

Wiley, H.S., Shvartsman, S.Y., Lauffenburger, D.A., 2003. Computational modeling of the EGF-receptor system: a paradigm for systems biology. Trends Cell Biol. 13, 43–50.

Winston, J.T., Strack, P., Beer-Romero, P., Chu, C.Y., Elledge, S.J., Harper, J.W., 1999. The SCFbeta-TRCP-ubiquitin ligase complex associates specifically with phosphorylated destruction motifs in IkappaBalpha and beta-catenin and stimulates IkappaBalpha ubiquitination in vitro. Genes Dev. 13, 270–283.

Wong, Y.H., Lee, T.Y., Liang, H.K., et al., 2007. KinasePhos 2.0: a web server for identifying protein kinase-specific phosphorylation sites based on sequences and coupling patterns. Nucleic. Acids Res. 35, W588–W594.

Wong, D.J., Liu, H., Ridky, T.W., Cassarino, D., Segal, E., Chang, H.Y., 2008. Module map of stem cell genes guides creation of epithelial cancer stem cells. Cell Stem. Cell 2, 333–344.

Woolf, P.J., Prudhomme, W., Daheron, L., Daley, G.Q., Lauffenburger, D.A., 2005. Bayesian analysis of signaling networks governing embryonic stem cell fate decisions. Bioinformatics 21, 741–753.

Wright, G., Tan, B., Rosenwald, A., Hurt, E.H., Wiestner, A., Staudt, L.M., 2003. A gene expression-based method to diagnose clinically distinct subgroups of diffuse large B cell lymphoma. Proc. Natl. Acad. Sci. USA 100, 9991–9996.

Wu, J.W., Hu, M., Chai, J., et al., 2001. Crystal structure of a phosphorylated Smad2. Recognition of phosphoserine by the MH2 domain and insights on Smad function in TGF-beta signaling. Mol. Cell 8, 1277–1289.

Xue, Y., Li, A., Wang, L., Feng, H., Yao, X., 2006. PPSP: prediction of PK-specific phosphorylation site with Bayesian decision theory. BMC Bioinformatics 7, 163.

Yaffe, M.B., 2002. Phosphotyrosine-binding domains in signal transduction. Nat. Rev. Mol. Cell Biol. 3, 177–186.

Yaffe, M.B., Cantley, L.C., 2000. Mapping specificity determinants for protein-protein association using protein fusions and random peptide libraries. Methods Enzymol. 328, 157–170.

Yaffe, M.B., Elia, A.E., 2001. Phosphoserine/threonine-binding domains. Curr. Opin. Cell. Biol. 13, 131–138.

Yaffe, M.B., Rittinger, K., Volinia, S., et al., 1997. The structural basis for 14-3-3:phosphopeptide binding specificity. Cell 91, 961–971.

Yaffe, M.B., Leparc, G.G., Lai, J., Obata, T., Volinia, S., Cantley, L.C., 2001. A motif-based profile scanning approach for genome-wide prediction of signaling pathways. Nat. Biotechnol. 19, 348–353.

Yeyati, P.L., Bancewicz, R.M., Maule, J., van Heyningen, V., 2007. Hsp90 selectively modulates phenotype in vertebrate development. PLoS Genet. 3, e43.

Yu, X., Chini, C.C., He, M., Mer, G., Chen, J., 2003. The BRCT domain is a phospho-protein binding domain. Science 302, 639–642.

Zhang, Y., Wolf-Yadlin, A., Ross, P.L., et al., 2005. Time-resolved mass spectrometry of tyrosine phosphorylation sites in the epidermal growth factor receptor signaling network reveals dynamic modules. Mol. Cell Proteomics 4, 1240–1250.

Zhao, Z., Tavoosidana, G., Sjolinder, M., et al., 2006. Circular chromosome conformation capture (4C) uncovers extensive networks of epigenetically regulated intra- and inter-chromosomal interactions. Nat. Genet. 38, 1341–1347.

Zhou, Q., Brown, J., Kanarek, A., Rajagopal, J., Melton, D.A., 2008. In vivo reprogramming of adult pancreatic exocrine cells to beta-cells. Nature 455, 627–632.

Zhu, H., Bilgin, M., Bangham, R., et al., 2001. Global analysis of protein activities using proteome chips. Science 293, 2101–2105.

Zimmermann, J., Buchdunger, E., Mett, H., Meyer, T., Lydon, N.B., 1997. Potent and selective inhibitors of the Abl-kinase: phenylamino-pyrimidine (PAP) derivatives *Bioorg*. Med. Chem. Lett. 7, 187–192.

CHAPTER 5

The Interface of MicroRNAs and Transcription Factor Networks

Wai-Leong Tam[1], and Bing Lim[1,2]

[1] Stem Cell and Developmental Biology, Genome Institute of Singapore, Singapore
[2] Center for Life Science, Beth Israel Deaconess Medical Center, Harvard Medical School, Boston, MA, USA

OUTLINE

Summary	109
Definitions	110
Transcription Network in Cellular Systems	110
MicroRNA Biogenesis and Function	111
A Stem Cell Model for the Transcriptional Control of miRNAs	113
Lessons from the miRNA Regulatory Landscape	115
One mRNA is Targeted by Several miRNAs	115
Predicting miRNA Targets	117
Engineering miRNA Networks	119
Coordinated Regulation of Target Genes	120
Distributing the Load Across Regulatory Fabrics	122
Autoregulation	124
Molecular Switches	126
Deciphering the Rules for a miRNA Switch	128
The Roadmap to Systems Biology: Deconvoluting Complexities	129
Concluding Remarks	130

Summary

Transcription factors are important determinants of cellular identity where their expression can shift the balance of cell fate. A recent class of small non-coding RNAs discovered, microRNAs (miRNAs), also appears to have determining roles in the control of cellular phenotypes, development and disease. While the transcriptional network has been well-elucidated in several clinically important cell types such as stem cells, we are only beginning to understanding the network of individual miRNAs in terms of their regulatory effects on other genes including transcription factors. However, the networks comprised of transcription factors and miRNAs are largely disconnected. It is unclear how the transcription of miRNA genes and the feedback of miRNAs into transcription hierarchies are regulated. This review attempts to provide timely insights into the interface between transcription and translational networks, and discuss some lessons we have gained from deciphering the reciprocal interplay between the different regulatory mechanisms. In particular, we will use the stem cell model to understand how miRNAs coordinately targets many common genes, the usefulness of an integrated miRNA–transcription factor regulation, the types and significance of network motifs employed and how miRNAs behave as molecular switches for translational control.

Definitions

Genome-wide transcription factor location analysis Chromatin immunoprecipitation (ChIP) is a technique used in identifying the DNA binding sites of transcription factors in the cell. When combined with whole genome analyses such as microarray and sequencing, it can potentially be used to map all previously unknown binding loci in an unbiased manner.

RNA interference A double-stranded RNA-induced gene silencing mechanism that is dependent on sequence homology. The double-stranded RNA is processed to a short interfering RNA (siRNA), which becomes incorporated into the RNA-induced silencing complex (RISC) and guide the endonucleolytic cleavage of the target mRNA. MicroRNAs also utilize this machinery by non-perfect base pairing which typically leads to translation repression rather than mRNA cleavage.

MicroRNA seed The seven or eight nucleotides at the 5′ end of a miRNA that has been postulated to serve as the primary determinant of target specificity.

MicroRNA target A messenger RNA, which encodes a protein, contains the binding sites for specific miRNAs. This leads to a regulatory response that may be translational inhibition or mRNA degradation.

Network motif These are patterns that recur within a network more frequently than expected at random. In the cellular context, these are the basic features of gene regulatory mechanics. Common motifs referred in this review are the feed-forward and feedback loops, autoregulatory loop, coherent and incoherent loops.

TRANSCRIPTION NETWORK IN CELLULAR SYSTEMS

Biological systems are maintained by gene regulatory networks tightly coupled to protein activity and function. As organisms evolve from simple unicellular entities that include bacteria and yeast, to higher order multicellular organisms such as plants and metazoans, additional regulatory modules are required for the coordinated response of distinct cellular processes within an organism, and for responding to the external environment. All classically defined living systems depend on the precise coordinated expression of gene products which interact and specify cellular phenotypes and function. Within the same species, all organisms possess near-exact DNA sequences, but each cell type in the body is specific in its role. Increasing complexity has demanded additional layers of regulation to cope with an increasing genomic complexity, as well as for the precise control of molecular determinants within each cell type.

One of the most important cellular process that determine the levels of gene products is transcription. The binding of transcription factors, together with the basal components of the transcription machinery on DNA largely determines the production of unspliced messenger RNA (mRNA) molecules or transcripts.

Transcription factors can act as activators or repressors in a tissue- or condition-specific manner. This may involve the recruitment of other protein components which help titer the expression of a gene. The roles of transcription factor complexes in regulating the levels of protein-coding genes that includes ligands, receptors, signaling molecules, cell adhesion proteins, basic cellular components and other downstream transcription regulators have been well-elucidated in many cell types.

Transcription factors have defining roles in conferring cellular identities. For example, the myogenic differentiation factor *MyoD* is required for specifying the skeletal muscle lineage (Edmondson and Olson, 1989), whereas the neurogenic differentiation factor *Neurogenin* is necessary for the induction of neurogenesis (Ma et al., 1996). Cumulative studies have revealed that these master regulators are necessary for the downstream control of other protein-coding genes which, in a synergistic manner, define the molecular characteristics of a cell. Notably, stem or progenitor cells are well-suited for dissecting mechanisms that govern the transcriptional and post-transcriptional regulation of gene expression. These unique cells are characterized by their dual abilities to self-renew and give rise to functional cell types when stimulated. Hence, stem cells provide a useful window for understand how cellular networks are constructed, maintained and destabilized when subjected to perturbations.

Embryonic stem cells (ESCs), derived from the inner cell mass of the early mammalian embryos of mouse and human, are capable of and primed to lineage-specific differentiation through either genetic manipulations or extracellular ligand-mediated signals. At the heart of molecular networks which govern ESCs self-renewing and pluripotent capabilities is a core set of transcription factors that exerts far-reaching effects. The pluripotency-associated factors, *Oct4*, *Sox2*, *Nanog*, *Sall4* and *Tcf3*, amongst others are essential for the ESC "stemness" state as the depletion of any single factor dramatically affects the stem cell phenotype. Several lessons have emerged from our studies of these transcription factors (Tam and Lim, 2008). Firstly, a high-order regulator has the tendency to control a wide repertoire of protein-coding genes. Secondly, a core set of several transcription factors may act in synergy to bind and regulate common genes downstream. Thirdly, key regulators commonly autoregulate their own expression, as well as the expression of other transcription factors, thus forming localized and tightly interconnected feedback loops. While extensive studies have focused on protein-coding genes which singly or synergistically maintain the "stemness" state, very little is understood regarding the role of small non-coding RNAs, which includes small interfering RNAs (siRNAs) (Doench et al., 2003), piwi-interacting RNAs (piRNAs) (Aravin et al., 2006) and microRNAs (miRNAs) (Lee et al., 1993; Reinhart et al., 2000). Since miRNAs constitute an entire layer of the regulatory fabric, it is useful for us to uncover their significance, function and interaction within the hierarchy of other cellular networks.

MICRORNA BIOGENESIS AND FUNCTION

In order to understand why miRNAs might be distinctively regulated as an integral part of the transcription machinery, we need to define: (i) what are miRNAs, (ii) why are they important for cellular processes and (iii) what is their mode of action? Several reviews provide an in-depth discussion on miRNA biogenesis and their function (Ambros, 2004; Bushati and Cohen, 2007; Filipowicz et al., 2008; Stefani and Slack, 2008). Briefly, miRNAs constitute a unique family of short, approximately 22-nucleotide length non-coding RNAs that have emerged as important post-transcription modulators of gene expression in metazoans and plants. The founding members of the miRNA family *lin-4* and *let-7* were first identified in the nematode *Caenorhabditis elegans* in a classical forward genetics screen through loss-of function analyses. They are required for the control of developmental timing (Lee et al., 1993; Reinhart et al., 2000). Subsequently, at least a few hundred miRNAs are found to be expressed in lower metazoans and plants, and several hundreds to thousands are detected or predicted to operate in mice and humans (Berezikov et al., 2006a; Lagos-Quintana et al., 2001), and these numbers are increasing.

A large proportion of miRNAs are transcribed by RNA polymerase II to produce a primary miRNA (pri-miRNA) transcript which contains a stem-loop. Depending on the number of miRNAs occurring on this secondary structure, the pri-miRNA may range from hundreds of bases to tens of kilobases (Lee et al., 2004). The pri-miRNA is processed within the nucleus by the Microprocessor protein complex composed of the RNase III enzyme Drosha and the double-stranded RNA-binding domain protein DGCR8 (Gregory et al., 2004; Han et al., 2004). The cleavage of the pri-miRNA stem produces a hairpin precursor miRNA (pre-miRNA) approximately 70 nucleotides in length (Han et al., 2006), which is then exported into the cytoplasm by Exportin-5 (Lund et al., 2004). Next, the pre-miRNA is cleaved by another RNase II enzyme Dicer to produce the mature miRNA duplex approximately 22 nucleotides in length (Hutvagner et al., 2001; Ketting et al., 2001). The functional strand of the mature miRNA becomes incorporated into the ribonucleoprotein RNA-induced silencing complex (RISC) whereas the passenger strand becomes degraded (Chendrimada et al., 2005; Gregory et al., 2005; Maniataki and Mourelatos, 2005). The incorporated miRNA guides the RISC–miRNA complex to its mRNA targets in part through base pairing interactions.

As regulators of gene expression, miRNAs exert their effects in two modes. In plants, miRNAs recognize the target mRNAs by perfect or near-perfect sequence complementarity, resulting in the cleavage and destruction of mRNA through the RNA interference (RNAi) machinery (Rhoades et al., 2002; Tang et al., 2003). By contrast, miRNAs appear to pair with imperfect complementarity to their target mRNAs in most instances observed in metazoan, and they inhibit protein synthesis through translational inhibition using unknown mechanisms that preserve the mRNA targets (Meister et al., 2004; Meister and Tuschl, 2004). It is widely speculated that the 2nd to 8th nucleotide on the 5' end of the miRNA, also known as the "seed," is a major determining factor in its pairing with potential target mRNAs, and may be complemented by extensive base pairing to the 3' end (Lewis et al., 2003, 2005). However, other evidence point that some miRNA target sites are 3' compensatory regions that have extensive pairing to the 3' end of the miRNA to compensate for imperfect base pairing to the seed (Brennecke et al., 2005). Base pairing rules, in addition to other parameters such as binding energies, pattern discovery and species sequence conservation, form important bases for the development of several miRNA target prediction algorithms presently employed for identifying putative targets.

MicroRNAs are necessary for many aspects of metazoan development, cellular function and stem cell maintenance. For instance, *lsy-6* and *mir-273* controls neuronal cell fate determination in *C. elegans* (Chang et al., 2004; Johnston and Hobert, 2003), *bantam* and *mir-14* regulates apoptosis in *Drosophila* (Brennecke et al., 2003; Xu et al., 2003) and *mir-181* modulates the differentiation of hematopoietic stem cells in mice (Chen et al., 2004). As a cluster, the *mir-17,92* series of miRNAs, which is transcribed as a single pri-miRNA and gets processed to individual miRNAs, has extensive roles in the development of the heart, lungs and immune system (Koralov et al., 2008; Ventura et al., 2008; Xiao et al., 2008; Yu et al., 2007). MiRNAs are also implicated in disease by behaving as oncogenes and tumor suppressors. It has been observed that the levels of certain miRNAs are dramatically altered in primary tumors (Calin et al., 2004, 2005), and global miRNA expression is lower in cancer tissues than in normal tissues (Lu et al., 2005). In many cases of chronic lymphocytic leukemia, *mir-15a* and *mir-16-1* is deleted along with large segments of chromosome 13 (Calin et al., 2005), and the pathogenesis is thought to occur through the loss of inhibition on the anti-apoptotic gene *Bcl2* which is targeted by the miRNAs (Cimmino et al., 2005). Remarkably, *mir-372* and *mir-373*, specific to testicular germ cell tumors, have further been shown to be able to overcome oncogenic *Ras*-mediated arrest and induce tumorigenesis in primary human fibroblasts transduced with the miRNAs (Voorhoeve et al., 2006). These, and other studies, highlight the dominant roles miRNAs might have in exerting dramatic phenotypic effects.

A STEM CELL MODEL FOR THE TRANSCRIPTIONAL CONTROL OF MIRNAS

MicroRNAs can have roles that recapitulate the gain or loss-of-function of transcription factors. This revelation supports the rationale for a deeper investigation into the global and local architecture of miRNA–transcription factor interactions. In order to appreciate the reasons for the precise regulation of miRNA expression, an obvious starting point would be to understand its transcription. The stem cell model presents an attractive strategy because many crucial stem cell-specific transcription factors have been identified, along with extensive mapping of their binding sites to gene promoters. The hierarchy of core transcription factors that control protein-coding gene expression has been well-characterized (Boyer et al., 2005, 2006; Jiang et al., 2008; Kim et al., 2008; Lee et al., 2006; Loh et al., 2006; Tam et al., 2008), but little is known regarding the regulation of miRNAs.

Several lines of evidence suggest that miRNAs contribute to the control of self-renewal, pluripotency and differentiation of ESCs. Since miRNAs can alter the expression of a significant portion of genes in mammalian cell types (Lewis et al., 2005; Lim et al., 2005), it is clearly conceivable that they have regulatory roles in ESCs. ESCs deficient in components of the miRNA processing machinery, either *Dicer* or *DGCR8*, show defects in differentiation and proliferation, indicating an absolute requirement of miRNAs for proper stem cell function (Kanellopoulou et al., 2005; Murchison et al., 2005). In other progenitor cell types, *Dicer* is also essential for the survival of B lymphocyte lineage and its antibody diversification (Koralov et al., 2008), proper development of T cell (Muljo et al., 2005), oocyte maturation and genomic integrity of female germline (Murchison et al., 2007) and maintenance of hair follicle stem cells (Andl et al., 2006), further underscoring the requirement of miRNAs. Specific miRNAs have been attributed roles in stem cells. For instance, the skin miRNA *mir-203*, represses the transcription factor *p63* necessary for stratified epithelial stem cells, hence promoting their differentiation (Yi et al., 2008b). In mouse ESCs, *mir-134* and *mir-1* induce differentiation into the neuroectoderm and cardiac muscle lineage, respectively (Ivey et al., 2008; Li and Gregory, 2008; Tay et al., 2008b).

Genome-wide expression profiling studies have revealed that a subset of miRNAs is preferentially expressed in ESCs or embryonic stages (Houbaviy et al., 2003, 2005; Laurent et al., 2008; Suh et al., 2004). While there are differences between miRNAs expressed in human and mouse ESCs, striking conservations of certain miRNA families are detected. The mouse *mir-290-295* family is homologous to the *mir-371/2/3* family in human, and members of *mir-302* family are present in both species. Many of these miRNAs manifest dynamic changes during differentiation which suggests a contribution to the stem cell state. In response to differentiation regimes that include retinoic acid treatment, embryoid body formation, depletion of transcription factors and cytokine-induced differentiation, the expression of some miRNAs becomes rapidly downregulated. As ESC-associated transcription factors are also greatly altered during the process, the results suggest that miRNAs may be under the influence of transcription regulators, and *vice versa*.

One direct approach to identify all transcriptionally regulated miRNAs is through genome-wide transcription factor location analysis. The stem cell factors, Oct4, Sox2, Nanog and Tcf3, are found to reside at the promoters of a large number of miRNA genes (Marson et al., 2008). Significantly, all four factors co-occupy the promoters of 55 distinct miRNA transcription units which include three large polycistronic clusters of miRNAs (Marson et al., 2008). MiRNAs which may have roles in either directing differentiation or conferring "stemness" appear to be regulated by a combination of key transcription factors (Fig. 5.1). Examples of such highly regulated miRNAs are also referred to as miRNA hubs. One of these co-regulated clusters, *mir17-92*, is crucial for animal development. Two other clusters, *mir-290-295* and *mir-302*, have not been assigned function in the ESCs, but they respond to differentiation signals (Houbaviy et al., 2003; Suh et al., 2004; Tay et al., 2008b). In contrast, many tissue-specific miRNAs are of low abundance in ESCs. It was found that Polycomb group proteins, which are repressors of gene expression, co-occupy the promoter regions of these miRNAs (Marson et al., 2008). However, one caveat is that the occupancy of miRNA promoters by transcription factors does not necessarily equate to regulation. The levels of miRNAs between different cell types cannot directly account for whether specific categories of miRNAs are directly regulated by transcription factors. While the study has provided valuable information on the annotation of miRNA promoters and expression profiles in different cell types (Marson et al., 2008), there is a critical lack of functional evidence to support the significance of miRNA activation or repression in ESCs.

A more relevant strategy to address the issue of direct transcriptional regulation is the systematic

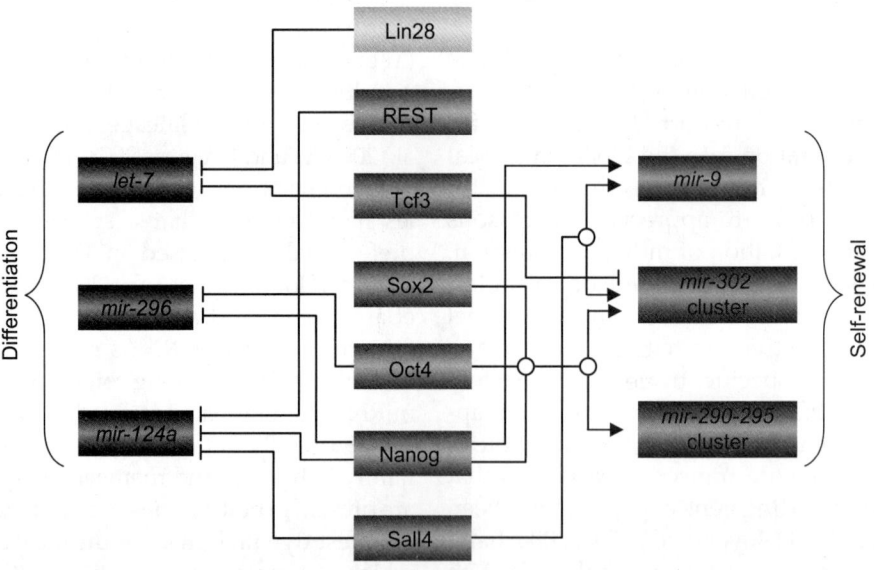

FIGURE 5.1 MicroRNA Hubs.
In ESCs, functionally important miRNAs involved in either self-renewal or differentiation are common transcriptional targets of key transcription factors. *Note*: Lin28 is a RNA binding protein.

I. FOUNDATIONS OF SYSTEMS BIOLOGY

perturbation of transcription factor abundance followed by analyses of alterations in miRNA expression patterns (Fig. 5.2). The intersection between transcription factor occupancy on miRNA promoters and regulation of miRNA levels will support a causal relationship. Based on the depletion of a wide repertoire of ESC factors involved in pluripotency, self-renewal and re-programming, we could identify differentially regulated miRNAs bound by each transcription factor. MiRNAs upregulated upon transcription factor depletion are likely repressed, and those downregulated may be activated in the ESC state. Presumably, repressed miRNAs could induce ESC differentiation when overexpressed while activated miRNAs would cause ESCs to lose pluripotency when depleted. Our test on several of these miRNAs indeed show that the integrated approach has yielded positive findings on miRNAs which maintain stem cell properties and those that cause differentiation (unpublished observations).

LESSONS FROM THE MIRNA REGULATORY LANDSCAPE

One miRNA Targets Many mRNAs

We have a good understanding of transcription factor regulation and the repertoire of network motifs involved, but very little is known about the features of a miRNA network and its interface with the transcriptional factors. Several features observed in transcriptional factor network are recapitulated in the miRNA landscape. One observation is that a single miRNA has the potential to target many genes (Fig. 5.3A). As metazoan miRNAs do not require perfect base pair complementarity with cognate mRNA sites, one miRNA can target many genes with no overall sequence homology except in short segments of the 3′ untranslated region (UTR). This ingenious mechanism allows the coordinated control of many genes by a miRNA. However, this has made the algorithms for predicting miRNA targets complicated, with many *in silico* prediction models being developed and tested, each showing progressively the impressive reach of miRNAs in gene regulation. Using the rna22 algorithm (Miranda et al., 2006), a large number of candidate miRNA targets was examined. One miRNA, *mir-134*, is predicted to be active against over 5000 mRNA species. Out of 160 putative binding sites tested, suppression of 114 sites (71%) is observed. More importantly, when the endogenous protein and mRNA levels of selected predicted *mir-134* target genes are examined, *mir-134* induces translation downregulation in these genes that include Nanog, Sox2 and LRH1 which are important for directing ESC growth (Tay et al., 2008a, 2008b). This study demonstrated the surprising breadth of impact conferred by miRNA–mRNA interactions.

Lessons learnt from the stem cell model suggest that, a miRNA network is not isolated. It is often linked and interlocked with several networks centered upon other miRNAs (Fig. 5.4). The miRNAs, *mir-134*, *mir-296* and *mir-21*, can independently induce a moderate degree of ESC differentiation (Singh et al., 2008; Tay et al., 2008a, 2008b). Surprisingly, all three share a common target, Nanog; and *mir-134* and *mir-21* also target Sox2. The targeting of pluripotency factors by these miRNAs provides a logical explanation as to why they are silent in ESCs. Furthermore, the expression of several miRNAs simultaneously may not necessarily induce a more dramatic differentiation phenotype than any single one. This result presents the challenging task of understanding how the targeting of multiple genes by a single miRNA, and the intersection of networks, can lead to a cellular effect.

One mRNA is Targeted by Several miRNAs

Another key observation is that a single mRNA gene may be targeted by several miRNAs (Fig. 5.3B). Since the 3′ UTR of mRNAs

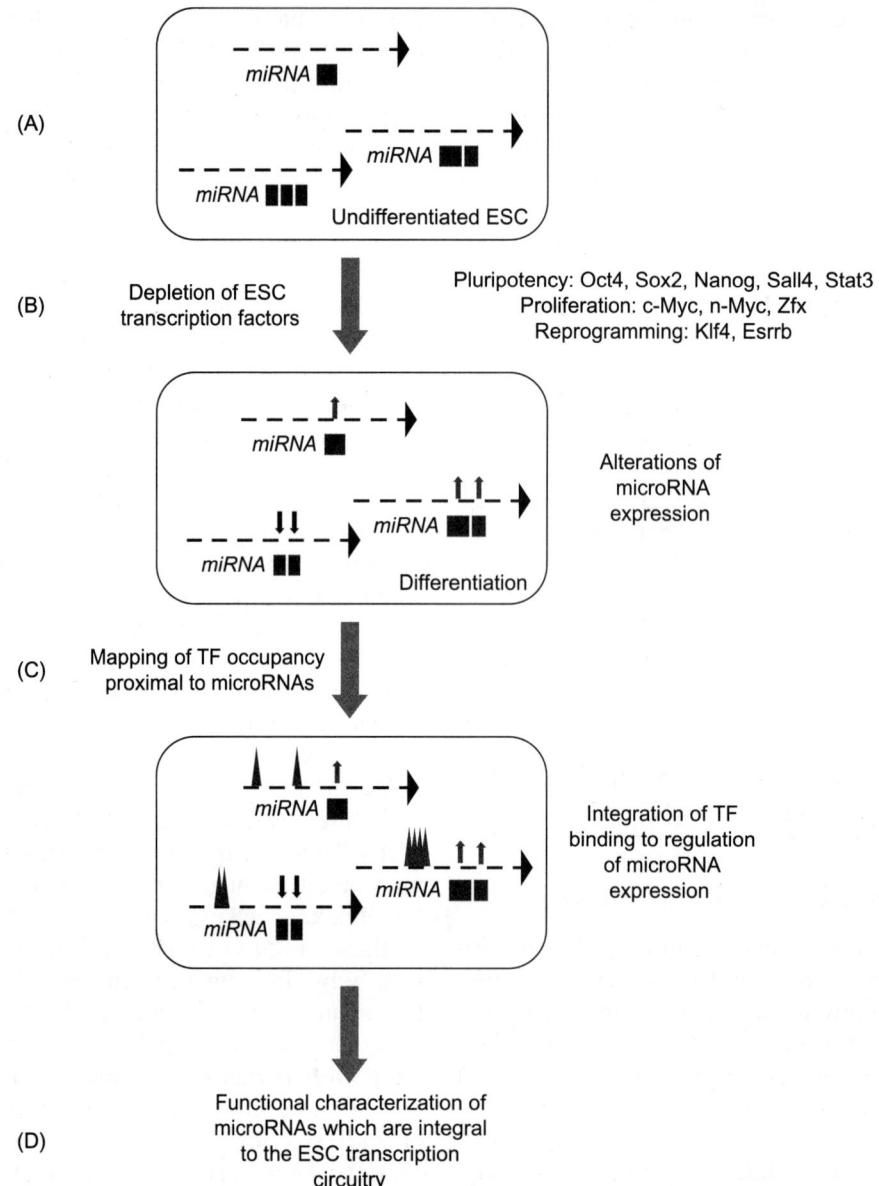

FIGURE 5.2 Schematic for Building miRNA–Transcription Factor Network.
A systematic approach to dissect the transcription regulation of miRNA involves: (A) an assessment of basal miRNA expression in undifferentiated ESCs, (B) alterations to the levels upon depletion of key transcription factors, (C) mapping of transcription factor bind sites to miRNA promoters infers direct regulation and (D) functional characterization of candidate miRNAs.

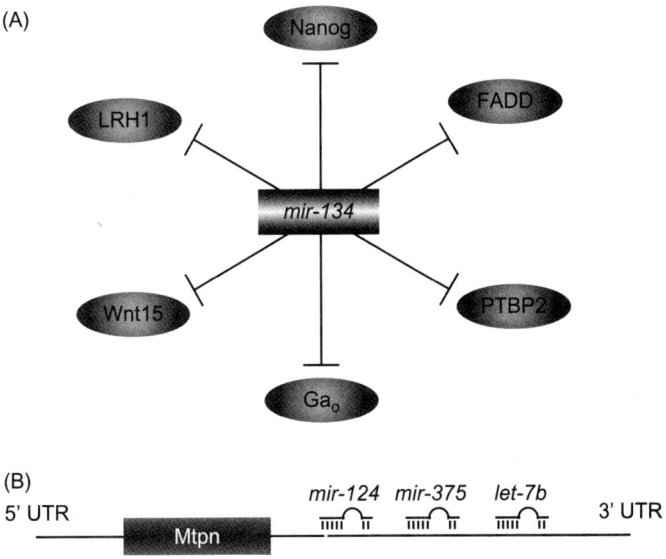

FIGURE 5.3 Target Gene Regulation by miRNAs.
(A) One miRNA targets many genes. Mir-134 translationally repress many target mRNAs in ESCs, several of which are involved in the maintenance of pluripotency. (B) Many miRNAs target a single gene. The mRNA of a single gene, for example *Mtpn*, can contain several binding sites for the different miRNAs or the same miRNA.

vary considerably in length and sequence, they carry numerous potential binding sites for the same or different miRNAs. Just as transcription factors recognize short sequences on DNA which partially results in their recruitment to specific chromosome loci, miRNAs likewise utilize sequence complementarity to its target for recognition. This specificity-determining region is often short, comprising seven or eight nucleotides (Lewis et al., 2003). In one study, experimental validation of the myotrophin mRNA *Mtpn* showed that it is targeted, and translationally inhibited, by three miRNAs, *mir-124*, *mir-375* and *let-7b* (Krek et al., 2005). The simultaneous action of all three miRNAs likely allows a blocking of translation more efficiently. This suggests that their high expression in certain tissues has a direct role in moderating the protein level of at least one major mRNA target. Direct experimental evidence of such synergistic regulation of translation is currently lacking, but various computational programs predict the prevalence of such a mechanism in which several miRNAs bind simultaneously and co-regulate their target. This is analogous to transcription regulation whereby several transcription factors tend to work in synergism through assembly as a protein complex to regulate the promoters and enhancers of target genes (Chen et al., 2008; Wang et al., 2006).

Predicting miRNA Targets

The accurate identification of miRNA targets is a crucial step in unraveling their contributions to biological pathways. Of the miRNAs identified in mouse and human, only a small handful

118   5. THE INTERFACE OF MICRORNAS AND TRANSCRIPTION FACTOR NETWORKS

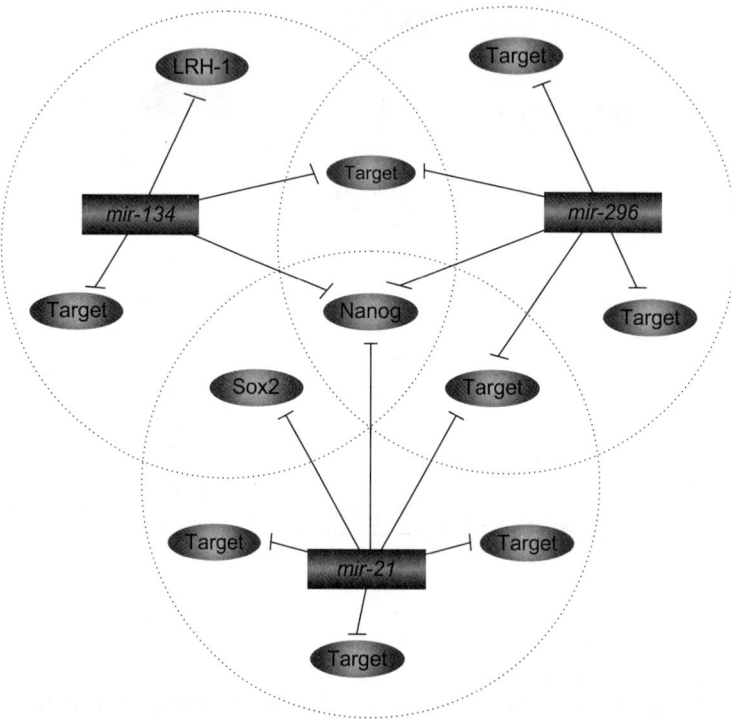

FIGURE 5.4 Intersection of miRNA Targeting Networks.
Each miRNA forms a network through its regulation of many genes. Different miRNA networks may become intersected when there is an overlap of common genes targeted.

has been experimentally linked to specific functions. The precise determination of the full range of targets is a major bottleneck in functional analysis. Since 2003, numerous miRNA target prediction programs are publicly available: MiRanda (Enright et al., 2003), TargetScan (Lewis et al., 2003), TargetScanS (Lewis et al., 2005), PicTar (Krek et al., 2005), rna22 (Miranda et al., 2006) and others (Table 5.1). The classic features of the majority of these programs fulfill two operations. The first step involves identification of potential miRNA binding sites according to base pairing rules. While TargetScanS requires perfect complementarity to the miRNA seed, PicTar tolerates targets with imperfect seed matches if they satisfy a defined binding energy threshold. In the second step, these programs utilize cross-species conservation requirements where TargetScanS and PicTar require conservation between at least five species for the mRNA target site that is complementary to the seed sequence. MiRanda requires only for conservation between human and mouse for an entire mRNA target site that has at least 90% sequence similarity.

Interestingly, rna22 relies on patterns derived from known and predicted miRNA sequences to identify putative binding sites for a target mRNA without the need for cross-species comparisons (Miranda et al., 2006). And since rna22 is not heavily dependent on recognition of the seed region, it can identify putative miRNA binding sites without a need to know the identity of the targeting miRNA. This permits the identification of binding sites even if the targeting miRNA is not among those currently known,

I. FOUNDATIONS OF SYSTEMS BIOLOGY

TABLE 5.1 Major Publicly Available microRNA Target Prediction Programs

Program	Web site	Reference
DIANA-microT	http://diana.cslab.ece.ntua.gr/	(Kiriakidou et al., 2004)
"EMBL"	http://www.russell.embl.de/miRNAs/	(Stark et al., 2005)
GenMiR++	http://www.psi.toronto.edu/genmir/	(Huang et al., 2007a)
MicroInspector	http://www.imbb.forth.gr/microinspector/	(Rusinov et al., 2005)
MiRanda	http://www.microrna.org/	(John et al., 2004)
MirWIP	http://mirtargets.org/	(Hammell et al., 2008)
PicTar	http://pictar.mdc-berlin.de/	(Krek et al., 2005)
PITA	http://genie.weizmann.ac.il/pubs/mir07/index.html	(Kertesz et al., 2007)
rna22	http://cbcsrv.watson.ibm.com/rna22.html	(Miranda et al., 2006)
RNAhybrid	http://bibiserv.techfak.uni-bielefeld.de/rnahybrid/	(Rehmsmeier et al., 2004)
TargetScan	http://www.targetscan.org/	(Lewis et al., 2005)

that is novel miRNAs. Rna22 is the only program that has been shown to be experimentally robust *in vitro* as the binding of miRNA to their targets has been validated on an extensive scale. This is not performed in a similar manner with other programs. The emergence of miRNA–mRNA target prediction programs such as rna22 has challenged conventional wisdom that seed sequence of a miRNA is the defining region, and created new avenues for increased understanding of miRNA interaction with mRNAs.

Recent attempts to identify physiologically active miRNA targets with greater accuracy have involved simultaneous profiling of miRNA and mRNA expressions. Since miRNAs can cause degradation of their targets and a large number of mRNAs appear to be regulated in this manner (Farh et al., 2005; Lim et al., 2005), the expression profiling of miRNAs and their putative targets should reveal an inverse relationship. Indeed, the inverse correlation between expression patterns for targets of widely expressed miRNAs and tissue-specific miRNAs has been observed (Huang et al., 2007b; Lim et al., 2005). Using a Bayesian-based data analysis algorithm, GenMiR++, we can identify a network of high-confidence target predictions for ~100 human miRNAs. It relies on support from mRNA expression data across multiple tissue and cell types, sequence complementarity and comparative genomics information (Huang et al., 2007a). Although GenMiR++ has been suggested to improve the accuracy of sequence-based miRNA-target predictions, as empirically demonstrated for a single miRNA *let-7b*, it is difficult to rule out whether the inverse expression patterns between miRNAs and their predicted targets arose from indirect regulation through other pathways. Another caveat is that GenMiR++ only predicts which mRNA targets are regulated by transcript degradation, but cannot account for candidates subject to translational repression since these are not linearly correlated to alterations in mRNA levels.

ENGINEERING MIRNA NETWORKS

The endpoint of transcription and translational regulation is to precisely define protein output. However, our current understanding of these regulatory aspects is largely incomplete. There is a critical gap in our understanding of how the networks of miRNAs and transcription factors are connected. A vast amount of genomic information has been gathered for both protein-coding and miRNA gene expression in many cell types. Computational efforts have helped to deconvolute the massive amount of information and decipher patterns of correlation between transcription factors and miRNAs. Prediction programs for miRNA targets are now more sophisticated and encompass a wider range of biological parameters. Pattern discovery algorithms are also being employed to examine the connectivity among related gene categories, and for the *de novo* prediction of yet undiscovered miRNAs and other small RNAs. Certain ground rules for gene regulation and interaction have been uncovered; leading to the revelation that miRNA is an inseparable component of the overall gene regulatory fabric.

Coordinated Regulation of Target Genes

A feature of gene regulatory network is that genes belonging to the same regulon, that is genes sets which are coordinately regulated, will be co-regulated not only at the transcription level, but also post-transcriptionally (Shalgi et al., 2005). One example is differentiating ESCs where the global increase in transcript levels is accompanied by an enhancement of protein translation efficiency, perhaps to cope with an increase in cellular complexity (Sampath et al., 2008). The simplest motif of co-regulation is observed when a common gene is coordinately targeted by a transcription factor and a miRNA. A common downstream target Z may be regulated by an upstream transcription factor X, and repressed by a miRNA *mir-A*. If X is a repressor, the overall function of the motif is to silence the target (Fig. 5.5A, left panel). This class of motif is termed "coherent" because both upstream regulators act synergistically in the same direction. In contrast, X may be an activator where the target is actively transcribed, only to be translationally dampened by *mir-A* (Fig. 5.5A, right panel). The negative interaction between the transcription activator and miRNA creates an "incoherent" motif where antagonism may be useful in certain circumstances. The parallel and separate function of both regulators targeting the same gene assumes no direct interaction between them. It is observed that transcription factor–miRNA pairings are abundant, but each is also involved in the regulation of a larger set of targets (Shalgi et al., 2007).

The regulation of common target genes in which upstream regulators also have an impact on each other, is reminiscent of feed-forward loops established within a transcription factor-based hierarchy. In the latter, the control of a downstream target Z may occur through the synergism of upstream factors X and Y, where X is upstream of Y (Fig. 5.5B). As all components in this motif are found at the transcription level, an integrative framework that accounts for transcriptional and post-transcriptional activities will need to incorporate both classes of regulators, that is transcription factors and miRNAs. The resultant feed-forward circuit straddles across two layers of regulatory fabric. The motif in which the transcription of miRNAs and their common downstream target gene is oppositely regulated is a coherent circuit (Mangan and Alon, 2003; Milo et al., 2002; Shen-Orr et al., 2002; Tsang et al., 2007). For example, the upstream transcription factor could activate the production of a miRNA and simultaneously repress the transcription of a common target gene (Fig. 5.5C, left panel), or the upstream factor could repress the production of a miRNA, whilst activating a target which is repressed by the miRNA (Fig. 5.5C, right panel). This design could minimize the effects of leaky gene transcription when their expression is not desired. Coherent circuits are prevalent, and supported by genome scale studies which show an inverse

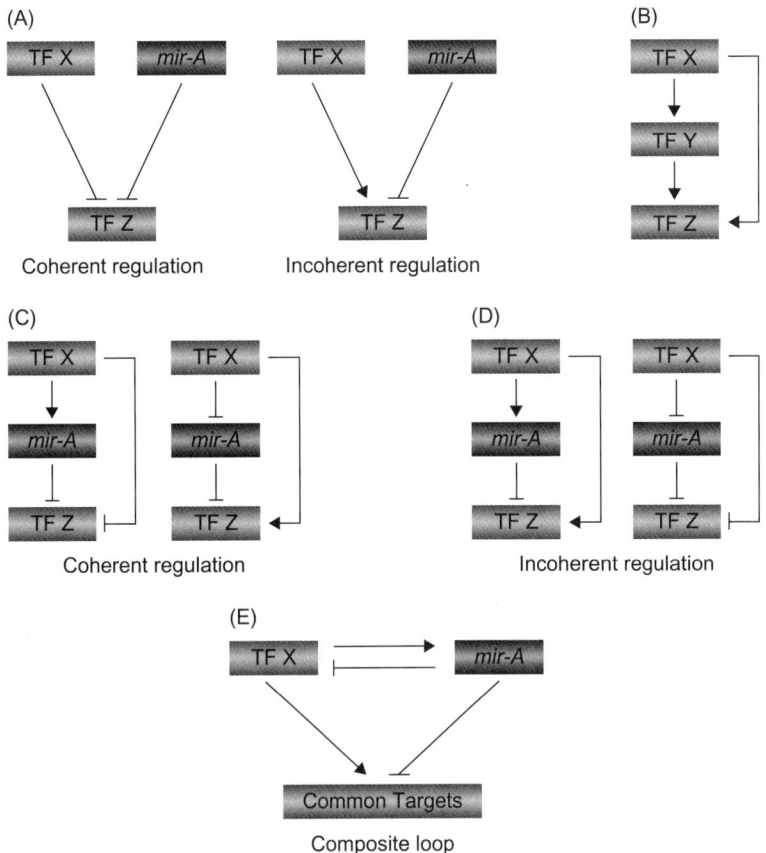

FIGURE 5.5 Network Motifs Comprised of miRNA and Transcription Factor.
(A) The basic feature of co-regulation comprised of a miRNA and a transcription factor pair regulating a common target. When the effect is synergistic, the motif is coherent; when the effect is antagonistic, it is incoherent. (B) Feed-forward loop comprised of transcription factors. (C) and (D) Feed-forward motifs that integrate the function of a miRNA with transcription factors. (E) Composite motif whereby the upstream transcription factor and miRNA pair regulating common targets, also mutually regulates each other.

relationship between the predicted mRNA targets of several tissue-specific miRNAs which tend to be lower in tissues where the miRNAs are expressed (Farh et al., 2005; Sood et al., 2006). Alternatively, a motif may comprise of a miRNA which represses target genes, and at the same time, silences a transcription activator for these common downstream targets (Fig. 5.5E). This forms a composite loop, discussed later.

In contrast, incoherent circuits in which the transcription of miRNAs and their targets are positively (or negatively) co-regulated appear counterintuitive. What is the functional significance of such a design? This form of regulation would appear inefficient because the activation of genes by a transcription factor would be offset by the silencing effects of miRNA (Fig. 5.5D, left panel). If X is repressing the miRNA and downstream target at the same time, the effects of the miRNA would also be antagonized (Fig. 5.5D, right panel). Surprisingly, incoherent circuits seem prevalent, particularly during neural development (Tsang et al., 2007). For instance, the transcription repressor REST, which inhibits the expression of neuronal genes in non-neuronal cells and in neuronal progenitors prior to differentiation (Chong et al., 1995), targets the miRNAs *mir-29* and *mir-135b* (Conaco et al., 2006; Mortazavi et al., 2006). These miRNAs, in turn, are predicted to silence many brain-enriched genes with REST binding sites (Tsang et al., 2007). A logical interpretation would argue that the simultaneous repression of REST-targeted protein-coding genes and the miRNAs which silence these genes is inefficient. However, the absolute requirement for precise temporal control of gene expression levels during the initiation of differentiation whereby a threshold must be maintained could render incoherent circuits useful. As *REST* levels gradually decrease during progenitor differentiation into neuronal phenotypes, it may be possible that functional targets of REST become activated and the transcriptions of *mir-29* and *mir-135b* are subsequently necessary for thresholding the appropriate protein levels of these neuronal genes. The difference in expression timing between the immediate transcription of neuronal mRNAs, and the delayed production and targeting by miRNA, provides a temporal gap. This is relevant during a transition whereby the levels of transcription factor-targeted genes accumulate, and the delayed activation of the miRNA may be timed to obtain a desired thresholding of regulated protein production. In support of this, thresholding has also been observed in circuits comprised solely of transcription factors. In ESCs, *Oct4* is highly expressed. The increased or decreased levels of *Oct4* beyond physiological levels can result in ESCs differentiation into the endoderm or trophectoderm lineages, respectively. Tcf3, another ESC-associated transcription factor, plays a role in repressing and moderating the appropriate levels of *Oct4* (Cole et al., 2008; Tam et al., 2008; Yi et al., 2008a). Interestingly, Oct4 is primarily responsible for activating *Tcf3*, and thereby leading to its own regulation. Such a complex and seemingly counterintuitive mechanism is crucial in determining cell fate, as the loss of *Tcf3* dramatically blocks the ability of ESCs to differentiate (Pereira et al., 2006; Tam et al., 2008).

The intracellular environment of the eukaryotic cell is noisy where transcription occurs in a burst-like manner, causing the mRNA transcript numbers to fluctuate significantly (Blake et al., 2006; Golding et al., 2005; Tsang et al., 2007). And since other regulatory control measures such as mRNA degradation and protein translation are also stochastic, protein levels may fluctuate considerably (Kaern et al., 2005; Raj et al., 2006). The initial burst of transcription events thus produces cumulative fluctuations which are propagated in a ripple-like manner, compromising stability. Hence, miRNAs in incoherent circuits may help determine and maintain protein steady states by buffering the propagation of fluctuations beyond translation. The additional opportunity for gene control created by the emergence of miRNAs appears to represent the evolution of another layer of regulatory mechanism.

Distributing the Load Across Regulatory Fabrics

In feed-forward circuits, multiple inputs as exemplified by transcription factors provide positive signals for ensuring consistent activity in regulating a common gene. This renders it insensitive to transient changes in individual input strength (Mangan and Alon, 2003; Mangan et al., 2003). When target genes are also co-regulated by a miRNA, it has been suggested that such an interaction is crucial for "canalizing" noise in gene expression especially during animal development (Hornstein and Shomron, 2006). Similar to transcription factor-based feed-forward loops comprised of activators and repressors, the integration of miRNAs provides a negative input thus enabling the circuit to behave as a sensor that can respond to the balance of signals. These distal transcription-based and proximal translation-based regulatory features located within gene regulatory networks acts as a "transistor" for receiving and moderating the signals in an overall framework (Fig. 5.6).

What is the advantage of an integrated distal and proximal network compared to distal-only regulation represented by transcription activators and repressors? Feed-forward loops are particularly vital for stem cells to respond rapidly and appropriately to external signals. Emerging evidence has revealed that protein translation and post-translational modifications are important mechanisms that have been overlooked. There are currently unresolved discrepancies between the mRNA and protein profiles of undifferentiated ESCs and their differentiated progeny as the level of gene expression does not necessarily correlate with protein levels observed in the same population (Chang and Stanford, 2008). For instance, the mRNA level of *Wnt1*, involved in the maintenance of several stem cell types, does not alter upon ESC differentiation, but its protein level is reduced (Sampath et al., 2008). A similar discrepancy is observed for *ATF5* and *DCC*, involved in neural development and axonal guidance respectively, whereby protein levels become upregulated while their transcript levels stay constant (Sampath et al., 2008). Part of the explanation may be the differential loading of certain mRNAs to ribosomes which are key components of the translational machinery. However, the basis for preferential mRNA selection remains unclear. Transcript loading of ribosome does not fully support the view that full-length protein production will occur as inhibition can occur downstream during translation. It then becomes interesting to address whether miRNAs have a role in mediating either the loading of specific transcripts to ribosomes or could block their translation progression, as has been postulated. Indeed, during transcription, a parallel observation can be made. Even as most genes experience transcriptional initiation marked epigenetically by the trimethylation of histone 3 lysine 4 (H3K4me3) at DNA promoters,

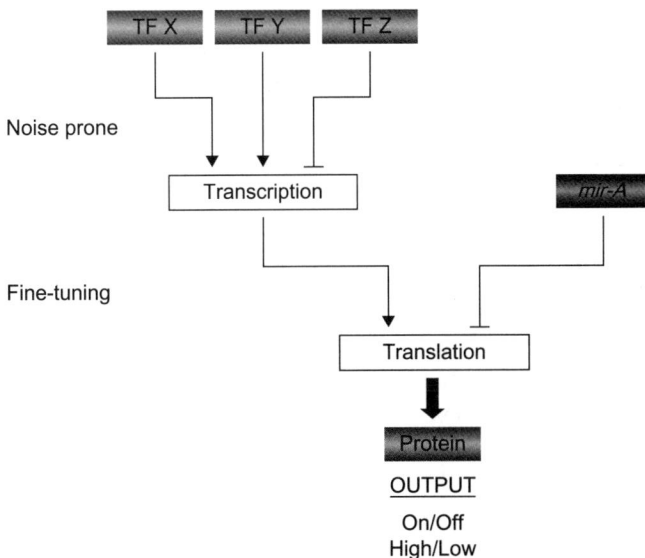

FIGURE 5.6 Fine-Tuning of Protein Output.
Coordinated activity at the levels of mRNA transcription and protein translation precisely control the output of protein either in an on/off or graded manner.

only a subset of these genes produce detectable full-length transcripts (Guenther et al., 2007). The production of these transcripts will require proper elongation which is associated with another epigenetic mark, H3K36me3, along the entire gene.

The production of active proteins, which are the ultimate functional blocks, ensues after transcription. The transcriptional control of gene expression may not respond quickly enough for certain cellular processes. MiRNAs, on the other hand, can directly dictate the levels of protein production and provide a proximal effector. Although miRNA levels are also subject to transcriptional control, several lines of evidence suggest that the combination of distal and proximal regulatory modes is superior. Firstly, the production of miRNA is rapid as these are mature products immediately functional after post-transcriptional processing. This process is rapid compared to the requirement and assembly of the protein translation machinery involving at least dozens of proteins. In ESCs, there is a surplus of free ribosomes actively recruited into translating polysomes during differentiation, supporting the view that the protein synthesis capacity is poised to allow for rapid increment in translation rate (Sampath et al., 2008). This reinforces the notion that post-transcriptional effectors such as miRNAs would be important features for swift response to differentiation signals. Secondly, some observations have suggested that miRNAs may be sequestered in discrete cellular foci termed the P-bodies (Eulalio et al., 2007; Parker and Sheth, 2007). There is a good correlation between miRNA-mediated translational repression, the accumulation of mRNAs and localization of RISC components in these structures (Liu et al., 2005b). The proximal location of miRNAs, mRNAs and P-bodies within the cytoplasm is efficient in coordinating direct protein translation and mRNA decay activities, reducing the lag time between cell stimuli and response. Thirdly, the mode of action conferred by miRNA is mostly reversible, at least in the mammalian system (Bhattacharyya et al., 2006; Schratt et al., 2006). Since miRNA bind their cognate target mRNA with non-perfect complementarity, the transcript remains productive when the corresponding miRNA becomes depleted. In some instances, micro-ribonucleoproteins (miRNPs) which are associated with the miRNA–mRNA complex may even act as translational activators (Vasudevan and Steitz, 2007). This ability to disengage miRNPs from the repressed mRNA, or render them activated, makes the regulatory effects of miRNA more dynamic and wide-ranging. Furthermore, the recycling of miRNA following its interaction with mRNA may be energetically favorable since it potentially skips the requirement for continuous turnover resulting from synthesis and degradation.

Autoregulation

A gene which is regulated through multiple control mechanisms can be tuned at a higher level of precision than what may be achieved from a single mechanism alone (Shalgi et al., 2007). In network motifs, miRNAs and transcription factors may form interconnected loops whereby each mutually regulates the other, in addition to common downstream targets (Fig. 5.5E). These targets may, in turn, feedback into the regulation of upstream factors. When the interaction is activating, it forms a positive feedback that reinforces the circuit; if repressive, a negative feedback that moderates the strength of the input is generated. Therefore, in such complex motifs, can we distinguish the regulator from the regulon?

In ESCs, one example of an autoregulatory motif comprised of the *mir-21* and the transcription factors Nanog and REST. Nanog activates REST, which in turn is responsible for the repression of *mir-21* (Fig. 5.7A). *Mir-21* has been postulated to target *Nanog* for translational inhibition (Singh et al., 2008). Since the depletion of *Nanog* or *REST*, or the overexpression of *mir-21* could result in differentiation, what is the trigger point

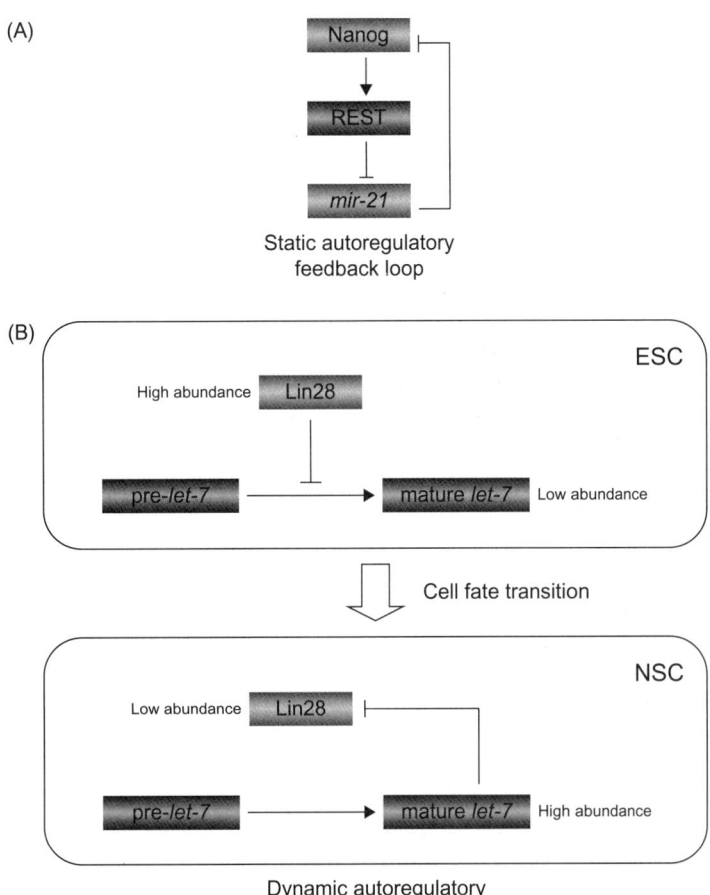

FIGURE 5.7 Autoregulation.
(A) A positive feedback loop where the downstream target *mir-21* regulates the expression of its upstream transcription factor Nanog. "Static" refers the maintenance of the motif in a homeostatic cellular state. The motif breaks down when differentiation is induced as the level of *Nanog* mRNA is depleted. (B) A dynamic autoregulatory loop is formed among the RNA binding protein Lin28, precursor stem-loop *let-7* and mature *let-7*. "Dynamic" refers to the shift in properties of the motif when present in different cell types, or during their transition.

for the cascade of reaction? Based on experimental evidence, the loss of *Nanog* could induce very severe and rapid differentiation whereas the depletion of *REST* or forced expression of *mir-21* causes milder differentiation phenotypes that are not readily noticeable. Nanog is known to activate the expression of many well-known ESC factors which individually is essential for pluripotency. The function of REST, however, appears to be primarily for the repression of neuronal genes; while *mir-21* has been predicted to target other genes such as *Sox2*. Mechanistically, the depletion of *REST* does not induce dramatic downregulation of pluripotency-associated genes since this is not its main function, and *mir-21* is capable of inducing only moderate decrements of *Nanog* and *Sox2*. Therefore, in this network, Nanog is likely the dominant regulator while both REST and *mir-21* are components of the overall pluripotency framework.

Another autoregulatory loop between the RNA binding protein *Lin28* and miRNA *let-7* exists in ESCs and neural stem cells (NSCs) (Fig. 5.7B). ESCs are highly abundant in Lin28, the first reported factor to specifically bind and block the processing of miRNA; in this case, the *let-7* stem-loop precursor (pre-miRNA) (Piskounova et al., 2008; Viswanathan et al., 2008). Interestingly, in NSCs, the opposite is observed. *Lin28* is downregulated by *let-7*, an NSC-specific miRNA, allowing the processing of pre-*let-7* to proceed (Rybak et al., 2008). The suppression of *let-7* leads to the upregulation of *Lin28* and loss of pre-*let-7* processing activity, thus *let-7* and *Lin28* participate in an autoregulatory circuit that controls miRNA processing during ESC commitment to NSC. The dynamic nature of this interaction makes it is difficult to precisely determine whether any trigger point exists. As either overexpressing *let-7* in the presence of *Lin28* or the loss of *Lin28* does not have any apparent effect on ESCs, further tests involving the concomitant depletion of *Lin28* and induction of *let-7*, and *vice versa*, may be required. Possibly, the mediation of a transition state from ESC to NSC could involve a transcription regulator that would trigger the shift of balance in *let-7* levels which occurs through *Lin28*.

Molecular Switches

Combinatorial interaction is a fundamental feature of transcription networks, and prevalent in many metazoans (Yuh et al., 1998). Combinatorial interaction among miRNAs is likely to allow for more accurate control of translation rates. As observed with transcription factors, combinatorial control allows multiple inputs, represented by individual miRNAs, to be integrated into the post-transcriptional regulation of target mRNAs. One approach to decipher this interaction is the analysis of pairs of co-regulating miRNAs which show a high rate of co-occurrence in the 3' UTR of the same target genes. Surprisingly, based on the intersection of the expression data for miRNAs and their predicted regulatory interactions shows a tendency for co-expressed miRNAs to have a high probability of co-occurrence on the same gene (Shalgi et al., 2007).

MicroRNAs can titer the levels of mRNAs and proteins through the graded increase in mRNA degradation or blockade of translation. Since several miRNAs may bind to one mRNA, understanding the extent of combinatorial interactions among miRNAs will provide clues toward the differential control of protein expression. A logical starting point is to identify mRNAs which are extensively targeted by miRNAs, also known as miRNA target hubs (Fig. 5.4). One approach to uncover these "hotspots" is an examination of the number of miRNAs which potentially bind to a common target gene. Based on TargetScan and PicTar predictions, several hundreds of miRNA target hubs can be detected. Gene annotation analyses revealed that many of these are commonly involved in a wide repertoire of developmental processes as well as transcription regulation (Shalgi et al., 2007). This confirms functional studies which point to miRNAs performing roles largely associated with many aspects of development ranging from embryogenesis and cellular differentiation to tissue organization and organogenesis. Parallel to what we know about key transcription factors being heavily regulated by other transcription factors, it is also observed that for these miRNAs target hubs containing genes that exert extensive regulation on crucial process, they themselves are also heavily regulated (Borneman et al., 2006; Shalgi et al., 2007).

The architecture of several miRNAs regulating an mRNA have been coined as a "rheostat" whereby miRNAs fine-tunes the degree of protein translation (Bartel and Chen, 2004). As metazoan miRNAs employ only short stretches of complementarity sequences (Doench and Sharp, 2004;

Lewis et al., 2003), multiple miRNAs might need to be recruited to a particular 3' UTR region for repression. In the rheostat model, each miRNA recognition site represents an individual dimmer switch, which collectively forms an adjustable resistor along the entire UTR (Bartel and Chen, 2004) (Fig. 5.3B). Empirical data in plants and metazoans have shown that target protein expression decreases in response to the presence of a miRNA (Brennecke et al., 2003; Lee et al., 1993; Reinhart et al., 2000; Tay et al., 2008b). In many of these earlier reported instances, the protein levels in metazoan decrease whereas the mRNA levels do not alter in a significant manner, thus resembling a resistor which dampens the flow of current along the electric circuit, but does not extinguish it.

MicroRNA functions were initially discovered through forward genetic approaches that favor dominant phenotypes as these miRNAs such as *lin-4*, can target to seven binding site on the 3' UTR of the *lin-14* mRNA (Lee et al., 1993; Wightman et al., 1993). However, this represents an atypical miRNA–target relationship as the set of miRNAs identified through an obvious loss-of-function phenotype is very small. The majority of mRNAs typically do not have more than one binding site for the same miRNA; fewer than 2% of these targets contain more than two sites (Hornstein and Shomron, 2006; Stark et al., 2005). This requires a re-evaluation to what we perceive the primary function of miRNA to be, and an effort to broadly classify miRNAs according to their ultimate mode of action. Bartel and Chen proposed that miRNAs fall into three categories in terms of their final effects on target gene protein abundance (Bartel and Chen, 2004). The first group comprised of miRNAs which directly act as "on/off" switches for target gene protein production. For example, the translation of *lin-14* is completely blocked by *lin-4* in *C. elegans*, rendering the absence of *lin-14* protein for proper transition of developmental stages. The second class is made up of miRNAs that pair with mRNA by chance. In these interactions, the consequent downregulation of proteins is either tolerated without adverse cellular effects, or the levels are compensated through other routes. These are "neutral" targets that are not subjected to selective pressure in the co-evolution of miRNA–mRNA pairing. The third class consists of miRNAs that dampens protein production, rather than completely eliminating them. This may apply to proteins which are lowly or moderately expressed in specific cell types. Here, the combinatorial use of miRNAs is potentially most interesting.

We can find parallel observations in the epigenetic regulation of transcription activity. The chromatin is made up of DNA coiled around nucleosomes composed of histone octamers. The covalent modifications on histone tails play a major role in determining the transcriptional output of a gene. The diverse combinations of different modifications (methylation, ubiquitination, acetylation and phosphorylation) on the specific amino acid residue of the tail on a particular histone subunit specify the "histone code." In this mechanism, a specific combination of modifications is strongly correlated with the transcription activities of a gene. With transcription, it has also been postulated that various combinations of transcription activators or repressors along the promoter and enhancer elements of a gene help determine the overall output. However, given the large number of transcription factors in a cell type, there exist enormous possibilities on how they may interact either synergistically or antagonistically along a promoter that typically can contain tens to hundreds of transcription factor binding motifs. Furthermore, individual transcription factors often function as part of a larger protein complex, and the different combinations of factors within this complex could have an influence on the activity of a binding site. With the exponential permutations that can be conferred by the combination and interaction amongst transcription factors on the *cis*-regulatory region of genes, a "code" or "set of rules" for predicting transcriptional activity and output has not been forthcoming. This is discussed in this volume (Chapter 7) by Ng et al.

Deciphering the Rules for a miRNA Switch

With our extensive knowledge of epigenetic and transcription regulation, can we begin to formulate any general rules for the combinatorial outcome of miRNA silencing? Several notions being unraveled about miRNA activities provide interesting possibilities. In comparison to transcription factors which may be activating or repressive, the effect of miRNA on the mRNA is largely repressive. Although one report suggests that a miRNA can upregulate translation in very specific instances (Vasudevan et al., 2007), this appears to be an exception. The association of one or multiple miRNAs on an mRNA will accordingly cause translational repression, or mRNA degradation, leading to a net loss in protein production. The degree of complementarity of miRNA to target sequences helps determine whether transcript degradation will occur. Several examples have shown that near-perfect complementarity of at least one miRNA on the 3'UTR is sufficient to cause transcript elimination, resulting in a drastic fall in protein output. It is unclear how the net repressive effect is determined when multiple miRNAs pair an mRNA with non-perfect complementarity, but numerous experimental instances support the view that a single pairing event is sufficient to block translation. Therefore, a *bona fide* miRNA–mRNA pairing will at least result in blockade of translation.

In contrast to transcription factors which have the ability to form larger complexes that interact in *trans* with DNA, miRNAs are not known to associate with each other. Each RISC carries one miRNA molecule, reducing the complexity in which it becomes specifically recruited to mRNA. As most mRNAs contain a distinct 3' UTR, the amount of potential regulatory material is limited. This differs from the DNA promoter of most genes which are poorly characterized, and further confounded by enhancers which may lie at vast distances away from the regulated gene. Not surprisingly, it has been observed that the length of 3' UTR is somewhat correlated to the number of miRNA binding sites, although high densities of these sites have also been found for a handful of shorter UTRs (Shalgi et al., 2007). This, again, supports the notion that certain classes of genes especially developmental and transcription regulators, which can exert far-reaching effects, are themselves extensively regulated.

There remain several outstanding questions pertaining to the discovery of ground rules for miRNA-mediated gene regulation. Firstly, does the nucleotide distance between two miRNA binding sites affect the degree of translational repression? As some sequence-specific transcription factors which dimerize require recognition motifs at a definite number of base pairs separations on DNA, it becomes relevant to determine whether the proximity of several miRNA binding sites is more efficient at blocking translation. Furthermore, whether translational inhibition occurs through the blockade of translational initiation (Humphreys et al., 2005), elongation (Nottrott et al., 2006), sequestration of Argonaute-bound mRNA into P-body (Liu et al., 2005a, 2005b), or other mechanisms, remains an area of controversy. Secondly, what is the link between miRNPs and their recognition to specific miRNAs, as well as their subsequent influence on the translational machinery? MiRNAs have been described to be associated with RNP complexes in several cell types, but the function of these complexes is unclear (Barbee et al., 2006; Dostie et al., 2003; Mourelatos et al., 2002). Given the uncharacterized function of most RNPs, investigations into their interaction with miRNAs, and the systematic dissection of components present in these complexes through methods such as miRNP immunopurification

(Easow et al., 2007; Keene et al., 2006), will help advance our understanding on miRNA-mediated translational inhibition. Thirdly, is the secondary structure of the mRNA, particularly of the 3′ UTR, relevant to the efficient recruitment of miRNA? A wealth of studies has indicated that in the context of chromatin, covalent modifications to nucleotides on the DNA or histones affect the permissiveness of recruiting transcription factors and the basal transcription machinery. It will be important to investigate if a parallel scenario exists for miRNA recruitment to mRNA in a structure-dependent manner. mRNAs contain structural elements that are involved in specifying post-transcriptional regulations such as differential mRNA decay rates (Wang et al., 2002). This may be mediated through binding preferences of RNA binding proteins as exemplified by the iron-responsive element, a secondary structure RNA motif located on the UTRs of genes involved in iron metabolism (Hentze et al., 2004). Secondary structure contributes to target recognition because it involves an energetic cost to freeing base pairing interactions within mRNA so as to make the target site accessible to miRNA (Long et al., 2007; Robins et al., 2005; Vella et al., 2004). It has indeed been reported that site accessibility has a significant effect on miRNA interactions as miRNA seed regions show a preference for highly accessible regions along the mRNA (Kertesz et al., 2007).

THE ROADMAP TO SYSTEMS BIOLOGY: DECONVOLUTING COMPLEXITIES

The roadmap toward understanding the intricacies of miRNA and transcription regulation has numerous unresolved challenges. Even as the conventional thinking prescribes that miRNAs have roles restricted to 3′ UTR silencing, emerging evidence suggests they could target other portions of the mRNA. Exploiting the sensitivity of ESCs to perturbations in mRNAs of key pluripotency-associated genes, one study has postulated that miRNA binding sites could occur in the coding region of *Nanog*, *Oct4* and *Sox2* (Tay et al., 2008a). The use of rna22 to predict binding sites for *mir-296*, *mir-470* and *mir-134* on these mRNAs is ideal because the algorithm does not require validated targets for training and does not rely on cross-species conservation for prediction (Miranda et al., 2006). Consistent with the possibility of multiple miRNA binding sites on 3′ UTR, it is shown that both *mir-296* and *mir-470* could simultaneously target the *Nanog* mRNA coding region in as many as two and six binding sites, respectively. There are three *mir-470* sites on *Oct4* and five *mir-134* sites on *Sox2*. Individual or simultaneous introduction of miRNAs into ESCs dramatically blocked the translation of the targeted gene, and resulted in ESC differentiation. This observation of a broader and far-reaching effect of miRNA action is supported by another study highlighting miRNA binding to 5′ UTR binding sites, and repressing translation as efficiently as 3′ UTR (Lytle et al., 2007). However, a recent report examining the impact of miRNA on global protein output reveals that translationally repressed mRNAs show strong enrichment for seed-matched motif in the 3′ UTRs, but not 5′ UTRs or coding regions (Baek et al., 2008). The reason for this discrepancy is unclear. One possibility could be both 3′ and 5′ UTRs are utilized but there is a predominance for target repression associated with 3′ UTR. It is not known for this particular miRNA if the 3′ UTR targeted mRNAs also contain binding sites for other regions, and not confined to the seed sequence.

Another confounding question which adds complexity is the spatial and temporal control of miRNA interaction on an mRNA. Although mRNAs contain a range of recognition sequences for different miRNAs, not all miRNAs will be expressed at the same time. This composition of miRNAs in different cell types expressing a subset of common mRNAs also differs. Therefore, how is the differential use of miRNA target sites determined? One factor could be the co-occurrence of miRNAs with their targets. However, as one mRNA may be targeted by several miRNAs, it is unclear what subset of miRNAs is needed to achieve repression. On a global level, it becomes harder to determine dominant vs. weak interactions as a result of constant flux in the expression of both miRNAs and their targets. For example, during cell fate transition when mRNA populations shift in abundance from high to low, do the targeting miRNAs which remain subsequently alter their preference for binding sites on other genes? This is an important experimental consideration because the majority of biological studies have relied on the artificial introduction of synthetic miRNAs into cells at dosages beyond physiological thresholds to elicit a phenotypic change. It is argued that such "misexpression" has the potential to regulate many targets that it might never encounter in its endogenous expression domain (Bushati and Cohen, 2007). Perhaps, a more precise approach would be the conditional deletion of a miRNA by gene targeting in tissues of interest, exemplified in several studies (Couzin, 2007; Johnnidis et al., 2008; Rodriguez et al., 2007; van Rooij et al., 2007; Xiao et al., 2007).

A comprehensive understanding of miRNA function and its interaction with transcription factors cannot be obtained without clear knowledge of the complete number of miRNAs. There is indeed a growing number of previously unreported miRNAs in the different organisms (Griffiths-Jones, 2004). The discovery of novel miRNAs traditionally relied on cloning of cDNA libraries from small RNAs supported by genomic analysis and detection through northern blotting (Berezikov et al., 2006c; Kloosterman et al., 2006; Lagos-Quintana et al., 2001, 2003). The advent of sequencing technologies and more comprehensive genome maps has accelerated the pace of reporting new miRNA species (Berezikov et al., 2006b; Landgraf et al., 2007). Computation approaches have also been employed to predict novel miRNAs through pattern discovery and surveying the genomic landscape to recognize a set of distinctive miRNA features (Bentwich et al., 2005; Miranda et al., 2006). Given the increasing number of miRNAs, the emerging challenge then is to verify whether these are physiologically relevant, or at least respond to cellular perturbation. We further need to consider the extent of mRNA regulation by these miRNAs, as well as the regulation of their expression by transcription factors.

Finally, the recent discovery that the production of a mature miRNA from the precursor miRNA is exclusively controlled provides important insights into a new level of miRNA regulation. Since Lin28 can bind specifically to *let-7* at the stem-loop sequence and block processing (Viswanathan et al., 2008), are other miRNAs similarly regulated by the vast repertoire of RNA binding proteins? It would be worthwhile to compare the profiles of precursor and mature miRNAs, along with the expression of RNA binding proteins. Perhaps, in our attempt to understand the transcription regulation of mature miRNA expression, we could be missing an entire layer of control mechanism. And, since several miRNAs appear associated with disease, the selective blockade of their processing to mature functional miRNA could have significant therapeutic potential. This strategy would be superior to the use of miRNA anti-sense molecules that may behave as short interfering RNA which targets biologically important genes in a non-specific manner.

CONCLUDING REMARKS

The interface between miRNAs and transcription factor networks presents a new frontier toward the comprehensive understanding of the molecular architecture of the cell. Over the next decade, we will begin to appreciate the significance of miRNA–transcription network interactions in several clinically important areas. What is the extent of miRNA contribution to human disease? The miRNA gene signatures in diseases that affect the cardiovascular (Care et al., 2007; Yang et al., 2007), nervous (Kim et al., 2007) and immune systems(Baltimore et al., 2008; Xiao et al., 2008) have been reported. The association of miRNA with cancers remains an intensively studied area. The *mir-17~92* cluster (Dews et al., 2006; He et al., 2005), *mir-372/373* (Voorhoeve et al., 2006) and *mir-155* (Tam and Dahlberg, 2006) are implicated as oncogenes in lymphomas and testicular cancers while the deletion of *mir-15* and *mir-16* is frequent in cases of chronic lymphatic leukemia (Calin et al., 2005). The *let-7* family appears to have extensive tumor suppressive roles in many cancers (Johnson et al., 2005; Mayr et al., 2007). The tumor suppressor *p53* has been at the center of a complex molecular network regulating responses to the initiation and progression of cancer. This network previously consisted of solely protein-coding genes that act upstream or downstream of p53 activity (Vogelstein et al., 2000; Zhao et al., 2000). Recent investigations has connected *mir-34* family to the p53 network, and provided a glimpse into the interplay between transcription regulators and miRNAs in oncogenesis. Findings revealed that members of *mir-34* family are direct transcriptional targets of p53, and significantly, *mir-34* activation can recapitulate elements of p53 activity that includes cell cycle arrest and apoptosis (Chang et al., 2007; He et al., 2007; Raver-Shapira et al., 2007). Consistent with miRNA function, the induction of *mir-34* downregulates hundreds of mRNAs enriched for cell cycle genes, directly or indirectly through other pathways. This model creates a useful framework for which the connectivity of miRNAs into the oncogenic pathway can be examined.

In regenerative medicine, a major challenge is the generation of patient-compatible stem cells for cell therapy. The use of existing stem cell lines presents the risks of immune-incompatibility, exposure to xeno-pathogens and chromosome instability as a result of long-term culture. In a major breakthrough, the induction of pluripotent stem (iPS) cells directly from primary somatic cells using a defined cocktail of factors, comprised mainly of transcription regulators, has been demonstrated. The generation of iPS cells entails viral integration of genes with oncogenic potential such as *c-Myc*, *n-Myc*, *Klf4* and *Oct4* (Park et al., 2008; Takahashi et al., 2007; Takahashi and Yamanaka, 2006; Yamanaka, 2007). Viral-based gene therapy further exposes patients to the risk of leukemia and represents a bottleneck for the treatment of other diseases as well. Hence, ongoing efforts have focused on the identification of small molecules that includes miRNA, for the re-programming of somatic cells to stem cells. A starting point would be to identify miRNAs which are activated by these re-programming transcription factors. Remarkably, the *mir-302* family, which is under the influence of key ESC regulators, could re-program human skin cancer cells into an ESC-like state (Lin et al., 2008). Presumably, the deciphering of other similarly regulated miRNAs could improve the process.

The use of miRNAs as anti-tumorigenic agents in cancer and as re-programming factors for generating stem cells highlights the value of miRNAs as therapeutic agents. The major advantage is that these small molecules can be chemically synthesized and modified to have long half-life. They may also be easier to administer owing to their size and stability. Even as more effective methods for overexpressing or ablating miRNAs, and their *in vitro* delivery are being developed, there are instances of efficient delivery of "anti-miRs" *in vivo* either systematically or locally that resulted in silencing of targeted miRNAs (Esau et al., 2006; Krutzfeldt et al., 2005, 2007). Arguably, the side effects associated with miRNA as a drug may be easier to predict because these are sequence-specific molecules. A refined understanding of the rules that governs miRNA targeting of transcription regulators will be valuable in overcoming off-target effects.

This will also require us to distinguish real physiological interactions from non-specific ones resulting from miRNA misexpression. The miRNA–transcription factor interface forms only one component of gene regulation. How this interface interacts with cellular processes that include epigenetic regulation, protein–protein network, post-translational modification of protein activity and specificity of miRNA processing, are crucial areas where deeper understanding is needed.

References

Ambros, V., 2004. The functions of animal microRNAs. Nature 431, 350–355.

Andl, T., Murchison, E.P., Liu, F., et al., 2006. The miRNA-processing enzyme dicer is essential for the morphogenesis and maintenance of hair follicles. Curr. Biol. 16, 1041–1049.

Aravin, A., Gaidatzis, D., Pfeffer, S., et al., 2006. A novel class of small RNAs bind to MILI protein in mouse testes. Nature 442, 203–207.

Baek, D., Villen, J., Shin, C., Camargo, F.D., Gygi, S.P., Bartel, D.P., 2008. The impact of microRNAs on protein output. Nature 455, 64–71.

Baltimore, D., Boldin, M.P., O'Connell, R.M., Rao, D.S., Taganov, K.D., 2008. MicroRNAs: new regulators of immune cell development and function. Nat. Immunol. 9, 839–845.

Barbee, S.A., Estes, P.S., Cziko, A.M., et al., 2006. Staufen- and FMRP-containing neuronal RNPs are structurally and functionally related to somatic P bodies. Neuron 52, 997–1009.

Bartel, D.P., Chen, C.Z., 2004. Micromanagers of gene expression: the potentially widespread influence of metazoan microRNAs. Nat. Rev. Genet. 5, 396–400.

Bentwich, I., Avniel, A., Karov, Y., et al., 2005. Identification of hundreds of conserved and nonconserved human microRNAs. Nat. Genet. 37, 766–770.

Berezikov, E., Cuppen, E., Plasterk, R.H., 2006a. Approaches to microRNA discovery. Nat. Genet. 38 (Suppl.), S2–S7.

Berezikov, E., Thuemmler, F., van Laake, L.W., et al., 2006b. Diversity of microRNAs in human and chimpanzee brain. Nat. Genet. 38, 1375–1377.

Berezikov, E., van Tetering, G., Verheul, M., et al., 2006c. Many novel mammalian microRNA candidates identified by extensive cloning and RAKE analysis. Genome Res. 16, 1289–1298.

Bhattacharyya, S.N., Habermacher, R., Martine, U., Closs, E.I., Filipowicz, W., 2006. Relief of microRNA-mediated translational repression in human cells subjected to stress. Cell 125, 1111–1124.

Blake, W.J., Balazsi, G., Kohanski, M.A., et al., 2006. Phenotypic consequences of promoter-mediated transcriptional noise. Mol. Cell 24, 853–865.

Borneman, A.R., Leigh-Bell, J.A., Yu, H., Bertone, P., Gerstein, M., Snyder, M., 2006. Target hub proteins serve as master regulators of development in yeast. Genes Dev. 20, 435–448.

Boyer, L.A., Lee, T.I., Cole, M.F., et al., 2005. Core transcriptional regulatory circuitry in human embryonic stem cells. Cell 122, 947–956.

Boyer, L.A., Plath, K., Zeitlinger, J., et al., 2006. Polycomb complexes repress developmental regulators in murine embryonic stem cells. Nature 441, 349–353.

Brennecke, J., Hipfner, D.R., Stark, A., Russell, R.B., Cohen, S.M., 2003. Bantam encodes a developmentally regulated microRNA that controls cell proliferation and regulates the proapoptotic gene hid in Drosophila. Cell 113, 25–36.

Brennecke, J., Stark, A., Russell, R.B., Cohen, S.M., 2005. Principles of microRNA-target recognition. PLoS Biol. 3, e85.

Bushati, N., Cohen, S.M., 2007. microRNA functions. Annu. Rev. Cell Dev. Biol. 23, 175–205.

Calin, G.A., Sevignani, C., Dumitru, C.D., et al., 2004. Human microRNA genes are frequently located at fragile sites and genomic regions involved in cancers. Proc. Natl. Acad. Sci. U.S.A. 101, 2999–3004.

Calin, G.A., Ferracin, M., Cimmino, A., et al., 2005. A microRNA signature associated with prognosis and progression in chronic lymphocytic leukemia. N. Engl. J. Med. 353, 1793–1801.

Care, A., Catalucci, D., Felicetti, F., et al., 2007. MicroRNA-133 controls cardiac hypertrophy. Nat. Med. 13, 613–618.

Chang, W.Y., Stanford, W.L., 2008. Translational control: a new dimension in embryonic stem cell network analysis. Cell Stem Cell 2, 410–412.

Chang Jr., S., Johnston, R.J., Frokjaer-Jensen, C., Lockery, S., Hobert, O., 2004. MicroRNAs act sequentially and asymmetrically to control chemosensory laterality in the nematode. Nature 430, 785–789.

Chang, T.C., Wentzel, E.A., Kent, O.A., et al., 2007. Transactivation of mir-34a by p53 broadly influences gene expression and promotes apoptosis. Mol. Cell 26, 745–752.

Chen, C.Z., Li, L., Lodish, H.F., Bartel, D.P., 2004. MicroRNAs modulate hematopoietic lineage differentiation. Science 303, 83–86.

Chen, X., Xu, H., Yuan, P., et al., 2008. Integration of external signaling pathways with the core transcriptional network in embryonic stem cells. Cell 133, 1106–1117.

Chendrimada, T.P., Gregory, R.I., Kumaraswamy, E., et al., 2005. TRBP recruits the Dicer complex to Ago2 for

REFERENCES

microRNA processing and gene silencing. Nature 436, 740–744.

Chong, J.A., Tapia-Ramirez, J., Kim, S., et al., 1995. REST: a mammalian silencer protein that restricts sodium channel gene expression to neurons. Cell 80, 949–957.

Cimmino, A., Calin, G.A., Fabbri, M., et al., 2005. mir-15 and mir-16 induce apoptosis by targeting BCL2. Proc. Natl. Acad. Sci. U. S. A. 102, 13944–13949.

Cole, M.F., Johnstone, S.E., Newman, J.J., Kagey, M.H., Young, R.A., 2008. Tcf3 is an integral component of the core regulatory circuitry of embryonic stem cells. Genes Dev. 22, 746–755.

Conaco, C., Otto, S., Han, J.J., Mandel, G., 2006. Reciprocal actions of REST and a microRNA promote neuronal identity. Proc. Natl. Acad. Sci. U. S. A. 103, 2422–2427.

Couzin, J., 2007. Genetics. Erasing microRNAs reveals their powerful punch. Science 316, 530.

Dews, M., Homayouni, A., Yu, D., et al., 2006. Augmentation of tumor angiogenesis by a Myc-activated microRNA cluster. Nat. Genet. 38, 1060–1065.

Doench, J.G., Sharp, P.A., 2004. Specificity of microRNA target selection in translational repression. Genes Dev. 18, 504–511.

Doench, J.G., Petersen, C.P., Sharp, P.A., 2003. siRNAs can function as miRNAs. Genes Dev. 17, 438–442.

Dostie, J., Mourelatos, Z., Yang, M., Sharma, A., Dreyfuss, G., 2003. Numerous microRNPs in neuronal cells containing novel microRNAs. RNA 9, 180–186.

Easow, G., Teleman, A.A., Cohen, S.M., 2007. Isolation of microRNA targets by miRNP immunopurification. RNA 13, 1198–1204.

Edmondson, D.G., Olson, E.N., 1989. A gene with homology to the myc similarity region of MyoD1 is expressed during myogenesis and is sufficient to activate the muscle differentiation program. Genes Dev. 3, 628–640.

Enright, A.J., John, B., Gaul, U., Tuschl, T., Sander, C., Marks, D.S., 2003. MicroRNA targets in Drosophila. Genome Biol. 5, R1.

Esau, C., Davis, S., Murray, S.F., et al., 2006. mir-122 regulation of lipid metabolism revealed by in vivo antisense targeting. Cell Metab. 3, 87–98.

Eulalio, A., Behm-Ansmant, I., Izaurralde, E., 2007. P bodies: at the crossroads of post-transcriptional pathways. Nat. Rev. Mol. Cell Biol. 8, 9–22.

Farh, K.K., Grimson, A., Jan, C., et al., 2005. The widespread impact of mammalian microRNAs on mRNA repression and evolution. Science 310, 1817–1821.

Filipowicz, W., Bhattacharyya, S.N., Sonenberg, N., 2008. Mechanisms of post-transcriptional regulation by microRNAs: are the answers in sight?. Nat. Rev. Genet. 9, 102–114.

Golding, I., Paulsson, J., Zawilski, S.M., Cox, E.C., 2005. Real-time kinetics of gene activity in individual bacteria. Cell 123, 1025–1036.

Gregory, R.I., Yan, K.P., Amuthan, G., et al., 2004. The Microprocessor complex mediates the genesis of microRNAs. Nature 432, 235–240.

Gregory, R.I., Chendrimada, T.P., Cooch, N., Shiekhattar, R., 2005. Human RISC couples microRNA biogenesis and posttranscriptional gene silencing. Cell 123, 631–640.

Griffiths-Jones, S., 2004. The microRNA registry. Nucleic Acids Res. 32, D109–D111.

Guenther, M.G., Levine, S.S., Boyer, L.A., Jaenisch, R., Young, R.A., 2007. A chromatin landmark and transcription initiation at most promoters in human cells. Cell 130, 77–88.

Hammell, M., Long, D., Zhang, L., et al., 2008. mirWIP: microRNA target prediction based on microRNA-containing ribonucleoprotein-enriched transcripts. Nat. Methods.

Han, J., Lee, Y., Yeom, K.H., Kim, Y.K., Jin, H., Kim, V.N., 2004. The Drosha-DGCR8 complex in primary microRNA processing. Genes Dev. 18, 3016–3027.

Han, J., Lee, Y., Yeom, K.H., et al., 2006. Molecular basis for the recognition of primary microRNAs by the Drosha–DGCR8 complex. Cell 125, 887–901.

He, L., Thomson, J.M., Hemann, M.T., et al., 2005. A microRNA polycistron as a potential human oncogene. Nature 435, 828–833.

He, L., He, X., Lim, L.P., et al., 2007. A microRNA component of the p53 tumour suppressor network. Nature 447, 1130–1134.

Hentze, M.W., Muckenthaler, M.U., Andrews, N.C., 2004. Balancing acts: molecular control of mammalian iron metabolism. Cell 117, 285–297.

Hornstein, E., Shomron, N., 2006. Canalization of development by microRNAs. Nat. Genet. 38 (Suppl.), S20–S24.

Houbaviy, H.B., Murray, M.F., Sharp, P.A., 2003. Embryonic stem cell-specific microRNAs. Dev. Cell 5, 351–358.

Houbaviy, H.B., Dennis, L., Jaenisch, R., Sharp, P.A., 2005. Characterization of a highly variable eutherian microRNA gene. RNA 11, 1245–1257.

Huang, J.C., Babak, T., Corson, T.W., et al., 2007a. Using expression profiling data to identify human microRNA targets. Nat. Methods 4, 1045–1049.

Huang, J.C., Morris, Q.D., Frey, B.J., 2007b. Bayesian inference of microRNA targets from sequence and expression data. J. Comput. Biol. 14, 550–563.

Humphreys, D.T., Westman, B.J., Martin, D.I., Preiss, T., 2005. MicroRNAs control translation initiation by inhibiting eukaryotic initiation factor 4E/cap and poly(A) tail function. Proc. Natl. Acad. Sci. U. S. A. 102, 16961–16966.

Hutvagner, G., McLachlan, J., Pasquinelli, A.E., Balint, E., Tuschl, T., Zamore, P.D., 2001. A cellular function for the RNA-interference enzyme Dicer in the maturation of the let-7 small temporal RNA. Science 293, 834–838.

Ivey, K.N., Muth, A., Arnold, J., et al., 2008. MicroRNA regulation of cell lineages in mouse and human embryonic stem cells. Cell Stem Cell 2, 219–229.

Jiang, J., Chan, Y.S., Loh, Y.H., et al., 2008. A core Klf circuitry regulates self-renewal of embryonic stem cells. Nat. Cell Biol. 10, 353–360.

John, B., Enright, A.J., Aravin, A., Tuschl, T., Sander, C., Marks, D.S., 2004. Human microRNA targets. PLoS Biol. 2, e363.

Johnnidis, J.B., Harris, M.H., Wheeler, R.T., et al., 2008. Regulation of progenitor cell proliferation and granulocyte function by microRNA-223. Nature 451, 1125–1129.

Johnson, S.M., Grosshans, H., Shingara, J., et al., 2005. RAS is regulated by the let-7 microRNA family. Cell 120, 635–647.

Johnston, R.J., Hobert, O., 2003. A microRNA controlling left/right neuronal asymmetry in Caenorhabditis elegans. Nature 426, 845–849.

Kaern, M., Elston, T.C., Blake, W.J., Collins, J.J., 2005. Stochasticity in gene expression: from theories to phenotypes. Nat. Rev. Genet. 6, 451–464.

Kanellopoulou, C., Muljo, S.A., Kung, A.L., et al., 2005. Dicer-deficient mouse embryonic stem cells are defective in differentiation and centromeric silencing. Genes Dev. 19, 489–501.

Keene, J.D., Komisarow, J.M., Friedersdorf, M.B., 2006. RIP-Chip: the isolation and identification of mRNAs, microRNAs and protein components of ribonucleoprotein complexes from cell extracts. Nat. Protoc. 1, 302–307.

Kertesz, M., Iovino, N., Unnerstall, U., Gaul, U., Segal, E., 2007. The role of site accessibility in microRNA target recognition. Nat. Genet. 39, 1278–1284.

Ketting, R.F., Fischer, S.E., Bernstein, E., Sijen, T., Hannon, G.J., Plasterk, R.H., 2001. Dicer functions in RNA interference and in synthesis of small RNA involved in developmental timing in C. elegans. Genes Dev. 15, 2654–2659.

Kim, J., Inoue, K., Ishii, J., et al., 2007. A microRNA feedback circuit in midbrain dopamine neurons. Science 317, 1220–1224.

Kim, J., Chu, J., Shen, X., Wang, J., Orkin, S.H., 2008. An extended transcriptional network for pluripotency of embryonic stem cells. Cell 132, 1049–1061.

Kiriakidou, M., Nelson, P.T., Kouranov, A., et al., 2004. A combined computational–experimental approach predicts human microRNA targets. Genes Dev. 18, 1165–1178.

Kloosterman, W.P., Steiner, F.A., Berezikov, E., et al., 2006. Cloning and expression of new microRNAs from zebrafish. Nucleic Acids Res. 34, 2558–2569.

Koralov, S.B., Muljo, S.A., Galler, G.R., et al., 2008. Dicer ablation affects antibody diversity and cell survival in the B lymphocyte lineage. Cell 132, 860–874.

Krek, A., Grun, D., Poy, M.N., et al., 2005. Combinatorial microRNA target predictions. Nat. Genet. 37, 495–500.

Krutzfeldt, J., Rajewsky, N., Braich, R., et al., 2005. Silencing of microRNAs in vivo with "antagomirs". Nature 438, 685–689.

Krutzfeldt, J., Kuwajima, S., Braich, R., et al., 2007. Specificity, duplex degradation and subcellular localization of antagomirs. Nucleic Acids Res. 35, 2885–2892.

Lagos-Quintana, M., Rauhut, R., Lendeckel, W., Tuschl, T., 2001. Identification of novel genes coding for small expressed RNAs. Science 294, 853–858.

Lagos-Quintana, M., Rauhut, R., Meyer, J., Borkhardt, A., Tuschl, T., 2003. New microRNAs from mouse and human. RNA 9, 175–179.

Landgraf, P., Rusu, M., Sheridan, R., et al., 2007. A mammalian microRNA expression atlas based on small RNA library sequencing. Cell 129, 1401–1414.

Laurent, L.C., Chen, J., Ulitsky, I., et al., 2008. Comprehensive microRNA profiling reveals a unique human embryonic stem cell signature dominated by a single seed sequence. Stem Cells 26, 1506–1516.

Lee, R.C., Feinbaum, R.L., Ambros, V., 1993. The C. elegans heterochronic gene lin-4 encodes small RNAs with antisense complementarity to lin-14. Cell 75, 843–854.

Lee, T.I., Jenner, R.G., Boyer, L.A., et al., 2006. Control of developmental regulators by Polycomb in human embryonic stem cells. Cell 125, 301–313.

Lee, Y., Kim, M., Han, J., et al., 2004. MicroRNA genes are transcribed by RNA polymerase II. EMBO J. 23, 4051–4060.

Lewis, B.P., Shih, I.H., Jones-Rhoades, M.W., Bartel, D.P., Burge, C.B., 2003. Prediction of mammalian microRNA targets. Cell 115, 787–798.

Lewis, B.P., Burge, C.B., Bartel, D.P., 2005. Conserved seed pairing, often flanked by adenosines, indicates that thousands of human genes are microRNA targets. Cell 120, 15–20.

Li, Q., Gregory, R.I., 2008. MicroRNA regulation of stem cell fate. Cell Stem Cell 2, 195–196.

Lim, L.P., Lau, N.C., Garrett-Engele, P., et al., 2005. Microarray analysis shows that some microRNAs downregulate large numbers of target mRNAs. Nature 433, 769–773.

Lin, S.L., Chang, D.C., Chang-Lin, S., et al., 2008. Mir-302 reprograms human skin cancer cells into a pluripotent ES-cell-like state. RNA 14, 2115–2124.

Liu III., J., Rivas, F.V., Wohlschlegel, J., Yates, J.R., Parker, R., Hannon, G.J., 2005a. A role for the P-body component GW182 in microRNA function. Nat. Cell Biol. 7, 1261–1266.

Liu, J., Valencia-Sanchez, M.A., Hannon, G.J., Parker, R., 2005b. MicroRNA-dependent localization of targeted mRNAs to mammalian P-bodies. Nat. Cell Biol. 7, 719–723.

Loh, Y.H., Wu, Q., Chew, J.L., et al., 2006. The Oct4 and Nanog transcription network regulates pluripotency in mouse embryonic stem cells. Nat. Genet. 38, 431–440.

Long, D., Lee, R., Williams, P., Chan, C.Y., Ambros, V., Ding, Y., 2007. Potent effect of target structure on microRNA function. Nat. Struct. Mol. Biol. 14, 287–294.

Lu, J., Getz, G., Miska, E.A., et al., 2005. MicroRNA expression profiles classify human cancers. Nature 435, 834–838.

Lund, E., Guttinger, S., Calado, A., Dahlberg, J.E., Kutay, U., 2004. Nuclear export of microRNA precursors. Science 303, 95–98.

Lytle, J.R., Yario, T.A., Steitz, J.A., 2007. Target mRNAs are repressed as efficiently by microRNA-binding sites in the 5′ UTR as in the 3′ UTR. Proc. Natl. Acad. Sci. U. S. A. 104, 9667–9672.

Ma, Q., Kintner, C., Anderson, D.J., 1996. Identification of neurogenin, a vertebrate neuronal determination gene. Cell 87, 43–52.

Mangan, S., Alon, U., 2003. Structure and function of the feed-forward loop network motif. Proc. Natl. Acad. Sci. U. S. A. 100, 11980–11985.

Mangan, S., Zaslaver, A., Alon, U., 2003. The coherent feed-forward loop serves as a sign-sensitive delay element in transcription networks. J. Mol. Biol. 334, 197–204.

Maniataki, E., Mourelatos, Z., 2005. A human, ATP-independent, RISC assembly machine fueled by pre-miRNA. Genes Dev. 19, 2979–2990.

Marson, A., Levine, S.S., Cole, M.F., et al., 2008. Connecting microRNA genes to the core transcriptional regulatory circuitry of embryonic stem cells. Cell 134, 521–533.

Mayr, C., Hemann, M.T., Bartel, D.P., 2007. Disrupting the pairing between let-7 and Hmga2 enhances oncogenic transformation. Science 315, 1576–1579.

Meister, G., Tuschl, T., 2004. Mechanisms of gene silencing by double-stranded RNA. Nature 431, 343–349.

Meister, G., Landthaler, M., Dorsett, Y., Tuschl, T., 2004. Sequence-specific inhibition of microRNA- and siRNA-induced RNA silencing. RNA 10, 544–550.

Milo, R., Shen-Orr, S., Itzkovitz, S., Kashtan, N., Chklovskii, D., Alon, U., 2002. Network motifs: simple building blocks of complex networks. Science 298, 824–827.

Miranda, K.C., Huynh, T., Tay, Y., et al., 2006. A pattern-based method for the identification of MicroRNA binding sites and their corresponding heteroduplexes. Cell 126, 1203–1217.

Mortazavi, A., Leeper Thompson, E.C., Garcia, S.T., et al., 2006. Comparative genomics modeling of the NRSF/REST repressor network: from single conserved sites to genome-wide repertoire. Genome Res. 16, 1208–1221.

Mourelatos, Z., Dostie, J., Paushkin, S., et al., 2002. miRNPs: a novel class of ribonucleoproteins containing numerous microRNAs. Genes Dev. 16, 720–728.

Muljo, S.A., Ansel, K.M., Kanellopoulou, C., Livingston, D.M., Rao, A., Rajewsky, K., 2005. Aberrant T cell differentiation in the absence of Dicer. J. Exp. Med. 202, 261–269.

Murchison, E.P., Partridge, J.F., Tam, O.H., Cheloufi, S., Hannon, G.J., 2005. Characterization of Dicer-deficient murine embryonic stem cells. Proc. Natl. Acad. Sci. U. S. A. 102, 12135–12140.

Murchison, E.P., Stein, P., Xuan, Z., et al., 2007. Critical roles for Dicer in the female germline. Genes Dev. 21, 682–693.

Nottrott, S., Simard, M.J., Richter, J.D., 2006. Human let-7a miRNA blocks protein production on actively translating polyribosomes. Nat. Struct. Mol. Biol. 13, 1108–1114.

Park, I.H., Zhao, R., West, J.A., et al., 2008. Reprogramming of human somatic cells to pluripotency with defined factors. Nature 451, 141–146.

Parker, R., Sheth, U., 2007. P bodies and the control of mRNA translation and degradation. Mol. Cell 25, 635–646.

Pereira, L., Yi, F., Merrill, B.J., 2006. Repression of Nanog gene transcription by Tcf3 limits embryonic stem cell self-renewal. Mol. Cell Biol. 26, 7479–7491.

Piskounova, E., Viswanathan, S.R., Janas, M., et al., 2008. Determinants of microRNA processing inhibition by the developmentally regulated RNA-binding protein Lin28. J. Biol. Chem. 283, 21310–21314.

Raj, A., Peskin, C.S., Tranchina, D., Vargas, D.Y., Tyagi, S., 2006. Stochastic mRNA synthesis in mammalian cells. PLoS Biol. 4, e309.

Raver-Shapira, N., Marciano, E., Meiri, E., et al., 2007. Transcriptional activation of mir-34a contributes to p53-mediated apoptosis. Mol. Cell 26, 731–743.

Rehmsmeier, M., Steffen, P., Hochsmann, M., Giegerich, R., 2004. Fast and effective prediction of microRNA/target duplexes. RNA 10, 1507–1517.

Reinhart, B.J., Slack, F.J., Basson, M., et al., 2000. The 21-nucleotide let-7 RNA regulates developmental timing in *Caenorhabditis elegans*. Nature 403, 901–906.

Rhoades, M.W., Reinhart, B.J., Lim, L.P., Burge, C.B., Bartel, B., Bartel, D.P., 2002. Prediction of plant microRNA targets. Cell 110, 513–520.

Robins, H., Li, Y., Padgett, R.W., 2005. Incorporating structure to predict microRNA targets. Proc. Natl. Acad. Sci. U. S. A. 102, 4006–4009.

Rodriguez, A., Vigorito, E., Clare, S., et al., 2007. Requirement of bic/microRNA-155 for normal immune function. Science 316, 608–611.

Rusinov, V., Baev, V., Minkov, I.N., Tabler, M., 2005. MicroInspector: a web tool for detection of miRNA binding sites in an RNA sequence. Nucleic Acids Res. 33, W696–W700.

Rybak, A., Fuchs, H., Smirnova, L., et al., 2008. A feedback loop comprising lin-28 and let-7 controls pre-let-7 maturation during neural stem-cell commitment. Nat. Cell Biol. 10, 987–993.

Sampath, P., Pritchard, D.K., Pabon, L., et al., 2008. A hierarchical network controls protein translation during murine embryonic stem cell self-renewal and differentiation. Cell Stem Cell 2, 448–460.

Schratt, G.M., Tuebing, F., Nigh, E.A., et al., 2006. A brain-specific microRNA regulates dendritic spine development. Nature 439, 283–289.

Shalgi, R., Lapidot, M., Shamir, R., Pilpel, Y., 2005. A catalog of stability-associated sequence elements in 3′ UTRs of yeast mRNAs. Genome Biol. 6, R86.

Shalgi, R., Lieber, D., Oren, M., Pilpel, Y., 2007. Global and local architecture of the mammalian microRNA–transcription factor regulatory network. PLoS Comput. Biol. 3, e131.

Shen-Orr, S.S., Milo, R., Mangan, S., Alon, U., 2002. Network motifs in the transcriptional regulation network of Escherichia coli. Nat. Genet. 31, 64–68.

Singh, S.K., Kagalwala, M.N., Parker-Thornburg, J., Adams, H., Majumder, S., 2008. REST maintains self-renewal and pluripotency of embryonic stem cells. Nature 453, 223–227.

Sood, P., Krek, A., Zavolan, M., Macino, G., Rajewsky, N., 2006. Cell-type-specific signatures of microRNAs on target mRNA expression. Proc. Natl. Acad. Sci. U. S. A. 103, 2746–2751.

Stark, A., Brennecke, J., Bushati, N., Russell, R.B., Cohen, S.M., 2005. Animal MicroRNAs confer robustness to gene expression and have a significant impact on 3′UTR evolution. Cell 123, 1133–1146.

Stefani, G., Slack, F.J., 2008. Small non-coding RNAs in animal development. Nat. Rev. Mol. Cell Biol. 9, 219–230.

Suh, M.R., Lee, Y., Kim, J.Y., et al., 2004. Human embryonic stem cells express a unique set of microRNAs. Dev. Biol. 270, 488–498.

Takahashi, K., Yamanaka, S., 2006. Induction of pluripotent stem cells from mouse embryonic and adult fibroblast cultures by defined factors. Cell 126, 663–676.

Takahashi, K., Tanabe, K., Ohnuki, M., et al., 2007. Induction of pluripotent stem cells from adult human fibroblasts by defined factors. Cell 131, 861–872.

Tam, W., Dahlberg, J.E., 2006. mir-155/BIC as an oncogenic microRNA. Genes Chromosomes Cancer 45, 211–212.

Tam, W.L. Lim, B. 2008. Genome-wide transcription factor localization and function in stem cells. In: Bernstein, B.E. (Ed.), StemBook. The Stem Cell Research Community.

Tam, W.L., Lim, C.Y., Han, J., et al., 2008. T-cell factor 3 regulates embryonic stem cell pluripotency and self-renewal by the transcriptional control of multiple lineage pathways. Stem Cells 26, 2019–2031.

Tang, G., Reinhart, B.J., Bartel, D.P., Zamore, P.D., 2003. A biochemical framework for RNA silencing in plants. Genes Dev. 17, 49–63.

Tay, Y., Zhang, J., Thomson, A.M., Lim, B., Rigoutsos, I., 2008a. MicroRNAs to Nanog, Oct4 and Sox2 coding regions modulate embryonic stem cell differentiation. Nature 455(7216), 1124–1128.

Tay, Y.M., Tam, W.L., Ang, Y.S., et al., 2008b. MicroRNA-134 modulates the differentiation of mouse embryonic stem cells, where it causes post-transcriptional attenuation of Nanog and LRH1. Stem Cells 26, 17–29.

Tsang, J., Zhu, J., van Oudenaarden, A., 2007. MicroRNA-mediated feedback and feedforward loops are recurrent network motifs in mammals. Mol. Cell 26, 753–767.

van Rooij, E., Sutherland, L.B., Qi, X., Richardson, J.A., Hill, J., Olson, E.N., 2007. Control of stress-dependent cardiac growth and gene expression by a microRNA. Science 316, 575–579.

Vasudevan, S., Steitz, J.A., 2007. AU-rich-element-mediated upregulation of translation by FXR1 and Argonaute 2. Cell 128, 1105–1118.

Vasudevan, S., Tong, Y., Steitz, J.A., 2007. Switching from repression to activation: microRNAs can up-regulate translation. Science 318, 1931–1934.

Vella, M.C., Reinert, K., Slack, F.J., 2004. Architecture of a validated microRNA:target interaction. Chem. Biol. 11, 1619–1623.

Ventura, A., Young, A.G., Winslow, M.M., et al., 2008. Targeted deletion reveals essential and overlapping functions of the mir-17 through 92 family of miRNA clusters. Cell 132, 875–886.

Viswanathan, S.R., Daley, G.Q., Gregory, R.I., 2008. Selective blockade of microRNA processing by Lin28. Science 320, 97–100.

Vogelstein, B., Lane, D., Levine, A.J., 2000. Surfing the p53 network. Nature 408, 307–310.

Voorhoeve, P.M., le Sage, C., Schrier, M., et al., 2006. A genetic screen implicates miRNA-372 and miRNA-373 as oncogenes in testicular germ cell tumors. Cell 124, 1169–1181.

Wang, J., Rao, S., Chu, J., et al., 2006. A protein interaction network for pluripotency of embryonic stem cells. Nature 444, 364–368.

Wang, Y., Liu, C.L., Storey, J.D., Tibshirani, R.J., Herschlag, D., Brown, P.O., 2002. Precision and functional specificity in mRNA decay. Proc. Natl. Acad. Sci. U. S. A. 99, 5860–5865.

Wightman, B., Ha, I., Ruvkun, G., 1993. Posttranscriptional regulation of the heterochronic gene lin-14 by lin-4 mediates temporal pattern formation in C. elegans. Cell 75, 855–862.

Xiao, C., Calado, D.P., Galler, G., et al., 2007. Mir-150 controls B cell differentiation by targeting the transcription factor c-Myb. Cell 131, 146–159.

Xiao, C., Srinivasan, L., Calado, D.P., et al., 2008. Lymphoproliferative disease and autoimmunity in mice with increased mir-17-92 expression in lymphocytes. Nat. Immunol. 9, 405–414.

Xu, P., Vernooy, S.Y., Guo, M., Hay, B.A., 2003. The Drosophila microRNA Mir-14 suppresses cell death and is required for normal fat metabolism. Curr. Biol. 13, 790–795.

Yamanaka, S., 2007. Strategies and new developments in the generation of patient-specific pluripotent stem cells. Cell Stem Cell 1, 39–49.

Yang, B., Lin, H., Xiao, J., et al., 2007. The muscle-specific microRNA mir-1 regulates cardiac arrhythmogenic potential by targeting GJA1 and KCNJ2. Nat. Med. 13, 486–491.

Yi, F., Pereira, L., Merrill, B.J., 2008a. Tcf3 functions as a steady-state limiter of transcriptional programs of mouse embryonic stem cell self-renewal. Stem Cells 26, 1951–1960.

Yi, R., Poy, M.N., Stoffel, M., Fuchs, E., 2008b. A skin microRNA promotes differentiation by repressing 'stemness'. Nature 452, 225–229.

Yu, F., Yao, H., Zhu, P., et al., 2007. let-7 regulates self renewal and tumorigenicity of breast cancer cells. Cell 131, 1109–1123.

Yuh, C.H., Bolouri, H., Davidson, E.H., 1998. Genomic cis-regulatory logic: experimental and computational analysis of a sea urchin gene. Science 279, 1896–1902.

Zhao, R., Gish, K., Murphy, M., et al., 2000. Analysis of p53-regulated gene expression patterns using oligonucleotide arrays. Genes Dev. 14, 981–993.

CHAPTER 6

Protein Networks in Integrin-Mediated Adhesions

Ronen Zaidel-Bar, Shalev Itzkovitz and Benjamin Geiger
Weizmann Institute of Science, Rehovot

OUTLINE

Summary	139	Interrelationships Between the Functional Protein Families	144
Definitions	140	Resolving Functional Subnets	145
Introduction	140	Identifying Molecular Entourages	147
Problem	141	Protein Domains and Switchable Links Enriched in the Adhesome Net	147
Solution	141		
A Holistic View of the Adhesome	141	Conclusion	150
Constructing the Adhesome Network	141	Acknowledgements	151
Functional Families of the Adhesome	142		

Summary

In this chapter we address the molecular complexity of integrin-mediated adhesions to the extracellular matrix. We constructed, by means of a systematic literature search, a comprehensive "adhesome" network, consisting of the diverse components of integrin-mediated adhesions and the multitude of interactions between them. Here, we present the network at several distinct levels. These range from an examination of the entire network, via a survey of specific families of components, to the characterization of functional subnets, then to individual protein entourages and, finally, to specific domains of adhesome constituents. We then discuss how these domains can be modified by signaling molecules, each of which can act as a "switch" that "turns on" or "turns off" the molecular interactions within the adhesion structure. By deconstructing the entire adhesome network into functional subnetworks, we gain insight into the structural and functional organization of integrin adhesions.

Definitions

Integrin adhesome Defined (Zaidel-Bar et al., 2007) as the collective of molecules participating in the formation, stabilization and signaling activity of all types on integrin-mediated adhesions, including focal adhesions, focal complexes, fibrillar adhesions and podosomes (Geiger et al., 2001). In this article, we address their molecular complexity.

Intrinsic components of the adhesome Defined as molecules physically associated with adhesions (based on morphological criteria).

Associated components Defined as molecules that are not stable residents of adhesion sites, but have been shown to interact with the intrinsic adhesome components **and** affect their function.

Interactions between adhesome constituents Can be non-directional *binding interactions*, as well as directional *signaling interactions* between specific signaling molecules and their downstream molecular targets. These interactions were operationally defined as *activating interactions* (e.g. phosphorylation, G-protein, the GTPase modulator, GEF) and *inhibitory interactions* (e.g. dephosphorylation, proteolysis, the GTPase modulator, GAP). Additional details are provided below.

INTRODUCTION

Interactions of living cells with each other and with the extracellular matrix are mediated by a variety of structurally and molecularly defined adhesion sites. These membrane-bound compartments consist of multimolecular complexes containing specific adhesion receptors, cytoskeletal components and interconnecting adapter proteins. In addition to these scaffolding elements, adhesion sites host a wide variety of signaling molecules that regulate their formation and turnover and participate in adhesion-mediated signaling events (Burgeson and Christiano, 1997; Burridge et al., 1988; Hynes, 1992; Simon and Goodenough, 1998; Stevenson and Keon, 1998; Yap et al., 1997).

Current thinking supports the view that adhesion structures serve, not only as means to link cells physically into functional tissues and organs, but also as a means by which cells learn about the nature of their environment, thereby triggering diverse responses that affect cell growth, viability, differentiation, morphogenesis and migration (Danen and Sonnenberg, 2003; Gumbiner, 2005; Kaverina et al., 2002; Watt, 2002). It appears that, via these adhesions, cells sense several features of their neighborhood, including the molecular composition of the matrix, its geometry and its physical properties (e.g. rigidity). This information is then integrated and translated into specific adhesion-mediated signaling events, that drive physiological cellular responses (Geiger and Bershadsky, 2002). Particularly relevant in this context are recent findings indicating that adhesion sites are highly mechanosensitive, and respond to both external and internal forces by altering their assembly dynamics and signaling activity (Katsumi et al., 2004; Zaidel-Bar et al., 2005). The molecular mechanisms underlying such responses are still poorly understood (Bershadsky et al., 2003), yet they appear to involve forced changes in the conformation of specific adhesion-associated molecules, which leads to their phosphorylation and "switching-on" their signaling activity (Geiger, 2006; Sawada et al., 2006).

In recent years, much effort has been invested in deciphering the composition and molecular architecture of integrin adhesions, and the complex interactions between their numerous constituents (Lo, 2006; Zamir and Geiger, 2001). Our current understanding of the molecular structure of diverse adhesion sites and of their signaling responses is primarily based on a combination of cellular localization data yielded by immunofluorescence microscopy, and biochemical studies, mostly consisting of protein-binding data. These data revealed that adhesions formed via a single class of receptors (integrin-mediated adhesions) can be structurally and functionally heterogeneous, consisting of at least four types of adhesion sites: focal complexes, focal adhesions, fibrillar adhesions and podosomes. Each of these structures can play distinct roles in the initiation of adhesions, stress fiber formation, matrix fibrillogenesis and matrix degradation (Geiger et al., 2001; Linder and Aepfelbacher, 2003; Nobes and Hall, 1995; Zamir et al., 2000). Although all these structures are similar in molecular composition, they differ greatly in such features as subcellular localization, morphology and dynamics, which are of critical functional importance.

PROBLEM

Overall, most studies of adhesion sites have focused on the in-depth characterization of individual proteins, and the signaling pathways affecting their activity (e.g. Brown and Turner, 2004; Legate et al., 2006)]. However, attempts to assign specific biological functions to individual molecules have proven to be difficult, probably because of the enormous complexity of adhesion sites and their diversity. Deciphering the function of particular proteins is further complicated by the tendency of adhesion components to function as multi-protein modules (Hartwell et al., 1999). Recent inventories of adhesion proteins (Lo, 2006; Zamir and Geiger, 2001) were an important prerequisite for system approaches, but analysis of the adhesome at the network level is still lacking.

SOLUTION

A Holistic View of the Adhesome

Adhesion sites, like many other cellular systems, can be studied in a "bottom-up" approach, "reconstructing" multimolecular function units from their individual constituents, or "top-down," starting with the complex, unperturbed structure. During the past few years, knowledge of the molecular underpinnings of the "integrin adhesome" and its constituents has greatly expanded. As a result, we are now able to combine bottom-up and top-down views, and construct an all-inclusive, mostly protein-based model of this "global molecular network." By subsequently dividing the adhesome into smaller modules, or "subnets," we can then explore the inner workings of this complex molecular ensemble.

Constructing the Adhesome Network

The definition of the integrin adhesome, its intrinsic and associated components and the nature of links and interactions between them are admittedly artificial, yet they enable us to distinguish between these molecules and the interactions between them in a clear and convenient manner. That said, many of the "associated" proteins may in fact reside, under certain conditions or for a limited period of time, in the adhesome proper, and could simply be evading detection. Conversely, some of the "intrinsic" proteins might reside only temporarily in the adhesion site, carrying out their tasks and then leaving.

The actual data used to compile the list of components of the integrin adhesome, and our description of the relationships between them, were derived from virtually thousands of publications that have appeared to date in the scientific literature. Our search, based on the criteria outlined above, indicated that the number of "intrinsic components" of this adhesome is close to 90, and the number of "associated components" that interact with the endogenous molecules and affect their activity and fate is over 60 (Zaidel-Bar et al., 2007). It should be emphasized that in this survey we refrained, insofar as was possible, from validating or questioning statements made in the different publications, or from overemphasizing data that received more attention or appeared to be more extensively substantiated. It is, perhaps, inevitable that certain components or interactions have escaped our notice. For this, we apologize.

The vast body of literature concerning cell adhesion documents more than 680 direct interactions between the various components of the adhesome. More than half of these represent direct binding between components; the others are directional "signaling interactions" that can either activate (i.e., positive input) or inhibit (i.e., negative input) the target molecule. Given that the same modification may activate certain molecular functions and inhibit others, we will refer here to specific modifications as "activating" or "inhibitory" according to the type of modification rather than the actual activity of the target (see below). In such instances, the signaling molecules consist of enzymes such as kinases, phosphatases, proteases, or Rho-family GTPases and their modulators (GEFs and GAPs). On average, each adhesome component can interact with about nine other components, making the adhesome a highly interconnected network (Fig. 6.1). However, the distribution of interactions is highly non-uniform: many proteins have few connections and a few have many, as is characteristic of biological networks (Barabasi and Oltvai, 2004).

Critical examination of the crude global network comprising the adhesome is a far from trivial task, and identification of the internal order among its components is hardly straightforward. It is important to bear in mind that not all components are always present in any given cell or adhesion, and all signaling pathways linking them are not active at all times (see below). To gain a deeper understanding of the functional interactions within the global network, one needs to examine the network more specifically, at the level of its segmentation into simpler structural or functional subnets.

Functional Families of the Adhesome

Functional annotation of the adhesome resulted in the classification of 18 families of components, based on their primary biological activity (Fig. 6.2). The three largest families consist of adapter, adhesion/receptor and actin-associated proteins. The main function of the adapter family is to form a robust structural scaffold, which anchors several signaling molecules, thus facilitating and directing their activity. The adhesion/receptor family contains, in addition to integrins, a dozen or so other transmembrane molecules, all of which are associated with, and affect, integrin-mediated interactions (Humphries et al., 2005). The actin-associated components are involved in linking the adhesion site to the cytoskeleton, and for their mechanical coupling. Most other families of adhesome components consist of enzymes, which regulate the formation and turnover of the adhesion complex, and participate in the generation, amplification and transduction of adhesion-mediated environmental cues. These include molecules such as protein and lipid kinases or phosphatases, in addition to Rho-family GTPases and their modulators, GEFs and GAPs. Notably, among the adhesome components, there also exist a single protease (calpain) and a single E3-ligase (Cbl), and a small, yet intriguing, group of proteins that are involved in RNA or DNA regulation and presumably shuttle between the nucleus and the adhesion site. Another small group of proteins, the function of which in integrin adhesions remains unclear, consists of three ion channels. Moreover, in addition to the approximately 150 intrinsic and associated proteins, the adhesome also contains three non-protein components: the

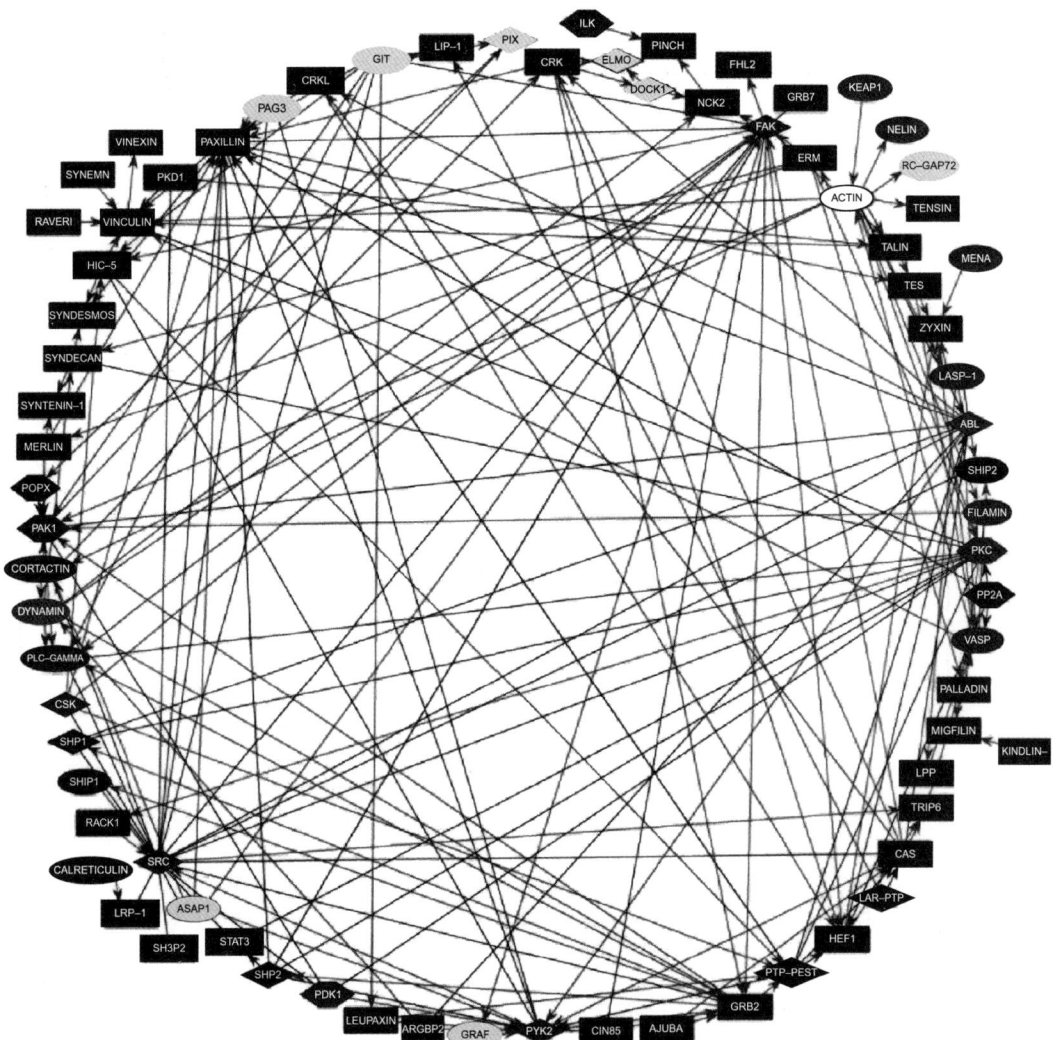

FIGURE 6.1 The Adhesome Network.
Illustration of the interactions between the intrinsic components of the adhesome. Directional interactions are depicted by arrows, red for positive inputs and blue for negative inputs; black lines denote binding interactions. The shape and color of each protein symbolizes its function, according to the scheme presented in Figure 6.2.

lipid derivatives phosphatidylinositol bisphosphate (PIP2) and phosphatidylinositol triphosphate (PIP3) and calcium ions.

As the number of proteins in each family varies greatly, so, too, does the number of interactions each family has with other proteins, indicating that their tendency to interact depends on the protein's specific function. For example, each component of the 46-member family of adapter proteins interacts, on average, with seven different proteins, whereas the phosphatidylinositol (PtdIns) kinase family, with only three members, takes part in an average of 16 interactions per protein (Fig. 6.2).

Protein type	Example symbol	Number of proteins in adhesome	Number of interactions (range)
Adapter	TENSIN	46	7 (1–35)
Adhesion/Receptor	INTEGRIN-B	14	6 (1–33)
Actin regulation	VASP	12	6 (1–16)
S/T kinase	ILK	11	9 (4–36)
Tyrosine kinase	FAK	9	22 (12–48)
GEF	VAV	9	7 (3–18)
Tyrosine phosphatase	SHP1	9	8 (1–16)
GAP	GRAF	9	6 (2–10)
GTPase	ARF1	5	11 (4–17)
RNA/DNA regulation	STAT3	4	3 (1–7)
PtdIns kinase	PI3K	3	16 (6–24)
PtdIns phosphatase	SHIP1	3	6 (5–6)
S/T phosphatase	POPX	3	4 (1–8)
Chaperone	HSP27	3	2 (2–2)
Ion-channel	HERG	3	2 (1–3)
Actin	ACTIN	1	23
E3-ligase	CBL	1	25
Cysteine-protease	CALPAIN	1	21

FIGURE 6.2 Classification of Adhesome Components.
Classification of 18 families of adhesome components, based on their primary biological activity.

Interrelationships Between the Functional Protein Families

Are there ground rules that determine the nature of the cross-talk between the protein families of the adhesome? If the probability that any two given proteins will interact with each other is independent of their function, we would expect the number of interactions between any two functional families of proteins to be simply proportional to the total number of interactions of their family members. Significantly higher or lower numbers of reported interactions between the components of two functional families, as compared with the calculated random interaction value, would indicate that the two are specifically "connected" or "non-connected," respectively. Indeed, using a hypergeometric test, we detected pairs of protein families that had a high tendency to interact (P value $<T$) or not to interact (P value $>1 - T$). (We used $T = 4 \times 10^{-3}$, taking into account a false discovery rate of 20% for multiple-hypothesis testing.) Our results, illustrated in Figure 6.3, indicate that the interactions between certain protein families are favored, whereas interactions between other protein families are strongly discouraged. Not surprisingly, actin regulators regulate actin, adhesion/receptor

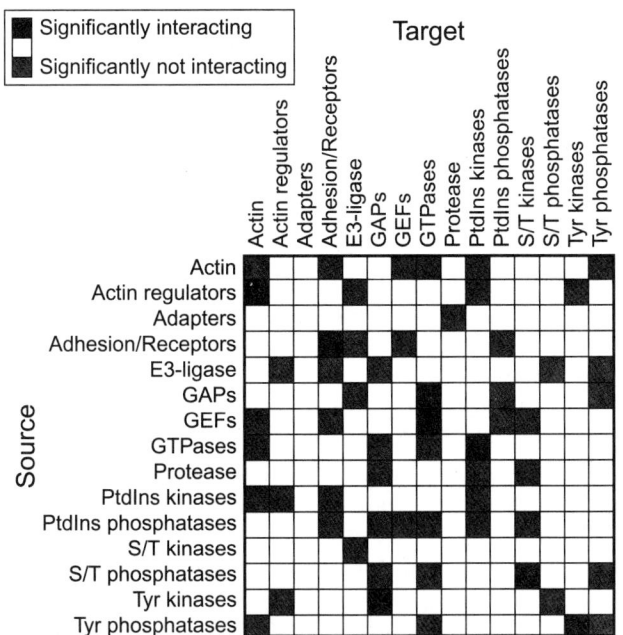

FIGURE 6.3 Interaction Between Functional Protein Families.
The probability that any two families of proteins will interact was calculated according to their total number of interactions, compared with the actual number of interactions between them (see text for details). Families that tend to interact significantly more than expected are marked by a blue square at their intersection in the matrix; families that interact significantly less than expected—i.e., tend not to interact—are marked by a green square. Note that the matrix is not symmetrical, because interactions are directional between a source (on the left) and target family (top). PtdIns, phosphatidylinositol; Tyr, tyrosine.

proteins interact with each other, and GAPs and GEFs modulate the activity of GTPases. Less obvious, *a priori*, are our discoveries concerning the enzyme protein families: GTPases, for example, tend to regulate PtdIns kinases, tyrosine kinases regulate GAPs, and serine/threonine (S/T) and tyrosine phosphatases dephosphorylate S/T and tyrosine kinases, respectively.

The strong tendency of certain protein families not to interact is also a matter of interest. As already indicated, adhesion receptors do not interact with actin, and GTPases do not interact with themselves. Interestingly, the E3 ligase (Cbl) does not target actin regulators or adhesion/receptors, nor does it target GAPs or S/T or tyrosine phosphatases. Furthermore, the protease (calpain) does not target GAPs or PtdIns kinases, and tyrosine kinases do not phosphorylate actin regulators. It should be emphasized that these calculations reflect general tendencies of cross-family interactions; thus a few of the components in non-interacting families may, in fact, interact; similarly, not all proteins in significantly interacting families necessarily interact.

Resolving Functional Subnets

Another approach for resolving functionally relevant modules within the integrin adhesome is the bottom-up construction of functional subnets, based on a specific type of protein modification. For example, one could focus on all the reported phosphorylation events (e.g. on S/T or on tyrosine) within the adhesome, mark the targets of such events, define the kinases and phosphatases involved and determine which proteins regulate their activity. Using the interaction database of the adhesome, one could also construct subnets for different regulatory pathways, involving, for example, proteases, GTPases, actin regulators and the like (Zaidel-Bar et al., 2007). Such subnets are of a considerably simpler nature than that of the global network of the adhesome, and can be more readily used by both experimentalists and modelers.

As an example, take the case of a "lipid subnet" that contains two main effector molecules, PIP2 and PIP3 (Fig. 6.4). The formation of PIP2 and PIP3 is regulated by PtdIns kinases and phosphatases, which in turn are primarily regulated by GTPases and tyrosine, as well as S/T kinases. The lipids themselves are mostly involved in the regulation of the actin-binding capabilities of adapter proteins (e.g. talin or vinculin), and in the control of actin bundling and cross-linking proteins such as filamin and alpha-actinin. In some cases, the lipids activate the effects on actin; in others, they inhibit such activity. PIP2 and/or PIP3 also regulate the S/T kinases of the adhesome, although, interestingly enough, they have no effect on tyrosine kinases. PIP2 and PIP3 do not have common substrates within the adhesion sites, with the exception of AKT. Naturally, one may proceed further "upstream" of these functional subnets, and extend the spectrum of regulatory components to additional hierarchical levels, or to interconnections with other subnets, inevitably rendering the subnet much more comprehensive—but, on the other hand, less specific. We consider functional subnets to be useful tools in planning perturbation experiments, using drugs or specific short interfering RNA (siRNA) to determine how different effector molecules modulate the cellular function of choice.

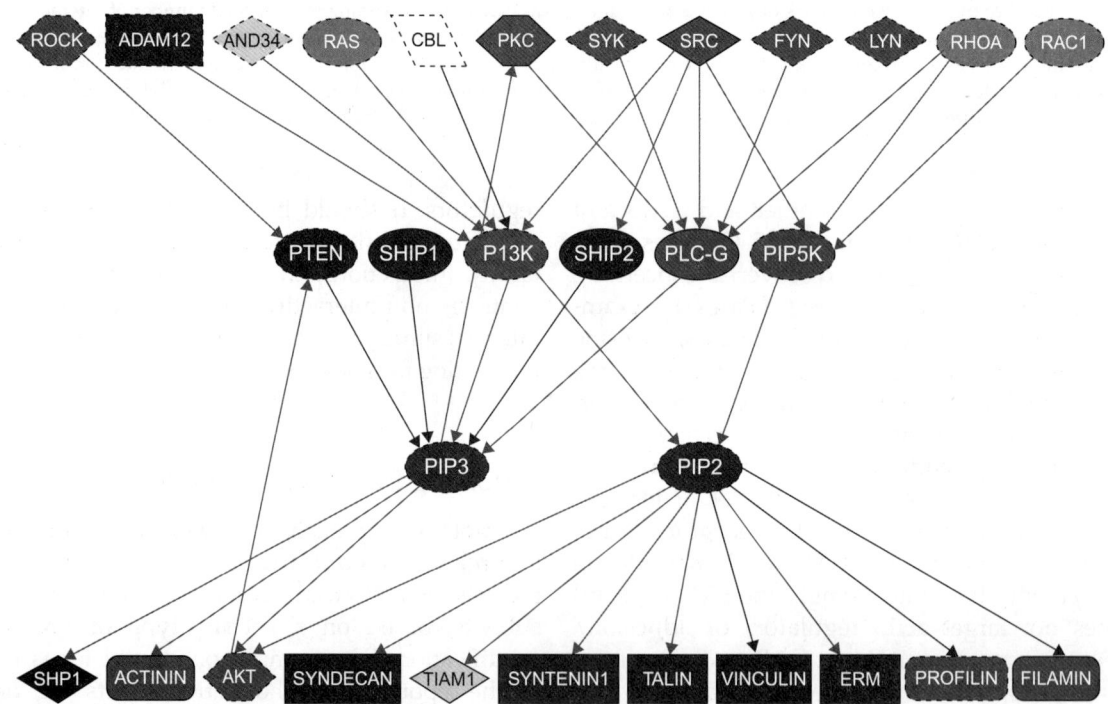

FIGURE 6.4 Lipid Subnet.
The lipid derivatives PIP2 and PIP3, their targets and their regulators, two hierarchical levels up. Only directional interactions are depicted: red for activating and blue for inhibiting. See text for further discussion.

I. FOUNDATIONS OF SYSTEMS BIOLOGY

Identifying Molecular Entourages

Zooming in on individual adhesome components can provide additional functional insights into the direct effectors and targets of key adhesome components. For example, one could examine the individual protein connections of actin (Fig. 6.5A) and of protein kinase C (Fig. 6.5B). What can we learn from such schemes? As mentioned above in the section on interrelationships, actin interacts with actin regulators and adapter proteins. However, it also clearly interacts with certain kinases, and in some cases (Abl, PLD1) it inhibits their enzymatic activity. Another example, namely protein kinase C (PKC) (all isoforms combined), reveals that these enzymes not only bind to adapter proteins and actin, but also regulate tyrosine kinases and phosphatases. Moreover, several, very different signaling pathways (including lipids, Rho GTPases, tyrosine and S/T phosphorylation) converge on their regulation. Such information can also be useful in the of planning perturbation experiments (e.g. siRNA suppression of gene expression, or the use of specific inhibitors).

Protein Domains and Switchable Links Enriched in the Adhesome Net

A search of the adhesome for specific protein domains reveals several domains that are significantly enriched within the adhesome, as compared with their presence in the entire human proteome (Table 6.1). These include the Pleckstrin homology (PH) and FERM domains, both of which target proteins to the plasma membrane, and the Calponin homology (CH) domain, which is an F-actin-binding motif. The importance of tyrosine phosphorylation for the regulation of protein–protein interactions is manifested by the enrichment of the tyrosine kinase and phosphatase domains, in addition to the Src homology 2 (SH2) domain, all of which mediate interactions with phosphorylated tyrosine residues. Protein–protein interactions, which are a hallmark of the adhesome, are also mediated by Src homology 3 (SH3), FERM and LIM domains, which mediate binding among specific proteins.

It is noteworthy that, within the adhesome, many of the links connecting the various protein components are not constitutive, but rather can be switched on or switched off by corresponding signaling components. The proteins talin and Crk demonstrate these functional transitions (Fig. 6.6). Both proteins can exist in two conformational states: a folded, inactive state, in which some of the binding domains are unavailable for interaction; and an active, extended form, in which most or all of the binding domains are exposed (Critchley, 2005; Feller, 2001). Crk, for example, is locked in a folded state by an interaction between its C-terminal SH2 domain, and phosphorylated tyrosine 221, located close to its N-terminus. This tyrosine residue is phosphorylated by Abl, which can also bind to Crk in the folded conformation. Dephosphorylation of Crk by phosphotyrosine phosphatase (PTP)-1B opens up the protein, rendering its SH2 domain available for binding to one of several phosphoproteins, including paxillin, cas and cortactin. This binding depends on the phosphorylation states of these proteins, which, in turn, are regulated by specific tyrosine kinases (e.g. Src, FAK, Abl) and phosphatases (e.g. PTP-PEST, SHP2). At the same time, the SH3 domain of Crk can bind to one of several GEFs for Rac, Rho or Ras, or to Abl or JNK (Feller, 2001).

It is likely that, following the same principle, unlocking of the pivotal adapter protein talin has major effects on its activity. In its conceived folded conformation, talin would still be able to bind PIP5K, which, when localized to the membrane, catalyzes the formation of PIP2. Following PIP2 binding, talin would undergo a conformational change, revealing binding sites for actin, vinculin and integrin, which are essential for its localization in the adhesion site and for integrin activation (Critchley, 2005). The binding of talin to PIP5K, integrin or layilin, through its FERM domain, is mutually exclusive, whereas its binding to FAK and actin can co-exist with any of the

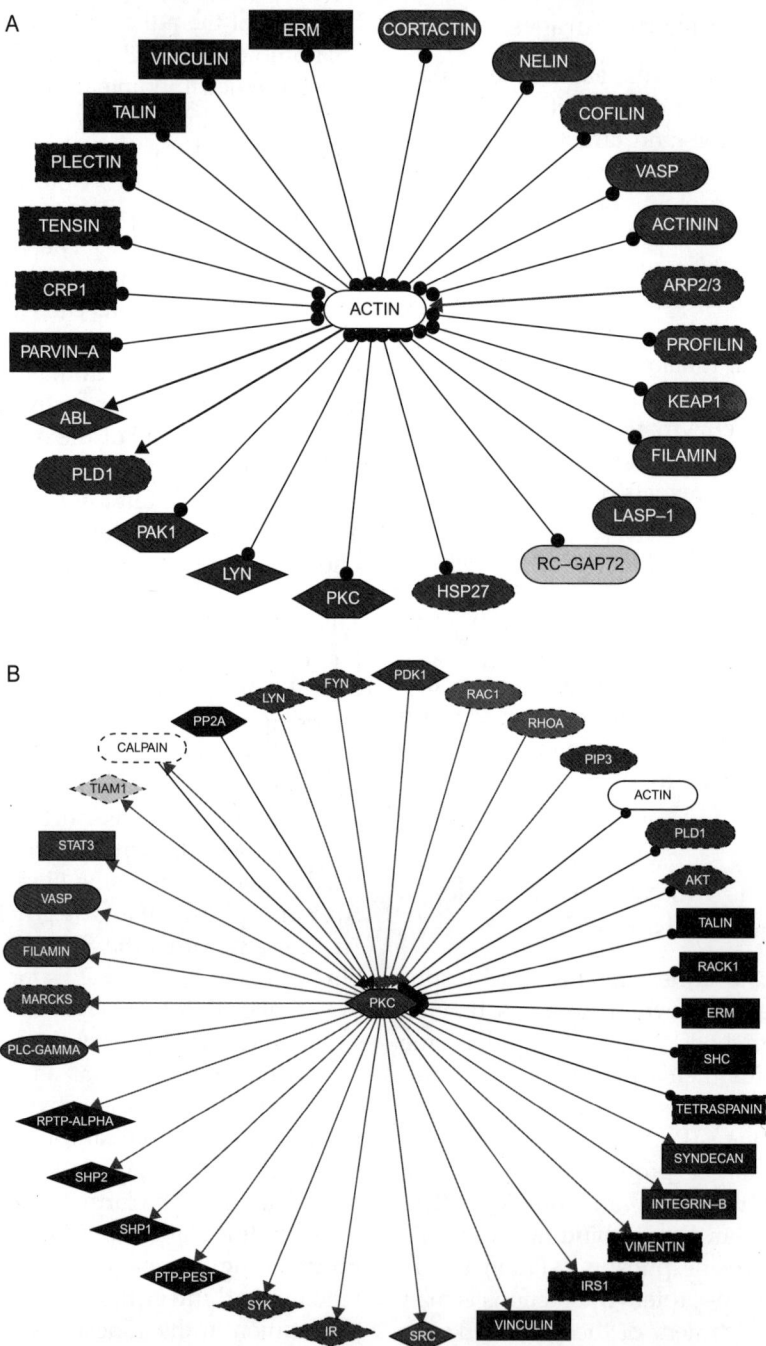

FIGURE 6.5 Protein Entourages of Actin and PKC.
Depicting the direct partners of a single component, in this case (A) actin or (B) protein kinase C (PKC). As in Figure 6.1, directional interactions are depicted by arrows, red for positive inputs and blue for negative inputs; black lines denote binding interactions.

TABLE 6.1 Domains Associated with Adhesome Components

Domain	Function	P-value enrichment in: Intrinsic Adhesome proteins	Associated Adhesome proteins
SH3 (Src homology 3) IPR001452	Mediates specific protein–protein interactions, by binding to PXXP-containing sequence motifs in target proteins	1.01E-10***	0.02170***
PH (Pleckstrin homology) IPR011993	Recognizes phosphoinositide headgroups and can target its host protein to the plasma membrane through its association with phosphoinositides	6.64E-05***	0.19098
SH2 (Src homology 2) IPR000980	Interacts with high affinity to phosphotyrosine-containing target peptides in a fashion that differs from one SH2 domain to another, and is strictly phosphorylation-dependent	1.42E-09***	0.00055***
LIM IPR001781	A zinc-binding, cysteine-rich motif consisting of two tandemly repeated zinc fingers. Appears to mediate protein–protein interactions	7.66E-09***	0.26090
Tyrosine kinase IPR008266	This signature contains the active site aspartate residue, which is specific to tyrosine protein kinases	0.02917***	0.00388***
Tyrosine phosphatase IPR000242	Tyrosine-specific protein phosphatase	0.00973***	0.00113***
FERM IPR009065	Responsible for PIP2-regulated membrane binding of proteins, and is also postulated to mediate PIP2-dependent protein–protein interactions	2.63E-07***	1
CH (Calponin homology) IPR001715	Two CH domains in tandem form an F-actin binding region and cross-link actin filaments into bundles and networks. A subset of CH domains act as regulatory domains or protein–protein interaction scaffolds to modulate the activity of proteins in which they are present	0.00293***	0.21320

The eight domains that appear in adhesome proteins significantly more than in the annotated human genome. This was calculated as follows: the number of times a domain appears in intrinsic or associated adhesome proteins was compared with the number of times the same domain appears in the 12 600 human genes in the Uniprot database
PIP2, phosphatidylinositol bisphosphate.
***Domain regarded as significantly enriched (P value less than 0.0292, which corresponds to a false discovery rate of 10%).

aforementioned interactions. Talin can also be cleaved by calpain (Critchley, 2005).

All in all, the enzymatic and binding activity of almost every protein in the adhesome is regulated by other components. For example, the binding of adapters containing SH2 domains (e.g. Grb2, Nck2, Shc) to phosphoproteins (e.g. Cas, HEF1, Gab1) is regulated by tyrosine kinases and phosphatases (e.g. Src, Csk, Shp2, RPTP-alpha), which in turn are regulated by S/T kinases (e.g. PKA, PKC), which themselves can be activated by Rho GTPases. Rho GTPases also activate PtdIns kinases, the products of which, PIP2 and PIP3, affect the actin-binding capabilities of proteins (e.g. vinculin, filamin, ERM) and regulate the enzymatic activity of kinases and phosphatases (e.g. AKT, SHP1). On the whole, more than half of the scaffold

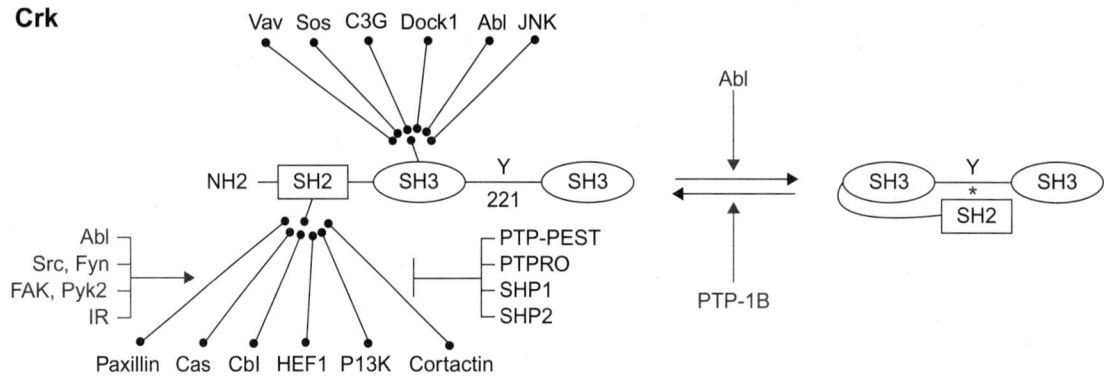

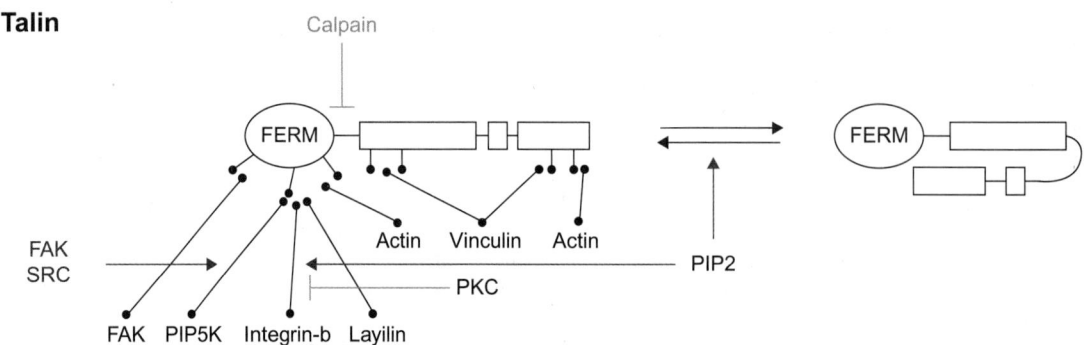

FIGURE 6.6 Protein Domains and Switchable Links of Crk and Talin.
The domains and potential interactions of two adapter proteins, Crk and talin, are presented. Many of their potential interactions can be turned on or off by regulatory modifications ("switches"), which are depicted in color (red = positive, blue = negative).

proteins in the adhesome are subjected to modification by their signaling partners, suggesting that such modifications can play a critical role in regulating the formation and turnover of the adhesion machinery.

CONCLUSION

In this chapter, we have explored the literature available on the molecular constituents of integrin adhesions and their interactions, in order to construct a global molecular network, consisting of more than 150 protein components and 680 links, defined as the integrin adhesome. Our objective was to divide the adhesome into simpler functional subnets and model their possible interactions at several hierarchical levels. In the adhesome, these interactions are dominated by links that can be switched on or switched off by associated signaling elements. This modular view of the adhesome reveals novel design principles that govern the molecular and functional architecture of these adhesions, and open up new possibilities for their controlled perturbation. We propose that the dissection of complex molecular circuits into functional, interacting units might serve as a general tool for understanding the integrative activity of complex biological networks.

ACKNOWLEDGEMENTS

This chapter is based on data collected within the framework of NIGMS, the National Institutes of Health Cell Migration Consortium (Grant U54 GM64346). Additional data on the adhesome can be found in the Cell Migration Knowledgebase (http://data.cellmigration.org/cmckb).

B. G. holds the Erwin Neter Professorial Chair in Cell and Tumor Biology.

References

Barabasi, A.L., Oltvai, Z.N., 2004. Network biology: understanding the cell's functional organization. Nat. Rev. Genet. 5, 101–113.

Bershadsky, A.D., Balaban, N.Q., Geiger, B., 2003. Adhesion-dependent cell mechanosensitivity. Annu. Rev. Cell Dev. Biol. 19, 677–695.

Brown, M.C., Turner, C.E., 2004. Paxillin: adapting to change. Physiol. Rev. 84, 1315–1339.

Burgeson, R.E., Christiano, A.M., 1997. The dermal-epidermal junction. Curr. Opin. Cell Biol. 9, 651–658.

Burridge, K., Fath, K., Kelly, T., Nuckolls, G., Turner, C., 1988. Focal adhesions: transmembrane junctions between the extracellular matrix and the cytoskeleton. Annu. Rev. Cell Biol. 4, 487–525.

Critchley, D.R., 2005. Genetic, biochemical and structural approaches to talin function. Biochem. Soc. Trans. 33, 1308–1312.

Danen, E.H., Sonnenberg, A., 2003. Integrins in regulation of tissue development and function. J. Pathol. 201, 632–641.

Feller, S.M., 2001. Crk family adaptors-signalling complex formation and biological roles. Oncogene 20, 6348–6371.

Geiger, B., 2006. A role for p130Cas in mechanotransduction. Cell 127, 879–881.

Geiger, B., Bershadsky, A., 2002. Exploring the neighborhood: adhesion-coupled cell mechanosensors. Cell 110, 139–142.

Geiger, B., Bershadsky, A., Pankov, R., Yamada, K.M., 2001. Transmembrane crosstalk between the extracellular matrix–cytoskeleton crosstalk. Nat. Rev. Mol. Cell Biol. 2, 793–805.

Gumbiner, B.M., 2005. Regulation of cadherin-mediated adhesion in morphogenesis. Nat. Rev. Mol. Cell Biol. 6, 334–622.

Hartwell, L.H., Hopfield, J.J., Leibler, S., Murray, A.W., 1999. From molecular to modular cell biology. Nature 402, C47–C52.

Humphries, M.J., Mostafavi-Pour, Z., Morgan, M.R., Deakin, N.O., Messent, A.J., Bass, M.D., 2005. Integrin-syndecan cooperation governs the assembly of signalling complexes during cell spreading. Novartis Found. Symp. 269, 178–188 discussion 188–192, 223–230.

Hynes, R.O., 1992. Integrins: versatility, modulation, and signaling in cell adhesion. Cell 69, 11–25.

Katsumi, A., Orr, A.W., Tzima, E., Schwartz, M.A., 2004. Integrins in mechanotransduction. J. Biol. Chem. 279, 12001–12004.

Kaverina, I., Krylyshkina, O., Small, J.V., 2002. Regulation of substrate adhesion dynamics during cell motility. Int. J. Biochem. Cell Biol. 34, 746–761.

Legate, K.R., Montanez, E., Kudlacek, O., Fassler, R., 2006. ILK, PINCH and parvin: the tIPP of integrin signalling. Nat. Rev. Mol. Cell Biol. 7, 20–31.

Linder, S., Aepfelbacher, M., 2003. Podosomes: adhesion hot-spots of invasive cells. Trends Cell Biol. 13, 376–385.

Lo, S.H., 2006. Focal adhesions: what's new inside. Dev. Biol. 294, 280–291.

Nobes, C.D., Hall, A., 1995. Rho, rac, and cdc42 GTPases regulate the assembly of multimolecular focal complexes associated with actin stress fibers, lamellipodia, and filopodia. Cell 81, 53–62.

Sawada, Y., Tamada, M., Dubin-Thaler, B.J., Cherniavskaya, O., Sakai, R., Tanaka, S., Sheetz, M.P., 2006. Force sensing by mechanical extension of the Src family kinase substrate p130Cas. Cell 127, 1015–1026.

Simon, A.M., Goodenough, D.A., 1998. Diverse functions of vertebrate gap junctions. Trends Cell Biol. 8, 477–483.

Stevenson, B.R., Keon, B.H., 1998. The tight junction: morphology to molecules. Annu. Rev. Cell Dev. Biol. 14, 89–109.

Watt, F.M., 2002. Role of integrins in regulating epidermal adhesion, growth and differentiation. Embo. J. 21, 3919–3926.

Yap, A.S., Brieher, W.M., Gumbiner, B.M., 1997. Molecular and functional analysis of cadherin-based adherens junctions. Annu. Rev. Cell Dev. Biol. 13, 119–146.

Zaidel-Bar, R., Kam, Z., Geiger, B., 2005. Polarized downregulation of the paxillin-p130CAS-Rac1 pathway induced by shear flow. J. Cell Sci. 118, 3997–4007.

Zaidel-Bar, R., Itzkovitz, S., Ma'ayan, A., Iyengar, R., Geiger, B., 2007. Functional atlas of the integrin adhesome. Nat. Cell Biol. 9, 858–867.

Zamir, E., Geiger, B., 2001. Molecular complexity and dynamics of cell-matrix adhesions. J. Cell Sci. 114, 3583–3590.

Zamir, E., Katz, M., Posen, Y., et al., 2000. Dynamics and segregation of cell-matrix adhesions in cultured fibroblasts. Nat. Cell Biol. 2, 191–196.

CHAPTER 7

Systems Biology and Stem Cell Biology

Huck-Hui Ng[1,2], Sheng Zhong[3,4], and Bing Lim[1,5]

[1]Stem Cell and Developmental Biology, Genome Institute of Singapore, Singapore
[2]Department of Biological Sciences, National University of Singapore, Singapore
[3]Department of Bioengineering
[4]Institute for Genomic Biology, University of Illinois at Urbana-Champaign, IL, USA
[5]Harvard Institutes of Medicine, Harvard Medical School, Boston, MA, USA

OUTLINE

Summary	154
Definitions	154
Introduction	154
Pluripotent Embryonic Stem Cells	155
Stem Cells for Systems Biology (Defining Molecular Networks, Interactions and Functionality)	155
Transcription Networks	156
Mapping Transcription Factor and DNA Interactions	157
Computational Tools for Network Construction and Modeling	161
Regulatory Module	162
Bayesian Network	162
Network Dynamics	163
Genetic Perturbation of the ES Cell Systems to Dissect Regulatory Pathways	163
Epigenetic and Chromatin Features of Pluripotent Stem Cells	166
MicroRNAs Provide Another Layer of Regulatory Control	168
MicroRNAs in Stem Cells	168
Computational Approach to miRNAs and their Target mRNAs	169
Forwarding Engineering of ES Cell Regulatory Network	169
Concluding Remarks	170

Summary

Stem cells are specialized progenitor cells that have the ability to develop into different somatic cell types in the body. Among the different stem cells, embryonic stem (ES) cells are considered the most pluripotent as they have the potential to form every cell type, including other somatic stem cells. ES cells also possess the capability for extensive self-renewing division in culture. Understanding the unique biological properties of these cells has captured intense interests in recent years, propelled by high expectations of their great potential in regenerative medicine and by advances in technologies for studying these cells using systems approaches. Genetic and epigenetic characterization of ES cells has been extensively carried out. The generation of large datasets, the availability of robust tools to perturb biological function and the application of computational methods have enabled new discoveries at an unprecedented pace. The new knowledge garnered will provide new strategies for engineering cell fate. The concerted effort in studying ES cells makes them a good cellular model for systems biology.

Definitions

Stem cells Stem cells are unspecialized and undifferentiated cells that retain the ability to differentiate into specialized cell types.
Pluripotency Pluripotency is defined as the developmental potential of stem cells to differentiate into various specific cell types of the embryo and adult. The inner cell mass (ICM) of a blastocyst is pluripotent, and serves as precursor of mouse embryonic stem cells that can be propagated in culture infinitely given appropriate conditions. During normal embryogenesis, pluripotency is lost upon cell differentiation into the different lineages.
Self-renewal Self-renewal is the process of continuous cell divisions without differentiation to generate daughter cells identical to the mother cell.
ChIP Chromatin immunoprecipitation is a technique used to study protein/DNA interactions in live cells. Formaldehyde cross links protein to DNA and this preserves the interaction which can be enriched by immunoprecipitation with a specific antibody.

INTRODUCTION

Stem Cells

Stem cells are undifferentiated cells that can give rise to other cell types with specialized functions. Stem cells found in the adult organism are referred to as somatic stem cells. In the absence of appropriate signals, somatic stem cells will remain in a non-cycling state (also known as G_0) or, given specific stimulation, undergo multiple divisions without differentiation, also known as self-renewal. The ability to expand somatic stem cells in the laboratory would make them an attractive renewable source for applications in medicine and biological research. The process of becoming specialized cell types is known as differentiation. With appropriate stimulations, different types of somatic stem cells can be induced to differentiate along desired lineage paths to eventually form a relatively pure population of progenies. Differentiation has conventionally been thought to be non-reversible because differentiated progenies no longer possess the special characteristics of stem cells. Genetic and epigenetic changes accompany this specialization of cell fate.

Many human diseases are caused by either a loss of specific cell types or tissues (neuromuscular degenerative diseases, anemias, diabetes and arthritis) or malfunction of specific cell types (immunological disorders and cancers). Supplementing the body with stem cells or their differentiated progenies would be one way to correct the deficiency that leads to the disease or provide a means for replacement with normal cells after ablation of malfunctioning cells.

Pluripotent Embryonic Stem Cells

Somatic stem cells differ from each other in terms of their potential to become different cell types. For example, neural stem cells cannot differentiate into blood cells and hematopoietic stem cells ("blood" stem cells) cannot form neurons. A separate class of stem cell is the pluripotent embryonic stem (ES) cell, first isolated from the inner cell mass (ICM) of early mouse embryos more than 20 years ago (Solter, 2006). When reintroduced into an animal, these cells are able to form the three major embryonic lineages, namely endoderm, mesoderm and ectoderm and contribute to the tissues of the entire animal. Derivatives of these tissues contribute to the bulk of the body. Endoderm progenies form the digestive system and part of the respiratory system. The mesoderm develops into connective tissues, muscles, bones and the urogenital and circulatory systems. Epidermal and nervous tissues originate from ectoderm. Thus the spectrum of cells that can be developed from ES cells is much more diverse than somatic stem cells and essentially, ES cells can give rise to all other somatic stem cells. Furthermore, unlike somatic stem cells that normally remains resting but poised to undergo self-renewal division when needed, ES cells proliferate and self-renew infinitely when maintained under the proper *in vitro* growth condition.

The isolation of human embryo-derived stem cells has lagged significantly behind their mouse counterpart. This is partly due to the difficulties involved in obtaining suitable human embryonic material as well as legal and ethical constraints. It was not until 1998 that the derivation of cell lines directly from the human blastocysts (human ES cells) was achieved (Solter, 2006). Human ES cells share many features of the mouse ES cells. For example, both human and mouse ES cells express alkaline phosphatase and transcription factors such as Oct4, Sox2 and Nanog. However, there are also considerable differences between the two ES cells. For instance, in contrast to human ES cells, mouse ES cells retain their undifferentiated state in serum-containing medium supplemented with leukemia inhibitory factor (LIF) via the Signal Transducer and Activator of Transcription-3 (STAT-3) pathway (Boiani and Schöler, 2005). Bone morphogenetic proteins (BMPs) in combination with LIF can replace the requirement for feeder cells and serum entirely for mouse ES cells, but not for human ES cells. Human ES cells are however supported by different growth factors such as basic fibroblast growth factor (bFGF) and activin. Therefore, from the beginning, there was an understanding that the "wiring" characteristics of mouse and human ES cells were different despite the ability of these cells to differentiate into cells of the three major embryonic lineages.

Stem Cells for Systems Biology (Defining Molecular Networks, Interactions and Functionality)

Systems biology requires comprehensive and quantitative measurements of the molecular events in the cells. Regulation of gene expression has been heavily studied using systems approaches. Since the initial derivation of mouse ES cells in 1981, culture conditions have been well defined and they have been extensively utilized for gene targeting experiments in numerous laboratories throughout the world. Mouse ES cells can easily be maintained in an undifferentiated state and sufficient amounts can be routinely obtained for large-scale experimentation. Although human ES cells are more difficult to maintain in culture, recent progress has made it possible to expand and to manipulate these cells. Hence, the ability to propagate sufficient numbers of ES cells for detailed quantitative experiments makes the ES cell system an ideal model for systems studies. In contrast, the use of somatic stem cells for large-scale experimentations has lagged behind largely because of the difficulty of identifying and isolating them from different tissues and, most importantly, current poor knowledge for propagating and expanding somatic stem cells in large quantity in culture. For these reasons, the ideas and issues addressed in the rest of this chapter are largely based on investigations and findings using ES cells.

TRANSCRIPTION NETWORKS

A major challenge in the study of ES cells is to explain how the complex gene network is "wired" to control their properties of pluripotency (i.e., the ability to generate all cell types) and self-renewal. It appears that the master regulatory switches that trigger ES cell differentiation are transcription factors. These regulatory proteins and their relevant target genomic sequences work together to precisely tune the expression levels of thousands of target genes in ES cells. The interactions among these regulatory proteins and their interactions with particular genomic sequences collectively define a transcription network. The elucidation of the components, architecture and dynamic properties of the network demands integrated research from high throughput measurements, intervention and perturbation of the network, mathematical modeling, simulation studies and biological validations. These studies have revealed a number of aspects of the transcription network, including the identification of (1) upstream signals, regulatory proteins and target genes (2) cis-regulatory elements and chromatin modification codes and (3) dynamic properties of the network. A comprehensive understanding of all these aspects might lead to understanding of how the undifferentiated state of ES cells is maintained, and how it can be disrupted to initiate and proceed into lineage-specific differentiation. The same research principles and tools might be applicable to the study of other cellular and developmental processes.

The transcriptome of ES cells has been interrogated extensively. DNA microarray based and sequencing based technologies (SAGE, MPSS, EST) have been utilized to probe the expressed genetic constituents of these cells and to provide a semi-quantitative measure of gene expression. Moreover, ES cell-specific transcripts have been readily identified through comparison with differentiated cells.

An initial interest of analyzing ES cell gene expression data is to identify genes that mark "stemness"—pluripotency and self-renewal. ES cell expression data have been compared to that of adult stem cells, differentiated ES cells and preimplantation embryos (Fortunel et al., 2003; Ivanova et al., 2002; Ramalho-Santos et al., 2002). The data generated from different biological samples within one laboratory can be easily compared to each other using classical two-sample comparison techniques, including T-test, SAM analysis and others. It is well known that the overlaps of the ES cell-specific genes identified from independent studies are small (Fortunel et al., 2003; Ivanova et al., 2002; Ramalho-Santos et al., 2002). Such differences can be contributed to the difference of biological samples, lab protocols, microarray platforms and statistical approaches. To normalize these differences, a Reproducibility Probability Score was developed to identify differentially expressed genes and maximize the chances for the identified genes to be reproducible by later independent studies conducted by other laboratories (Lin et al., 2006). A meta-analysis approach was further exploited to jointly analyze multiple gene expression datasets, despite the different experimental designs (Glover et al., 2006). In such a study, a meta-analysis of gene expression data from three ES cell lines identified 88 genes whose expression consistently changed when ES cells were induced to differentiate. Seven of these (*103728_at*, *8430410A17Rik*, *Klf2*, *Nr0b1*, *Sox2*, *Tcl1* and *Zfp42*) showed a rapid decrease in expression concurrent with a decrease in frequency of undifferentiated cells and remained predictive when evaluated in additional maintenance and differentiating protocols.

A common practice to address the functional importance of a set of genes identified from expression analysis is to test in this set of genes for enrichment of functional categories, often in terms of Gene Ontology (GO). GoSurfer www.gosurfer.org) is an interactive software tool, which is applied to search for enriched GO terms in various gene clusters identified from ES cell differentiation data (Zhong and Xie, 2007). GoSurfer provides a statistical test to account for the multiple hypothesis testing issue that is naturally entailed in GO enrichment tests. In this study, five gene clusters were identified, representing upregulation, downregulation and other patterns in the differentiation time course. Taking the five gene clusters as input data, "cell adhesion" and "muscle contraction" were noted to be significant GO terms for the upregulated cluster, "amino acids metabolism" as a significant GO term for the downregulated gene cluster and GO terms related to RNA processing and RNA transport as significantly associated with a gene cluster that is upregulated in both early and late time-points.

Mapping Transcription Factor and DNA Interactions

In the pioneering work done by Davidson and colleagues, a framework based on the systems approach was used to build a genomic regulatory network model for a complex developmental process in sea urchin embryos (Davidson et al., 2002). The goal is to construct a model that describes key features for endomesoderm specification. One of the cardinal steps in building the knowledge base for *cis*-regulatory elements is to define the inputs and outputs of genes in a comprehensive manner. Perturbation analyses that involve RNA interference-mediated suppression of protein expression, usage of transcription factor with altered specificity and alternation of signaling processes were used to probe the spatial and temporal changes in gene expression. Quantitative PCR and whole mount *in situ* hybridization effectively captured the key information in these analyses. Key *cis*-regulatory elements are inferred from conserved sequences that impart identical gene expression of a homologous gene from a different species of sea urchin. An iterative process of model building and hypothesis testing refines the eventual network model. This sophisticated work also underscores the need for large-scale experimentation (large-scale perturbation and *cis*-regulatory element analyses) with quantitative measurements.

In the context of mammalian systems, a rather powerful approach has been developed to study regulatory elements in living cells. This methodology is known as chromatin immunoprecipitation (ChIP). Sequence-specific transcription factors interact with genomic DNA in a specific manner. These interactions can be preserved by formaldehyde which cross links the protein to DNA. Using specific antibodies toward the transcription factor, these complexes which occur in the living cell can be enriched. By capturing these protein–DNA complexes, one will be able to define the molecular constituents of the transcriptional regulatory networks and investigate how transcription regulators are wired to the genome.

Recent advances in technologies enable survey of transcription factor binding sites throughout the genome. Two major platforms are currently available. The first platform utilizes DNA microarray to detect ChIP-enriched DNA through hybridization. Increasing feature density has allowed DNA microarray to tackle the challenge of covering the large mammalian genomes. The second platform utilizes high throughput sequencing to capture the locations of ChIP-enriched DNA. There has been rapid development in the use of massively parallel technology to sequence DNA fragments . In contrast to Sanger method-based capillary sequencing, the new generation of sequencing technology offers a cost-effective way of sequencing millions of short DNA tags. An unbiased survey of transcription factor binding sites is important as different transcription factors exhibit distinct binding profiles.

Mouse ES cells are maintained in pluripotent state by several key regulators. They include DNA binding factors such as Oct4, Sox2 and Nanog (Boiani and Schöler, 2005). Oct4 is a POU domain transcription factor with an octamer consensus binding site, ATGCAAAT. Sox2 belongs to the Sox family of transcription factor and recognizes a 7bp binding motif. Nanog is a homeodomain-containing transcription factor that binds to ATTA motif. These regulators are highly expressed in ES cells and their depletion leads to differentiation (Fig. 7.1A). Along with other genes upregulated in ES cells, the expression of these genes

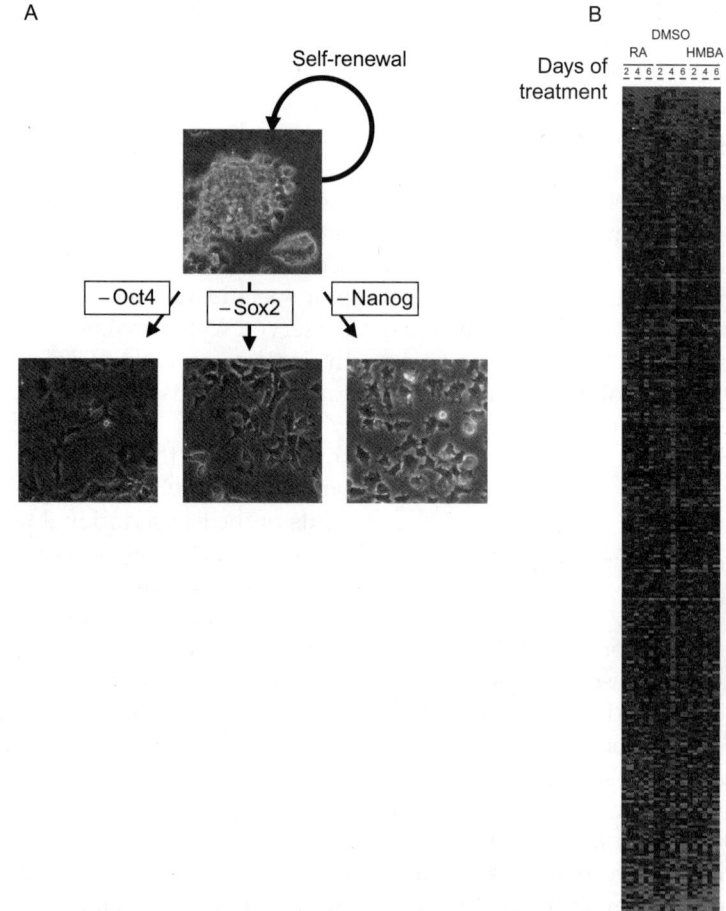

FIGURE 7.1 Properties of ES Cells.
(A) Mouse ES cells propagated under feeder-free culture condition show characteristic colony morphology. Self-renewing division expands the size of the colony and maintains the pluripotency of ES cells. Depletion of key transcriptional factors such as Oct4, Sox2 or Nanog by RNA interference induces differentiation. These cells undergo morphological changes and exit the self-renewal state. (B) Heatmaps showing the changes in gene expression after ES cells were induced to differentiate using three different chemical treatments (retinoic acid, DMSO and HMBA). RNA samples were harvested at different days after treatment and were analyzed by DNA microarray. The gene expression profiles were clustered based on changes relative to undifferentiated ES cells. Red denotes upregulation and green denotes downregulation.

gives rise to the unique transcriptome of ES cells. ES cells can be triggered to differentiate and ES cell-specific gene expression is lost (Fig. 7.1B).

How do the key transcription factors control gene expression and specify the transcriptome in ES cells? Studies to address this question have been performed in mouse and human ES cells (Boyer et al., 2005; Loh et al., 2006). Loh and colleagues mapped out the binding sites of Oct4 and Nanog using ChIP coupled to a paired-end ditag (PET) sequencing technology. Instead of direct sequencing the entire genomic DNA fragments obtained from ChIP, this PET sequencing technology captures the 5′ and 3′ ends of genomic DNA and fuses them as a single PET unit. The PET units are further concatenated for efficient sampling. After sequencing, the information on each PET unit is then mapped back to the genome to demarcate the location of ChIP-enriched DNA. The ChIP–PET method of mapping transcription factor binding site is unbiased and offers high resolution in locating the binding motifs. Indeed, the DNA binding motif for Oct4 can be inferred from the ChIP–PET cluster using *de novo* motif discovery algorithms that detect over-represented motifs. The ChIP–PET analysis reveals approximately 1000 and 3000 high confident binding loci for Oct4 and Nanog, respectively. The majority of the binding loci are found within the gene body, indicating that Oct4 and Nanog do not preferentially bind to promoter regions and potentially regulate gene expression from distal genomic sites.

ChIP analyses for OCT4, SOX2 and NANOG were performed using promoter arrays for human ES cells (Boyer et al., 2005). NANOG binds to at least 60% of the OCT4 bound or SOX2 bound promoters. The extensive co-occupancies led to the proposal that these three factors form a core transcriptional regulatory circuitry in human ES cells. A comparison between the human and mouse datasets shows limited overlap, suggesting that the OCT4 and NANOG circuitries may differ between the two species.

With the advent of next sequencing technologies such as the Solexa sequencing method, it is now feasible to do deep sampling of ChIP-enriched DNA to enable a comprehensive survey of transcription factor binding sites with even higher precision (Fig. 7.2A, B). Chen et al. (2008b) have used ChIP-seq to map the locations of 13 sequence-specific transcription factors (Nanog, Oct4, STAT3, Smad1, Sox2, Zfx, c-Myc, n-Myc, Klf4, Esrrb, Tcfcp2l1, E2f1 and CTCF) and two co-regulators (p300 and Suz12) in ES cells. A key finding is the discovery of transcription factor co-localization hotspots co-occupied by multiple transcription factors. A total of 3583 multiple transcription factor binding loci (MTL) are bound by 4 or more transcription factors (Chen et al., 2008b). The high degree of evolution conservation of these MTL suggests functional importance. Two major clusters of MTL can be segregated. The first cluster consists of Oct4, Sox2 and Nanog, and is enriched with Smad1, STAT3 and Esrrb. The second cluster is made up of c-Myc, n-Myc, Zfx and E2f1. MTL from the Oct4 cluster are associated with ES cell-specific enhancer activity. The densely bound genomic loci may serve several functions. First, these loci are proposed to act as enhanceosomes where the multiple transcription factors congregate to generate a platform for the recruitment of co-activator complexes (Fig. 7.2C) (Panne et al., 2007). Second, these loci may serve as the focal point for communication between the signaling pathways (through Smad1 or STAT3) and the core transcription factors (Oct4, Sox2 and Nanog). Third, the assembly or maintenance of a stable complex may require multiple synergistic interactions. It is also of interest to note that an independent genome-wide mapping study of a slightly different set of transcription factors (Oct4, Sox2, Nanog, Klf4, and c-Myc, Dax1, Rex1, Zpf281 and Nac1) also reveals clustering of transcription factors at selective sites (Kim et al., 2008). Hence, transcription factor co-localization hotspots are likely to be a general feature of mammalian ES cells.

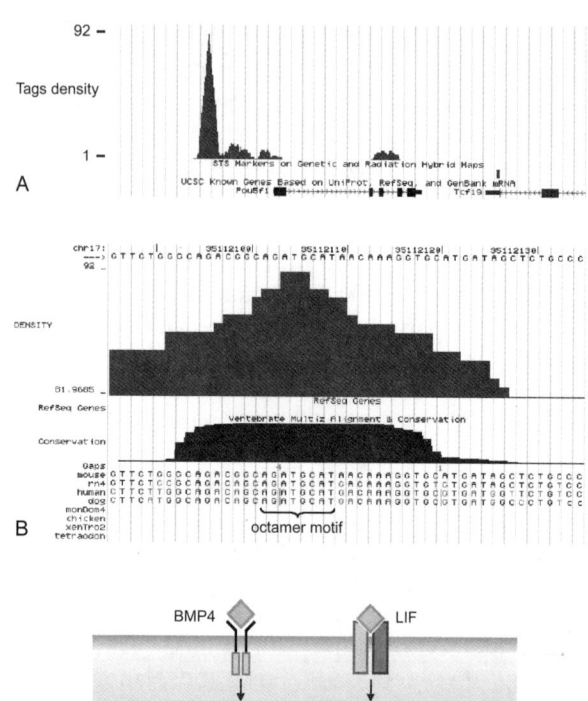

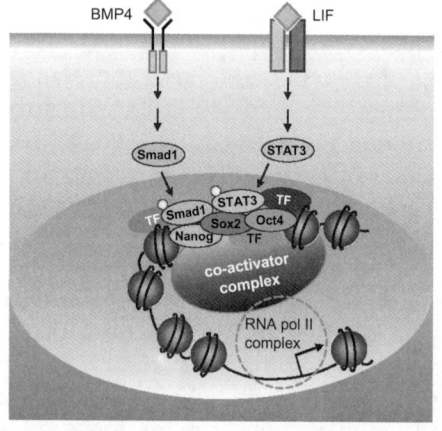

FIGURE 7.2 Mapping of Transcription Factor Binding Site and Profile Using Next Generation Sequencing Technology. (A) A screen shot of the genome browser showing the binding profile (colored in green) reconstructed using ChIP-seq analysis for Oct4 transcription factor. Instead of using PET to map the 5′ and 3′ end information of genomic DNA, ChIP-seq captures only the short tags of one end. High throughput sequencing using the Solexa technology enables a deep survey of DNA fragments and the profile of transcription factor binding can be reconstructed computationally. (B) A display of 50 bp sequence of the peak region identified by ChIP-seq. The location of the octamer motif corresponds to the peak of the binding profile. This region is also conserved among different mammals (shown by the blue conservation track). (C) A model for ES cell-specific enhanceosome. Transcription of genes specifically upregulated in ES cells requires the assembly of multiprotein complexes at enhancer sites. The interface created by multiple transcription factors may assist in the recruitment of co-activator complexes to enhance transcription.

Work done by several laboratories revealed several interesting features of the ES cell transcriptional regulatory network (Fig. 7.3) (Jaenisch and Young, 2008). This network contains extensive interconnected autoregulatory and feed-forward loops. Such design may help to stabilize the ES cell gene expression. The network also receives inputs from extracellular signaling

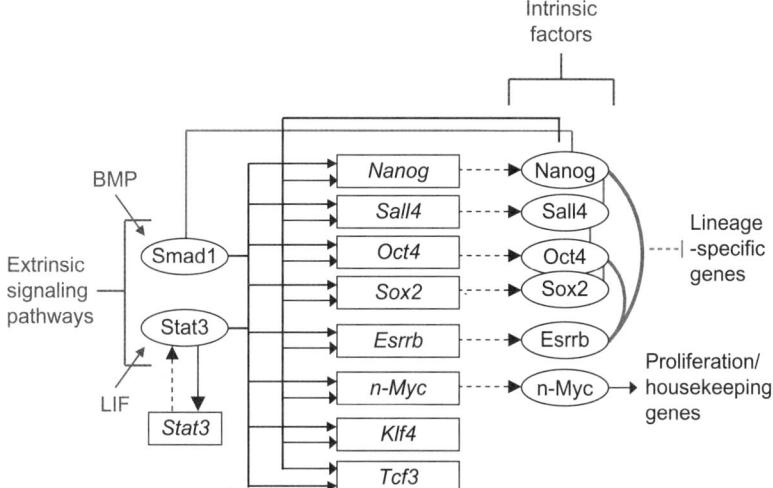

FIGURE 7.3 A Model of Transcriptional Regulatory Network in ES Cells.
Transcription factors are represented by ovals and the genes (printed in italics) are represented by rectangles. Nanog, Sall4, Oct4, Sox2, Esrrb, n-Myc are considered the intrinsic factors as they are not directly controlled by the extracellular signaling pathways. Stat3 and Smad1 are downstream effectors for the LIF and BMP pathways, respectively. A black arrow indicates a transcription factor binding to a gene. Dotted arrows denote the synthesis of gene products from their respective genes. Some of the intrinsic factors such as Oct4 are found to bind to lineage-specific genes suggesting that they may inhibit lineage-specific differentiation (denoted by orange inhibitory link). Protein–protein interactions between the transcription factors are shown as green connections.

pathways (LIF/STAT3 and BMP/Smad1), suggesting that these signaling pathways are likely to modulate the activity of the key nodes of the network. Interactions between the transcription factors are also common in this network. These transcription factors could be part of larger nucleoprotein complexes as discussed earlier.

COMPUTATIONAL TOOLS FOR NETWORK CONSTRUCTION AND MODELING

Computational approaches are often used to further characterize the transcription factor binding sites within binding regions determined by ChIP analysis. There are a number of computational algorithms that detect transcription factor binding motifs in *cis*-regulatory regions. These algorithms typically utilize the over-representation property of motifs for a set of co-expressed genes. A couple of recent developments have increased the accuracy of motif identification and shed light on the modular activities of multiple binding sites in the regulation of ES cell-specific expression. By simultaneously utilizing the representation property of a motif in co-expressed genes and the co-localization property of multiple motifs in a *cis*-regulatory module, Wong and co-workers identified a regulatory network composed of regulators of *Oct4, Sox2, Nanog, Esrrb, Stat3, Tcf7, Sall4* and *LRH-1* (Zhou et al., 2007).

Comparison of the human and the mouse genomes can identify conserved non-coding regions which are more likely to contain functional sequences. Moreover, the conservation of the DNA motif itself is another important indicator of its functional importance. CompMoby is a computational algorithm which analyzes both aligned and non-aligned sequences between different genomes with a probabilistic segmentation model to systematically predict short DNA motifs that regulate gene expression. CompMoby is used to identify conserved over-represented motifs in genes upregulated in pluripotent cells (Grskovic et al., 2007). It is shown that the motifs are preferentially active in undifferentiated mouse ES and embryonic germ cells in a sequence-specific manner, and that they can act as enhancers in the context of an endogenous promoter. Importantly, the activity of the motifs is conserved in human ES cells. It is also shown that the transcription factor NF-Y specifically binds to one of the motifs, is differentially expressed during ES cell differentiation, and is required for ES cell proliferation.

It is advisable to exercise caution in the comparative analysis of human and mouse genomes for identification of ES cell-specific motifs. Human and mouse ES cells, although sharing many properties, appear to sustain their transcriptional programs with very different network structures. Evidence for different transcriptional program being used in human and mouse lies in twofold. First, different transcription factors are involved in maintaining the self-renewal property. For example, transcription factor FoxD3 is required for self-renewal of mouse ES cells, but its expression appears to be non-essential in human ES cells. The expression of FoxD3 is also highly variable in different human ES cell lines. Second, different transcription factors participate in the initiation of early differentiation processes in human and mouse. For example, the transcription factor Ehox is essential for the early differentiation process of mouse ES cells, but no functional orthologue has been found in human. These evidences suggest that there are more than one network structure that are capable of maintaining a transcriptional program that constituently expresses genes for self-renewal and suppresses genes for differentiation.

Besides analysis of gene expression and ChIP–chip/ChIP–PET data, a number of more computationally demanding approaches have been proposed to reconstruct gene regulatory networks, including both transcription networks and signaling pathways in ES cells. These approaches include a regulatory module method, network mapping and Bayesian network.

Regulatory Module

A regulatory module refers to a set of co-regulated genes and their regulators. A co-clustering latent variable model has been applied to identify stem cell-specific regulatory modules from integrated experimental datasets (Joung et al., 2006). A latent variable is introduced to associate *cis*-regulatory motifs to subpopulations of cell types, where subpopulations are defined as different stages of differentiating ES cells and multiple adult stem cells. A data matrix is constructed by computing the matches of 360 position weight matrices (PWM) of the TRANSFAC database on the 5K upstream regions of 23 346 genes. The latent variable model simultaneously clusters stem cell subpopulations and putative transcription factor binding sites from PWM matches. Five regulatory modules have been identified. One module is regarded as a stemness module. Potential transcription regulators of this module include *Egr2*, *CREB*, *CRE-BP1* and *Ap2*.

Bayesian Network

Signaling events that direct ES cell self-renewal and differentiation are complex and accordingly difficult to understand in an integrated manner. This problem is addressed by adapting a Bayesian network learning algorithm to model proteomic signaling data for ES cell fate responses to external cues (Woolf et al., 2005). This model characterizes the signaling pathway influences as quantitative, logic-circuit type interactions. It has been demonstrated that the Bayesian networks can capture the linear, non-linear and multistate logic interactions that connect extracellular cues, intracellular signals and consequent cell functional responses.

In this study, an experimental dataset is compiled from measurements for 28 signaling protein phosphorylation states across 16 different factorial combinations of cytokine and matrix stimuli. The Bayesian network model recovers previously reported signaling activities related to mouse ES cell self-renewal, such as the roles of LIF and STAT3 in maintaining undifferentiated ES cell populations. Furthermore, the network predicts novel influences such as between ERK phosphorylation and differentiation, or RAF phosphorylation and differentiated cell proliferation. Visualization of the influences detected by the Bayesian network provides intuition about the underlying physiology of the signaling pathways.

Network Dynamics

Besides the static architecture of the transcriptional circuitry in ES cells, their kinetic and temporal properties are critical for understanding how cell fate is decided during the differentiation process. Two major approaches have been developed to investigate the kinetic properties of ES cell transcription networks.

In a "forward" approach, the architecture of a core transcription network is given, and a set of differential equations are set up to simulate the transcriptional responses of the target genes regulated by this core network (Chickarmane et al., 2006). In this study, simulation study demonstrates a bistable switch in the OCT4–SOX2–NANOG network, which arises due to several positive feedback loops, and is switched on/off by input environmental signals. The switch stabilizes the expression levels of the three genes, and through their regulatory roles on the downstream target genes, leads to a binary decision: when OCT4, SOX2 and NANOG are expressed and the switch is on, the self-renewal genes are on and the differentiation genes are off.

In a "backward" approach, temporal gene expression data are measured at multiple time-points along the differentiation time course. These data are used to infer the mode in which the transcription factors interact and how such modes of interaction affect the quantitative changes of the target transcripts (Chen et al., 2008a). For each mode of interaction, the theoretical equilibrium levels of the transcripts of the target gene are derived from the joint application of thermodynamic models that relate transcription factor binding to RNA polymerase (RNAP) binding and a kinetic model that relate RNAP binding to the equilibrium levels of the transcripts of the target gene. With a reverse-engineering approach, the modes of interaction can be searched and the mode that gives rise to a theoretical temporal transcriptional pattern that is closest to the measured responses can be identified (Fig. 7.4). In this study, the interaction modes of Oct4 and Nanog on *Zic3*, *Jarid2*, *Sall4*, *Rif1*, *Gbx2* and *Eomes* are identified as Oct4 being an activator and Nanog being a helper. The activator directly interacts with RNAP and the helper helps to stabilize the activator's binding with DNA. This study also suggests that Oct4 and Nanog assume two inhibition modes of interaction on the target genes of *Atbf1* and *Foxc1*.

GENETIC PERTURBATION OF THE ES CELL SYSTEMS TO DISSECT REGULATORY PATHWAYS

In the analysis of ES cells using the systems approaches, genetic perturbation plays a key role in understanding the role(s) of different molecules or pathways in this system. Two strategies (gain-of-function and loss-of-function) have been used to screen for gene products that affect ES cell phenotype (Fig. 7.5). In the first approach, Lemischka and colleagues performed a gain-of-function genetic screen (Pritsker et al., 2006). A cDNA expression library was transfected into ES cells. The transfected cells were cultured under two conditions. The first culture

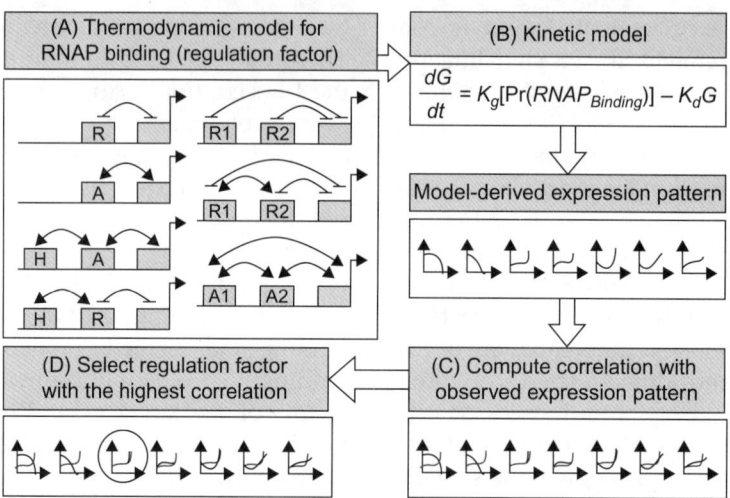

FIGURE 7.4 Flowchart of the Reverse-Engineering Algorithm for Identification of Modes of Interactions Between Two Transcription Factors.
(A) It begins by using a thermodynamic function, termed regulation factor, to predict the equilibrium probability that RNAP binds to the promoter of its targeted gene (P_{RNAP}) based on concentrations of associated transcription factors and interaction forms among transcription factors and RNAP. (B) It then utilizes systems of ordinary differential equations to simulate the dynamics of expression interested genes. (C) With measured time course gene expression data from microarray experiments, it computes the Pearson correlation coefficient between the observed expression pattern and the predicted expression pattern. Steps A, B and C are carried out for all potential interaction modes between transcription factors and promoters. (D) The regulation factor that predicts an expression pattern with highest correlation to the observed expression pattern is identified as most plausible interaction form that transcription factors take to regulate this target gene

condition has LIF and is permissive for propagation of ES cells. The second culture condition is without LIF and selects for cells that can be maintained upon overexpression of certain factors. Overexpression of 11 genes (*Akt1, Chop-10, Cited2, RhoJ, NCE, Nspc1, Prune, Asb6, Snx6, Ssbp4, Mm.41868*) maintain higher number of cells in the absence of LIF. These genes encode for proteins of diverse biological functions, including protein kinase, signaling molecule, enzymes and transcriptional regulators. The phenotype exhibited is similar to the overexpression of Nanog, albeit at a much lower efficiency. In fact, Nanog was originally identified as a factor that can sustain self-renewal of ES cells in the absence of LIF (Boiani and Schöler, 2005). The same study also leads to the discovery of 9 genes (*JunB, c-Fos, Nsbp1, Catna, Pum1, Nab1, Fin14, Fbox30, SpiC*) that drive differentiation upon overexpression.

The gene products include transcription factors, RNA-binding factors and signaling molecules. The ES cells underwent morphological change to become fibroblast-like and showed reduced proliferation rate. The gain-of-function analysis can potentially identify genes that drive ES cells into specific lineages. For instance, overexpression of Oct4 induces ES cell to differentiate mainly to extraembryonic endoderm. The mechanisms of rendering ES cells LIF-independent or promoting differentiation through overexpression of these genes remain to be studied. One major limitation of the gain-of-function analysis is that it cannot determine whether the gene is essential.

The second strategy that complements the gain-of-function analysis is to deplete the expression of candidate genes and examine the effect on ES cell properties. Several methods are available for depleting gene expression. Homologous

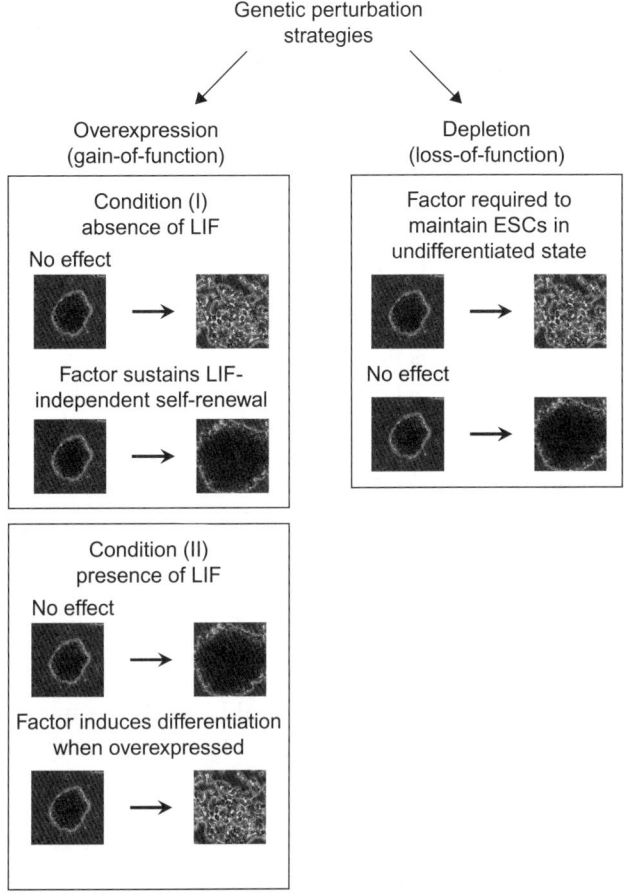

FIGURE 7.5 Genetic Perturbation Strategies to Identify New Regulators of ES Cells.
Gain-of-function assay involves the overexpression of gene product and examines the phenotypes of the cells. Withdrawal of the growth factor, LIF from the culture media induces ES cell to differentiate (condition I). The ES cells were stained for alkaline phosphatase (red coloration). Differentiation leads to change in morphology and the loss of alkaline phosphatase staining. It is found that overexpression of transcription factor such as Nanog promotes self-renewal of ES cells without the requirement of LIF. Certain factors such as Cdx2 are able to induce differentiation under the normal culture condition (condition II). Loss-of-function assay involves the depletion of gene product. A commonly used method is RNA interference.

recombination is a way to delete an allele in mouse ES cells and this technology has been routinely employed to generate gene-targeted animals. Homozygous null ES cells can be obtained from the ICM of the knockout animals or the second allele of the gene can be targeted. In the event that the gene of interest is important for the maintenance of ES cells, it will not be possible to derive homozygous null ES cells or to successfully generate ES cells with the targeted second allele. In order to achieve a higher throughput analysis of gene function, RNA interference (RNAi) is the platform of choice. Lemischka and colleagues set up a large-scale screen for genes required to maintain self-renewal in ES cells (Ivanova et al., 2006). In this study, 70 genes were selected for knockdown. These genes are among the 901 rapidly downregulated genes upon retinoic acid-induced differentiation. Lentiviruses harboring shRNA and *GFP* expression cassettes were used to achieve high transduction efficiency. The GFP expression marks the transduced cells for a fluorescence-based competition assay to measure self-renewal. GFP-positive cells which were transduced by the lentiviruses were mixed in a 4:1 ratio with GFP-negative non-transduced cells. The GFP-positive/GFP-negative ratios were measured in a time course experiment. Reduction of the GFP-positive/GFP-negative ratios could be due to a few causes. The differentiation of ES cells will reduce proliferation rate. There could be changes in cell cycle kinetics or cell adhesion. If depletion of a gene product leads to cell death, the GFP-positive cells will progressively be lost. All these are possible causes that will result in non-transduced cells out-competing the lentivirus-transduced GFP-positive cells. Downregulation of 8 genes (*Nanog*, *Oct4*, *Sox2*, *Tbx3*, *Esrrb*, *Tcl1*, *Dppa4*, *Mm.343880*) resulted in impaired self-renewal, morphological changes and loss of alkaline phosphatase activity. Further validation of shRNA specificity was obtained from rescue experiments. A rescue experiment is a genetic complementation strategy to determine if restoring the gene product of interest can prevent the loss-of-function phenotype. Apart from *Mm.343880*, knockdown of the other 7 genes could be complemented by co-expression of RNAi-immune open reading frame of the respective genes. Importantly, other laboratories have independently shown that knockdown of *Nanog*, *Oct4*, *Sox2*, *Esrrb* and *Tcl1* leads to ES cell differentiation (Loh et al., 2006; Matoba et al., 2006).

Using similar RNAi-mediated depletion approach, *Sall4*, *Zic3*, *Jmjd1a*, *Jmjd2c* and other genes have been shown to be required for the maintenance of ES cells. Sall4 and Zic3 are transcription factors while Jmjd1a and Jmjd2c are histone H3 lysine 9 demethylases. Depletion of these factors leads to change in ES cell morphology and loss of alkaline phosphatase activity. In contrast to this differentiation phenotype, the loss-of-function of another group of genes shows proliferation defect while maintaining pluripotency. ES cells with null mutation of *Eras* and *Zfx* are viable and can be propagated (Takahashi et al., 2003; Galan-Caridad et al., 2007). *Eras* is a Ras-like gene while *Zfx* encodes for a transcription factor. Both genes are upregulated in ES cells. The knockout cells show severely reduced growth rate, indicating that they are involved in promoting self-renewal of ES cells through a different mechanism. When transplanted into nude mice, *Eras*-deficient cells produced markedly smaller tumors than did wild-type cells. *Zfx*-deficient ES cells underwent spontaneous apoptosis.

The self-renewal regulators of ES cells identified to date included many transcription factors. These transcription factors contribute to the entire transcriptional regulatory network by targeting specific genes. The importance of the downstream targets in ES cells is emerging through loss-of-function analysis. In the context of the transcriptional regulatory circuitry governed by Oct4, Sox2 and Nanog, the key nodes are beginning to be elucidated. Future work should extend this network by mapping the targets of the downstream transcription factors. A combination of genetic perturbation and comprehensive survey of binding sites will enable the reconstruction of the network model that describes the ES cell transcriptome.

EPIGENETIC AND CHROMATIN FEATURES OF PLURIPOTENT STEM CELLS

Eukaryotic DNA is packaged with proteins that are primarily histones to form chromatin. Mammalian chromatin is subjected to different types of modifications on both the DNA and histones. Methylation of DNA at cytosine residue is known to be associated with transcriptional repression. Methyl-CpGs are the binding sites for a class of proteins known as methyl-CpG binding proteins. They are generally transcription repressors that associate with histone deacetylases.

Modifications of histones are however more complex as there are at least 40 types of modifications ranging from phosphorylation, acetylation, methylation to ubiquitylation. Modifications of DNA or histones have been shown to confer distinct properties to genes without altering the base composition of the DNA. This phenomenon is generally known as epigenetics.

Different histone modifications are associated with different states of chromatin. For example, methylation of lysine 4 residue of histone H3 is generally correlated with transcription while methylation of lysine 9 or lysine 27 residue of histone H3 is associated with silenced chromatin. The levels of gene expression are linked to the structure and conformation of the chromatin. Condensed chromatin regions are usually incompatible with transcription activity, while active chromatin adopts a structure that is accessible to nuclear processes such as transcription.

Chromatin structure plays a fundamental role in controlling the accessibility of DNA. An attractive hypothesis to explain the reduction in potentiality after cellular differentiation is the restriction in accessibility of chromatin to cell type-specific transcription factors. More recently, it has been shown that mouse ES cells possess a "looser" chromatin structure compared to differentiated cells. Differentiation of ES cells leads to an increase in the repressive marking, histone H3 lysine 9 trimethylation and a reduction in the active markings, histone H3 and H4 acetylations (Meshorer and Misteli, 2006). By examining the dynamic behavior of histones in undifferentiated but lineage-committed cells, it was shown that the hyperdynamic binding of chromatin-associated proteins is a hallmark of pluripotent cells and not just of an undifferentiated state. It is proposed that the loosely bound and soluble pool of structural proteins is crucial for maintaining pluripotency and for early differentiation. An attractive model to explain these observations is that the dynamic and plastic chromatin state is the key to keeping all differentiation options open. The importance of chromatin methylation is further highlighted by the findings that drastic reduction of DNA methylation blocks ES cell differentiation and ES cells cannot survive without a histone H3 lysine 9 methyltransferase, ESET. Hence, there is a clear link between histone methylation and stem cell biology.

Pioneering work has been carried out by Bernstein and colleagues on probing the histone H3 lysine 4 and lysine 27 trimethylations at highly conserved non-coding elements. These regions which cover less than 2% of the mouse genome are enriched for genes encoding for developmentally regulated transcription factors. Interestingly, key developmental genes are marked by both modifications and the term "bivalent domains" is coined to describe this phenomenon in mouse ES cells. These bivalent domains, which consist of large regions of H3K27 methylation flanking smaller regions of H3 lysine 4 methylation, are found to occur at genes that are expressed at very low levels. Upon ES cell differentiation, some of these bivalent domains are gradually resolved to either H3K27 or H3K4 methylation (Bernstein et al., 2006). As the bivalently marked genes are expressed at low level in ES cells, it is proposed that these domains silence developmental genes while keeping them poised for activation.

The prevalence of bivalent domains is next investigated in three independent studies that performed genome-wide survey using ChIP–chip, ChIP–PET and ChIP–Solexa (Mikkelsen et al., 2007; Sharov and Ko, 2007). All three findings in both human (Sharov and Ko, 2007) and mouse ES cells (Mikkelsen et al., 2007) had a high level of consistency in the localization of bivalent domains occurring in the genome. H3K4 methylation marks more than two-third of the human promoters, and is surprisingly not indicative of transcriptional activity. On the other hand, H3K27 methylation is less extensive and the majority of H3K27-methylated loci are co-modified by H3K4 methylation. Importantly, these studies also reveal that bivalent domains are not unique to pluripotent ES cells, but are also found in human lung fibroblast cells, and in mouse neural progenitor cells and embryonic fibroblasts.

MICRORNAs PROVIDE ANOTHER LAYER OF REGULATORY CONTROL

While there is mounting data and increased appreciation of the intricacies of networks of transcription factors involved in regulating the self-renewal and differentiation of ES and somatic stem cells, details of the molecular mechanisms by which the output of these factors are orchestrated in governing ES cell fate remain poorly understood. Post-transcriptional regulatory mechanisms provide another layer of modulation of expression of many genes and it is now clear that non-coding RNAs, including microRNAs (miRNAs), play major roles in regulating the output of mRNAs (He and Hannon, 2004). miRNAs are ~22nt non-coding RNAs that regulate other coding mRNAs by interfering with and suppressing translation and in some instances destabilizing target mRNAs. Nascent primary miRNA transcripts (pri-miRNAs) are processed sequentially by nuclear Drosha and cytoplasmic Dicer RNase III endonuclease-containing complexes to yield mature miRNAs, which are incorporated into the RNA interference silencing complex (RISC). The activated RISC–miRNA complexes bind to cognate mRNA cis-elements, and these complexes are directed to the P-bodies where mRNA degradation or translational repression occurs.

MicroRNAs in Stem Cells

Amongst the hundreds of, and possibly several thousands, microRNAs, the function of only a handful of them has been elucidated. This reflects a general difficulty in functionalizing miRNAs, partly because of a paucity of good assay system to test for miRNA function and partly because the functional effects of miRNAs may be subtle. In addition, the expression patterns of most miRNAs are still not known although recent large-scale studies have begun to generate a useful database for the expression of miRNAs in different tissues (Landgraf et al., 2007).

In mouse ES cells, the loss of mature miRNAs in *Dicer* 1−/− ES cells results in a failure of the ES cells to differentiate (Kanellopoulou et al., 2005), highlighting the importance of regulated miRNA expression in controlling ES cell growth and differentiation. This is likely to apply also to other stem cells. Comparative profiling of miRNA signatures between cell types and cell populations enriched for stem cells has been useful in uncovering candidate miRNAs that may be important for lineage development. For example, comparison of hematopoietic progenitor populations has resulted in the discovery of *miR-181* as a driver of B lymphoid (Chen et al., 2004) and T lymphocyte development (Li et al., 2007). Using similar approach, *miR-150* was also shown to be important and crucial for determining progression from ProB to B cells (Xiao et al., 2007). These results show not only the impact of miRNA levels on lineage development but also indicate that the same miRNA may have effect on different lineages. In ES cells, ES cell-specific miRNAs such as the *miR-290-296* cluster in murine ES cells (Houbaviy et al., 2003) and the human homologue, the *miR-371-373* cluster (Suh et al., 2004) have been identified but their functional significance remains to be determined. Intriguingly, this family of miRNAs are also highly expressed in germ cell cancer lines, and in human cells *miR-372* and *miR-373* have the ability to protect cells from oncogenic stress and transform primary human cells (Voorhoeve et al., 2006). This suggests that they may operate key regulatory networks conserved in pluripotent stem cells, germ cells and cancer cells. Expression profiling of miRNA expression pattern during differentiation of

ES cells have shown that many miRNAs are upregulated or downregulated with differentiation. The overexpression or knockdown of these miRNAs have shown little effect on ES cells and only a few have shown a dominant effect (Tay et al., 2008a). Other approaches have combined expression data with computational approach for targets of miRNAs (Miranda et al., 2006).

Computational Approach to miRNAs and Their Target mRNAs

A unique feature of miRNAs is that they do not require complete complementarity with their cognate mRNA cis-element, suggesting a sliding scale is required for predicting the mRNA target sequences of miRNAs (Stark et al., 2005). Therefore, a miRNA can target many mRNAs with no overall sequence homology except in short regions in the mRNA via microRNA recognizing elements (MREs). This is an ingenious mechanism allowing the co-ordinate control of many genes by a single miRNA. This however poses challenges to the algorithms for in silico prediction of miRNAs' target mRNAs. Consequently, a bottleneck to understanding the function of different miRNAs has been the ability to predict accurately the mRNA targets of miRNAs and MREs mediating their interaction. Several in silico predictive algorithms have been developed. All of which predict and show that a single miRNA can target from a few miRNAs to as many as hundreds of targets. Applying the rna22 algorithm to predict targets for three miRNAs, many candidate miRNA targets were tested (Miranda et al., 2006). For example, one miRNA studied, *miR-134*, was predicted to be active against over 5000 mRNA species. Out of 160 *cis*-elements tested, suppression of luciferase reporter activity with 114 *cis*-elements was observed. Most importantly, when the endogenous protein and mRNA levels of selected predicted *miR-134* target genes were examined, it was found that *miR-134* induced a translation downregulation in these genes, some of which are important in directing ES cell growth or differentiation including key pluripotency-associated transcription factors (Tay et al., 2008a). Furthermore, overexpression of *miR-134* alone appears to be capable of inducing differentiation of mouse ES cells to a primitive ectodermal phenotype, a precursor to neuronal differentiation. These results highlight the significant impact that a single miRNA may have on stem cells and the challenging task of understanding how the targeting of multiple targets by a single miRNA leads to a cellular effect.

Further demonstration of the power of computational approach is the recent important discovery that miRNAs can target not only the 3'UTRs of mRNAs but also the coding region of mRNAs (Tay et al., 2008b), thereby vastly expanding the domain of miRNA impact on mRNA targets. Recent large-scale proteomic studies confirmed that the expression of a single miRNA can result in subtle changes in levels of large number of proteins that are product of direct targets of the miRNAs (Baek et al., 2008; Selbach et al., 2008). The accumulating evidences therefore is pointing toward a regulatory system in stem cells of parallel modules of coding and non-coding RNAs, in which transcription networks provide the hard wiring for multiple pathways while a network of miRNAs superimpose their modulation of the protein output of the transcription networks (Marson et al., 2008). A deeper inquiry into how miRNAs intersect with the transcription network will be described in the chapter on miRNA in this book.

FORWARDING ENGINEERING OF ES CELL REGULATORY NETWORK

In somatic cells, the ES cell regulatory network is not present because many of the key pluripotency-associated transcription factors are not expressed. Conceptually, if we assume that transcription factors are key drivers of gene expression, then it will be feasible for cell fate to be altered by introducing transcription factor(s). The re-wiring of transcription factor/genome interactions could jump-start the ES cell regulatory network and consequently induces a pluripotent phenotype.

How many transcription factors are required to reconstruct this network in somatic cells? This question was empirically answered by a piece of pioneering work by Yamanaka and colleague (Takahashi and Yamanaka, 2006). Twenty-four ES cell-related factors were screened for their ability to convert terminally differentiated fibroblasts into pluripotent cells. Retrovirus was used to ectopically express these transcription factors in fibroblasts. Re-programming of fibroblasts is accompanied by a change in cellular morphology and the induction of ES cell-specific gene expression program. While each of the single factor had no activity, a combination of four transcription factors (Oct4, Sox2, Klf4, c-Myc) was able to induce the formation of pluripotent stem cells. Stem cells derived using this method are also known as induced pluripotent stem cells (iPSCs).

Besides these four transcription factors, are there other combinations of factors or novel transcription factors with re-programming activity? The acquisition of genome-scale location and gene expression datasets allows one to construct a mechanistic model of the ES cell regulatory network. Such model will illuminate the key nodes, which may represent contact points to ignite the ES cell-specific gene expression program. Future work will be able to determine whether the transcription factors at these key nodes have re-programming activity. In general, the wealth of knowledge generated from large-scale experimentations can be used in the engineering of biological systems to attain unique cellular fate.

CONCLUDING REMARKS

A measure of the usefulness of a systems biology approach to the integration and utilization of stem cell genomic information is whether it is possible to make accurate predictions of cellular responses upon manipulation of genes or extracellular signals. In the field of ES cell biology, one area where systems biology is beginning to make an impact is in revealing clues on what genes to genetically manipulate to induce ES cell differentiation or direct cell fate (Fig. 7.6). The intersection of network of top ES cell-specific transcriptional factors have revealed a list of core genes that include several that are clearly involved in regulating ES cell transitions to specific lineages as revealed by RNAi-validation studies.

Another area where systems biology has also made its impact and will likely continue to do so is in the area of re-programming. Historically, the discovery that differentiation is reversible was first demonstrated in somatic nuclear transfer into oocytes, first in *Xenopus* and later in mammals. In these experiments, the isolated nuclei of differentiated cells, when injected into enucleated ova, can be re-programmed into stem cells. With the derivation and rapid advances in the use of ES cells, fusion of ES with other cell types demonstrated the dominant phenotype of ES cells and strongly suggests the presence of factors that are capable of initiating re-programming. With recent rapid advances in genomic technologies, it became possible to deduce from the 30 000–40 000 total number of mammalian genes a reasonably short list of genes that appear to be strong candidates involved in conferring ES cell-stemness state. The accumulative literature on ES cell transcriptional regulatory network has clearly highlighted the dominant role of Oct4, Sox2 and Nanog in ES cells, even as new candidate "stemness" factors are being uncovered. Therefore, there is an increasing repertoire of prime candidates to consider in the choice of genes to select for re-programming by genetic factors. A systems approach may also continue to shed light on the mechanism for how re-programming is initiated to establish the epigenome of a pluripotent cell. The redundancy of the regulatory network in

ES cells for maintaining the ES state also suggest that different combination of factors may perform the same task. Because miRNAs have profound impact on the levels of protein and consequently their biological activities, one prediction would be that certain miRNAs may have significant impact on the efficiency of re-programming. Another possibility is that genetic factors can be used to re-program a terminally differentiated cell to other somatic stem cells. In all these experiments, the general observation is that transcriptional regulation appears to be the key level of control and that there are many redundant systems often affecting a broad range of factors that converge on the same functional output. Yet, these redundant systems may very well be genetic "buffers" that maintain a pluripotent state against stochastic cellular events until sufficient signals trigger a transition phase. Perturbation analyses, of the type that is common in systems experimentation, will help elucidate the components of such networked systems.

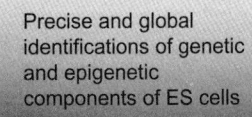

FIGURE 7.6 Stem cell as a model for systems biology. Intellectual framework for using ES cell as a model for systems biology is depicted. Research efforts were initially focused on defining the genetic and epigenetic components in a precise and comprehensive manner. Functional studies are carried out using genetic perturbation strategies. Integration of these datasets will provide new insights into the different networks (transcriptional regulatory network, protein–protein interaction network). With computational modeling, different models can be built to describe the networks in ES cell. One of the key goals is to model ES cell-specific gene expression in ES cell. This wealth of knowledge can be applied to cellular engineering to impart desired properties in other non-stem cells. Recently, it has been feasible to reconstruct ES cell regulatory network and induce pluripotency in non-stem cells.

References

Baek, D., Villén, J., Shin, C., Camargo, F.D., Gygi, S.P., Bartel, D.P., 2008. The impact of microRNAs on protein output. Nature 455 (7209), 64–71.

Bernstein, B.E., Mikkelsen, T.S., Xie, X., et al., 2006. A bivalent chromatin structure marks key developmental genes in embryonic stem cells. Cell 125 (2), 315–326.

Boiani, M., Schöler, H.R., 2005. Regulatory networks in embryo-derived pluripotent stem cells. Nat. Rev. Mol. Cell Biol. 6 (11), 872–884.

Boyer, L.A., Lee, T.I., Cole, M.F., et al., 2005. Core transcriptional regulatory circuitry in human embryonic stem cells. Cell 122 (6), 947–956.

Chen, C.C., Zhu, X.G., Zhong, S., 2008a. Selection of thermodynamic models for combinatorial control of multiple transcription factors in early differentiation of embryonic stem cells. BMC Genomics 9 (Suppl. 1), S18.

Chen, C.Z., Li, L., Lodish, H.F., Bartel, D.P., 2004. MicroRNAs modulate hematopoietic lineage differentiation. Science 303 (5654), 83–86.

Chen, X., Xu, H., Yuan, P., et al., 2008b. Cell 133 (6), 1106–1117.

Chickarmane, V., Troein, C., Nuber, U.A., Sauro, H.M., Peterson, C., 2006. Transcriptional dynamics of the embryonic stem cell switch. PLoS Comput. Biol. 2 (9), e123.

Davidson, E.H., Rast, J.P., Oliveri, P., et al., 2002. A genomic regulatory network for development. Science 295 (5560), 1669–1678.

Fortunel, N.O., Out, H.H., Ng, H.H., et al., 2003. Comment on "Stemness": transcriptional profiling of embryonic and adult stem cells"and"a stem cell molecular signature. Science 302 (5644), 393.

Galan-Caridad, J.M., Harel, S., Arenzana, T.L., et al., 2007. Zfx controls the self-renewal of embryonic and hematopoietic stem cells. Cell 129 (2), 345–357.

Glover, C.H., Marin, M., Eaves, C.J., Helgason, C.D., Piret, J.M., Bryan, J., 2006. Meta-analysis of differentiating mouse embryonic stem cell gene expression kinetics reveals early change of a small gene set. PLoS Comput. Biol. 2 (11), e158.

Grskovic, M., Chaivorapol, C., Gaspar-Maia, A., Li, H., Ramalho-Santos, M., 2007. Systematic identification of cis-regulatory sequences active in mouse and human embryonic stem cells. PLoS Genet. 3 (8), e145.

He, L., Hannon, G.J., 2004. MicroRNAs: small RNAs with a big role in gene regulation. Nat. Rev. Genet. 5 (7), 522–531.

Houbaviy, H.B., Murray, M.F., Sharp, P.A., 2003. Embryonic stem cell-specific MicroRNAs. Dev. Cell 5 (2), 351–358.

Ivanova, N.B., Dimos, J.T., Schaniel, C., Hackney, J.A., Moore, K.A., Lemischka, I.R., 2002. A stem cell molecular signature. Science 298 (5593), 601–604.

Ivanova, N., Dobrin, R., Lu, R., et al., 2006. Dissecting self-renewal in stem cells with RNA interference. Nature 442 (7102), 533–538.

Jaenisch, R., Young, R., 2008. Stem cells, the molecular circuitry of pluripotency and nuclear reprogramming. Cell 132 (4), 567–582.

Joung, J.G., Shin, D., Seong, R.H., Zhang, B.T., 2006. Identification of regulatory modules by co-clustering latent variable models: stem cell differentiation. Bioinformatics 22 (16), 2005–2011.

Kanellopoulou, C., Muljo, S.A., Kung, A.L., et al., 2005. Dicer-deficient mouse embryonic stem cells are defective in differentiation and centromeric silencing. Genes Dev. 19 (4), 489–501.

Kim, J., Chu, J., Shen, X., Wang, J., Orkin, S.H., 2008. Cell 132 (6), 1049–1061.

Landgraf, P., Rusu, M., Sheridan, R., et al., 2007. A mammalian microRNA expression atlas based on small RNA library sequencing. Cell 129 (7), 1401–1414.

Li, Q.J., Chau, J., Ebert, P.J., et al., 2007. miR-181a is an intrinsic modulator of T cell sensitivity and selection. Cell 129 (1), 147–161.

Lin, G., He, X., Ji, H., Shi, L., Davis, R.W., Zhong, S., 2006. Reproducibility probability score-incorporating measurement variability across laboratories for gene selection. Nat. Biotechnol. 24 (12), 1476–1477.

Loh, Y.H., Wu, Q., Chew, J.L., et al., 2006. The Oct4 and Nanog transcription network regulates pluripotency in mouse embryonic stem cells. Nat. Genet. 38 (4), 431–440.

Marson, A., Levine, S.S., Cole, M.F., et al., 2008. Connecting microRNA genes to the core transcriptional regulatory circuitry of embryonic stem cells. Cell 134 (3), 521–533.

Matoba, R., Niwa, H., Masui, S., et al., 2006. Dissecting Oct3/4-regulated gene networks in embryonic stem cells by expression profiling. PLoS ONE 1, e26.

Meshorer, E., Misteli, T., 2006. Chromatin in pluripotent embryonic stem cells and differentiation. Nat. Rev. Mol. Cell Biol. 7 (7), 540–546.

Mikkelsen, T.S., Ku, M., Jaffe, D.B., et al., 2007. Genome-wide maps of chromatin state in pluripotent and lineage-committed cells. Nature 448 (7153), 553–560.

Miranda, K.C., Huynh, T., Tay, Y., et al., 2006. A pattern-based method for the identification of MicroRNA binding sites and their corresponding heteroduplexes. Cell 126 (6), 1203–1217.

Panne, D., Maniatis, T., Harrison, S.C., 2007. An atomic model of the interferon-beta enhanceosome. Cell 129 (6), 1111–1123.

Pritsker, M., Ford, N.R., Jenq, H.T., Lemischka, I.R., 2006. Genomewide gain-of-function genetic screen identifies functionally active genes in mouse embryonic stem cells. Proc. Natl. Acad. Sci. U. S. A. 103 (18), 6946–6951.

Ramalho-Santos, M., Yoon, S., Matsuzaki, Y., Mulligan, R.C., Melton, D.A., 2002. "Stemness": transcriptional profiling of embryonic and adult stem cells. Science 298 (5593), 597–600.

Selbach, M., Schwanhäusser, B., Thierfelder, N., Fang, Z., Khanin, R., Rajewsky, N., 2008. Widespread changes in protein synthesis induced by microRNAs. Nature 455 (7209), 58–63.

Sharov, A.A., Ko, M.S., 2007. Human ES cell profiling broadens the reach of bivalent domains. Cell Stem Cell 1, 237–238.

Solter, D., 2006. From teratocarcinomas to embryonic stem cells and beyond: a history of embryonic stem cell research. Nat. Rev. Genet. 7 (4), 319–327.

Stark, A., Brennecke, J., Bushati, N., Russell, R.B., Cohen, S.M., 2005. Animal MicroRNAs confer robustness to gene expression and have a significant impact on 3'UTR evolution. Cell 123 (6), 1133–1146.

Suh, M.R., Lee, Y., Kim, J.Y., et al., 2004. Human embryonic stem cells express a unique set of microRNAs. Dev. Biol. 270 (2), 488–498.

Takahashi, K., Yamanaka, S., 2006. Induction of pluripotent stem cells from mouse embryonic and adult fibroblast cultures by defined factors. Cell 126 (4), 663–676.

Takahashi, K., Mitsui, K., Yamanaka, S., 2003. Role of ERas in promoting tumour-like properties in mouse embryonic stem cells. Nature 423 (6939), 541–545.

Tay, Y.M., Tam, W.L., Ang, Y.S., et al., 2008a. MicroRNA-134 modulates the differentiation of mouse embryonic stem cells where it causes post-transcriptional attenuation of nanog and LRH1. Stem Cells 26 (1), 17–29.

Tay, Y., Zhang, J., Thomson, A.M., Lim, B., Rigoutsos, I., 2008b. MicroRNAs to Nanog, Oct4 and Sox2 coding regions modulate embryonic stem cell differentiation. Nature [Epub ahead of print].

Voorhoeve, P.M., le Sage, C., Schrier, M., et al., 2006. A genetic screen implicates miRNA-372 and miRNA-373 as oncogenes in testicular germ cell tumors. Cell 124 (6), 1169–1181.

Woolf, P.J., Prudhomme, W., Daheron, L., Daley, G.Q., Lauffenburger, D.A., 2005. Bayesian analysis of signaling networks governing embryonic stem cell fate decisions. Bioinformatics 21 (6), 741–753.

Xiao, C., Calado, D.P., Galler, G., et al., 2007. MiR-150 controls B cell differentiation by targeting the transcription factor c-Myb. Cell 131 (1), 146–159.

Zhong, S., Xie, D., 2007. Gene ontology analysis in multiple gene clusters under multiple hypothesis testing framework. Artif. Intell. Med. 41 (2), 105–115.

Zhou, Q., Chipperfield, H., Melton, D.A., Wong, W.H., 2007. A gene regulatory network in mouse embryonic stem cells. Proc. Natl. Acad. Sci. U. S. A. 104 (42), 16438–16443.

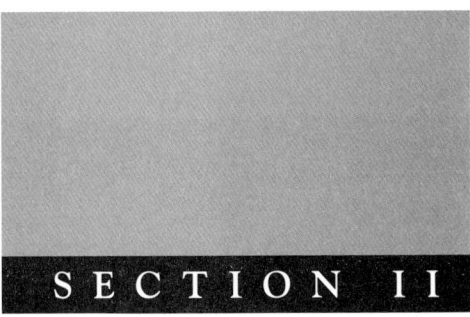

SECTION II

COMPUTATIONAL MODELING IN SYSTEMS BIOLOGY

CHAPTER

8

Computational Challenges in Systems Biology

Mano Ram Maurya and Shankar Subramaniam
University of California, San Diego

OUTLINE

Summary	177	Challenges in Building Computational Models	199
Introduction	178	Unknown Parameters	199
Different Levels of Models of Biochemical Systems	181	Variation in Local Concentrations and Multiple Scales of Distance and Time	201
Challenges in Building Biochemical Models	184	Cell-specific Variability and Subpopulational Variability	204
Complexity of Proteomic States and Interactions	184	Case Study: Modeling the Regulation of Calcium Dynamics in RAW 264.7 Cells	204
Integration of Diverse Data to Infer Biochemical Interactions	186	Mechanisms	204
Temporal State of Biochemical Models	188	Mathematical Representation of the Model	207
Challenges in Building Mathematical Models	190	Results for Simulation and Parameter Estimation Using Data from RAW 264.7 Cells	208
Incorporating Statistical/Probabilistic Information into Analytical Models	191	Future Directions and Concluding Remarks	211
Utilizing Qualitative Constraints in Mathematical Models	191	Acknowledgements	213
Incomplete Knowledge and Coarse-graining	193		

Summary

The "state" of a cell is defined by its components (their concentrations and locations, the interactions between components), which are modulated in space and time, and the complex circuitry, which involves a large number of interacting networks. The state represents a snapshot of the dynamic processes, such as gene expression, cell cycle, transport of components, that characterize the function of the cell. Advances in high-throughput genomic, metabolomic and proteomic technologies now allow study of the cellular components and their interactions in a quantitative manner. These technologies are aiding the development of predictive models by combining legacy knowledge and novel data. There are two paradigms in computational systems biology: (i) the iterative cycle of biochemical model–mathematical model–computational model, and (ii) integration of novel data and legacy knowledge to develop context-specific biochemical, mathematical and computational models. Challenges in building *biochemical models* include (a) the complexity of proteomic states and interactions, (b) integration of diverse data to infer biochemical interactions and (c) the temporal state of biochemical models. Challenges in building *mathematical models* include (i) incorporating statistical/probabilistic information into analytical models, (ii) utilizing qualitative constraints in mathematical models, and (iii) incomplete knowledge and coarse-graining. Challenges in *computational modeling* include: (a) the absence of knowledge about model parameters such as rate constants, (b) local versus global concentrations of species and multiple scales of distance and time, and (c) variation among different cell types and subpopulation variability, or variability among biological repeats. This chapter will review these challenges and some of the recent advances in computational systems biology.

INTRODUCTION

Cells and tissues function in context. Under a given growth or survival medium, they perform tasks, replicate and die. Given a stimulus, they respond by invoking myriad biomolecular networks that result in a specified cellular outcome. At any given instant, it can be argued that the cell is in a "state" defined by its components—their concentrations and locations; the interactions between components—that are modulated in space and time, and the complex circuitry that involves a large number of interacting networks and a snapshot of the dynamic processes such as gene expression, cell cycle and transport of components. During the past 10 years, research in cellular systems biology has been catalyzed by our ability to develop a detailed parts list based on genome annotations, and by the advances in high-throughput technologies that enable quantitative measurement of the cellular components such as mRNA levels (genomic data), signaling proteins and their phosphorylated states (proteomic data) and metabolites such as glucose, ATP and lipids (metabolomics and lipidomics). Collectively, these technologies are referred to as "omics" (Altman et al., 2004; Bouvier and Friedlander, 2006; Casciano, 2003; Dimond, 2003; Johnson et al., 2003; Joyce and Palsson, 2006; Kiechle et al., 2004; Lay et al., 2006; Merrill, 2007; Orphanides, 2004; Singh, 2007; Van den Bulcke et al., 2006).

Cellular processes are complex because they involve several interacting components, sometimes located in different organelles. Cellular events involve many scales of distance and time. In the case of cellular signaling, as depicted in Figure 8.1, various layers are involved. In the topmost layer, events such as activation of cell surface receptors and other individual signaling reactions are very fast, occurring within from a fraction of a second to several seconds. In the middle layer, cascades of individual intracellular signaling pathways, mostly within the cytosol, operate at the time scale of from several seconds to minutes. In the final layer, nuclear signaling events such as activation of transcription factors and translocation of such molecules to the nucleus also occur within minutes. Events such as gene expression, translation and protein translocation occur on a time scale of several hours, and sometimes days (Papin et al., 2005; Stephanopoulos et al., 1998). The secreted

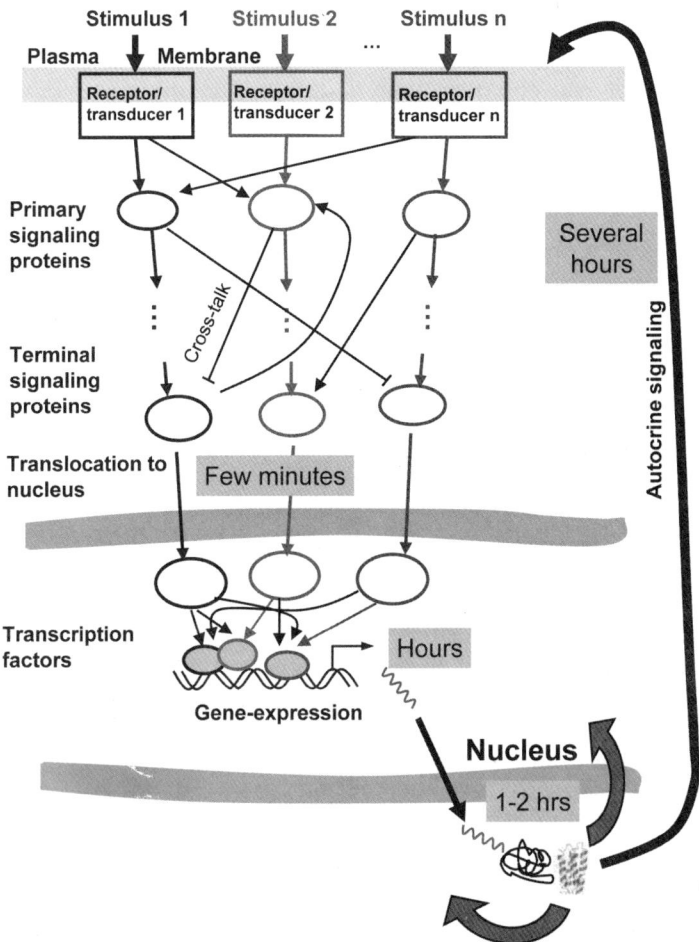

FIGURE 8.1 Various Levels of Cellular Signaling.

proteins can bind to the receptors on their own surface (autocrine signaling), travel short distances to bind to nearby cells (paracrine signaling) or travel over long distances to different organs in other parts of the body through the blood stream (endocrine system). The feedback loops and cross-talk between different signaling pathways make it very complex to decipher their interactions.

Systematic study of such complex processes requires a systems biology approach. The field of systems biology deals with the modeling and analysis of whole systems, as opposed to individual components, to decipher, model, understand and predict the phenotype of the entire system. Systems biology brings constructionist, quantitative and engineering perspectives to cell biology, and helps develop testable mechanistic hypotheses for complex cellular phenotypes. Modeling is at its core. The modeling cycle starts with an initial formulation of a model based on the knowledge about the physical and biochemical processes involved. The formulated model is simulated and the results are analyzed and validated against available data. Specific predictions can be made that assist in developing new hypotheses requiring new experiments and often lead to modifications and improvements in the model. Thus the cycle of model development, validation and refinement can run iteratively until the underlying process has been understood at a suitable level of detail as required by the intended application of the model.

Using the parts list and high-throughput data, it is now possible to decipher the interactions between the components and reconstruct the underlying cellular network. In many cases, concomitant with the process of deciphering the interactions from data, a computational model may be developed that will have some predictive power. In other cases, if the network is built using legacy data such as a list of known reactions, a computational model may nevertheless not be developed because of a lack of parameters, although the structure of the computational model—or more precisely, a mathematical model—may be developed. The networks and models developed are generally context specific, as they are based on structural, qualitative and quantitative data generated under specific conditions in specific cells or tissues.

Systems-level Modeling

The main theme of systems biology is systems-level modeling and analysis. Many researchers have contributed to promoting this theme by developing reasonably large-scale mathematical models of different biochemical systems, such as signaling, metabolic and regulatory pathways. A detailed review of research in this area is not intended here. Some of the significant contributions have come from the laboratories of Iyengar [mitogen-activated protein kinase (MAPK) pathway, G-protein pathway and other pathways (Bhalla and Iyengar, 1999; Bhalla et al., 2002; Ma'ayan et al., 2007; Neves and Iyengar, 2002; Neves et al., 2002); other models of the MAPK pathway (Kholodenko, 2000; Markevich et al., 2004; Schoeberl et al., 2002)], Bhalla [calcium regulation in neuronal and generic cell types (Bhalla, 2004a, 2004b; Bhalla and Iyengar, 1999; Bhalla et al., 2002; Mishra and Bhalla, 2002)], Lauffenburger [mechanistic and data-driven modeling (Hua et al., 2006), epidermal growth factor (EGF) receptor activation (Joslin et al., 2007), ErbB receptor phosphorylation (Hendriks et al., 2006) and the interleukin-2 (IL-2) pathway (Fallon and Lauffenburger, 2000)], Tyson [models of cell cycle (Allen et al., 2006; Calzone et al., 2007; Novak et al., 2007; Sible and Tyson, 2007; Zwolak et al., 2005) and circadian rhythm (Hong et al., 2007)], Arkin [stochastic simulation of gene regulatory networks (Alm and Arkin, 2003; Weinberger et al., 2005) and cellular signaling pathways (Gilman et al., 2002; Hucka et al., 2003; Rao and Arkin, 2003)], Davidson [developmental gene regulatory networks (Bolouri and Davidson, 2002; Longabaugh et al., 2005; Materna and Davidson, 2007; Revilla-i-Domingo and Davidson, 2003; Smith et al., 2007)], Winslow [deterministic, stochastic and spatial modeling of calcium regulation of cardiac myocytes (Hinch et al., 2004; Jafri et al., 1998; Tanskanen et al., 2007; Winslow et al., 2006)], Palsson [large-scale models of signaling and metabolic pathways (Becker et al., 2007; Jamshidi et al., 2001; Resendis-Antonio et al., 2007; Yeung et al., 2007)], Doyle [chemotaxis (Park et al., 2007), circadian rhythm (Kronauer et al., 2007; Liu et al., 2007; Stelling et al., 2004; To et al., 2007; Zeilinger et al., 2006) and blood glucose control modeling (Dua et al., 2006; Parker and Doyle, 2001; Parker et al., 1999)], Stephanopoulos [modeling and analysis relevant to metabolic engineering, such as metabolic flux analysis and modeling of isotopomer labeling (Antoniewicz et al., 2007; Koffas and Stephanopoulos, 2005; Misra et al., 2007; Stafford et al., 2002; Young et al., 2007)], Hunter [physiology-based organ-level spatially resolved models and their parameter estimation (Crampin et al., 2004; Jor et al., 2007; Niederer et al., 2006; Schmid et al., 2008)] and Gilles [signaling and regulatory pathways, reduction of modular complexity (Ederer and Gilles, 2007; Hucka et al., 2003; Koschorreck et al., 2007;

Saez-Rodriguez et al., 2007; Schoeberl et al., 2002; Stelling and Gilles 2004)]. These contributions are paving the way for more advanced and larger-scale studies of integrated modeling and analysis of pathways.

DIFFERENT LEVELS OF MODELS OF BIOCHEMICAL SYSTEMS

A majority of the systems biology models have implicitly or explicitly used the concept of a three-level modeling strategy. As shown in Figure 8.2, an experimentally driven biochemical model (often a connected set of biochemical components) is developed and this is cast into a mathematical model such as a set of differential equations representing reactions; ultimately, this is converted into a computational model that also describes the parameters of the model. The computational model can be numerically solved to predict the response of the system using a suitable computational methodology and numerical solution techniques.

A biochemical model consists of the mechanistic description of the system and usually consists of a network-based description.

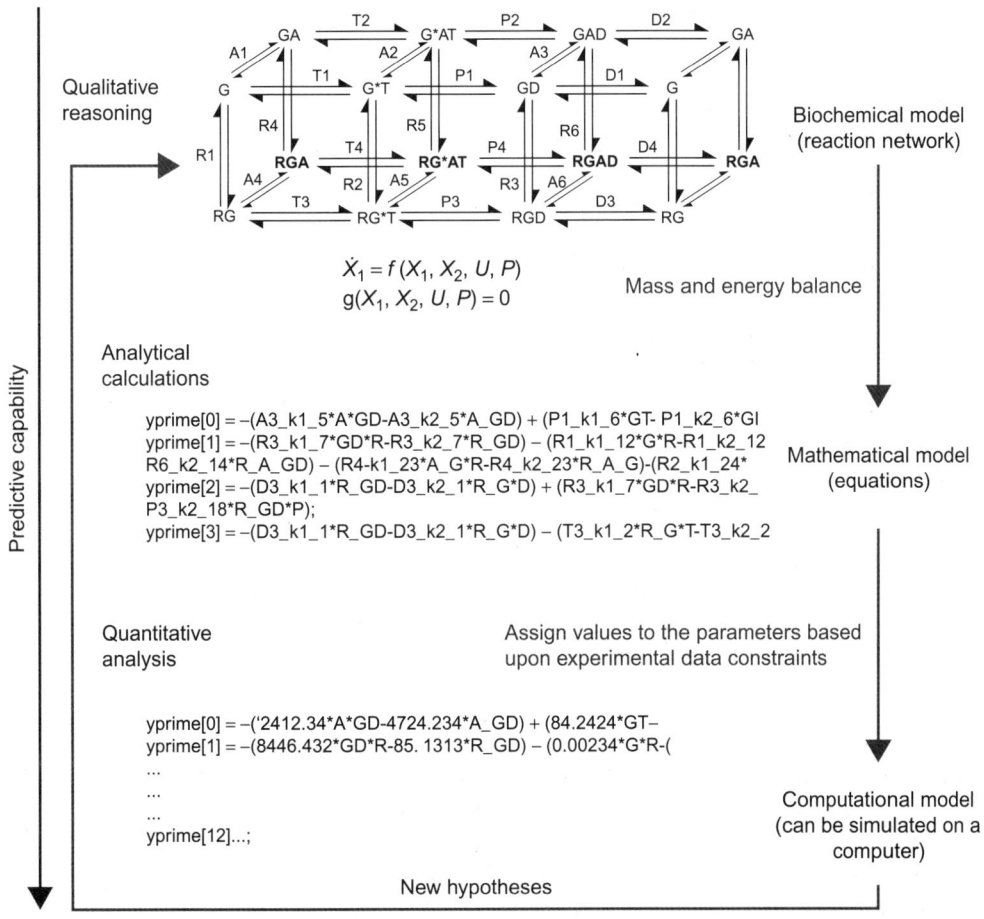

FIGURE 8.2   Three Levels of the Models of Biochemical Systems.

One example is a network of reactions in the GTPase-cycle module of G-protein signaling (Bornheimer et al., 2004; Maurya et al., 2005). Another example is a metabolic pathway—for example the glycolysis pathway—in which some of the transport processes across the plasma membrane and reactions of glucose metabolism may be depicted. Such models, by themselves, can at best be used for predicting qualitative behavior; however, for an experimentalist, they are a useful starting point from which to think more analytically about the system and to design "what if" experiments. For instance, it can be inferred, on the basis of the glycolysis pathway, that an increase in the glucose concentration in the extracellular media will result in increased production of ATP. Such qualitative reasoning becomes very difficult with biochemical models if complex feedback is involved. A biochemical model is specified by two types of information: the components of the network (i.e., the relevant parts list) and the interaction between the components. Although substantial progress has been made in developing the parts list on the basis of legacy knowledge and genome annotation, progress in the discovery of novel interactions (documented or verified in the literature), which invariably requires context-specific data, is happening at a much slower rate.

Once a biochemical model is available, an analytical description of the system can be developed by applying the principles of mathematical modeling (mass, energy and charge balance). Such a mathematical model can be in the form of a set of ordinary or partial differential algebraic equations, which, when necessary, can be converted into a form suitable for probabilistic analysis. Such models encapsulate more information than a biochemical model, and hence they can be used for limited analytical calculations. Although a mathematical model contains a precise description of how state variables and the model parameters such as rate constants and transport coefficients are coupled to each other, exact analytical calculations are limited to smaller systems, because of the inherently non-linear nature of biochemical processes.

When the parameters and other appropriate variables in a mathematical model are assigned numerical values, they can be simulated on a computer. Such a description—a mathematical model with concomitant detail on the parameter values—is called a "computational model." A computational model can be used to make actual quantitative predictions about the behavior of the system, and can be used for a numerical assessment of the results of what-if experiments. As we go from a biochemical to a mathematical to a computational model, the amount of information required increases, but so does our ability to make more detailed and quantitative predictions. Based on the predictions made by a computational model, new hypotheses are derived that are usually utilized to refine the biochemical model, thus making a cycle of the three levels of the system description. In other words, during model refinement, a biochemist will generally think at the level of mechanisms of a biochemical model, rather than at the level of a mathematical or a computational description. Any alterations at the level of a biochemical model result in broader changes in the system response compared with those at a computational level. The development of models at each level has specific challenges, as described below.

Despite the advances in genomic and other experimental technologies, the parts-list databases are usually incomplete for the intended context. As stated in another review, "Constructing biomolecular networks for new systems will require significant resources and expertise, and even when one works with a biomolecular network database the systemic picture may be incomplete or only partially accurate" (Rigoutsos and Stephanopoulos, 2007). Even with a complete parts-list database for a specific pathway or module, the component interactions are only partially known, because it is rare that a small number of experiments can explicitly decipher the network. It is reasonable to say that network discovery is data intensive and requires a large number of experiments under diverse conditions in order to probe the network in detail.

Recently, numerous systems biology software products have been developed that translate mechanistic descriptions into some form of a mathematical model. A non-exhaustive list includes: GEPASI (Mendes and Kell, 1998; Mendes and Kummer, 2006), COPASI (Mendes and Kummer, 2006), Simmune (Meier-Schellersheim et al., 2006), Virtual Cell (VCell, http://www.nrcam.uchc.edu/; Mace et al., 2004; Moraru et al., 2002), CellML (CellML, http://www.cellml.org; Cuellar et al., 2003), Simpheny (Mahadevan et al., 2005), Systems Biology Workbench (SBW, http://sbw.kgi.edu/; Sauro et al., 2003), JDesigner (Sauro et al., 2003) and Kinetikit (Vayttaden and Bhalla, 2004). Some of these tools allow models to be exported in systems biology markup language (SBML) format (Hucka et al., 2003). Models based on ordinary or partial differential equations are generated by a majority of these tools. In studies in which the biochemical network is barely known or only partially known, simple input–output models or probabilistic networks such as Bayesian networks (Jordan, 1999; Werhli and Husmeier, 2007; Werhli et al., 2006) are more realistic to build. Bayesian networks have predictive capability and allow the inclusion of a priori knowledge about the system (Jansen et al., 2003; Pandey et al., 2007; Sachs et al., 2005; Stetter et al., 2003; Sun and Zhao, 2004; Woolf et al., 2005; Zou and Conzen, 2005). As our knowledge about the components and their interactions increases, we are able to build more comprehensive and larger mathematical models. As the size of the model increases, so does the demand on the amount of data required to compute the model parameters and to interpret the large volumes of simulation and prediction results that can be generated from such models. When the models become large, it becomes essential to simplify (coarse-grain) the biochemical and mathematical models contextually, so that reliable models with sufficient predictive capability and the desired mechanistic information can be developed. Such models are more stable with respect to parametric fluctuations, and are less likely to predict unrealistic behavior for novel and multidimensional perturbations than are the very detailed models. When experimental data on parameters of the model are limited, legacy knowledge and qualitative constraints are useful in building and understanding the model. Challenges in integrating qualitative constraints into mathematical models and coarse-graining will be discussed further, and results from recent work in our laboratory and elsewhere will be highlighted.

A computational model requires complete details of parameters such as steady-state or initial conditions of the components and rate constants in a signaling or metabolic network, and the weights and probability distributions in a Bayesian network. In certain modeling philosophies, such as input–output models and probabilistic networks (broadly classified as data-driven models), many of the network/model parameters are derived in the process of identifying the network topology itself, because the connections between the components are parameterized by the assigned weights. Thus the three levels of description of the model described previously are highly linked. In other types of model, which are mostly based on differential algebraic equations, the derivation or formulation of the mathematical model does not require values of the parameters. In contrast to data-driven models, in purely mechanism-driven models such as reaction networks there is a general tendency to not restrict the size of the model, because of the rich biochemistry that is detailed. Hence, the eventual simulation of such models requires knowledge of a large number of parameters. Thanks to advances in computing technologies, simulation of the model is not computationally expensive; however, estimation of the parameters and interpretations of the results are prohibitively difficult for models of large networks. This is because the complexity of parameter estimation for non-linear models can increase at least semi-exponentially. For a comprehensive prediction of the behavior of the system under many different conditions, the number of simulations required can be combinatorial (e.g. single and paired perturbations in all independent variables, including initial states and model parameters). Intrinsic parameters such as those related to mass action kinetics are relatively constant across various cell types, but others such as lumped rate constants, which are actually a function of the enzyme concentrations, can vary substantially across different cell types. Thus cell-specific constraining of parameters is necessary, even if their values may be available from a different cell type. Another challenge that shows up in the numerical simulation as well as in the interpretation of the simulation results is the presence of multiple time scales. These issues will be discussed further.

CHALLENGES IN BUILDING BIOCHEMICAL MODELS

One of the challenges in building biochemical networks is the complexity of protein interactions. A majority of proteins interact with two or more other proteins. This implies that the number of states in which a protein can exist as protein complexes (with other proteins or small molecules, or with one or more of its residues modified covalently) is very large (Li et al., 2002). For example, phospholipase C beta (PLCβ) can bind to both the alpha and the beta subunits of G-proteins, and it can also bind to calcium ions (Mishra and Bhalla, 2002). Furthermore, various complexes of PLCβ catalyze hydrolysis of phosphatidylinositol 4,5-bisphosphate (PIP2). This requires binding of PIP2 onto several enzymatic complexes. In all, the total number of possible states is eight or more. Modeling each of these states into the networks is challenging even for the most sophisticated software and graphical network design tools. Another challenge is the integration of diverse types of data generated using different experimental techniques such as gene microarray, mass spectrometry, chromatin-immunoprecipitation, gene knockout, RNA interference and yeast two-hybrid assays (Papin et al., 2007) to infer the biochemical interactions between various components. An important challenge concerns the temporal state of the entire biochemical model. At different times, different parts of the network may be active, and the concentrations of components can change dynamically, so that interpretation of experimental data in model building becomes dependent on the state of the network.

Complexity of Proteomic States and Interactions

A state of a protein can be uniquely defined by using a 0/1 tag for each of its binding sites for different protein partners, depending upon whether or not a particular site is occupied or not. On the basis of this philosophy, several researchers have developed approaches to modeling the multiple states of proteins in signaling networks (Hlavacek et al., 2006; Kremling and Saez-Rodriguez, 2007; Saez-Rodriguez et al., 2005). Some small molecules such as calcium ions can bind to proteins at several sites. This adds additional complexity to the task of accurately capturing all the unique states of the protein. A classic example is the binding of calcium and inositol 1,4,5-trisphosphate (IP3) to the IP3 receptor (IP3R) proteins on the endoplasmic reticulum membrane. On the IP3R there are three sites, one for IP3 and two for calcium ions (Ca^{2+}), resulting in eight possible states for IP3R. Further, for the receptor channel to open for the release of calcium into the cytosol, IP3 must be bound to at least three of the four subunits of IP3R (De Young and Keizer, 1992; Li and Rinzel, 1994). If one were to treat the joint complex of the four subunits as one entity, there are potentially 4096 ($=2^{12}$; $12 = 3 \times 4$) states. Given that the protein under consideration is one of several hundreds of proteins even for one signaling pathway—namely, calcium regulation in the cytosol—for modeling purposes, all the four subunits are generally treated identically (De Young and Keizer, 1992). The size and the complexity of the model are further reduced by considering time-scale decomposition (Li and Rinzel, 1994). The simplified flux expression thus developed is the most widely used model for the activation of IP3R. If the story is this complex for the binding of just two small signaling molecules (Ca^{2+} and IP3) to one protein (IP3R), one can only imagine the mathematical complexity of interactions between three or more proteins in conjunction with the binding of small molecules and other substrates, including possibly the binding of the resulting complex to DNA (Amoutzias et al., 2007; Ideker et al., 2001; Komurov and White, 2007; LaCount et al., 2005; Rhodes et al., 2005; Scott et al., 2006; Shannon et al., 2003; Sharan and Ideker, 2006). It is accurate to say that the combinatorial complexity of proteomic states is the most daunting challenge that directly affects the size and complexity of any model developed, and affects the development of models at all levels.

A group of researchers have developed formal rules for protein–protein interactions to represent the binding and enzymatic activities of proteins in cellular signaling (Hlavacek et al., 2006). A mathematical model can be generated by processing the rule-based description of the pathway. To update the model, instead of changing the model equations directly, new interactions can be added by introducing a new rule about the protein and interaction of interest. Graphical visualization of rules is also facilitated (Blinov et al., 2006; Hlavacek et al., 2006). Another group of researchers have developed a novel approach to tackle the complexity that arises as a result of the explicit modeling of each and every state of protein complexes (Saez-Rodriguez et al., 2005). In this approach, the authors use the absence of retroactivity as a criterion to define modules. These modules can be made up of several proteins and metabolites or only a subset of all the possible states of the protein of interest (Conzelmann et al., 2006). Instead of modeling every possible state, lumped (macro) states (e.g. total occupancy of binding sites) are used. These macro states are considered as outputs, because they can be realistically measured. To simplify the overall network, first a detailed mechanistic description is developed, followed by the introduction of macro states based on a state space transformation. In the next step, the equations having no effect on the output (usually the collection of macro states) are eliminated. Although the formal procedure is new in a qualitative way, these approaches have been used in developing the simplified model for IP3 receptor dynamics (Li and Rinzel, 1994). A computational modeling software, called Simmune (Meier-Schellersheim et al., 2006) has been developed that specifically allows the physical interaction between proteins and other molecules to be defined. The user is still required to draw all the interactions (unlike the previous two approaches, in which the development of the mechanistic descriptions is somewhat automated), but Simmune is very useful for biologists and biochemists, because they are traditionally used to thinking in terms of biomolecular binding and interactions. Another pathway drawing tool, Biopathways Workbench (http://www.biopathwaysworkbench.org/), is centered around state-based representation of molecules in biochemical networks. This software does not allow automatic generation of all the proteomic states, but the object definitions, such as those for nodes and interactions, allow for explicit modeling of molecular interactions, enzymatic effects and biochemical transformations.

Integration of Diverse Data to Infer Biochemical Interactions

There has been substantial progress is developing network models using data of a particular type—for example, gene microarray data for clustering networks and yeast two-hybrid data for protein interaction networks—, but they provide only a partial, and generally a static, picture of the entire system, comprised of signaling, gene regulatory and metabolic events. Data generated using different experimental techniques allow us to learn different aspects of the system and they can have advantages and disadvantages such as false positives and negatives. Thus data integration has the potential to provide maximum information about the system. In addition, some of the drawbacks of different approaches can be compensated by others (Hwang et al., 2005b). Moreover, in the case of conflict, they serve to propose additional hypotheses and experiments. Research on data-driven network reconstruction and the development of predictive quantitative systems biology models includes the contributions by Bonneau et al. (2006), Janes et al. (2005) and Pradervand et al. (2006). Bayesian approaches also have been used to reconstruct biochemical networks from data; examples include studies by Sachs et al. (2005), Hartemink et al. (2002) and Yu et al. (2004). As discussed in a recent review by Camacho et al. (2007), many other approaches such as partial correlation analysis and other statistical and systems engineering methods have been developed (Arkin and Ross, 1995; Bansal et al., 2007; de la Fuente et al., 2004, 1995; Laubenbacher and Stigler, 2004; Lezon et al., 2006; Ross and Arkin, 2009; Sontag et al., 2004). Matrix-based approaches also have been proposed (Famili et al., 2005; Karnaukhov et al., 2007). These efforts underline the importance of applying systems approaches to deciphering and reconstructing cellular networks using high-throughput data. Although the research efforts stated above are very significant, only a few have attempted to integrate different types of experimental data. An approach based on partial least squares has been used to identify the interaction of apoptotic and pro-survival signals in cellular apoptosis (Janes et al., 2005). Deciphering these relationships is complex, because any given stimulus activates more than one pathway, and any given pathway can be usually activated by several stimuli. In turn, the signaling pathways act together as a module or network to elicit specific responses. Janes et al. (2005) used high-throughput data on signaling activations and apoptotic or survival phenotypes to construct a canonical network linking signaling to apoptosis.

Recently, we have developed a novel algorithm to perform input–output mapping using steady-state or time-averaged data, wherein, to identify the lumped networks from signaling pathways to cytokines in macrophages, the levels of activation of the signaling pathway acted as inputs and the levels of cytokine release acted as the outputs (Pradervand et al., 2006). Upon application of Toll-like receptor (TLR) ligands and non-TLR ligands, the release of cytokines during the inflammatory response is mediated by a complex signaling network in which multiple stimuli produce different signals that generate different cytokine responses. The current state of the art does not provide a complete picture of all the signaling pathways, but specific markers of these pathways, such as signaling proteins, allowed us to develop lumped input–output relationships between pathway activation and cytokine release. From this model we were able to decipher common regulatory modules for various cytokines. Accurate deciphering of these mappings was made possible because of the large amount of data made available by the Alliance for Cellular Signaling (http://www.signaling-gateway.org/). Principal component regression was used for input–output mapping. The significance of the identified relationships of the inputs to a chosen output was estimated using statistical significance tests of the model coefficients. Thus, besides using two different types of data to decipher the lumped structure of the signaling and gene regulatory network, the methodology integrated several types of mathematical analyses such as regression, combinatorial optimization and statistical significance testing. Although regression and optimization approaches have been successfully used in network structure identification, statistical testing is necessary to control the rate of false positives. Our algorithm was specifically designed to reduce the false-positive rate while ensuring a low false-negative rate. It can be noted that in costly experiment design a very low false-positive rate is desired, whereas in diagnosis a very low false-negative rate is accepted. The methodology identified required signaling factors necessary and sufficient to predict the release of seven cytokines (granulocyte-colony stimulating factor [G-CSF]; interleukins [IL]-1α, -6 and -10; macrophage inflammatory protein [MIP])-1α; regulated on activation normal T cells expressed and secreted [RANTES]; tumor necrosis factor [TNF]α) in response to selected ligands. This study provided a model-based quantitative estimate of cytokine release and identified 10 signaling components involved in cytokine production. The models captured many of the known signaling pathways involved in cytokine release and predicted potentially important novel signaling components, such as p38 MAPK for G-CSF release, interferon (IFN)γ and IL-4-specific pathways for IL-1α release, and a macrophage-colony stimulating factor (M-CSF)-specific pathway for TNFα release.

Recent efforts at the Institute for Systems Biology (Bonneau et al., 2006; Hwang et al., 2005a, 2005b) have also spearheaded research in this area. A software package named POINTILLIST has been developed. The data integration methodology can deal with several datasets, which can differ in type, size and information content. The data may also span different or all parts of the network. The aim has been to develop a robust framework for data integration that can handle data generated using both existing and future technologies. The hallmarks of the methodology are weighted integration of the P value (statistical significance) and the selection of a joint-significance threshold, improvement of the threshold using mixture distribution models, and the use of nonparametric decision boundaries. While the main focus of the software package is to test the overall statistical significance of differential changes on the basis of several types of data, by combining the results with information gleaned from other data analysis techniques such as protein–protein interaction networks and protein–DNA interaction networks, the researchers were able to capture most of the known mechanisms in galactose metabolism and derived novel results for further experimental validation.

Approaches based on hybrid intelligent systems also under development allow modeling of complex biochemical dynamics using rule-based models to capture expert knowledge, which can be qualitative, quantitative or semi-quantitative in nature (Bosl, 2007). A web browser tool to integrate data and information from various bioinformatics resources has been developed that can also exchange data with Cytoscape, the R statistics package and several other popular desktop software tools. The application known as Firegoose facilitates querying popular databases such as Kyoto Encyclopedia of Genes and Genomes (KEGG) and other bioinformatics resources. Recently, another multivariate statistical method, called co-inertia analysis (CIA), has been used in conjunction with principal component analysis to integrate proteomic and gene expression data collected from the same samples (Fagan et al., 2007). As the two types of data are from the same set of samples, some of the variability inherent to data collected from different subjects is reduced. A recent review on integration of heterogeneous data in the context of biomedical and clinical research provided interesting ideas as to how computational biology can help advance clinical research through unified approaches to data preprocessing, integration and storage (Mathew et al., 2007). Some of these efforts are not tailored towards mining the interactions and connectivity, but they will be indispensable tools for deriving new network models.

Temporal State of Biochemical Models

Biochemical systems are inherently dynamic in nature. If a biochemical model is developed using legacy knowledge about the mechanisms and other annotations which directly describe the mechanisms of metabolic reactions and signaling and regulatory interactions, then mass and energy balance can be applied to formulate dynamic models from which a steady-state description can also be derived (Murray, 2002). Such a biochemical model or mechanistic description is not tied to a static (at one or more specific time-points), steady-state or dynamic view of the process. Hence, one need not worry about the issue of the temporal state of the biochemical model. However, if the network topology is derived using high-throughput data such as gene microarray data, the issue of temporal causality captured in such networks becomes relevant.

Correlation Networks

If connections are inferred on the basis of clustering or correlation analysis of high-dimensional data, the connections are bidirectional between nodes (correlation) or modules (clustering) and multidirectional or coupled within modules (clustering). In this case, regardless of whether data from just one time-point or many time-points (vectorial correlation/clustering) is used, the issue of temporal causality does not arise, as a result of the absence of directionality between the nodes or the modules. An example of such a network is shown in Figure 8.3A for eight genes that are clustered in three groups. The within-cluster correlations are high,

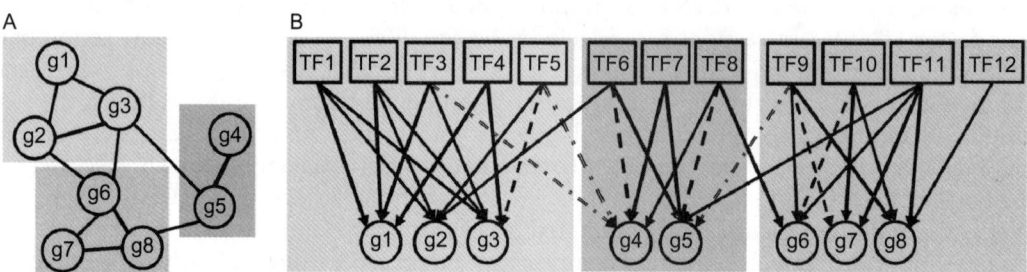

FIGURE 8.3 Various Types of Network Generated Using Data-driven Approaches.
(A) Correlation/clustering-based gene network. The connections are undirected and contain no causal information. For simplicity, signs of correlations are not shown, as the main interest is in the topology. (B) Non-causal and causal networks derived using input–output mapping of data. The network is essentially a bipartite directed graph (no connections within the input or output nodes themselves). The non-causal network comprises all nodes and all connections except those shown with double lines in dash-dot style; the causal network comprises all nodes and connections except those shown by dashed lines. Thus there is substantial overlap in their topologies. Sign information is suppressed for simplicity, and the sign of a connection present in both networks could potentially be different in each. The thickness of the arrows indicates the absolute value of the connection weight. More details are provided in the text. TF, transcription factor.

whereas between-cluster correlations are low, as indicated by the thickness of the connections (signs not shown).

Static Pseudocausal Directional Networks

Static pseudocausal directional networks have directional connections. Directional connections are usually obtained when input–output mapping is performed. The choice of the inputs and outputs is decided by the expert modeler, and usually requires some biochemical knowledge—for example, it is well established that the level of transcription factors regulates the level of gene expression, and not *vice versa* (feedback effects are part of a super-network in this context). It is possible to have common components in inputs and outputs: for example, the cross-talk of feedback effects between signaling pathways or interactions between transcription factors. Mapping from transcription factors to genes in a gene regulatory network is an example in which the components in the inputs and outputs are different. In input–output mapping, if the connections are inferred from data at just one time-point (or at several time-points individually or the average of all time-points), the network only provides a snapshot (or a lumped picture) of the process and, hence, it may not capture the temporal causality of the dynamic process. Such a network provides a static view of the process.

It can be noted that some of the directional connections may overlap with the causal connections derived using a dynamic system identification approach or otherwise. Here, the issue of directional correlation and causation arises. Their overlap can depend on several factors, such as how non-linear is the process, how much the features change with time and whether or not the true network has a positive-feedback loop. The presence of a positive-feedback loop is interesting, and has been explored extensively. There is considerable literature on the directed-graph based qualitative modeling of chemical processes showing that, in a dynamic system, if there are positive-feedback loops or zero-self cycles on state variables (e.g. an integrator), the directed graph corresponding to steady-state behavior can be substantially different from that for the dynamic model (Maurya et al., 2003a; Oyeleye and Kramer, 1988).

An example of a transcription factor–gene mapping network is shown in Figure 8.3B. To make a comparison with the network shown in Figure 8.3A, the modularity has been preserved so that three groups of transcription factors regulate three groups of co-regulated genes, although some additional transcription factors may be regulating a chosen gene, as indicated by the cross connections between the modules. Both non-causal and causal networks are illustrated in this example. The non-causal network, derived using data at one time-point, or time-averaged data for transcription factor activation levels and gene expression, consists of all connections except those shown by double lines in dash-dot style. There is an implicit sense of some sort of causation in input–output mapping, because it is assumed that the inputs affect the output; however, in a strict sense it is not temporally causal, as the time information was never used or was masked during averaging. One could develop such non-causal or pseudocausal networks using either linear input–output modeling or Bayesian networks (Janes et al., 2004, 2005; Pradervand et al., 2006; Sachs et al., 2005), using data at many time-points, and monitor how the connections change in terms of appearing and disappearing, and their sign and strengths.

Dynamic and Temporally Causal Networks

By definition, dynamic and temporally causal networks are derived by mapping the input data at a previous (current) time-point to the output data at the current (future) time-point, to capture the temporal causality explicitly (Iwasaki and Simon, 1986; Maurya et al., 2003a;

Uckun, 1992). In recent years, many approaches for constructing dynamic networks have been developed. These include (i) techniques based on state space representation (Bonneau et al., 2006; Ma and Chan, 2007; Yeung et al., 2002), and (ii) dynamic Bayesian networks (Cho et al., 2007; Geier et al., 2007). In one approach, a linear dynamic Bayesian network is trained using the F-statistic and nearly exhaustive searching on the possible combinations of transcription factors that could be the putative regulators of a chosen gene (Geier et al., 2007). The use of such networks, and the associated computational models, is not restricted to the prediction of the dynamic response of the system: the significant connections in such networks are more likely to be the true cause–effect links in the actual biological process. An example of such a causal network is shown in Figure 8.3B: the subnetwork comprised of all nodes and connections except those shown by dashed lines. One can see that, while there is much overlap between the causal and non-causal network, some of the connections are present or absent in one of them. If the non-causal network was based on time-averaged data, the common connections (present in both with same signs of the weights) between the causal and non-causal network are very likely to be true. Others may be false-positives, and such conflicts motivate for further experimentation to probe the specific connections by genetic or chemical perturbation studies. In essence, although a temporally causal network capturing the dynamic behavior should ideally contain information on static (non-causal) networks at different time-points, it is important to analyze both, to reconcile any differences. Also, most approaches intended for utilizing dynamic data for network identification can also handle steady-state data by setting the time-rate of change of the output or the state nodes to zero (Bonneau, 2007). One such algorithm uses regression coupled with a search based on a genetic algorithm to utilize both static and dynamic data on gene expression (Ferrazzi et al., 2006). Some of the limitations of using gene expression data for identifying gene regulatory networks have been discussed recently (Margolin and Califano, 2007). Many other researchers have contributed to this exciting and challenging research area (Galbraith et al., 2006; Lezon et al., 2006; Liao et al., 2003; Rogers and Girolami, 2005; Wang et al., 2006, 2007b), and an exhaustive coverage is not intended here.

CHALLENGES IN BUILDING MATHEMATICAL MODELS

With the development of several algorithms and software packages for building models based on ordinary differential equations, partial differential equations, stochastic descriptions (www.sbml.org), Boolean networks (Akutsu et al., 2000; Ching et al., 2007; Covert et al., 2004; Kauffman, 1993; Kauffman et al., 2004; Kim et al., 2007; Lahdesmaki et al., 2006; Mehra et al., 2004; Thomas, 1973; Willadsen and Wiles, 2007) and Bayesian networks (Hartemink et al., 2002; Sachs et al., 2005; Yu et al., 2004), computational systems biology has made good progress. When the mechanisms and the topology of the biochemical network are only partially known, input–output models or probabilistic networks such as Bayesian networks (Jordan, 1999; Werhli et al., 2006; Werhli and Husmeier, 2007) can be used. The main challenge there is how to incorporate precisely known *a-priori* information into the probabilistic model, or *vice versa*; that is, if most interactions are known, how one can model the unknown interactions in a probabilistic manner. When the mechanisms and interactions are completely known, as the size of the model increases, it becomes essential to contextually simplify and coarse-grain the biochemical and mathematical model to facilitate interpretation. Effective use of prior heterogeneous knowledge and data in building computational models also requires the integration of qualitative constraints into mathematical models.

Incorporating Statistical/Probabilistic Information into Analytical Models

Bayesian networks have predictive capability and allow the inclusion of *a-priori* knowledge about the system (Jansen et al., 2003; Pandey et al., 2007; Sachs et al., 2005; Stetter et al., 2003; Sun and Zhao, 2004; Woolf et al., 2005; Zou and Conzen, 2005). However, during the training of the Bayesian network using new data, some of the parameters based on the *a-priori* information can change. Although this is part of model refinement, it is not clear how to strictly retain the deterministic information. One approach is to apply constraints on the weights of such connections. Another approach is to develop a hybrid model in which the set of outputs is partitioned into two subsets: deterministic and probabilistic. In principle, this is similar to hybrid deterministic–stochastic multi-scale simulation of complex biochemical networks in which slowly evolving components and components in sufficient number (e.g. greater than ~100) can be treated in a deterministic fashion, whereas others can be treated as a stochastic process or variable (Bhalla, 2004a, 2004b; Kaznessis, 2006; Li et al., 2007; Salis and Kaznessis, 2005; Salis et al., 2006; Scott et al., 2007). Stochastic behavior in genetic circuits has been described and studied, both theoretically and experimentally (Kepler and Elston, 2001; Raser and O'Shea, 2005). One study aimed at bridging the gap between stochastic and deterministic regimens in biochemical kinetics (Puchalka and Kierzek, 2004). A recent review compared models based on mechanistic and statistical networks (Price and Shmulevich, 2007).

Bayesian network learning—that is, identification of the causal connections from data—is computationally very intensive. Usually, pseudoglobal optimization, stochastic search and heuristic approaches are used, because the complexity of exhaustive search is superexponential with regard to the number of total possible values of all the nodes (when nodes hold discrete values) (Pe'er, 2005; Sachs et al., 2005). Recent articles described relationships between correlation and Bayesian and other types of network for gene regulation (Markowetz and Spang, 2007; Markowetz and Troyanskaya, 2007). The authors observed that, for gene regulatory networks, the number of samples (i.e., the different experiments), is usually much fewer than the number of genes of interest, so the full conditional probability of a Bayesian network cannot be accurately estimated; in other words, many networks and corresponding parameter values can result. Hence, *a-priori* information (e.g. that a given gene is usually regulated by no more than 10 other genes or transcription factors) is used, and heuristic approaches are often used to obtain suboptimal but insightful solutions (Bonneau et al., 2006).

Utilizing Qualitative Constraints in Mathematical Models

With increase in the size of the model, the amount of data required for complete parameter specification of the model increases superlinearly. Because such a huge amount of quantitative data cannot be generated even by high-throughput technologies, there is a need to be able to incorporate qualitative constraints on the parameters and variables of the model. Conceptually, data serve as constraints. In machine learning and parameter estimation, the optimization problem is posed as minimization of fit-error between experimental data and model predictions. The objective function and the constraints are mutually interconvertible to some extent. That is why, in approaches to optimization that are based on stochastic searches, it is possible to handle constraints by adding a weighted term to penalize for violation of constraints (Katare et al., 2004a, 2004b; Lin et al., 2004; Maurya and Subramaniam, 2007a; Yan et al., 2004). Stated differently, if one knows a safe limit on the optimal value of the objective function, it can be imposed as a constraint. Fit-error limits on subsets of data also can be written as constraints. The concept of primal and dual problems in linear and non-linear programming is also related to mutual interconvertibility of objective function and constraints (Bertsekas, 2004; Bertsekas et al., 2003). By imposing the constraints, the parameter space (and the network structure space in the data-driven identification of network topology) is restricted to specific regimes. The greater the amount of data and other constraints used, the more restricted will be the parameter space that satisfies the constraints and fits the data.

As far as possible, quantitative constraints should be used, because they restrict the structure and parameter spaces to a greater extent than do qualitative and semi-quantitative constraints. However, if the information or legacy knowledge is known only qualitatively, it should not be ignored, as it still can restrict the search space, albeit to a lesser degree. If the network topology is poorly known and is to be refined through iterations guided by the mismatch between model predictions and experimental data, then such qualitative constraints are beneficial, even though the corresponding data are already included in the objective function. This is because, for large models, fitting all the data together is essentially a multi-objective optimization problem, and is the most difficult problem in optimization (Bot et al., 2007; Chinchuluun and Pardalos, 2007; Handl et al., 2007; Nagrath et al., 2007; Wang et al., 2007a). The fundamental reason why qualitative constraints are useful for refinement of incomplete models is that there can be many parameter-value combinations that can give the same fit-error but for which the corresponding temporal trends of components will differ from each other (Dash et al., 2004). Below, we exemplify several types of qualitative constraints and how they can be used in network learning and parameter estimation.

Qualitative Trend of Temporal Responses

An example of a qualitative constraint is the constraint on the qualitative trends of simulated responses of a component in response to a stimulus (Katare et al., 2004b). As qualitative-trend extraction is expensive, only the essential features expressed in a semi-quantitative fashion can be used. For example, retaining the specific sign of the first (and second) derivative in different segments of the signal is more important than accurately fitting the quantitative values, especially when the latter is difficult to achieve during the first few iterations of model refinement. The desired signs can be computed from experimental data, which may or may not have been measured in the same units (dimensions) as the units used in the numerical / quantitative simulation: in most mathematical models, concentration is expressed in mole/liter or its variants but, experimentally, it is measurable only in terms of fluorescence intensity, moles per cell count or weight of DNA (Fahy et al., 2005, 2007). The qualitative trends are preserved in linear or moderately non-linear (but monotonic) scaling.

Semi-quantitative Constraints

Consider the temporal response of the concentration of cytosolic calcium, in which the first peak is obtained within 10–40 seconds of applying a stimulus to the cell. This can be imposed as a constraint: $10 \leq \arg\max_t(\max([Ca^{2+}](t))) \leq 40$ where arg is argument (the exact formulation could slightly differ, to check for the first peak only) (Maurya and Subramaniam, 2007a, and associated on-line supporting material). Evaluation of this constraint will require computing the maximum of the temporal response over a time window, but at least it will exclude the parameter space corresponding to the very fast and the slow modes. Similar constraints can be imposed on other quantities derived from the model outputs. An important example for the case of cytosolic calcium regulation is that the fraction of free calcium ions in the endoplasmic reticulum is greater than that in the cytosol.

Additional Simulations for Validation of Qualitative Constraints

Inclusion of qualitative constraints may require computation of additional quantities that were otherwise not required. This is the case for the constraint on the location of the first peak of the calcium response, as explained above. If the qualitative behavior of some components under novel perturbations is known, then such perturbations can be quantitatively simulated and used to evaluate the qualitative constraints. It is imperative that the additional simulations increase the computational complexity of a single iteration (evaluation of the objective function and the constraints). However, it is expected that more of the unfeasible or the undesired network structure and parameter space is excluded compared with simulations in which the (additional) qualitative and semi-quantitative constraints were not used. Thus, overall, fewer iterations will be needed during each refinement. Also, the total number of refinements will be potentially reduced, although the overall computational time for model development and refinement will increase. As model refinement usually requires substantial human intervention, fewer iterations are desired over shorter computing time. Furthermore, because the resulting model would be based on more constraints and unstructured legacy knowledge, it will be more realistic and robust for making predictions.

Incomplete Knowledge and Coarse-graining

With unavailability of data and constraints commensurate with the size of a detailed biochemical and mathematical model, estimated parameter values are just one of the many degenerate parameter value sets that can satisfy a computational model. The chosen parameter values, despite satisfying the available data and constraints, may not be even close to the true values. In such a case, predicted responses of novel scenarios could be completely unrealistic, not only quantitatively, but also qualitatively. Hence, parsimonious models are desired that have little degeneracy, and sizes commensurate with the amount of data and knowledge used in their training. With a simplified model, it is easier to understand the underlying systemic design and control principles of the system. Thus it is desirable to develop reduced-order (simplified) models starting from detailed biochemical and mathematical models. This is not so much to reduce the complexity of simulating the model a few times, but to reduce the complexity of parameter estimation and to facilitate meaningful interpretation of simulation results.

Modularity of networks is an additional advantage of coarse-graining. As the first step in the simplification, the networks can be broken down into distinct modules (Ashburner et al., 2000; Asthagiri and Lauffenburger, 2000; Hartwell et al., 1999; Hofestadt and Thelen, 1998; Lauffenburger, 2000; Neves and Iyengar, 2002; Ravasz et al., 2002; Rumbaugh et al., 1991). In fact, it is the modularity of biochemical networks that makes it amenable to develop models of complex processes by re-wiring the models of individual modules. Substantial contributions to the study of the modularity of cellular pathways in the context of computational modeling have come from Bhalla and Iyengar (Bhalla and Iyengar, 1999; Neves and Iyengar, 2002; Neves et al., 2002); in the context of motif discovery and topological complexity, Alon (Alon, 2007a, 2007b; Geva-Zatorsky et al., 2006; Itzkovitz et al., 2005; Kashtan and Alon, 2005; Reigl et al., 2004; Rosenfeld et al., 2007; Yeger-Lotem et al., 2004) and Barabasi (Barabasi and Oltvai, 2004; Balazsi et al., 2005; Goh et al.,

2007; Lim et al., 2006; Oltvai and Barabasi, 2002) have been major contributors. The modules themselves can be quite complex. For example, Hoffmann et al. (2002) have developed a detailed quantitative model of the I kappa B (IκB)–nuclear factor kappa B (NF-κB) signaling module involved in gene activation. This single module alone consists of about 20 ordinary differential equations and 50 parameters.

One approach to model simplification is to ignore biochemical processes that are very fast or very slow compared with the characteristic time-scale of interest (Stephanopoulos et al., 1998). For most networks, we do not have experimentally characterized time constants and parameters, and this makes it difficult to carry out model simplification through knowledge-driven elimination of reactions. However, a biochemical model can be coarse-grained by systematically eliminating reactions and species that are unimportant in the given context. The coarse-grained model must retain the important reactions. The mechanisms encapsulated in such a simpler model could be putative coarse-grained descriptions of corresponding detailed biochemical mechanisms. Regardless of the methodology chosen, in the process of coarse-graining, care should be taken to maintain all the important context-specific biochemically and physiologically relevant species, and constraints. Examples of constraints include: (i) thermodynamic constraints imposed on rate constants involved in thermodynamic cycles (second law of thermodynamics), (ii) the range of values of rate constants as dictated by diffusion limits, and (iii) constraints (e.g. on rate constants) gleaned from measurements available in the literature.

The generation of reduced-order models (ROMs) for linear systems is well studied (Green and Limebeer, 1995); however, the process is not as straightforward for non-linear systems (Petzold and Zhu, 1999; Vora and Daoutidis, 2001). The main factors leading to complexity in biological systems are the presence of several reactions and processes, multiple time-scales, and many species. Based on Tikhonov's theorem (Tikhonov, 1952), a well known principle of model reduction in this context is to eliminate biochemical processes that are very fast (use quasi-steady-state approximation) or very slow (assume constant) compared with the characteristic time-scale of interest of a biochemical system (Stephanopoulos et al., 1998). A number of methods have been proposed to reduce models of chemical systems. Edwards et al. (1998) used a genetic algorithm for the reduction of kinetic models that include bimolecular and trimolecular rate expressions. Parametric sensitivity analysis can be helpful to identify important parameters in complex models, but Petzold and Zhu (1999) have stressed that parametric sensitivity analysis can sometimes be misleading, particularly for stiff systems with a wide range of time-scales. They proposed an optimization-based approach for reaction elimination. The drawback is that the user must decide the number of reactions to be retained. Okino and Mavrovouniotis (1998) have reviewed several approaches, such as species/parameter lumping, sensitivity analysis and time-scale analysis for order reduction when starting with a detailed model. Vora and Daoutidis (2001) proposed a method for reducing non-linear kinetic models with more than one time-scale. The fast dynamics and stiffness are restricted to a single or few parameters using singular perturbation, and the ROM is derived by retaining the slow dynamics. The drawback is that lumping terms in this manner may result in species or reactions that do not correspond to actual species or reactions in the biochemical network. Androulakis (2000) proposed a two-step approach, based on integer-programming, to reduce the number both of species and of reactions in a reaction network. Conzelmann et al. (2004) concluded that the existing approaches for model reduction are inadequate, and they have presented a simulation-based approach for model reduction.

Maurya et al. (2006) proposed a bottom-up strategy for modeling of reaction networks; this is not a model reduction method: instead it *builds* models in three hierarchical steps, starting from a skeletal model using minimal knowledge about the system. The steps closely correspond to the hierarchy of biochemical, mathematical and computational models— namely, updating network structure by adding or deleting mechanisms, updating the expressions for reactions, fluxes and other processes, and tuning the model parameters through parameter estimation. Other recent efforts aiming to achieve coarse-graining include a macro or lumped state formalism for highly complex biochemical networks with combinatorial proteomic states (Conzelmann et al., 2006; Kremling and Saez-Rodriguez, 2007; Saez-Rodriguez et al., 2005) and a graph-theoretic approach to reduce the structural complexity (Blinov et al., 2006; Hlavacek et al., 2006).

Most existing methods assume that all parameters are known. However, for biochemical reaction networks, often no more is known than upper and/or lower limits of the parameters. Hence, computational analysis tools such as parameter estimation and sensitivity analysis are required for reduced-order modeling of such systems. Maurya et al. (2005) proposed a MultiParametric Variability Analysis (MPVA) strategy for reduced-order modeling of reaction networks. Starting with a detailed model, we systematically explored the importance and sensitivity of parameters and used this to guide model reduction. The most attractive feature of the MPVA-based approach is that the result (information) obtained during the parameter estimation for the detailed model itself is used to drive the elimination of reactions. Maurya et al. (2009) have also proposed a mixed-integer non-linear programming/optimization (MINLP) approach for model reduction. We will discuss these two approaches and a graph-theoretic approach to model simplification in more detail below.

MultiParametric Variability Analysis for Coarse-graining of Biochemical Networks

In the MPVA strategy, the importance of parameters is characterized on the basis of simultaneous perturbations in all the parameters, as opposed to sensitivity analysis on single parameters, so that non-linear parametric interactions can be effectively taken into account. Multiple-parameter perturbation can be performed either explicitly or implicitly. In the explicit approach, such as latin hypercube sampling (McKay et al., 1979) or the Fourier amplitude sensitivity test (Fang et al., 2003; Gueorguieva et al., 2006; Koda et al., 1979; Xu and Gertner, 2007), multiple random combinations of parameter values are selected from a set of specified possible values for each parameter, and the overall averaged sensitivity is computed for each parameter. This approach is generally used when the base values of the parameters are known. In the implicit approach, when a technique based on stochastic searching (such as genetic algorithms) is applied for parameter estimation, the pool of good parameter value sets that satisfy the data and constraints are analyzed, in addition to the optimal parameter values. We have followed the implicit approach. Coarse-graining involves three steps: (i) parameter estimation, (ii) multiparametric variability analysis, and (iii) generation of reduced-order models. Parameter estimation is described in detail in the section on Challenges in Building Computational Models. The two other steps are summarized below.

MultiParametric Variability Analysis

MPVA is motivated by the idea that small changes in important parameters have large impacts on the system (i.e., there is a high sensitivity of the system with respect to these parameters), whereas even large changes in unimportant parameters have small or negligible effects (low system sensitivity with respect to these parameters) (Maurya et al., 2005). To implement our MPVA method, we have used an optimization method based on a hybrid genetic algorithm (developed by Katare et al., 2004a) to search the entire parameter space and generate a pool of near-optimal parameter sets that fit the experimental data well (MPVA pool). These sets are used as a basis to determine, for each parameter, the minimum (MIN) and maximum (MAX) values and the range (the ratio MAX/MIN) of values. Parameters with narrow range are potentially more important for predicting the data at hand, whereas those with wide range are potentially less important. The parameters are ordered according to increasing MAX/MIN in a sorted list. Thus, during the model-reduction procedure, the reactions with parameters with wider range are more likely to be eliminated.

Generation of Reduced-order Models

Reactions/parameters are eliminated either one at a time or in groups, starting with the parameter with highest MAX/MIN in the sorted list. A crucial step after each knockout is the verification of the structural integrity of the remaining model. Once this is satisfied, the parameters of the ROM are re-estimated within their constraints, to reflect the fact that parameter values found for the detailed model may not be optimal for the ROM. If the ROM shows satisfactory performance (i.e., fits the experimental data well and predicts the essential features), additional parameters are knocked out. Analysis of biochemical systems is still limited by the amount of experimental data available. Hence, to avoid over-reduction of the model as a result of limited data, qualitative constraints and other biochemical knowledge are useful here. If the ROM is not acceptable, then the previous reaction elimination is invalid, the corresponding reaction/parameter is retained, and the next reaction in the sorted list is eliminated. This can happen because less importance (low sensitivity) does not imply that such a parameter can always be eliminated (Petzold and Zhu, 1999).

Implementation and Case Study

The elimination of parameters and the generation of ROMs have been carried out using Matlab® (MathWorks, 1994) for simplicity of implementation. Quantitative simulation and parameter estimation are performed in a C++ programming environment to achieve computational efficiency (Katare et al., 2004a; Maurya et al., 2005). We have tested the MPVA approach by developing a reduced-order model of the GTPase cycle module of the m1 muscarinic acetylcholine receptor, G_q, and regulator of G-protein signaling 4 (RGS4, a GTPase activating protein [GAP]), starting from a detailed model proposed by Bornheimer et al. (2004). The detailed model consisted of 17 ordinary differential equations and 48 reaction-rate parameters. The measurable outputs from the model were the fraction of G-protein in the active state (i.e., bound to GTP) and the rate of GTP turnover. The detailed model satisfied experimental data on rate of turnover (Biddlecome et al., 1996) and predicted four limiting signaling regimens characterized by very low or high values of the active receptor concentration and GAP concentration. Using the MPVA approach, a ROM was developed which retained only 17 reactions, captured the data and predicted the four limiting signaling regimens. The ROM and the intermediate networks all retained an active ternary complex of G-protein bound to GTP, active receptor and GAP. Thus the ROM shed light on the importance of the ternary complex, which had been proposed by other researchers (Biddlecome et al., 1996; Ross and Wilkie, 2000). This was the first computational evidence for the requirement of the ternary complex. Thus, as mentioned before, the main purpose of coarse-graining is not centered on reducing the complexity of simulation, but on deriving meaningful interpretations and hypotheses.

A Mixed-integer Non-linear Programming Approach to Coarse-graining

Simultaneous Determination of Network Structure and Estimation of Parameters

The MPVA approach presented above is useful, but the method is recursive and hence time consuming, in that the size of the model is reduced in several rounds by eliminating few parameters in each round. In addition, the parameter elimination space is not searched well, even in a pseudoglobal sense. We therefore developed a mixed-integer non-linear optimization approach to model reduction (Maurya et al., 2009), in which the structure (e.g. reaction network) and the parameters of the ROM are determined simultaneously by solving the optimization problem using a genetic algorithm (Goldberg, 1989). In principle, this is a parameter elimination approach. A brief description follows.

Basic Concept

In a general parameter estimation problem, model parameters (p_i) are estimated by minimizing the fit-error between experimental data and model predictions while satisfying appropriate constraints. For model reduction, the parameter estimation problem is extended by including binary variables (u_i) to indicate whether or not a parameter is retained in the ROM. The key idea is to substitute each parameter, say, p_i (that can be possibly eliminated) by the expression $u_i^* p_i$, and then to minimize a suitable objective function with respect to both p_i and u_i, with $u_i = 1$ or 0 implying that the parameter is retained or eliminated, respectively. Complex expressions in which some parameters should be retained or should be eliminated simultaneously can be handled by introducing appropriate constraints case by case. As an example, in a Michaelis–Menten flux expression, both V_{max} and K_M should be either retained or eliminated. The essential idea is to focus on mechanisms. In fact, even though the MINLP approach is general enough, it is more suitable for reducing modules comprised of mostly detailed—as opposed to lumped—reaction mechanisms. Complex rate expressions correspond to lumped reactions, which themselves are reduced representations of underlying several detailed reactions. To avoid potential side-effects, it is best to deal at the level of mechanisms. This also makes the translation of mathematical results into the network structure transparent. As a general rule, binary variables should be directly multiplied with only parameters such as V_{max}, k_{cat} or k_f and k_b, and not with K_M.

Formulation of the Mixed-integer Non-linear Program (MINLP)

In the resulting optimization problem, the objective function is composed of two terms: (i) the number of retained parameters, and (ii) an expression to reflect the fit-error so as to differentiate between ROMs with an equal number of retained parameters but different structures. The procedure is as follows:

1. Given the model equations, substitute each parameter p_i by $u_i^* p_i$.
2. Transform the constraints (if any) appropriately.
3. Develop the MINLP:

$$\min_{(\{p_i\}, \{u_j\})} obj = \sum_j u_j + \alpha^* e(\{p_i\}, \{u_j\}, \Omega)$$

Constraints: $e(\{p_i\}, \{u_j\}, \Omega) \leq e_{th}$
$h_k(\{p_i\}, \{u_j\}) = 0, \quad k = 1, \ldots, m_1$
$g_l(\{p_i\}, \{u_j\}) \leq 0, \quad l = 1, \ldots, m_2$
$p_{i,LB} \leq p_i \leq p_{i,UB}, \quad i = 1, \ldots, n_1;$
$u_j = 0/1, j = 1, \ldots, n_2$ \hfill (8.1)

where Ω denotes the model, n_1 is the number of parameters to be optimized, n_2 is the total number of parameters that can be eliminated, m_1 is the number of equality constraints, m_2 is the number of inequality constraints, $i - l$ are generic indices, h and g denote functions and LB and UB are lower and upper bounds respectively. α is a factor used to adjust the relative weight of the fit-error, e. Different indices, i and j on p and u, respectively, are used to indicate that some of the fixed parameters can also possibly be eliminated, and that some of the estimated parameters can be specifically retained if appropriate. The fit-error, e, is usually a weighted sum of squared errors between model prediction and experimental data. e_{th} is the threshold on fit-error and is usually decided on the basis of acceptable fit-error for the detailed model and error or noise in experimental data.

4. Solve the resulting constrained MINLP using the hybrid stochastic-search-based optimizer, GA–DE–PSO (genetic algorithm [GA], differential evolution [DE] and particle-swarm optimization [PSO]), or any other suitable software such as COPASI (Mendes and Kummer, 2006), individual algorithms such as genetic algorithms (Maurya et al., 2005 ; Goldberg, 1989) or a deterministic approach (Tawarmalani and Sahinidis, 2004).

The values of the retained parameters are used for computational purposes. The estimates of values of other parameters may not be used without appropriate justification, as they did not play a part in fitting the experimental data, even if they satisfied all the constraints on the parameters. This approach is much faster than the MPVA approach. The computational complexity of the MINLP approach is little more than twice that of the parameter estimation problem when a stochastic-search approach is used.

Graph-theoretic Approach to Coarse-graining

If the network structure for the detailed model is sparsely connected, considerable model reduction can only be achieved either by state space transformation or by replacing several connections (reactions) in series/parallel by a single connection. Methods of state space reduction have the disadvantage that a biochemist cannot easily relate the states (components) of the reduced network model to the detailed network model (Okino and Mavrovouniotis, 1998). For biological systems, state elimination is most useful but equally challenging, whereas reaction (connection or mechanism) elimination is easier but less effective for whole networks (Androulakis, 2000; Bhattacharjee et al., 2003; Edwards et al., 1998). To reduce the model for sparsely connected networks or modules, concepts from simplification of graphical networks can be useful (Cormen et al., 2001; Maurya et al., 2003a, 2003b). There are two types of simplification: (i) on a long path, if an intermediate node is not connected to other nodes, it can be eliminated, and (ii) if there are several reaction paths from a source species node to a product or intermediate species node, the paths with relatively much lesser fluxes can be eliminated. If an intermediate species node is highly connected—that is, it is formed in many reactions, consumed in many reactions or directly affects many other reactions—such nodes should be retained. This logic fits well with the rule that highly connected nodes are potentially more important (Venkatasubramanian et al., 2004). A clear understanding about important effects to be captured by the reduced network is necessary to increase the robustness of the reduction technique in a given context. We present below an example of the use of a shorter pathway to replace a long unbranched pathway, and the collapsing of two short parallel pathways into a lumped reaction.

Figure 8.4A shows a two-step mechanism for the activation of heterotrimeric G-proteins. In the first step, GDP (D) dissociates. In the next step, GTP (T) binds to G-protein (G_i) and the $G_{\alpha i}$ (bound to T) and $G_{\beta \gamma}$ subunits dissociate almost instantly. The simplified mechanism contains just one reaction. Figure 8.4B shows simplification of the PLCβ and IP3 generation module of cytosolic calcium regulation (Maurya and Subramaniam, 2007a, and associated on-line supporting material). This simplification

is achieved in two steps. In step 1, the four reversible reactions of the binding of $G_{\beta\gamma}$ and Ca_i (intracellular calcium) to the binding sites on PLCβ (an enzyme) are converted to one reaction (not shown). To maintain all the reactants involved, the simplified reaction could potentially be written as $G_{\beta\gamma} + Ca_i + PLC\beta \rightarrow PLC\beta.G_{\beta\gamma}.Ca$. The rate expression will still be complex. In the second step of simplification, we combine the reaction $G_{\beta\gamma} + Ca_i + PLC\beta \rightarrow PLC\beta.G_{\beta\gamma}.Ca$ with the reaction $PIP2 \rightarrow IP3 + DAG$. As PLCβ.$G_{\beta\gamma}$.Ca is the most potent, form catalysis of PIP2 hydrolysis by PLCβ.$G_{\beta\gamma}$ and PLCβ.Ca is ignored. To incorporate the complexity of the effective rate of hydrolysis, the following lumped reaction is used: $PIP2 + Ca_i + G_{\beta\gamma} + PLC\beta \rightarrow IP3 + DAG + Ca_i + G_{\beta\gamma} + PLC\beta$ In the process of merging, essentially, PLCβ.$G_{\beta\gamma}$.Ca has been replaced by PLCβ, $G_{\beta\gamma}$ and Ca_i. The resulting rate expression is:
Rate = $k_{cat} \times PLC\beta_{tot} \left[[Ca_i]/(K_2' + [Ca_i]) \right] ([G_{\beta\gamma}]/(K_1' + [G_{\beta\gamma}]))$.
This expression is equivalent to $k_{cat} \times$ [PLCβ.$G_{\beta\gamma}$.Ca] for $f = 1$. Generally, $f < 0.5$ ($f = 0.1$

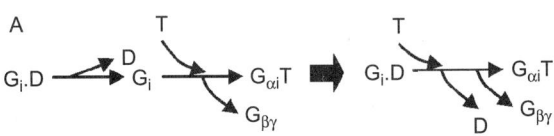

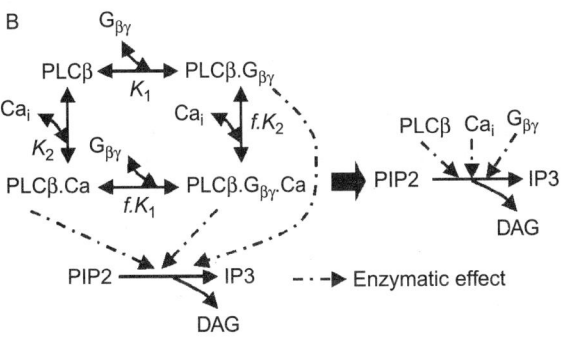

FIGURE 8.4 Examples of Lumping Reactions. (A) Two-steps in the activation of heterotrimeric G-protein (G_i) are lumped into a single step. (B) Reduction of the PLCβ module and generation of IP3 into a single lumped reaction.

was used by Mishra and Bhalla, 2002). These simplified representations are actually utilized in the model for calcium dynamics presented later (Maurya and Subramaniam, 2007a, and associated on-line supporting material).

CHALLENGES IN BUILDING COMPUTATIONAL MODELS

The purpose of a computational model is to be able to simulate and predict, under novel conditions, the behavior of the biological process or system to be modeled. In such a model, the value of the parameters should be precisely known. Thus the foremost challenge in developing a computational model is the unavailability of model parameters such as rate constants and initial concentrations of the myriad components. The next challenge in their development is how to account for variations in the local concentrations of cellular components; this issue is also related to the scales of distance involved. The third challenge is to account for the variation in the parameters and concentrations of the components across different cell types and across different subpopulations drawn from a large batch of a chosen cell type.

Unknown Parameters

Computational analysis of large biochemical networks is impractical because of the lack of availability of data and the computational complexity of simulation required for the estimation of unknown parameters. The complexity of such computational models of biochemical networks is exemplified by a detailed model for the activation of the MAPK pathway by platelet-derived growth factor (PDGF) proposed by Bhalla et al. (2002). This model consists of about 100 non-linear ordinary differential equations and algebraic equations, and about 200 parameters. Similarly, a detailed model for calcium signaling consists of about 200 equations and an even greater number of parameters (Mishra and Bhalla, 2002). Although, thanks to the availability of affordable computing power, simulating these subsystems when all the parameter values are known is not difficult, the same is not true if some of the parameters are unknown. This is because estimating a single unknown parameter may require several hundreds of simulations, and the total number of simulations required increases with the number of unknown parameters in a quadratic or more extensive manner. Except for a few well studied systems such as those stated above, mathematical descriptions of most systems lack parameter values. In some circumstances, the limits on the parameters can be gleaned on the basis of known values in comparable cell or tissue types; however, in many cases, the limits span more than two orders of magnitude, which, coupled with the characteristic non-linearity of biochemical systems, makes reliable parameter estimation a challenging task. The complexity of parameter estimation becomes even more appreciable when a computational model corresponding to the entire cell, possibly composed of tens of thousands of non-linear mixed (both continuous and discrete variables) equations with a similar number of parameters, needs to be developed. This still generally requires the model to treat the cell as a well mixed system (a property that is unphysiologic).

The level of attention to the precise values of parameters also depends on the objectives of the study being performed. If one is interested only in gross qualitative features or the range of qualitative features across many cell types, the parameter space can be scanned using latin hypercube sampling (McKay et al., 1979) or the Fourier amplitude sensitivity test (Fang et al., 2003; Gueorguieva et al., 2006; Koda et al., 1979; Xu and Gertner, 2007), which have traditionally been used for multiparametric global sensitivity analysis,. Even in this case, if the limits on the unknown parameters are too wide—for example, more than two orders of magnitude—some parameter constraining is desired. Global sensitivity analysis can identify the parameters to which the system is more sensitive. The limits on such parameters can be narrowed to improve the accuracy of qualitative predictions. If one is interested in capturing the fine qualitative features or semi-quantitative features, substantial constraining of the parameters is required. As an example, in our recent study on calcium dynamics, which will be detailed later in this section, the effective time constants of the temporal responses predicted using parameter values obtained from the literature were substantially different from those observed in the data used for our studies. Although precise quantitative comparisons/predictions of fine features such as peak height are not essential to the calculations, it is essential to capture overall temporal variations such as effective time constants and oscillatory versus non-oscillatory behavior for a model to be accurate and be of predictive value. Thus some cell-specific constraining of the parameters may be necessary. One way to carry out constraining of the parameters is to "tweak" each parameter in a trial-and-error fashion. The alternative, and arguably the best, way is to use cell-specific *in vivo* data to develop a systems-level model. The known biochemistry and other constraints from legacy data must be included to maintain the qualitative generality of the results. It is reasonable to expect differences in the values of some of the lumped/effective kinetic parameters besides the differences in the species concentrations in various cell types. Cell-specific modeling, including the estimation/measurement of parameters, is quite important for real-life applications such as drug dose–response effects, and applications of systems biology.

Approaches to Parameter Estimation

There is a vast literature on constrained non-linear optimization using approaches based on deterministic searches (Chang and Sahinidis,

2005; Esposito and Floudas, 2000; Famili et al., 2005; Floudas et al., 2005; Lall and Voit, 2005; Marquardt, 1963; Papamichail and Adjiman, 2005; Singer et al., 2006; Tawarmalani and Sahinidis, 2004; Zwolak et al., 2005), stochastic searches (Al-Kazemi and Mohan, 2005; Goldberg, 1989; Hu et al., 2003; Kennedy and Eberhart, 1995; Liang et al., 2004; Moles et al., 2003; Ozcan and Mohan, 1998; Robinson et al., 2002; Storn and Price, 1997; Summanwar et al., 2002; Sundaram and Venkatasubramanian, 1998; Ji and Xu, 2006; Xiao et al., 2004; Yan et al., 2004) or their combination (Katare et al., 2004a; Lin et al., 2001; Mendes and Kell, 1998; Moles et al., 2003; Rodriguez-Fernandez et al., 2006). A detailed survey is not intended here.

In much of our own recent research, we have used stochastic search optimization strategies. The essential idea is that model parameters are estimated by minimizing the mismatch between the experimental data and the corresponding model prediction using the hybrid stochastic-search algorithm, GA–DE–PSO, which combines genetic algorithms (Back, 1996; Goldberg, 1989; Katare et al., 2004a), differential evolution (Lin et al., 2001; Storn and Price, 1997) and particle-swarm optimization (Al-Kazemi and Mohan, 2005; Hu et al., 2003; Kennedy and Eberhart, 1995). All three, GA, DE and PSO, are population-based optimization methods. In all three, the initial population is chosen randomly from parameters distributed uniformly on a normal or a log scale, depending upon the specific parameter ranges. In the genetic algorithm, candidates/members are represented as a genome and the population evolves into the next generation by transferring good candidates from the current generation (elitism) (Back, 1996) and generating new members by applying crossover and/or mutation operators to parents; one parent genome is selected on the basis of fitness, and the other randomly. Thus a more fit member is more likely to be used for crossover. The offspring genomes are evaluated (objective function is calculated) and included in the next generation. Finally, the population is sorted (members are rank ordered) according to fitness. This process is repeated for a fixed number of generations. In differential evolution, given a chosen parent, its weighted difference with another randomly chosen member is added to another parent and the resulting candidate undergoes crossover with a trial vector to create an offspring (step 1). If the offspring is better than the chosen parent, the parent is replaced by the offspring (step 2). This ensures that every member of the next generation is at least as good as the corresponding member in the previous generation. In the case of particle-swarm optimization, the population (swarm) is updated by moving each member towards the best member of the swarm. The movement of each member is tracked, so that it can also move to its best location so far. The overall algorithm is still biased towards the GA component, but the concepts from DE and PSO are used appropriately. A class of algorithms similar to genetic algorithms, known as evolutionary search/computation (Ji and Xu, 2006; Liang et al., 2004; Lin et al., 2004; Rodriguez-Fernandez et al., 2006), is also quite popular and successful in the optimization of biochemical systems. However, approaches based on evolutionary algorithms are not really very different from genetic algorithms, at least at a conceptual level. In fact, most evolutionary algorithms can be seen as elitist genetic algorithms (Katare et al., 2004a; Liang et al., 2004; Rodriguez-Fernandez et al., 2006) or a minor variant.

Variation in Local Concentrations and Multiple Scales of Distance and Time

Deterministic simulation based on ordinary differential equations is accurate only if large reaction volumes (and hence a large number of molecules) are considered. As stated earlier, most models of biochemical reaction systems assume a well mixed system. Such models are sufficient for making comparisons with measurements based on populations of cells, because cell-to-cell variations are averaged out. For the purpose of predictive modeling while still fully capturing the biochemical mechanisms, the discrepancy between the model outputs and the populational measurements can generally be compensated by slight variations in the parameter values. However, nowadays, data at the level of single cells can be collected using high-throughput imaging and flow cytometry techniques (Alliance for Cellular Signaling (a); Sachs et al., 2005; Zheng et al., 2006). Such imaging data have revealed that the concentration of various components even within the same compartment of the cell (e.g. the plasma membrane or the cytosol) can vary substantially; naturally, the local concentrations can widely differ from the average or the global concentration. Many of the cellular functions are strongly dependent on the spatial variation of chemical species inside the cell. For example, the density of receptors on the cell surface of a cell is not uniform; instead, patches of high receptor density are found. Similarly, variations in local concentrations of IP3 in oocytes are responsible for setting the calcium wave and polarity with respect to the site of sperm entry (Wagner et al., 1998; Yi et al., 2005), and the sensing of concentration gradients underlies cell motility (Subramanian and Narang, 2004). Local variations in the concentrations of components also allow the cell to elicit a wide range of responses as needed.

For accurate modeling of the behavior at the level of small subcellular volumes, stochastic simulations are required, to account for diffusion effects and small copy numbers of molecules (Bhalla, 2004a; Brinkerhoff et al., 2004). A computational study on calcium waves during egg fertilization considered spatial effects in the model (Bugrim et al., 2003). At the level of single cells, stochastic simulation can generate many realizations of the temporal response, some of which would be both qualitatively and quantitatively distinct. Thus stochastic simulation plays an important part in our understanding of the biological variability observed at the level of single cells or small populations of cells. Although solutions based on partial differential equations and finite-element methods can be used to model spatial variation, it is important to account for the stochastic effects, because the copy number of molecules becomes small (e.g. of the order of 1–10 as opposed to 100 or 1000) in small mesh volumes. Thus, in the context of cell biology, to a large extent spatial variation and stochastic behavior are coupled. A brief account of the research in stochastic simulation and recent advances is presented below.

Methods for Stochastic Simulation

Since the pioneering work of Gillespie (1976) and several other researchers, recently several methods have been developed to tackle the complexity of stochastic simulation. One approach is the tau-leap method, in which a larger time-step is taken and many reactions are fired in the chosen time interval (Gillespie, 2001). A variant of this method is the binomial tau-leap method to avoid negative populations (Chatterjee and Vlachos, 2006; Chatterjee et al., 2005). In another method, approaches based on deterministic simulation, stochastic simulation and the Markov model are used in an integrated manner (Kaznessis, 2006). Yet a third approach partitions the reactions and species as "slow" and "fast", with the partial equilibrium assumption that the population of slow species is not altered by the fast reactions (Cao et al., 2005).

Stochastic Simulation in Parameter Estimation Studies

It may be necessary to account for stochastic effects during parameter estimation. Similar to deterministic simulation, stochastic simulation also requires that the reaction rate parameters be known. As elaborated in the previous section, this is seldom the case, especially for processes that are not yet fully understood but are becoming understood through the integration of computational modeling and experimental research. Given that any of the realizations of stochastic simulation do not individually correspond to the experimental results in single cells, at best, the average of many (thousands of) realizations can be compared with that of a small population of cells. This will result in a more accurate description of the system than that provided by deterministic simulation. However, the computational complexity is enormous, thus requiring methods for accelerated stochastic simulation. In our view, the best approach to this is to obtain an approximation to the satisfactory parameter regions through deterministic simulation that relies on population-based measurements. Stochastic simulation should then be performed using those parameter values. If the average response from the stochastic simulation is similar to that obtained by the deterministic simulation, there is no need to use stochastic simulation in parameter estimation. Otherwise, parameter estimation must be carried out by using stochastic simulation; that is, the average of many realizations will be used for each evaluation of the objective function (e.g. sum of squares errors). The limits on the parameters in this second optimization can be obtained by slightly relaxing the range of good parameter values obtained using deterministic simulation. As these limits would be narrower than the original limits used in the deterministic simulation, the overall complexity of parameter estimation will be reduced considerably.

Multiple Scales of Distance and Time

Various cellular processes in entire systems span several scales of distance. At one extreme, local diffusion from cytosol to membrane deals with less than one-tenth of a micron, and intracellular cytosolic and nuclear events and autocrine signaling involve up to a few microns. At the other extreme, endocrine signaling and paracrine signaling can require molecular movements of from millimeters (secretion of insulin) to several meters (central nervous system). In general, the scales of distance are closely related to the size of the organelles, cells, tissues or body parts in question. Besides multiple distance-scales, cellular process also encompass multiple time-scales. Some events such as cell surface receptor activation and other individual signaling reactions are very fast and occur within a fraction of a second; some events such as allosteric control and protein modifications are slow, with characteristic time spans of a few seconds to minutes, and yet others such as gene expression, translation, translocation, and cell division and growth take from several minutes to several hours (Papin et al., 2005; Stephanopoulos et al., 1998). The presence of several time-scales makes the dynamic model a stiff system, which slows down the computation speed, for example in numerical integration. A generic approach with which to develop simple and reliable computational models is to model in detail the events occurring at the time-scale of interest. Reactions and other processes occurring at much faster rates can be assumed to be in equilibrium and in a quasi-steady state, whereas much slower processes can be assumed to be constant. More formal mathematical approaches to simplification include decomposition of time-scales using Eigenvalue analysis of the Jacobian matrix of the linearized system (Moore, 1981; Palsson and Lightfoot, 1985; Palsson et al., 1987). Methods of simplifying non-linear reaction systems, also known as computational singular perturbation, have been developed which also address time-scale decomposition to some extent (Vora and Daoutidis, 2001). A recent review highlighted the research in time-scale decomposition and model simplification (Kremling and Saez-Rodriguez, 2007).

Cell-specific Variability and Subpopulational Variability

As different tissues are involved in different and specific functions, it is no surprise that the internal compositions of the cells from different organs and tissues will be somewhat different: for example, adipocytes contain large amount of fats, whereas myocytes contain many myofibrils, the filamentous contractile unit of muscles. Macrophages and B cells are specialized for the production of cytokines and antibodies. Neuronal and muscle cells (excitable cells) have generally much higher concentrations of cytosolic calcium ions (0.2–0.5 micromoles per liter (μM) (Mishra and Bhalla, 2002) as compared with non-excitable cells such as macrophages (0.03–0.1 μM) (Alliance for Cellular Signaling (b); Letari et al., 1991). Besides the cell-type-specific differences, which are inherent, from the point of view of experimental and computational studies, differences across different subpopulations of the same cell type have been observed. In recent experiments conducted by the Alliance for Cellular Signaling it was observed that, when triggered by the same strength of a stimulus, different cell populations (cloned from the same parent cell) exhibited responses that differed both quantitatively and qualitatively (different peak heights, rise time, etc.). According to our current understanding, the underlying reason is the variation in the unmeasurable concentrations of hundreds of species (components) inside the cells, arising from variation in the overall state of the cell. This variability could result from both intrinsic sources such as noise in gene expression (Raser and O'Shea, 2005) and extrinsic noise such as unsynchronized cell cycles in different experiments. Although some of these fluctuations across cells are averaged out in cell populations, a non-trivial variation is still observed from one population to another. This variability is an inevitable fact concerning biological systems (Babnigg et al., 2000), and cannot be explained by using a single set of values of reaction parameters and the initial conditions, because concentrations and fluxes vary across subpopulations.

CASE STUDY: MODELING THE REGULATION OF CALCIUM DYNAMICS IN RAW 264.7 CELLS

Cytosolic calcium is a second messenger and plays an important role in intracellular signaling (Carafoli, 2002). It is involved in regulating numerous cellular functions by regulating the activity of proteins such as calmodulin, calreticulin and calcineurin. Dynamic changes in intracellular calcium serve both as an important indicator of cellular events and a quantitative measure of cellular responses to stimuli. In our laboratory, a simplified model has been developed for calcium signaling in RAW 264.7 cells, incorporating most of the relevant mechanisms included in the published models (Fig. 8.5). In the calcium model for RAW 264.7 cells, the stimulus is the complement protein, C5a, which activates G-protein, G_i. Most of the mechanisms are generic, and they can be easily tailored for another stimulus in a non-excitable cell. We have included some mechanisms explicitly so that knockdown of important proteins, such as G-protein-coupled receptor (GPCR) kinase (GRK), Arrestin, $G_{\beta\gamma}$ and $G_{\alpha i}$, can be modeled quantitatively. Below, we present a concise schematic and mathematical model and the main findings. A detailed description of the model and the related results are presented elsewhere (Maurya and Subramaniam, 2007a, 2007b).

Mechanisms

In a eukaryotic cell, the average cytosolic calcium concentration ($[Ca^{2+}]_i$) is maintained low (0.05–0.5 μM), whereas Ca^{2+} concentrations in

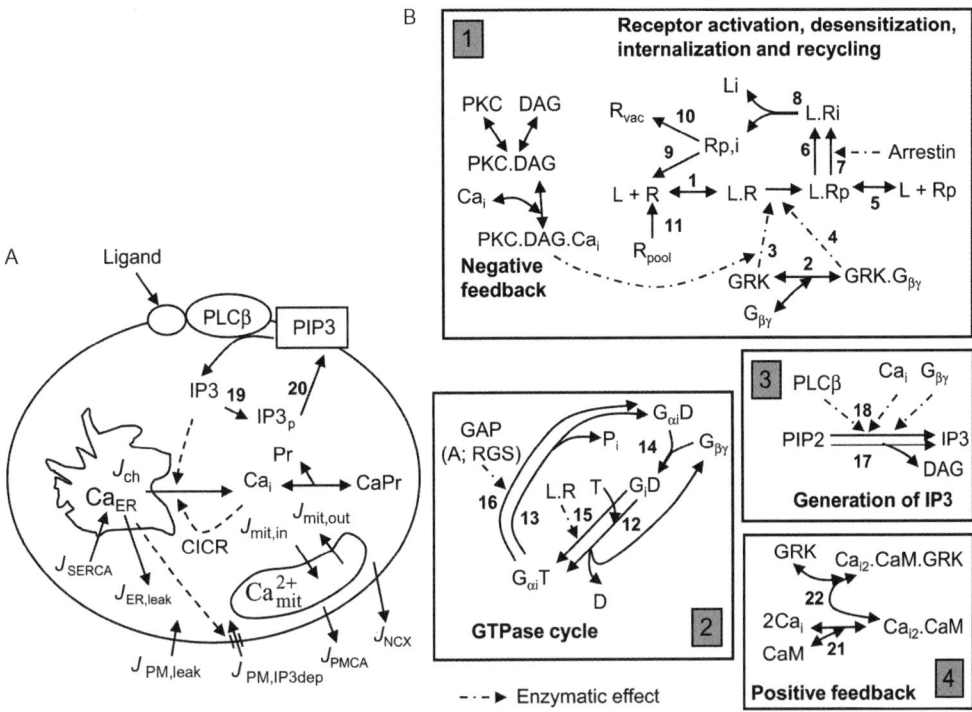

FIGURE 8.5 A Simplified Model for Calcium Signaling Including Calcium Influx, and ER and Mitochondrial Exchange and Storage, Used in Computations Based on the Conceptual Model.
(A) Overall schematic model. The ligand C5a (L) binds to its receptor C5aR (R) on the plasma membrane (PM) activating G-protein, Gi. The free subunit $G_{\beta\gamma}$ binds to and activates PLCβ, which hydrolyses PIP2 to IP3 and DAG. IP3 binds to its receptor on the ER membrane and the IP3R channels open to release calcium into the cytosol. Other calcium fluxes—for example between mitochondria and extracellular space—are also shown. CICR, calcium-induced calcium release; $IP3_p$, IP3 product; J_{ch}, rate of Ca^{2+} flux from ER to cytosol through the Ca^{2+} releasing channel; $J_{mit,in}$ and $J_{mit,out}$, rates of Ca^{2+} uptake and release by mitochondria; $J_{PM,IP3dep}$, flux through IP3-dependent channels on the PM; $J_{PM,leak}$, leakage flux; J_{PMCA} and J_{NCX}, extrusions of Ca^{2+} to the extracellular space by the plasma-membrane calcium ATPase (PMCA) pump and the Na^+–Ca^{2+} exchanger (NCX) on the plasma membrane; J_{SERCA}, rate of Ca^{2+} pumping by the sarco(endo)plasmic reticulum calcium ATPase (SERCA) pump; PM, plasma membrane; Pr, protein. (B) Modules and reactions. The mechanisms for the receptor module (panel [1]), GTPase cycle module (panel [2]), IP3-generation module (panel [3]), and the feedback effects (panels [1] and [4]). Ca_i, cytosolic Ca^{2+}; CaM, calmodulin; CICR, calcium-induced calcium release; D, GDP; DAG, diacylglycerol; ER, endoplasmic reticulum; $G_{\alpha i}$, $G_{\beta\gamma}$, G-protein subunits; GAP, (A) GTPase activating protein; Gi, G-protein, GRK, G-protein coupled receptor (GPCR) kinase; IP3, inositol 1,4,5-trisphosphate; $IP3_p$, a lumped product of IP3 phosphorylation; IP3R, IP3 receptor; L, ligand C5a; Li, internalized ligand; L.R, ligand-bound active receptor; L.Ri, internalized ligand-bound phosphorylated receptor; mit, mitochondria; NCX, Na^+/Ca^{2+} exchanger; P_i, inorganic phosphate; PIP2, phosphatidylinositol 4,5-bisphosphate; PKC, protein kinase C; PLCβ, phospholipase C-β; PM, plasma membrane; PMCA, PM calcium ATPase; R, receptor C5aR; RGS, regulator of G-protein signaling; R_p, phosphorylated receptor; $R_{p,i}$, internalized phosphorylated receptor; Rpool, fresh receptor pool; SERCA: sarco(endo)plasmic reticulum calcium ATPase; T, GTP; vac, vocuole. Numbers 1–22 represent reaction numbers.
Reproduced from Maurya and Subramaniam (2007a) (Fig. 1), with permission.

the extracellular space ($[Ca^{2+}]_o$) and (sarcoplasmic or) endoplasmic reticulum (ER) ($[Ca^{2+}]_{ER}$) are several thousand times greater (Berridge et al., 2003). This large concentration gradient of Ca^{2+} between different cellular compartments is utilized by cells to generate rapid intracellular Ca^{2+} changes through receptor-mediated mechanisms. In non-excitable cells, such as macrophages, ligand-induced release of calcium from the endoplasmic reticulum is the main initiator of calcium dynamics. In excitable cells, other sources that initiate dynamics include the calcium influx through voltage-gated channels on the plasma membrane (Jafri et al., 1998). Both of these eventually lead to increased activation and opening of the IP3R channels on the endoplasmic reticulum membrane, through either increased hydrolysis of PIP2 to IP3 (Lemon et al., 2003) or a local increase in $[Ca^{2+}]_i$ leading to calcium-induced release of calcium (Berridge, 1992). Calcium release from the endoplasmic reticulum leads to increased Ca^{2+} in the cytosol. Most of the calcium released binds to various proteins—calmodulin among others. Calcium is also pumped back to the endoplasmic reticulum by the sarco(endo)plasmic reticulum calcium ATPase (SERCA) pump. Some calcium is also expelled to the extracellular space through the Na^+–Ca^{2+} exchanger (NCX) and the plasma membrane calcium ATPase (PMCA) pump; calcium exchange with the mitochondria also has been observed in the presence of high levels of $[Ca^{2+}]_i$. If the Ca^{2+} concentration in the endoplasmic reticulum becomes quite low, calcium can enter the cell as a calcium-release-activated current, through store-operated channels on the plasma-membrane (Dellis et al., 2006; Hofer et al., 2002).

Figure 8.5A shows an overall schematic of the ligand-induced release of calcium from the endoplasmic reticulum into the cytosol, the binding of calcium (Ca_i) to proteins (Pr) in the cytosol (shown) and in the endoplasmic reticulum (not shown), and other calcium-exchange fluxes to/from the endoplasmic reticulum, the extracellular space and the mitochondria. Figure 8.5B shows the modules and reactions (both simple and lumped) that have been modeled explicitly. The modules involved in the ligand-induced release of calcium from the endoplasmic reticulum are discussed below. In short, binding of the ligand (C5a, denoted by L) to its receptor (C5aR, denoted by R) leads to the activation of the receptor, which in turn leads to the activation of G-protein, G_i. Free $G_{\beta\gamma}$ binds with PLCβ and activates it, resulting in increased hydrolysis of PIP2 to IP3. The increase in IP3 concentration results in increased release of calcium from the endoplasmic reticulum.

Receptor Module (Fig. 8.5B, Panel 1)

Reaction 1 is activation through ligand binding. Reactions 3–5 lead to desensitization through phosphorylation of the ligand-bound active receptor (reaction 3 is catalyzed by GRK and reaction 4 is catalyzed by GRK. $G_{\beta\gamma}$) (Lemon et al., 2003; Riccobene et al., 1999; Woolf and Linderman, 2003). Reactions 6 and 7 are internalizations (reaction 7 is catalyzed by Arrestin). Reactions 8–10 are for recovery of the receptor (L.Ri: internalized ligand-bound phosphorylated receptor) (Sitaramayya and Bunnett, 1999). Hydrolysis of the phosphate of $R_{p,i}$ (internalized phosphorylated receptor) is lumped in both reactions 9 and 10 (Lemon et al., 2003; Hoffman et al., 1996). Reaction 11 is fresh receptor generation (Hoffman et al., 1996; Yi et al., 2003). In most existing models, GRK and Arrestin have not been explicitly included. Reaction 2 represents the binding of GRK to $G_{\beta\gamma}$ and is very fast. The rate constant for reaction 4 is much higher (about 100-fold) than that for reaction 3, so that most phosphorylation occurs through GRK.$G_{\beta\gamma}$ when ligand is present, and through GRK in the basal state. Similarly, internalization (reactions 6 and 7) is enhanced substantially by Arrestin (buffered). Reactions 3, 4 and 7 are lumped enzymatic reactions.

GTPase Cycle Module (Fig. 8.5B, Panel 2)

Reactions 12–16 depict the GTPase cycle. Reactions 12 and 13 are in the absence of active receptor and GAP, respectively. Reaction 15 is similar to reaction 12, but is catalyzed by L.R (ligand-bound active receptor) and reaction 16 is similar to 13 but is catalyzed by GAP (A, RGS). Reactions 15 and 16 model the G-protein activation (binding of the alpha subunit to GTP), and GTP hydrolysis catalyzed by GTPase activating protein (GAP), respectively (T is GTP, D is GDP, A is GAP (RGS)).

IP3 Module (Fig. 8.5B, Panel 3)

During the basal state, most of the IP3 is generated through the slow hydrolysis of PIP2 (reaction 17), because free $G_{\beta\gamma}$ is present in very small amounts. Upon G-protein activation, dissociated $G_{\beta\gamma}$ binds to PLCβ. Each of PLCβ.$G_{\beta\gamma}$, PLCβ.Ca$_i$ and PLCβ.$G_{\beta\gamma}$.Ca$_i$ catalyze hydrolysis of PIP2, but PLCβ.$G_{\beta\gamma}$.Ca$_i$ is the most potent. In our model, for simplification, a lumped enzymatic reaction is used to model the enhancement due to PLCβ.Ca$_i$ (reaction 18). Reactions 19 and 20 are simplified and highly lumped representations of IP3 metabolism (degradation/conversion to/from other inositol phosphates and back to PIP2), with only one intermediate pseudo-species (IP3$_p$, IP3 product) (Lemon et al., 2003). This representation is sufficient for both excitable and non-excitable cells, as the main mechanism responsible for calcium oscillation in muscle cells is the interaction between fluxes through IP3R, ryanodine receptor channels, the SERCA pump and the voltage-operated and store-operated channels. Marhl et al. (2000) have shown that interactions with the mitochondria (included in our model) can also result in oscillations, especially at values of cytosolic [Ca^{2+}] greater than 0.5 μM.

Feedback Effects from Calmodulin and PKC (Fig. 8.5B, Panel 4)

As shown in Figure 8.5B, calmodulin (CaM) binds with intracellular Ca^{2+} (Ca$_i$) (reaction 21) and the resulting complex binds with GRK (reaction 22), reducing the effective amount of free GRK that can bind $G_{\beta\gamma}$. The result is reduced phosphorylation of the active receptor, and thus this constitutes a functional positive feedback. In contrast (Panel 1), the PKC. DAG.Ca$_i$ complex enhances the activity of GRK and thus promotes phosphorylation, resulting in a negative feedback. This effect is modeled as enzymatic activation by calcium, to avoid explicit modeling of the complexes.

Mathematical Representation of the Model

In the model, the state variables are described by a set of ordinary differential equations (Schuster et al., 2002) involving the Ca^{2+} fluxes between different cellular compartments and other fluxes caused by reactions. Apart from the state variables used to model the details of ligand-induced generation of IP3, the four main state variables are [Ca^{2+}]$_i$, [Ca^{2+}]$_{ER}$, [Ca^{2+}]$_{mit}$, and [IP$_3$], which represent the Ca^{2+} concentrations in cytosolic (i), endoplasmic reticulum (ER) and mitochondrial (mit) compartments, and the IP3 concentration in cytosol, respectively. The differential equations for the state variables related to the reactions (including [IP3]) are automatically derived using a reaction parser developed in our laboratory. The expressions for other state variables and related fluxes, specified manually, are given below:

$$\frac{d[Ca^{2+}]_i}{dt} = \beta_i(J_{ch} + J_{ER,leak} + J_{PM,IP3dep} - J_{SERCA} - (J_{PMCA} + J_{NCX} - J_{PM,leak}) + (J_{mit,out} - J_{mit,in}) - 2v_{21}) \quad (8.2)$$

$$\frac{d[Ca^{2+}]_{ER}}{dt} = \frac{\beta_{ER}}{\rho_{ER}}(J_{SERCA} - J_{ch} - J_{ER,leak}) \quad (8.3)$$

$$\frac{d[Ca^{2+}]_{mit}}{dt} = \frac{\beta_m}{\rho_m}(J_{mit,in} - J_{mit,out}) \quad (8.4)$$

$$\frac{dh}{dt} = k_{on}(Q - ([Ca^{2+}]_i + Q)h) \quad (8.5)$$

where, β_i, β_{ER}, and β_m are the ratio of free calcium to free and bound calcium in the cytosol, endoplasmic reticulum and mitochondria, respectively, assuming fast buffering (equilibrium) with calcium binding proteins. ρ_{ER} and ρ_m are the ratio of the volume of the ER and the mitochondria, respectively, to the volume of the cytosol. The expressions for other terms are as follows:

$$J_{ch} = v_{max,ch}\left(\left(\frac{[IP3]}{[IP3]+K_{IP3}}\right)\left(\frac{[Ca^{2+}]_i}{[Ca^{2+}]_i+K_{act}}\right)h\right)^3$$
$$([Ca^{2+}]_{ER} - [Ca^{2+}]_i) \quad (8.6)$$

$$J_{ER,leak} = k_{ER,leak}([Ca^{2+}]_{ER} - [Ca^{2+}]_i) \quad (8.7)$$

$$J_{PM,IP3dep} = V_{max,PM,IP3dep}[IP3]^2 / (K_{m,PM,IP3dep}^2 + [IP3]^2) \quad (8.8)$$

$$J_{SERCA} = V_{max}([Ca^{2+}]_i^2 / ([Ca^{2+}]_i^2 + K_P^2)) \quad (8.9)$$

$$J_{PMCA} = \frac{V_{max,PMCA,l}[Ca^{2+}]_i^2}{[Ca^{2+}]_i^2 + K_{M,PMCA,l}^2} + \frac{V_{max,PMCA,h}[Ca^{2+}]_i^5}{[Ca^{2+}]_i^5 + K_{M,PMCA,h}^5}$$

$$J_{NCX} = \frac{V_{max,NCX}[Ca^{2+}]_i}{[Ca^{2+}]_i + K_{M,NCX}} \quad (8.10)$$

$$J_{PM,leak} = v_{pm,leak} \quad (8.11)$$

$$J_{mit,out} = (k_{out}([Ca^{2+}]_i^2 / (K_1^2 + [Ca^{2+}]_i^2)) + k_m)[Ca^{2+}]_{mit} \quad (8.12)$$

$$J_{mit,in} = k_{in}[Ca^{2+}]_i^4 / (K_2^4 + [Ca^{2+}]_i^4) \quad (8.13)$$

$$Q = K_{inh}([IP3] + d_1) / ([IP3] + d_3) \quad (8.14)$$

and v_{21} is the rate of reaction 21 (Fig. 8.5B).

Note that: (i) J_{ch}, the rate of Ca^{2+} flux from endoplasmic reticulum to cytosol through the Ca^{2+}-releasing channel, is based on the IP3R model of De Young and Keizer (1992) and Li and Rinzel (1994) (see also Fink et al., 2000), by implementing the calcium-induced calcium release (CICR) mechanism of the Ca^{2+}-releasing channel (h is the fraction of IP3R in which Ca^{2+} is not bound to the inhibitory site); (ii) J_{SERCA}, the rate of Ca^{2+} pumping by the SERCA pump, is expressed as a Hill-type equation with a Hill constant of 2, as observed in many cell types (Gill and Chueh, 1985; Lytton et al., 1992); (iii) $J_{mit,in}$ and $J_{mit,out}$, the rates of Ca^{2+} uptake and release by mitochondria, are from Marhl et al. (2000) and Haberichter et al. (2001), except that, for $J_{mit,in}$, a Hill coefficient of 4 is used instead of 8; (iv) J_{PMCA} and J_{NCX}, extrusions of Ca^{2+} to the extracellular space by the plasma-membrane calcium ATPase (PMCA) pump and Na^+–Ca^{2+} exchanger (NCX) on the plasma membrane are modeled as described by Wiesner et al. (1996), and $J_{PM,leak}$, the leakage flux from the extracellular space to the cytosol, is treated as described by Hofer et al. (2002); (v) the expression for $J_{PM,IP3dep}$, which includes store-operated channel flux, is also from Hofer et al. (2002).

Results for Simulation and Parameter Estimation Using Data from RAW 264.7 Cells

We have used four datasets (a control dataset, $G_{\alpha i}2,3$ knockdown data, the corresponding control data and PLCβ-3 knockdown data) on RAW 264.7 cells to constrain the rate parameters. In order to utilize multiple datasets corresponding to different subpopulations of cells, to avoid imposing unrealistic constraints, some of the extrinsic parameters—such as initial conditions of state variables, concentrations of buffered species, lumped rate parameters and the parameters related to the capacity and shape of the cell—were allowed to vary within a factor of 3 across the four datasets. Other parameters, such as those related to basic reactions, were maintained constant across all datasets. The independent control/basic dataset is later used for prediction of the dose response of the ligand C5a, and the knockdown response for several proteins. The results are shown in Figure 8.6. The optimizer is able to find parameter values that satisfy the data from all the four datasets

(Fig. 8.6A); hence, we have confidence in the structure/mechanisms of the model. The main results from the simulation of dataset 1 are: (i) activated receptor is quickly desensitized and remains internalized for a long time, (ii) negative-feedback regulation of receptor activity is mediated by the activated G-protein, (iii) peak IP3 concentrations are more than 5 times higher than the basal level, and (iv) mitochondrial uptake is slower compared with that by the endoplasmic reticulum. Distinct results from the simulation of dataset 2 are: (a) a higher PLCβ pool results in higher peak [IP3], (b) subpopulational variability is able to explain anomalous peak calcium responses, and (c) larger basal cytosolic calcium concentrations require larger calcium concentrations in the endoplasmic reticulum and mitochondria. Analysis of the simulations results for dataset 3 reveals that (i) a high dose results in depletion of the surface receptors, (ii) knockdown of $G_{\alpha i}$ results in higher basal and peak levels of $[G_{\beta \gamma}]$ and [IP3], and (iii) knockdown of $G_{\alpha i}$ results in partial depletion of the endoplasmic reticulum. Dataset 4 indicates that subpopulational variability is required, and that calcium oscillations are unlikely in macrophages.

Dose Response

The dose response of a ligand is one of the most useful and experimentally measurable indicators of the efficacy of the ligand for its target. For our system, the sigmoidal shape of the predicted dose–response curve (Fig. 8.6B, panel [2]) is as expected, the half-maximal concentration (EC_{50}) being about 18 nM (about half of the total surface receptor concentration). Other important results from the dose–response study are: (i) 75 nM C5a results in a full response, and with an increasing dose the rise time decreases; (ii) higher doses result in a bimodal response of the activated receptors; (iii) the total surface receptor, not the total $G_{\beta \gamma}$, is the limiting factor for the maximal response. The EC_{50} is about the

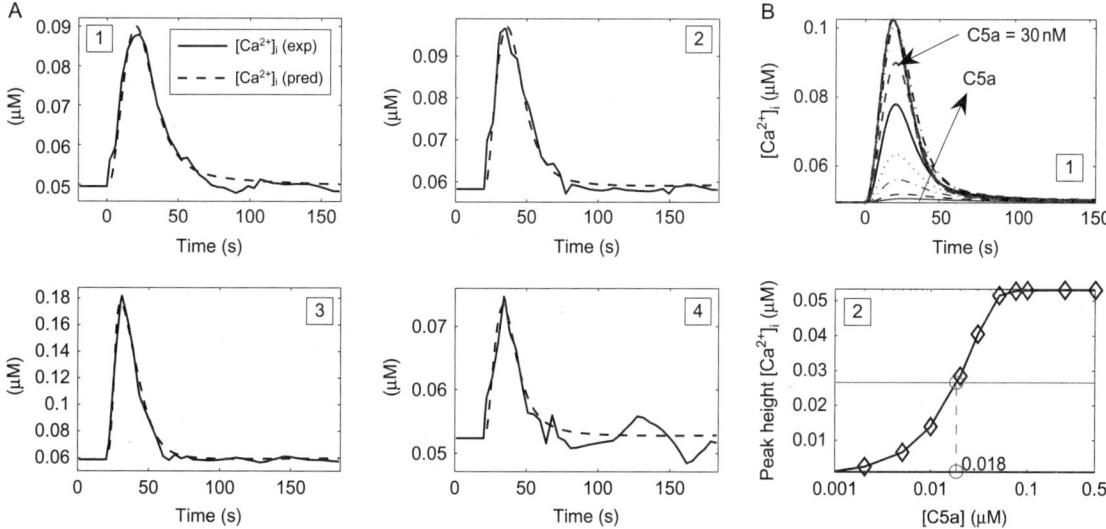

FIGURE 8.6 Results on Calcium Modeling: Expected (exp) Versus Predicted (pred).
(A) Fit to four datasets. Panel [1]: control for knockdown of RGS with 30 nM C5a. Panel [2]: control for knockdown of $G_{\alpha i}$ with 100 nM C5a. Panel [3]: 85% knockdown of $G_{\alpha i}$ with 100 nM C5a. Panel [4]: 83% knockdown of PLCβ with 100 nM C5a. (B) Panel [1]: time-course of $[Ca^{2+}]_i$ for increasing doses of C5a. Panel [2]: Predicted dose–response curve for C5a. EC_{50} is ~18 nM and the effective Hill coefficient is about 2.
Reproduced from Maurya and Subramaniam (2007c) (Fig. 5), with permission.

half of total surface receptors because of the 1:1 binding ratio of C5a and C5aR. Thus total surface receptor concentration can be computed using the EC_{50} value obtained from carefully controlled experiments, serving as a soft-sensor.

Sensitivity Analysis

Multiparametric variability analysis and single-parametric sensitivity analysis have been carried out. On the basis of multiparametric variability analysis, the four most constrained parameters are: IC:[$G_{\beta\gamma}$], IC:[$G_{\alpha i}D$], $k_{f,18}$ (the rate constant for reaction 18) and GRK_{tot}, in that order, where IC stands for initial condition. This makes sense, because any imbalance in $G_{\beta\gamma,tot}$ or $G_{\alpha i,tot}$ leads to large changes, as observed in dataset 3. $k_{f,18}$ directly affects the production of IP3, and hence it is a crucial parameter. Similarly, GRK_{tot} is important because GRK competes against $G_{\alpha i}D$ for binding to $G_{\beta\gamma}$. According to sensitivity analysis, the most sensitive parameters are IC:[$G_{\beta\gamma}$], IC:[$G_{\alpha i}D$], $k_{ER,leak}$ and K_P (the dissociation constant for the SERCA pump). Both $k_{ER,leak}$ and K_P exert strong control on the basal value because, during the basal state, the leakage flux from endoplasmic reticulum to cytosol is balanced mainly by the SERCA pump flux back to the endoplasmic reticulum. The response is also sensitive to the parameters related to the production of IP3 or the binding of IP3 to the IP3R channel. This is in agreement with the legacy knowledge about the crucial role of the endoplasmic reticulum and IP3 dynamics in regulating the cytosolic calcium (De Young and Keizer, 1992; Zhang et al., 2006). Mishra and Bhalla (2002) reported similar findings on the central role of IP3 dynamics.

Knockdown Response

Knockdown responses have the same role in quantitative modeling of a biochemical system as knockout in network structure (qualitative) modeling (Janes et al., 2005). The knockdown response can serve to characterize the efficacy of drugs that act through RNA interference (Clayton, 2004). The knockdown responses of most of the key players in the network shown in Figure 8.5 have been determined and have been qualitatively validated against Alliance for Cellular Signaling data. They have revealed the multiplicity of features in the calcium response. These include, with increasing knockdown: sharp initial decrease, increased basal level, increased rise time and increased response. The predicted knockdown response for PLCβ-3 (Fig. 8.7A), GRK2 (Fig. 8.7B), receptor, Arrestin, $G_{\beta\gamma}$ and RGS10 (not shown) is accurate. For example, upon knockdown of PLCβ-3 (Fig. 8.7A), the rate of generation of IP3 through hydrolysis of PIP2 is reduced, which results in a lower channel flux (J_{ch}) and hence a lower peak concentration. Similarly, knockdown of GRK2 leads to greater amounts of free $G_{\beta\gamma}$ for a longer time, resulting in greater quantities of IP3 and hence a larger peak concentration and a slower return to the basal state (Fig. 8.7B). The alterations resulting from these knockdowns have been observed in certain disease states, for example with respect to C5a in the systemic inflammatory response syndrome (SIRS) during infection with septicemia (Wikipedia, 2006) and decreased $G_{\alpha i}$ concentrations in Alzheimer's disease (Young et al., 1999). This suggests that a detailed understanding of these perturbations may suggest novel drug targets or lead to putative targets for treatment based on RNA interference (Clayton, 2004). More details are presented by Maurya and Subramaniam (2007a, 2007b).

Analysis of the Receptor Recovery System

A detailed study of receptor internalization and recycling has been carried out in the context of long-term responses. Many interesting findings have emerged, including the observation that, if a second dose is applied soon after the first dose, as a result of fast desensitization of the receptors, a lower second peak is obtained, whereas if the second dose is applied a sufficiently long time after the first dose, much of the response is recovered, because of the internalization and the subsequent recycling of the receptor. During long-term responses, only one peak is obtained for C5a doses below a certain threshold, but two peaks (or one peak and one plateau) are obtained for doses above the threshold (Fig. 8.8). After a dose that is somewhat higher than the threshold, it is not the height but the duration of the second peak that increases. This is because, once some receptor is recycled, any newly recycled receptor binds to the unused ligand immediately, until all the ligand is internalized. A third peak is never obtained. Sensitivity analysis of long-term responses also showed that the parameters related to receptor desensitization, internalization and recycling are important; this was not apparent from short-term responses. An interesting application for the characterization of the receptor recycle system would be the formulation of optimal doses of agonists and antagonists to avoid excessive desensitization of the receptor (Lanzara, 2005). Another potential application is in understanding drug addiction and tolerance, or loss of sensitivity (Nestler, 2005).

FUTURE DIRECTIONS AND CONCLUDING REMARKS

Computational systems biology has seen tremendous advances during this decade. In the past few years, research in computational systems biology has moved beyond interaction networks based simply on clustering and correlation. With respect to network identification, the emphasis is now on deriving networks that capture the

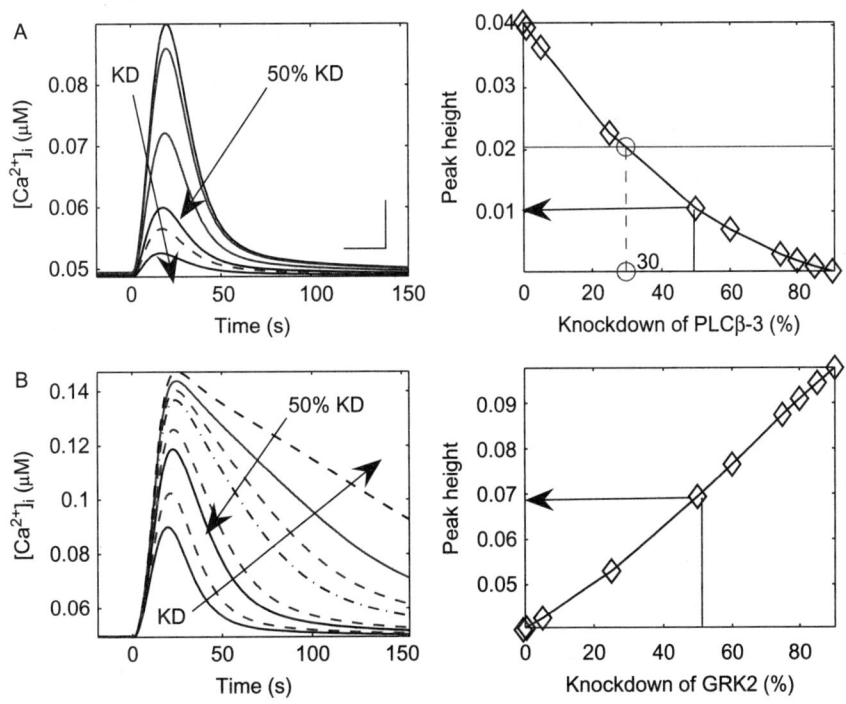

FIGURE 8.7 Predicted Knockdown Responses.
(A) Varying knockdown responses for knockdown of PLCβ-3. (B) Varying knockdown responses for knockdown of GRK2. Reproduced from Maurya and Subramaniam (2007c) (Fig. 6), with permission.

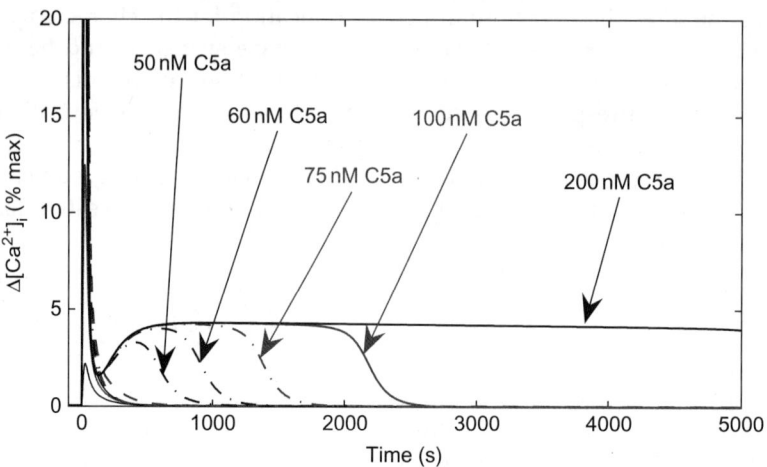

FIGURE 8.8 Long-term Dose Responses.
An increasing dose of C5a is initiated at time 0s and the system is simulated for 5000 seconds. The temporal response of $[Ca^{2+}]_i$ is expressed as deviation from the basal value as a percentage of the maximum peak height for the first peak across all doses. The temporal responses resulting in a second peak or plateau are labeled with the doses of C5a that produced them. The y-axis has been clipped at 20% to give a better view of the second peak. No second peak is observed for 40 nM C5a, but a clear second peak is obtained for 50 nM C5a. As the concentration of C5a is further increased, the height of the second peak remains unchanged, but it becomes a plateau.
Reproduced from Maurya and Subramaniam (2007a) (Fig. .5A), with permission.

causality and dynamics of interesting cellular processes such as regulation of gene transcription, cross-talk among signaling pathways, long-term feedback regulation and signaling among the cells of the immune system, and signaling and gene regulation relevant to stem-cell research. The number of journal articles published in 2007 that focused on identifying dynamic networks of biochemical systems using either state-space formalism or Bayesian network approaches was increased several-fold compared with previous years. Two challenges have become clear in the development of causal networks: (i) the requirement of huge amounts of data, and (ii) the superexponential complexity of network identification. Hence, more and more of the newer algorithms are focusing on finding ways to incorporate as much known information (legacy knowledge) in network modeling as possible.

Approaches are being developed to integrate different types of heterogeneous data on the chosen system. Bioinformatics and collaborative research have much to contribute in this endeavor. To deal with the prohibitive time complexity, stochastic search approaches, such as genetic algorithms and Markov-chain Monte Carlo searches are becoming more common for training the dynamic networks. There is a growing realization that, given the enormous complexity of biochemical interactions and paucity of data (compared with the amount required to uniquely identify the networks and parameters), unique networks would seldom be obtained in data-driven network identification. When manageable, this degeneracy is not bad, because it provides new and alternate hypotheses that can be further tested by knockout and pathway inhibition (intervention) studies, thus leading to the refinement of the network model. To date, most approaches to incorporate prior knowledge into network modeling have been based on the Bayesian network or its variants. Can prior knowledge be systematically included in deterministic approaches (e.g.

state-space formulation) also? In all likelihood, the answer is yes. Such a framework must be able to operate on the network topology and the parameters simultaneously. It will require the ability to manipulate the topology, the complex expressions for the postulated cause–effect relationships and the corresponding model parameters simultaneously. It is imperative that such an approach will require mixed binary / integer non-linear optimization. Given the complexity of non-linear optimization, approaches that are based on stochastic searches are expected to be more practical for such an application. Such a framework will be able to accommodate hybrid models—composed of continuous variables (differential algebraic equations) and discrete variables and constraints over them—which have been envisaged as the ultimate solution to modeling the complexity of hierarchical, multi-scale and multi-tiered processes that operate at the level of the entire cell.

After developing a model with a million differential equations, it is important to ask what the model yields. Does it account for spatial variations, and can it predict how an individual will respond to a drug? With the growing body of knowledge, as larger and larger models are being developed, interpretation and making sense of simulation results is becoming a challenge. Hence, some researchers have focused on developing approaches for coarse-graining the biochemical networks without compromising the predictive ability and the important mechanistic knowledge captured by the detailed model. Time-scale decomposition and state-space reduction hold promise in this research. Coarse-graining is also desired so that non-degenerate computational models can be developed using the limited data available. To achieve the delicate balance needed between controlling the complexity and retaining all the context-specific important mechanisms will be a challenge. In the context of coarse-graining, parameter estimation is a challenge. The availability of limited data is a further major challenge, and can be tackled to some extent by the systematic incorporation of qualitative constraints into modeling and parameter estimation. Concepts from artificial intelligence, such as the representation and processing of hybrid knowledge, can aid this process. Advanced research in coarse-graining will also pave the way for progress in the development of multi-scale multi-domain modeling that can connect fundamental research in network biology to clinical research.

ACKNOWLEDGEMENTS

We would like to acknowledge funding from the National Institutes of Health, the National Science Foundation and the Hilblom Foundation. Part of the case study presented was previously presented in the chapter 6 "Systems Biology of Macrophages" in the book "Current Topics in Innate Immunity" (Series: Advances in Experimental Medicine and Biology, Volume 598).

References

Akutsu, T., Miyano, S., Kuhara, S., 2000. Algorithms for identifying Boolean networks and related biological networks based on matrix multiplication and fingerprint function. J. Comput. Biol. 7, 331–343.

Al-kazemi, B. and Mohan, C.K., 2005. Discrete Multi-Phase Particle Swarm Optimization. In: M. Granã, R. Duro, A. d'Anjou and P. P. Wang (Eds.) Information Processing with Evolutionary Algorithms. London, Springer-Verlag, 305–327.

Allen, N.A., Chen, K.C., Shaffer, C.A., Tyson, J.J., Watson, L.T., 2006. Computer evaluation of network dynamics models with application to cell cycle control in budding yeast. IEE Proc. Syst. Biol. 153, 13–21.

Alliance for Cellular Signaling. (a). Alliance for Cellular Signaling (AfCS) Protocols. Available from http://www.signaling-gateway.org/data/ProtocolLinks.html. [Accessed 2006 Aug 16].

Alliance for Cellular Signaling. (b). The AfCS FXM signaling map. Available from http://www.signaling-gateway.org/data/fxm/query?type = map. [Accessed 2006 Aug 16].

Alm, E., Arkin, A.P., 2003. Biological networks. Curr. Opin. Struct. Biol. 13, 193–202.

Alon, U., 2007a. Network motifs: theory and experimental approaches. Nat. Rev. Genet. 8, 450–461.

Alon, U., 2007b. Simplicity in biology. Nature 446, 497.

Altman, R.B., Rubin, D.L., Klein, T.E., 2004. An "omics" view of drug development. Drug Dev. Res. 62, 81–85.

Amoutzias, G.D., Pichler, E.E., Mian, N., et al., 2007. A protein interaction atlas for the nuclear hormone receptors: properties and quality of a hub-based dimerisation network. BMC Syst. Biol. 1, 34.

Androulakis, I.P., 2000. Kinetic mechanism reduction based on an integer programming approach. AIChE J. 46, 361–371.

Antoniewicz, M.R., Kraynie, D.F., Laffend, L.A., Gonzalez-Lergier, J., Kelleher, J.K., Stephanopoulos, G., 2007. Metabolic flux analysis in a nonstationary system: fed-batch fermentation of a high yielding strain of E. coli producing 1,3-propanediol. Metab. Eng. 9, 277–992.

Arkin, A., Ross, J., 1995. Statistical construction of chemical-reaction mechanisms from measured time-series. J. Phys. Chem. 99, 970–979.

Ashburner, M., Ball, C.A., Blake, J.A., et al., 2000. Gene ontology: tool for the unification of biology. Nat. Genet. 25, 25–29.

Asthagiri, A.R., Lauffenburger, D.A., 2000. Bioengineering models of cell signaling. Ann. Rev. Biomed. Eng. 2, 31–53.

Babnigg, G., Heller, B., Villereal, M.L., 2000. Cell-to-cell variation in store-operated calcium entry in HEK-293 cells and its impact on the interpretation of data from stable clones expressing exogenous calcium channels. Cell Calcium. 27, 61–73.

Back, T., 1996. Evolutionary Algorithms in Theory and Practice: Evolution Strategies, Evolutionary Programming, Genetic Algorithms. Oxford University Press, Oxford.

Balazsi, G., Barabasi, A.L., Oltvai, Z.N., 2005. Topological units of environmental signal processing in the transcriptional regulatory network of Escherichia coli. Proc. Natl. Acad. Sci. USA 102, 7841–7846.

Bansal, M., Belcastro, V., Ambesi-Impiombato, A., di Bernardo, D., 2007. How to infer gene networks from expression profiles. Mol. Syst. Biol. 3, 78.

Barabasi, A.L., Oltvai, Z.N., 2004. Network biology: understanding the cell's functional organization. Nat. Rev. Genet. 5, 101–113.

Becker, S.A., Feist, A.M., Mo, M.L., Hannum, G., Palsson, B.O., Herrgard, M.J., 2007. Quantitative prediction of cellular metabolism with constraint-based models: the COBRA Toolbox. Nat. Protoc. 2, 727–738.

Berridge, M.J., 1992. Inositol trisphosphate and calcium oscillations. Adv. Second Messenger Phosphoprotein Res. 26, 211–223.

Berridge, M.J., Bootman, M.D., Roderick, H.L., 2003. Calcium signalling: dynamics, homeostasis and remodelling. Nat. Rev. Mol. Cell Biol. 4, 517–529.

Bertsekas, D.P., 2004. Nonlinear Programming. Athena Scientific, Nashua, NH.

Bertsekas, D.P., Nedic, A., Ozdaglar, A.E., 2003. Convex Analysis and Optimization. Athena Scientific, Nashua, NH.

Bhalla, U.S., 2004a. Signaling in small subcellular volumes. I. Stochastic and diffusion effects on individual pathways. Biophys. J. 87, 733–744.

Bhalla, U.S., 2004b. Signaling in small subcellular volumes. II. Stochastic and diffusion effects on synaptic network properties. Biophys. J. 87, 745–753.

Bhalla, U.S., Iyengar, R., 1999. Emergent properties of networks of biological signaling pathways. Science 283, 381–387.

Bhalla, U.S., Ram, P.T., Iyengar, R., 2002. MAP kinase phosphatase as a locus of flexibility in a mitogen-activated protein kinase signaling network. Science 297, 1018–1023.

Bhattacharjee, B., Schwer, D.A., Barton, P.I., Green, W.H., 2003. Optimally-reduced kinetic models: reaction elimination in large-scale kinetic mechanisms. Combustion Flame 135, 191–208.

Biddlecome, G.H., Berstein, G., Ross, E.M., 1996. Regulation of phospholipase C-beta 1 by Gq and m1 muscarinic cholinergic receptor. Steady-state balance of receptor-mediated activation and GTPase-activating protein-promoted deactivation. J. Biol. Chem. 271, 7999–8007.

Blinov, M.L., Yang, J., Faeder, J.R., Hlavacek, W.S., et al., 2006. Graph theory for rule-based modeling of biochemical networks. In: Priami, C., Ingolfsdottir, A., Mishra, B. (Eds.) Lecture Notes in Computer Science, Vol. 4230. Springer, Berlin/Heidelberg, pp. 89–106.

Bolouri, H., Davidson, E.H., 2002. Modeling transcriptional regulatory networks. Bioessays 24, 1118–1129.

Bonneau, R., Reiss, D.J., Shannon, P., et al., 2006. The Inferelator: an algorithm for learning parsimonious regulatory networks from systems-biology data sets de novo. Genome Biol. 7, R36.

Bornheimer, S.J., Maurya, M.R., Farquhar, M.G., Subramaniam, S., 2004. Computational modeling reveals how interplay between components of a GTPase-cycle module regulates signal transduction. Proc. Natl. Acad. Sci. USA 101, 15899–15904.

Bosl, W.J., 2007. Systems biology by the rules: hybrid intelligent systems for pathway modeling and discovery. BMC Syst. Biol. 1, 13.

Bot, R.I., Vargyas, E., Wanka, G., 2007. Conjugate duality for multiobjective composed optimization problems. Acta Math. Hungar. 116, 177–196.

Bouvier, M., Friedlander, G., 2006. To apprehend the complexity of living at the era of the "omics" [in French]. Med. Sci. (Paris) 22, 3–4.

Brinkerhoff, C.J., Woolf, P.J., Linderman, J.J., 2004. Monte Carlo simulations of receptor dynamics: insights into cell signaling. J. Mol. Histol. 35, 667–677.

Bugrim, A., Fontanilla, R., Eutenier, B.B., Keizer, J., Nuccitelli, R., 2003. Sperm initiate a Ca2+ wave in frog eggs that is more similar to Ca2+ waves initiated by IP3 than by Ca2 + . Biophys. J. 84, 1580–1590.

Calzone, L., Thieffry, D., Tyson, J.J., Novak, B., 2007. Dynamical modeling of syncytial mitotic cycles in Drosophila embryos. Mol. Syst. Biol. 3, 131.

Camacho, D., Vera-Licona, P., Mendes, P., Laubenbacher, R., 2007. Comparison of reverse engineering methods using an in silico network. Ann. NY Acad. Sci. 1115, 73–89.

Cao, Y., Gillespie, D., Petzold, L., 2005. Multiscale stochastic simulation algorithm with stochastic partial equilibrium assumption for chemically reacting systems. J. Comput. Phys. 206, 395–411.

Carafoli, E., 2002. Calcium signaling: a tale for all seasons. Proc. Natl. Acad. Sci. USA 99, 1115–1122.

Casciano, D.A., 2003. There is no place like ome: omics at the NCTR. Genomics–proteomics–metabonomics–bioinformatics. Neurotoxicology 24, 289.

Chang, Y.J., Sahinidis, N.V., 2005. Optimization of metabolic pathways under stability considerations. Comput. Chem. Eng. 29, 467–479.

Chatterjee, A., Vlachos, D.G., 2006. Multiscale spatial Monte Carlo simulations: multigriding, computational singular perturbation, and hierarchical stochastic closures. J. Chem. Phys. 124, 64110.

Chatterjee, A., Vlachos, D.G., Katsoulaki, M.A., 2005. Binomial distribution based tau-leap accelerated stochastic simulation. J. Chem. Phys. 122, 024112.

Chinchuluun, A., Pardalos, P.M., 2007. A survey of recent developments in multiobjective optimization. Ann. Oper. Res. 154, 29–50.

Ching, W.K., Zhang, S., Ng, M.K., Akutsu, T., 2007. An approximation method for solving the steady-state probability distribution of probabilistic Boolean networks. Bioinformatics 23, 1511–1518.

Cho, K.H., Choo, S.M., Jung, S.H., Kim, J.R., Choi, H.S., Kim, J., 2007. Reverse engineering of gene regulatory networks. IET Syst. Biol. 1, 149–163.

Clayton, J., 2004. RNA interference: the silent treatment. Nature 431, 599–605.

Conzelmann, H., Saez-Rodriguez, J., Sauter, T., Bullinger, E., Allgower, F., Gilles, E.D., 2004. Reduction of mathematical models of signal transduction networks: simulation-based approach applied to EGF receptor signaling. Syst. Biol. 1, 159–169.

Conzelmann, H., Saez-Rodriguez, J., Sauter, T., Kholodenko, B.N., Gilles, E.D., 2006. A domain-oriented approach to the reduction of combinatorial complexity in signal transduction networks. BMC Bioinformatics 7, 34.

Cormen, T.H., Leiserson, C.E., Rivest, R.L., Stein, C., 2001. Introduction to Algorithms. MIT Press, Cambridge, MA.

Covert, M.W., Knight, E.M., Reed, J.L., Herrgard, M.J., Palsson, B.O., 2004. Integrating high-throughput and computational data elucidates bacterial networks. Nature 429, 92–96.

Crampin, E.J., Smith, N.P., Hunter, P.J., 2004. Multi-scale modelling and the IUPS physiome project. J. Mol. Histol. 35, 707–714.

Cuellar, A.A., Lloyd, C.M., Nielsen, P.F., Bullivant, D.P., Nickerson, D.P., Hunter, P.J., 2003. An overview of CellML 1.1, a biological model description language. Simulation 79, 740–747.

Dash, S., Maurya, M.R., Rengaswamy, R., Venkatasubramanian, V., 2004. A novel interval-halving framework for automated identification of process trends. AIChE J. 50, 149–162.

de la Fuente, A., Bing, N., Hoeschele, I., Mendes, P., 2004. Discovery of meaningful associations in genomic data using partial correlation coefficients. Bioinformatics 20, 3565–3574.

De Young, G.W., Keizer, J., 1992. A single-pool inositol 1,4,5-trisphosphate-receptor-based model for agonist-stimulated oscillations in Ca2+ concentration. Proc. Natl. Acad. Sci. USA. 89, 9895–9899.

Dellis, O., Dedos, S.G., Tovey, S.C., Taufiq Ur, R., Dubel, S.J., Taylor, C.W., 2006. Ca2+ entry through plasma membrane IP3 receptors. Science 313, 229–233.

Dimond, P.F., 2003. Omics technologies forward life sciences—making progress on the long road between genes and drugs. Genet. Eng. News 23, 1.

Dua III, P., Doyle, F.J., Pistikopoulos, E.N., 2006. Model-based blood glucose control for type 1 diabetes via parametric programming. IEEE Trans. Biomed. Eng. 53, 1478–1491.

Ederer, M., Gilles, E.D., 2007. Thermodynamically feasible kinetic models of reaction networks. Biophys. J. 92, 1846–1857.

Edwards, K., Edgar, T.F., Manousiouthakis, .I., 1998. Kinetic model reduction using genetic algorithms. Comput. Chem. Eng. 22, 239–246.

Esposito, W.R., Floudas, C.A., 2000. Global optimization for the parameter estimation of differential-algebraic systems. Ind. Eng. Chem. Res. 39, 1291–1310.

Fagan, A., Culhane, A.C., Higgins, D.G., 2007. A multivariate analysis approach to the integration of proteomic and gene expression data. Proteomics 7, 2162–2171.

Fahy, E., Cotter, D., Byrnes, R., et al., 2007. Bioinformatics for lipidomics. Methods Enzymol. 432, 247–273.

Fahy, E., Subramaniam, S., Brown, H.A., et al., 2005. A comprehensive classification system for lipids. J. Lipid Res. 46, 839–862.

Fallon, E.M., Lauffenburger, D.A., 2000. Computational model for effects of ligand/receptor binding properties on interleukin-2 trafficking dynamics and T cell proliferation response. Biotechnol. Prog. 16, 905–916.

Famili, I., Mahadevan, R., Palsson, B.O., 2005. k-Cone analysis: determining all candidate values for kinetic parameters on a network scale. Biophys. J. 88, 1616–1625.

Fang, S.F., Gertner, G.Z., Shinkareva, S., Wang, G.X., Anderson, A., 2003. Improved generalized Fourier amplitude sensitivity test (FAST) for model assessment. Stat. Comput. 13, 221–226.

Ferrazzi, F., Magni, P., Sacchi, L., Bellazzi, R., 2006. Inferring gene expression networks via static and dynamic data integration. Stud. Health Technol. Inform. 124, 119–124.

Fink, C.C., Slepchenko, B., Moraru, I.I., Watras, J., Schaff, J.C., Loew, L.M., 2000. An image-based model of calcium waves in differentiated neuroblastoma cells. Biophys. J. 79, 163–183.

Floudas, C.A., Akrotirianakis, I.G., Caratzoulas, S., Meyer, C.A., Kallrath, J., 2005. Global optimization in the 21st century: A advances and challenges. Comput. Chem. Eng. 29, 1185–1202.

Galbraith, S.J., Tran, L.M., Liao, J.C., 2006. Transcriptome network component analysis with limited microarray data. Bioinformatics 22, 1886–1894.

Geier, F., Timmer, J., Fleck, C., 2007. Reconstructing gene-regulatory networks from time series, knock-out data, and prior knowledge. BMC Syst. Biol. 1, 11.

Geva-Zatorsky, N., Rosenfeld, N., Itzkovitz, S., et al., 2006. Oscillations and variability in the p53 system. Mol. Syst. Biol. 2, 0033.

Gill, D.L., Chueh, S.H., 1985. An intracellular (ATP + $Mg2+$)-dependent calcium pump within the N1E-115 neuronal cell line. J. Biol. Chem. 260, 9289–9297.

Gillespie, D.T., 1976. General method for numerically simulating stochastic time evolution of coupled chemical-reactions. J. Comput. Phys. 22, 403–434.

Gillespie, D.T., 2001. Approximate accelerated stochastic simulation of chemically reacting systems. J. Chem. Phys. 115, 1716–1733.

Gilman, A.G., Simon, M.I., Bourne, H.R., et al., 2002. Overview of the alliance for cellular signaling. Nature 420, 703–706.

Goh, K.I., Cusick, M.E., Valle, D., Childs, B., Vidal, M., Barabasi, A.L., 2007. The human disease network. Proc. Natl. Acad. Sci. USA 104, 8685–8690.

Goldberg, D.E., 1989. Genetic Algorithms in Search, Optimization and Machine Learning. Addison-Wesley, Reading, MA.

Green, M., Limebeer, D.J.N., 1995. Linear Robust Control. Prentice Hall, Englewood Cliffs, NJ.

Gueorguieva, I., Nestorov, I.A., Rowland, M., 2006. Reducing whole body physiologically based pharmacokinetic models using global sensitivity analysis: diazepam case study. J. Pharmacokin. Pharmacodyn. 33, 1–27.

Haberichter, T., Marhl, M., Heinrich, R., 2001. Birhythmicity, trirhythmicity and chaos in bursting calcium oscillations. Biophys. Chem. 90, 17–30.

Handl, J., Kell, D.B., Knowles, J., 2007. Multiobjective optimization in bioinformatics and computational biology. IEEE/ACM Trans. Comput. Biol. Bioinform. 4, 279–292.

Hartemink, A.J., Gifford, D.K., Jaakkola, T.S., Young, R.A., 2002. Bayesian methods for elucidating genetic regulatory networks. IEEE Intell. Syst. 17, 37–43.

Hartwell, L.H., Hopfield, J.J., Leibler, S., Murray, A.W., 1999. From molecular to modular cell biology. Nature 402, C47–C52.

Hendriks, B.S., Cook, J., Burke, J.M., Beusmans, J.M., Lauffenburger, D.A., de Graaf, D., 2006. Computational modelling of ErbB family phosphorylation dynamics in response to transforming growth factor alpha and heregulin indicates spatial compartmentation of phosphatase activity. IEE Proc. Syst. Biol. 153, 22–33.

Hinch, R., Greenstein, J.L., Tanskanen, A.J., Xu, L., Winslow, R.L., 2004. A simplified local control model of calcium-induced calcium release in cardiac ventricular myocytes. Biophys. J. 87, 3723–3736.

Hlavacek, W.S., Faeder, J.R., Blinov, M.L., Posner, R.G., Hucka, M., Fontana, W., 2006. Rules for modeling signal-transduction systems. Sci. STKE re6.

Hofer, T., Venance, L., Giaume, C., 2002. Control and plasticity of intercellular calcium waves in astrocytes: a modeling approach. J. Neurosci. 22, 4850–4859.

Hofestadt, R., Thelen, S., 1998. Quantitative modeling of biochemical networks. In. Silico. Biol. 1, 39–53.

Hoffman, J.F., Linderman, J.J., Omann, G.M., 1996. Receptor up-regulation, internalization, and interconverting receptor states. Critical components of a quantitative description of N-formyl peptide-receptor dynamics in the neutrophil. J. Biol. Chem. 271, 18394–18404.

Hoffmann, A., Levchenko, A., Scott, M.L., Baltimore, D., 2002. The I kappa B-NF-kappa B signaling module: temporal control and selective gene activation. Science 298, 1241–1245.

Hong, C.I., Conrad, E.D., Tyson, J.J., 2007. A proposal for robust temperature compensation of circadian rhythms. Proc. Natl. Acad. Sci. USA 104, 1195–1200.

Hu, X. H., Eberhart, R. C., Shi, Y. H., 2003. Engineering optimization with particle swarm. In "Proceedings of the IEEE Swarm Intelligence Symposium, April 24–26, Indianapolis, USA," 53–57. IEEE, Piscataway, NJ.

Hua, F., Hautaniemi, S., Yokoo, R., Lauffenburger, D.A., 2006. Integrated mechanistic and data-driven modelling for multivariate analysis of signalling pathways. J. R. Soc. Interface 3, 515–526.

Hucka, M., Finney, A., Sauro, H.M., et al., 2003. The systems biology markup language (SBML): a medium for representation and exchange of biochemical network models. IEEE, Piscataway, NJ. Bioinformatics 19, 524–531.

Hwang, D., Rust, A.G., Ramsey, S., et al., 2005a. A data integration methodology for systems biology. Proc. Natl. Acad. Sci. USA 102, 17296–17301.

Hwang, D., Smith, J.J., Leslie, D.M., et al., 2005b. A data integration methodology for systems biology: experimental verification. Proc. Natl. Acad. Sci. USA 102, 17302–17307.

Ideker, T., Thorsson, V., Ranish, J.A., et al., 2001. Integrated genomic and proteomic analyses of a systematically perturbed metabolic network. Science 292, 929–934.

Itzkovitz, S., Levitt, R., Kashtan, N., Milo, R., Itzkovitz, M., Alon, U., 2005. Coarse-graining and self-dissimilarity of complex networks. Phys. Rev. E Stat. Nonlin. Soft Matter Phys. 71, 016127.

Iwasaki, Y., Simon, H.A., 1986. Causality in device behavior. Artif. Intell. 29, 3–32.

Jafri, M.S., Rice, J.J., Winslow, R.L., 1998. Cardiac Ca2+ dynamics: the roles of ryanodine receptor adaptation and sarcoplasmic reticulum load. Biophys. J. 74, 1149–1168.

Jamshidi, N., Edwards, J.S., Fahland, T., Church, G.M., Palsson, B.O., 2001. Dynamic simulation of the human red blood cell metabolic network. Bioinformatics 17, 286–287.

Janes, K.A., Kelly, J.R., Gaudet, S., Albeck, J.G., Sorger, P.K., Lauffenburger, D.A., 2004. Cue–signal–response analysis of TNF-induced apoptosis by partial least squares regression of dynamic multivariate data. J. Comput. Biol. 11, 544–561.

Janes, K.A., Albeck, J.G., Gaudet, S., Sorger, P.K., Lauffenburger, D.A., Yaffe, M.B., 2005. A systems model of signaling identifies a molecular basis set for cytokine-induced apoptosis. Science 310, 1646–1653.

Jansen, R., Yu, H.Y., Greenbaum, D., et al., 2003. A Bayesian networks approach for predicting protein–protein interactions from genomic data. Science 302, 449–453.

Ji, X., Xu, Y., 2006. libSRES: a C library for stochastic ranking evolution strategy for parameter estimation. Bioinformatics 22, 124–126.

Johnson, C.D., Balagurunathan, Y., Tadesse, M., et al., 2003. From "omics" to insight: the use of a novel computational approach to study genegene interactions. Toxicol. Sci. 72, 93.

Jor, J.W., Nash, M.P., Nielsen, P.M., Hunter, P.J., 2007. Modelling the mechanical properties of human skin: towards a 3D discrete fibre model. Conf. Proc. IEEE Eng. Med. Biol. Soc. 1, 6641–6644.

Jordan, M.I. (Ed.),, 1999. Learning in Graphical Models. MIT Press, Cambridge, MA.

Joslin, E.J., Opresko, L.K., Wells, A., Wiley, H.S., Lauffenburger, D.A., 2007. EGF-receptor-mediated mammary epithelial cell migration is driven by sustained ERK signaling from autocrine stimulation. J. Cell Sci. 120, 3688–3699.

Joyce, A.R., Palsson, B.O., 2006. The model organism as a system: integrating "omics" data sets. Nat. Rev. Mol. Cell Biol. 7, 198–210.

Karnaukhov, A.V., Karnaukhova, E.V., Williamson, J.R., 2007. Numerical Matrices Method for nonlinear system identification and description of dynamics of biochemical reaction networks. Biophys. J. 92, 3459–3473.

Kashtan, N., Alon, U., 2005. Spontaneous evolution of modularity and network motifs. Proc. Natl. Acad. Sci. USA 102, 13773–13778.

Katare, S., Bhan, A., Caruthers, J.M., Delgass, W.N., Venkatasubramanian, V., 2004a. A hybrid genetic algorithm for efficient parameter estimation of large kinetic models. Comput. Chem. Eng. 28, 2569–2581.

Katare, S., Caruthers, J.M., Delgass, W.N., Venkatasubramanian, V., 2004b. An intelligent system for reaction kinetic modeling and catalyst design. Ind. Eng. Chem. Res. 43, 3484–3512.

Kauffman, S.A., 1993. Differentiation: the dynamical behaviors of genetic regulatory networks. In "The Origins of Order," 441–522. Oxford University Press, New York.

Kauffman, S., Peterson, C., Samuelsson, B., Troein, C., 2004. Genetic networks with canalyzing Boolean rules are always stable. Proc. Natl. Acad. Sci. USA 101, 17102–17107.

Kaznessis, Y.N., 2006. Multi-scale models for gene network engineering. Chem. Eng. Sci. 61, 940–953.

Kennedy, J., Eberhart, R.C., 1995. Particle swarm optimization. In "Proceedings of the IEEE International Conference on Neural Networks" 1942–1948. IEEE, Piscataway, NJ, Vol. 4.

Kepler, T.B., Elston, T.C., 2001. Stochasticity in transcriptional regulation: origins, consequences, and mathematical representations. Biophys. J. 81, 3116–3136.

Kholodenko, B.N., 2000. Negative feedback and ultrasensitivity can bring about oscillations in the mitogen-activated protein kinase cascades. Eur. J. Biochem. 267, 1583–1588.

Kiechle, F.L., Zhang, X.B., Holland-Staley, C.A., 2004. The -omics era and its impact. Arch. Pathol. Lab. Med. 128, 1337–1345.

Kim, H., Lee, J.K., Park, T., 2007. Boolean networks using the chi-square test for inferring large-scale gene regulatory networks. BMC Bioinformatics 8, 37.

Koda, M., McRae, G.J., Seinfeld, J.H., 1979. Automatic sensitivity analysis of kinetic mechanisms. Int. J. Chem. Kinet. 11, 427–444.

Koffas, M., Stephanopoulos, G., 2005. Strain improvement by metabolic engineering: lysine production as a case study for systems biology. Curr. Opin. Biotechnol. 16, 361–366.

Komurov, K., White, M., 2007. Revealing static and dynamic modular architecture of the eukaryotic protein interaction network. Mol. Syst. Biol. 3, 110.

Koschorreck, M., Conzelmann, H., Ebert, S., Ederer, M., Gilles, E.D., 2007. Reduced modeling of signal transduction—a modular approach. BMC Bioinformatics 8, 336.

Kremling, A., Saez-Rodriguez, J., 2007. Systems biology—an engineering perspective. J. Biotechnol. 129, 329–351.

Kronauer III, R.E., Gunzelmann, G., Van Dongen, H.P., Doyle, F.J., Klerman, E.B., 2007. Uncovering physiologic mechanisms of circadian rhythms and sleep/wake regulation through mathematical modeling. J. Biol. Rhythms. 22, 233–245.

LaCount, D.J., Vignali, M., Chettier, R., et al., 2005. A protein interaction network of the malaria parasite Plasmodium falciparum. Nature 438, 103–107.

Lahdesmaki, H., Hautaniemi, S., Shmulevich, I., Yli-Harja, O., 2006. Relationships between probabilistic Boolean networks and dynamic Bayesian networks as models of gene regulatory networks. Signal Proc. 86, 814–834.

Lall, R., Voit, E.O., 2005. Parameter estimation in modulated, unbranched reaction chains within biochemical systems. Comput. Biol. Chem. 29, 309–318.

Lanzara, R., 2005. Optimal agonist/antagonist combinations maintain receptor response by preventing rapid beta-1 adrenergic receptor desensitization. Intl. J. Pharmacol. 1, 122–131.

Laubenbacher, R., Stigler, B., 2004. A computational algebra approach to the reverse engineering of gene regulatory networks. J. Theor. Biol. 229, 523–537.

Lauffenburger, D.A., 2000. Cell signaling pathways as control modules: complexity for simplicity?. Proc. Natl. Acad. Sci. USA 97, 5031–5033.

Lay, J.O., Borgmann, S., Liyanage, R., Wilkins, C.L., 2006. Problems with the "omics". Trends Anal. Chem. 25, 1046–1056.

Lemon, G., Gibson, W.G., Bennett, M.R., 2003. Metabotropic receptor activation, desensitization and sequestration—I: modelling calcium and inositol 1,4,5-trisphosphate dynamics following receptor activation. J. Theor. Biol. 223, 93–111.

Letari, O., Nicosia, S., Chiavaroli, C., Vacher, P., Schlegel, W., 1991. Activation by bacterial lipopolysaccharide causes changes in the cytosolic free calcium concentration in single peritoneal macrophages. J. Immunol. 147, 980–983.

Lezon, T.R., Banavar, J.R., Cieplak, M., Maritan, A., Fedoroff, N.V., 2006. Using the principle of entropy maximization to infer genetic interaction networks from gene expression patterns. Proc. Natl. Acad. Sci. USA 103, 19033–19038.

Li, Y.X., Rinzel, J., 1994. Equations for InsP3 receptor-mediated [Ca2+]i oscillations derived from a detailed kinetic model: a Hodgkin–Huxley like formalism. J. Theor. Biol. 166, 461–473.

Li, J., Ning, Y., Hedley, W., et al., 2002. The Molecule Pages database. Nature 420, 716–717.

Li, H., Cao, Y., Petzold, L. R., Gillespie, D. T., 2007. Algorithms and software for stochastic simulation of biochemical reacting systems. *Biotechnol. Prog.*

Liang, Y., Leung, K.S., Mok, T.S.K., 2004. Evolutionary drug scheduling model for cancer chemotherapy. In: "Lecture Notes in Computer Science. Vol. 3103, pp. 1126–1137.

Liao, J.C., Boscolo, R., Yang, Y.L., Tran, L.M., Sabatti, C., Roychowdhury, V.P., 2003. Network component analysis: reconstruction of regulatory signals in biological systems. Proc. Natl. Acad. Sci. USA 100, 15522–15527.

Lim, J., Hao, T., Shaw, C., et al., 2006. A protein–protein interaction network for human inherited ataxias and disorders of Purkinje cell degeneration. Cell 125, 801–814.

Lin, Y.C., Hwang, K.S., Wang, F.S., 2001. Co-evolutionary hybrid differential evolution for mixed-integer optimization problems. Eng. Optim. 33, 663–682.

Lin, Y.C., Hwang, K.S., Wang, F.S., 2004. A mixed-coding scheme of evolutionary algorithms to solve mixed-integer nonlinear programming problems. Comput. Math. Applic. 47, 1295–1307.

Liu, A.C., Welsh, D.K., Ko, C.H., et al., 2007. Intercellular coupling confers robustness against mutations in the SCN circadian clock network. Cell 129, 605–616.

Longabaugh, W.J., Davidson, E.H., Bolouri, H., 2005. Computational representation of developmental genetic regulatory networks. Dev. Biol. 283, 1–16.

Lytton, J., Westlin, M., Burk, S.E., Shull, G.E., MacLennan, D.H., 1992. Functional comparisons between isoforms of the sarcoplasmic or endoplasmic reticulum family of calcium pumps. J. Biol. Chem. 267, 14483–14489.

Ma, P.C., Chan, K.C., 2007. An effective data mining technique for reconstructing gene regulatory networks from time series expression data. J. Bioinform. Comput. Biol. 5, 651–668.

Ma'ayan, A., Jenkins, S.L., Goldfarb, J., Iyengar, R., 2007. Network analysis of FDA approved drugs and their targets. Mt. Sinai J. Med. 74, 27–32.

Mahadevan, R., Burgard, A.P., Famili, I., Van Dien, S., Schilling, C.H., 2005. Applications of metabolic modeling to drive bioprocess development for the production of value-added chemicals. Biotechnol. Bioprocess Eng. 10, 408–417.

Margolin, A.A., Califano, A., 2007. Theory and limitations of genetic network inference from microarray data. Ann. NY Acad. Sci. 1115, 51–72.

Marhl, M., Haberichter, T., Brumen, M., Heinrich, R., 2000. Complex calcium oscillations and the role of mitochondria and cytosolic proteins. Biosystems 57, 75–86.

Markevich, N.I., Hoek, J.B., Kholodenko, B.N., 2004. Signaling switches and bistability arising from multisite phosphorylation in protein kinase cascades. J. Cell Biol. 164, 353–359.

Markowetz, F., Spang, R., 2007. Inferring cellular networks—a review. BMC Bioinformatics 8 (suppl 6), S5.

Markowetz, F., Troyanskaya, O.G., 2007. Computational identification of cellular networks and pathways. Mol. Biosyst. 3, 478–482.

Marquardt, D.W., 1963. An algorithm for least-squares estimation of nonlinear parameters. J. Soc. Ind. Appl. Math. 11, 431–441.

Materna, S.C., Davidson, E.H., 2007. Logic of gene regulatory networks. Curr. Opin. Biotechnol. 18, 351–354.

Mathew, J.P., Taylor, B.S., Bader, G.D., et al., 2007. From bytes to bedside: data integration and computational biology for translational cancer research. PLoS Comput. Biol. 3, e12.

Mathworks, 1994. The Mathworks, Inc., Natick, MA. Copyright © (1994–2004). Available from http://www.mathworks.com/.

Maurya, M.R., Rengaswamy, R., Venkatasubramanian, V., 2003a. A systematic framework for the development and analysis of signed digraphs for chemical processes. 1. Algorithms and analysis. Ind. Eng. Chem. Res. 42, 4789–4810.

Maurya, M.R., Rengaswamy, R., Venkatasubramanian, V., 2003b. A systematic framework for the development and analysis of signed digraphs for chemical processes. 2. Control loops and flowsheet analysis. Ind. Eng. Chem. Res. 42, 4811–4827.

Maurya, M.R., Bornheimer, S.J., Venkatasubramanian, V., Subramaniam, S. 2005. Reduced-order modeling of biochemical networks: application to the GTPase-cycle signaling module. IEE Proc. Syst. Biol. 152, 229–242.

Maurya, M.R., Bornheimer, S.J., Venkatasubramanian, V., Subramaniam, S., 2009. A mixed-integer nonlinear optimisation approach to coarse-graining biochemical networks. IET Systems Biology. 3, 24–39.

Maurya, M.R., Katare, S., Patkar, P.R., Rundell, A., Venkatasubramanian, V., 2006. A systematic framework for the design of reduced-order models for signal transduction pathways from a control theoretic perspective. Comput. Chem. Eng. 3, 437–452.

Maurya, M.R., Subramaniam, S., 2007a. A kinetic model for calcium dynamics in RAW 264.7 cells: 1. Mechanisms, parameters, and subpopulational variability. Biophys. J. 93, 709–728 [on-line supporting material also available].

Maurya, M.R., Subramaniam, S., 2007b. A kinetic model for calcium dynamics in RAW 264.7 cells: 2. Knockdown response and long-term response. Biophys. J. 93, 729–740.

Maurya, M.R., Benner, C., Pradervand, S., Glass, C., Subramaniam, S., 2007c. Systems biology of macrophages. Adv. Exp. Med. Biol. 598, 62–79.

McKay, M.D., Beckman, R.J., Conover, W.J., 1979. A comparison of three methods for selecting values of input variables in the analysis of output from a computer code. Technometrics 21, 239–245.

Mehra, S., Hu, W.S., Karypis, G., 2004. A Boolean algorithm for reconstructing the structure of regulatory networks. Metab. Eng. 6, 326–339.

Meier-Schellersheim, M., Xu, X.H., Angermann, B., Kunkel, E.J., Jin, T., Germain, R.N., 2006. Key role of local regulation in chemosensing revealed by a new molecular interaction-based modeling method. PLoS Comput. Biol. 2, 710–724.

Mendes, P., Kell, D., 1998. Non-linear optimization of biochemical pathways: applications to metabolic engineering and parameter estimation. Bioinformatics 14, 869–883.

Mendes, P., Kummer, U., 2006. COPASI: COmplex PAthway SImulator. Copyright © 2006. Available from http://www.copasi.org/.

Merrill, A., 2007. Sphingolipid metabolism from an omics perspective. Chem. Phys. Lipids 149, S8–S9.

Mishra, J., Bhalla, U.S., 2002. Simulations of inositol phosphate metabolism and its interaction with InsP(3)-mediated calcium release. Biophys. J. 83, 1298–1316.

Misra, J., Alevizos, I., Hwang, D., Stephanopoulos, G., Stephanopoulos, G., 2007. Linking physiology and transcriptional profiles by quantitative predictive models. Biotechnol. Bioeng. 98, 252–260.

Moles, C.G., Mendes, P., Banga, J.R., 2003. Parameter estimation in biochemical pathways: a comparison of global optimization methods. Genome Res. 13, 2467–2474.

Moore, B.C., 1981. Principal component analysis in linear-systems: controllability, observability, and model-reduction. IEEE Trans. Automat. Contr. 26, 17–32.

Moraru, I.I., Schaff, J.C., Slepchenko, B.M., Loew, L.M., 2002. The Virtual Cell—an integrated modeling environment for experimental and computational cell biology. Ann. NY Acad. Sci. 971, 595–596.

Murray, J.D., 2002. Mathematical Biology I. An Introduction. Springer-Verlag, Berlin/Heidelberg.

Nagrath, D., Avila-Elchiver, M., Berthiaume, F., Tilles, A.W., Messac, A., Yarmush, M.L., 2007. Integrated energy and flux balance based multiobjective framework for large-scale metabolic networks. Ann. Biomed. Eng. 35, 863–885.

Nestler, E.J., 2005. Is there a common molecular pathway for addiction?. Nat. Neurosci. 8, 1445–1449.

Neves, S.R., Iyengar, R., 2002. Modeling of signaling networks. Bioessays 24, 1110–1117.

Neves, S.R., Ram, P.T., Iyengar, R., 2002. G protein pathways. Science 296, 1636–1639.

Niederer, S.A., Hunter, P.J., Smith, N.P., 2006. A quantitative analysis of cardiac myocyte relaxation: a simulation study. Biophys. J. 90, 1697–1722.

Novak, B., Tyson, J.J., Gyorffy, B., Csikasz-Nagy, A., 2007. Irreversible cell-cycle transitions are due to systems-level feedback. Nat. Cell Biol. 9, 724–728.

Okino, M.S., Mavrovouniotis, M.L., 1998. Simplification of mathematical models of chemical reaction systems. Chem. Rev. 98, 391–408.

Oltvai, Z.N., Barabasi, A.L., 2002. Systems biology. Life's complexity pyramid. Science 298, 763–764.

Orphanides, G., 2004. Understanding mechanisms through "-omics" technology. Toxicology 202, 34–35.

Oyeleye, O.O., Kramer, M.A., 1988. Qualitative simulation of chemical process systems—steady-state analysis. AIChE J. 34, 1441–1454.

Ozcan, E., Mohan, C.K., 1998. Analysis of a simple particle swarm optimization system. In: Intelligent Engineering Systems Through Artificial Neural Networks. C.H. Dagli, M. Akay, AL. Buczak, O, Ersoy, B.R. Bernandez, (eds.). American Society of Mechanical Engineers (ASME) NewYork Vol. 8, pp. 253–258.

Palsson, B.O., Lightfoot, E.N., 1985. Mathematical-modeling of dynamics and control in metabolic networks. 4. Local stability analysis of single biochemical control loops. J. Theor. Biol. 113, 261–277.

Palsson, B.O., Joshi, A., Ozturk, S.S., 1987. Reducing complexity in metabolic networks—making metabolic meshes manageable. Fed. Proc. 46, 2485–2489.

Pandey, J., Koyuturk, M., Kim, Y., Szpankowski, W., Subramaniam, S., Grama, A., 2007. Functional annotation of regulatory pathways. Bioinformatics 23, I377–I386.

Papamichail, I., Adjiman, C.S., 2005. Proof of convergence for a global optimization algorithm for problems with ordinary differential equations. J. Global Optim. 33, 83–107.

Papin, J.A., Hunter, T., Palsson, B.O., Subramaniam, S., 2005. Reconstruction of cellular signalling networks and analysis of their properties. Nat. Rev. Mol. Cell Biol. 6, 99–111.

Papin, J.A., Gianchandani, E.P., Subramaniam, S., 2007. Mapping the genotype–phenotype relationship in cellular signaling networks: building bridges over the unknown. In: Rigoutsos, I., Stephanopoulos, G. (Eds.) Systems Biology: Volume II: Networks, Models, and Applications. Oxford University Press, New York, pp. 137–168.

Park III, M.J., Dahlquist, F.W., Doyle, F.J., 2007. Simultaneous high gain and wide dynamic range in a model of bacterial chemotaxis. IET Syst. Biol. 1, 222–229.

Parker III, R.S., Doyle, F.J., 2001. Control-relevant modeling in drug delivery. Adv. Drug Deliv. Rev. 48, 211–228.

Parker III, R.S., Doyle, F.J., Peppas, N.A., 1999. A model-based algorithm for blood glucose control in type I diabetic patients. IEEE Trans. Biomed. Eng. 46, 148–157.

Pe'er, D., 2005. Bayesian network analysis of signaling networks: a primer. Sci STKE p. 14.

Petzold, L., Zhu, W.J., 1999. Model reduction for chemical kinetics: an optimization approach. AIChE J. 45, 869–886.

Pradervand, S., Maurya, M.R., Subramaniam, S., 2006. Identification of signaling components required for the prediction of cytokine release in RAW 264.7 macrophages. Genome Biol. 7, R11.

Price, N.D., Shmulevich, I., 2007. Biochemical and statistical network models for systems biology. Curr. Opin. Biotechnol. 18, 365–370.

Puchalka, J., Kierzek, A.M., 2004. Bridging the gap between stochastic and deterministic regimes in the kinetic simulations of the biochemical reaction networks. Biophys. J. 86, 1357–1372.

Rao, C.V., Arkin, A.P., 2003. Stochastic chemical kinetics and the quasi-steady-state assumption: application to the Gillespie algorithm. J. Chem. Phys. 118, 4999–5010.

Raser, J.M., O'Shea, E.K., 2005. Noise in gene expression: origins, consequences, and control. Science 309, 2010–2013.

Ravasz, E., Somera, A.L., Mongru, D.A., Oltvai, Z.N., Barbasi, A.L., 2002. Hierarchical organization of modularity in metabolic networks. Science 297, 1551–1555.

Reigl, M., Alon, U., Chklovskii, D.B., 2004. Search for computational modules in the C. elegans brain. BMC Biol. 2, 25.

Resendis-Antonio, O., Reed, J.L., Encarnacion, S., Collado-Vides, J., Palsson, B.O., 2007. Metabolic reconstruction and modeling of nitrogen fixation in Rhizobium etli. PLoS Comput. Biol. 3, 1887–1895.

Revilla-i-Domingo, R., Davidson, E.H., 2003. Developmental gene network analysis. Int. J. Dev. Biol. 47, 695–703.

Rhodes, D.R., Tomlins, S.A., Varambally, S., et al., 2005. Probabilistic model of the human protein–protein interaction network. Nat. Biotechnol. 23, 951–959.

Riccobene, T.A., Omann, G.M., Linderman, J.J., 1999. Modeling activation and desensitization of G-protein coupled receptors provides insight into ligand efficacy. J. Theor. Biol. 200, 207–222.

Rigoutsos, I., Stephanopoulos, G. (Eds.), 2007. Systems Biology: Volume II: Networks, Models, and Applications. Oxford University Press, New York.

Robinson, J., Sinton, S., Rahmat-Samii, Y., 2002. Particle swarm, genetic algorithm, and their hybrids: optimization of a profiled corrugated horn antenna. In Proceedings of the IEEE Antennas and Propagation Society International Symposium. San Antonio, TX, USA, IEEE, Piscataway, NJ. June 16–21, Volume 1, pp. 314–317.

Rodriguez-Fernandez, M., Mendes, P., Banga, J.R., 2006. A hybrid approach for efficient and robust parameter estimation in biochemical pathways. Biosystems 83, 248–265.

Rogers, S., Girolami, M., 2005. A Bayesian regression approach to the inference of regulatory networks from gene expression data. Bioinformatics 21, 3131–3137.

Rosenfeld, N., Young, J.W., Alon, U., P Swain, S., Elowitz, M.B., 2007. Accurate prediction of gene feedback circuit behavior from component properties. Mol. Syst. Biol. 3, 143.

Ross, E.M., Wilkie, T.M., 2000. GTPase-activating proteins for heterotrimeric G proteins: regulators of G protein signaling (RGS) and RGS-like proteins. Ann. Rev. Bioch. 69, 795–827.

Ross, J., Arkin, A.P., 2009. Complex systems: From chemistry to systems biology. Proc. Natl. Acad. Sci. USA, 106, 6433–4.

Rumbaugh, J., Blaha, M., Premerlani, W., Eddy, F., Lorenson, W., 1991. Object Oriented Modeling and Design. Prentice-Hall, Englewood Cliffs, NJ.

Sachs, K., Perez, O., Pe'er, D., Lauffenburger, D.A., Nolan, G.P., 2005. Causal protein-signaling networks derived from multiparameter single-cell data. Science 308, 523–529.

Saez-Rodriguez, J., Kremling, A., Gilles, E.D., 2005. Dissecting the puzzle of life: modularization of signal transduction networks. Comput. Chem. Eng. 29, 619–629.

Saez-Rodriguez, J., Simeoni, L., Lindquist, J.A., et al., 2007. A logical model provides insights into T cell receptor signaling. PLoS Comput. Biol. 3, e163.

Salis, H., Kaznessis, Y., 2005. Accurate hybrid stochastic simulation of a system of coupled chemical or biochemical reactions. J. Chem. Phys. 122, 54103.

Salis, H., Sotiropoulos, V., Kaznessis, Y.N., 2006. Multiscale Hy3S: hybrid stochastic simulation for supercomputers. BMC Bioinformatics 7, 93.

Sauro, H.M., Hucka, M., Finney, A., et al., 2003. Next generation simulation tools: the Systems Biology Workbench and BioSPICE integration. OMICS 7, 355–372.

Schmid, H., O'Callaghan, P., Nash, M.P., et al., 2008. Myocardial material parameter estimation: a nonhomogeneous finite element study from simple shear tests. Biomech. Model Mechanobiol. 7, 161–173.

Schoeberl, B., Eichler-Jonsson, C., Gilles, E.D., Muller, G., 2002. Computational modeling of the dynamics of the MAP kinase cascade activated by surface and internalized EGF receptors. Nat. Biotechnol. 20, 370–375.

Schuster, S., Marhl, M., Hofer, T., 2002. Modeling of simple and complex calcium oscillations, from single-cell responses to intercellular signaling. Eur. J. Biochem. 269, 1333–1355.

Scott, J., Ideker, T., Karp, R.M., Sharan, R., 2006. Efficient algorithms for detecting signaling pathways in protein interaction networks. J. Comput. Biol. 13, 133–144.

Scott, M., Hwa, T., Ingalls, B., 2007. Deterministic characterization of stochastic genetic circuits. Proc. Natl. Acad. Sci. USA 104, 7402–7407.

Shannon, P., Markiel, A., Ozier, O., et al., 2003. Cytoscape: a software environment for integrated models of biomolecular interaction networks. Genome Res. 13, 2498–2504.

Sharan, R., Ideker, T., 2006. Modeling cellular machinery through biological network comparison. Nat. Biotechnol. 24, 427–433.

Sible, J.C., Tyson, J.J., 2007. Mathematical modeling as a tool for investigating cell cycle control networks. Methods 41, 238–247.

Singer, A.B., Taylor, J.W., Barton, P.I., Green, W.H., 2006. Global dynamic optimization for parameter estimation in chemical kinetics. J. Phys. Chem. A 110, 971–976.

Singh, O.V., 2007. Integrating "-omics" into biological processes and modeling for bioremediation. OMICS 11, 231–232.

Sitaramayya, A., Bunnett, N.W., 1999. Cell surface receptors: mechanisms of signaling and activation. In: Sitaramayya, A. (Ed.), Introduction to Cellular Signal Transduction. Birkhauser, Boston, MA, pp. 7–28.

Smith, J., Theodoris, C., Davidson, E.H., 2007. A gene regulatory network subcircuit drives a dynamic pattern of gene expression. Science 318, 794–797.

Sontag, E., Kiyatkin, A., Kholodenko, B.N., 2004. Inferring dynamic architecture of cellular networks using time series of gene expression, protein and metabolite data. Bioinformatics 20, 1877–1886.

Stafford, D.E., Yanagimachi, K.S., Lessard, P.A., Rijhwani, S.K., Sinskey, A.J., Stephanopoulos, G., 2002. Optimizing bioconversion pathways through systems analysis and metabolic engineering. Proc. Natl. Acad. Sci. USA 99, 1801–1806.

Stelling, J., Gilles, E.D., 2004. Mathematical modeling of complex regulatory networks. IEEE Trans, Nanobioscience 3, 172–179.

Stelling III, J., Sauer, U., Szallasi, Z., Doyle, F.J., Doyle, J., 2004. Robustness of cellular functions. Cell 118, 675–685.

Stephanopoulos, G., Aristidou, A., Nielsen, J., 1998. Review of cellular metabolism. In: "Metabolic Engineering: Principles and Methodologies. ?(eds.).? Academic Press, San Diego, USA, pp. 21–79.

Stetter, M., Deco, G., Dejori, M., 2003. Large-scale computational modeling of genetic regulatory networks. Artif. Intell. Rev. 20, 75–93.

Storn, R., Price, K., 1997. Differential evolution—a simple and efficient heuristic for global optimization over continuous spaces. J. Global. Optim. 11, 341–359.

Subramanian, K.K., Narang, A., 2004. A mechanistic model for eukaryotic gradient sensing: spontaneous and induced phosphoinositide polarization. J. Theor. Biol. 231, 49–67.

Summanwar, V.S., Jayaraman, V.K., Kulkarni, B.D., Kusumakar, H.S., Gupta, K., Rajesh, J., 2002. Solution of constrained optimization problems by multi-objective genetic algorithm. Comput. Chem. Eng. 26, 1481–1492.

Sun, N., Zhao, H.Y., 2004. Genomic approaches in dissecting complex biological pathways. Pharmacogenomics 5, 163–179.

Sundaram, A., Venkatasubramanian, V., 1998. Parametric sensitivity and search-space characterization studies of genctic algorithms for computer-aided polymer design. J. Chem. Inf. Comput. Sci. 38, 1177–1191.

Tanskanen, A.J., Greenstein, J.L., Chen, A., Sun, S.X., Winslow, R.L., 2007. Protein geometry and placement in the cardiac dyad influence macroscopic properties of calcium-induced calcium release. Biophys. J. 92, 3379–3396.

Tawarmalani, M., Sahinidis, N.V., 2004. Global optimization of mixed-integer nonlinear programs: a theoretical and computational study. Math. Progr. 99, 563–591.

Thomas, R., 1973. Boolean formalization of genetic control circuits. J. Theor. Biol. 42, 563–585.

Tikhonov, A.N., 1952. Systems of differential equations containing a small parameter in the derivatives. Mat. Sb. 31, 575–586.

To III, T.L., Henson, M.A., Herzog, E.D., Doyle, F.J., 2007. A molecular model for intercellular synchronization in the mammalian circadian clock. Biophys. J. 92, 3792–3803.

Uckun, S., 1992. Model-based reasoning in biomedicine. Crit. Rev. Biomed. Eng. 19, 261–292.

Van den Bulcke, T., Lemmens, K., Van de Peer, Y., Marchal, K., 2006. Inferring transcriptional networks by mining "omics" data. Current Bioinformatics 1, 301–313.

Vayttaden, S.J., Bhalla, U.S., 2004. Developing complex signaling models using GENESIS/Kinetikit. *Sci. STKE* 14.

Venkatasubramanian, V., Katare, S., Patkar, P.R., Mu, F. P., 2004. Spontaneous emergence of complex optimal networks through evolutionary adaptation. Comput. Chem. Eng. 28, 1789–1798.

Vora, N., Daoutidis, P., 2001. Nonlinear model reduction of chemical reaction systems. AIChE J. 47, 2320–2332.

Wagner, J., Li, Y.X., Pearson, J., Keizer, J., 1998. Simulation of the fertilization Ca2+ wave in Xenopus laevis eggs. Biophys. J. 75, 2088–2097.

Wang, Y., Joshi, T., Zhang, X.S., Xu, D., Chen, L., 2006. Inferring gene regulatory networks from multiple microarray datasets. Bioinformatics 22, 2413–2420.

Wang, Y., Cai, Z., Guo, G., Zhou, Y., 2007a. Multiobjective optimization and hybrid evolutionary algorithm to solve constrained optimization problems. IEEE Trans. Systems Man Cybernetics B 37, 560–575.

Wang, R.S., Wang, Y., Zhang, X.S., Chen, L., 2007b. Inferring transcriptional regulatory networks from high-throughput data. Bioinformatics 23, 3056–3064.

Weinberger, L.S., Burnett, J.C., Toettcher, J.E., Arkin, A. P., Schaffer, D.V., 2005. Stochastic gene expression in a lentiviral positive-feedback loop: HIV-1 Tat fluctuations drive phenotypic diversity. Cell 122, 169–182.

Werhli, A.V., Husmeier, D., 2007. Reconstructing gene regulatory networks with Bayesian networks by combining expression data with multiple sources of prior knowledge. *Stat. Appl. Genet. Mol. Biol.* 6:Article15.

Werhli, A.V., Grzegorczyk, M., Husmeier, D., 2006. Comparative evaluation of reverse engineering gene regulatory networks with relevance networks, graphical Gaussian models and Bayesian networks. Bioinformatics 22, 2523–2531.

Wiesner, T.F., Berk, B.C., Nerem, R.M., 1996. A mathematical model of cytosolic calcium dynamics in human umbilical vein endothelial cells. Am. J. Physiol. Cell Physiol. 39, C1556–C1569.

Wikipedia, 2006. Systemic Inflammatory Response Syndrome. Available from http://en.wikipedia.org/wiki/SIRS. [Accessed 2006 Aug 02].

Willadsen, K., Wiles, J., 2007. Robustness and state-space structure of Boolean gene regulatory models. J. Theor. Biol. 249, 749–765.

Winslow, R.L., Tanskanen, A., Chen, M., Greenstein, J.L., 2006. Multiscale modeling of calcium signaling in the cardiac dyad. Ann. NY Acad. Sci. 1080, 362–375.

Woolf, P.J., Linderman, J.J., 2003. Untangling ligand induced activation and desensitization of G-protein-coupled receptors. Biophys. J. 84, 3–13.

Woolf, P.J., Prudhomme, W., Daheron, L., Daley, G.Q., Lauffenburger, D.A., 2005. Bayesian analysis of signaling networks governing embryonic stem cell fate decisions. Bioinformatics 21, 741–753.

Xiao, X., Dow, E.R., Eberhart, R., Miled, Z.B., Oppelt, R.J., 2004. A hybrid self-organizing maps and particle swarm optimization approach. Concurrency and Computation 16, 895–915.

Xu, C., Gertner, G., 2007. Extending a global sensitivity analysis technique to models with correlated parameters. Comput. Stat. Data Anal. 51, 5579–5590.

Yan, L., Shen, K., Hu, S., 2004. Solving mixed integer nonlinear programming problems with line-up competition algorithm. Comput. Chem. Eng. 28, 2647–2657.

Yeger-Lotem, E., Sattath, S., Kashtan, N., et al., 2004. Network motifs in integrated cellular networks of transcription-regulation and protein-protein interaction. Proc. Natl. Acad. Sci. USA 101, 5934–5939.

Yeung, M.K., Tegner, J., Collins, J.J., 2002. Reverse engineering gene networks using singular value decomposition and robust regression. Proc. Natl. Acad. Sci. USA 99, 6163–6168.

Yeung, M., Thiele, I., Palsson, B.O., 2007. Estimation of the number of extreme pathways for metabolic networks. BMC Bioinformatics 8, 363.

Yi, T.M., Kitano, H., Simon, M.I., 2003. A quantitative characterization of the yeast heterotrimeric G protein cycle. Proc. Natl. Acad. Sci. USA 100, 10764–10769.

Yi, Y.B., Wang, H., Sastry, A.M., Lastoskie, C.M., 2005. Direct stochastic simulation of Ca2+ motion in Xenopus eggs. Phys. Rev. E Stat. Nonlin. Soft Matter Phys. 72, 021913.

Young, R.A., Talbot, K., Gao, Z.Y., Trojanowski, J.Q., Wolf, B.A., 1999. Phospholipase pathway in Alzheimer's disease brains: decrease in Galphai in dorsolateral prefrontal cortex. Brain Res. Mol. Brain Res. 66, 188–190.

Young, J.D., Walther, J.L., Antoniewicz, M.R., Yoo, H., Stephanopoulos, G., 2007. An elementary metabolite unit (EMU) based method of isotopically nonstationary flux analysis. Biotechnol. Bioeng. 99, 686–699.

Yu, J., Smith, V.A., Wang, P.P., Hartemink, A.J., Jarvis, E.D., 2004. Advances to Bayesian network inference for generating causal networks from observational biological data. Bioinformatics 20, 3594–3603.

Zeilinger III, M.N., Farre, E.M., Taylor, S.R., Kay, S.A., Doyle, F.J., 2006. A novel computational model of the circadian clock in Arabidopsis that incorporates PRR7 and PRR9. Mol. Syst. Biol. 2, 58.

Zhang, S.L., Yeromin, A.V., Zhang, X.H., et al., 2006. Genome-wide RNAi screen of Ca(2+) influx identifies genes that regulate Ca(2+) release-activated Ca(2+) channel activity. Proc. Natl. Acad. Sci. USA 103, 9357–9362.

Zheng, B., Tang, T., Tang, N., et al., 2006. Essential role of RGS-PX1/sorting nexin 13 in mouse development and regulation of endocytosis dynamics. Proc. Natl. Acad. Sci. USA 103, 16776–16781.

Zou, M., Conzen, S.D., 2005. A new dynamic Bayesian network (DBN) approach for identifying gene regulatory networks from time course microarray data. Bioinformatics 21, 71–79.

Zwolak, J.W., Tyson, J.J., Watson, L.T., 2005. Parameter estimation for a mathematical model of the cell cycle in frog eggs. J. Comput. Biol. 12, 48–63.

CHAPTER 9

High-level Modeling of Biological Networks

Kevin A. Janes[1], Peter J. Woolf[2] and Shayn M. Peirce[1]
[1]University of Virginia, Charlottesville
[2]University of Michigan, Ann Arbor

OUTLINE

Summary	225	Introduction	235
Introduction	226	Theory and Computational Algorithms	235
High-level Modeling	226	Application to Hedgehog Signaling	237
Morphogens and Shh Signal Transduction	226	Agent-based Modeling of Cellular Networks	239
Partial-least-squares Modeling of Signaling Networks	228	Introduction	239
Introduction	228	Agent-based Theory and Computational Algorithms	240
Theory and Computational Algorithms	228	Application to Multicell Morphogen-regulated Patterning	244
Application to the Shh Signaling Network	231		
Bayesian Modeling of Transcriptional Networks	235		

Summary

Many biological networks are not understood to the extent that they can be entirely modeled as a dynamic system of reaction–diffusion events at the molecular level. High-level models are useful systems tools for situations in which the important biological questions are defined but essential molecular detail is lacking. In place of differential equations, high-level modeling approaches draw from probability and linear algebra to analyze and predict experimental data. Here, we present three different types of high-level models: partial least squares,

Bayesian networks and agent-based models. To illustrate the breadth of applications and length scales that are amenable to high-level modeling, our examples span the signaling, transcriptional and cell-fate responses triggered by the morphogen, Sonic hedgehog.

INTRODUCTION

High-level Modeling

The preceding chapters have described mathematical techniques for completely elaborating the reaction and diffusion events of molecules in biological systems. Such "low-level" approaches are obviously preferred when there is detailed biochemical and biophysical understanding of the individual components comprising a network. Often, however, true quantitative estimates of the kinetic constants and initial conditions in low-level models are fragmented, and the exact connectivity between components can be highly uncertain. In addition, sometimes one is willing to sacrifice low-level detail for a model that is more easily interpreted or can be executed more rapidly. These situations call for "high-level" models, which can test biological hypotheses, incorporate prior knowledge and combine biological processes with less emphasis on the detailed molecular mechanisms.

How are high-level models useful as systems tools in the absence of complete molecular detail? Frequently, the reduction of molecular detail to a smaller number of biologically interpretable relationships is itself valuable. With low-level models, the number of parameters increases (at least) multiplicatively with the number of molecules (Janes and Lauffenburger, 2006). Assessing the individual and synergistic influences that these parameters exert on network function becomes daunting, even for moderately sized systems. Using high-level models, complex biological networks are simplified to a minimal description that is sufficient to explain and predict the available experimental data.

An important consequence of network simplification is that high-level models cannot be constructed from "first principles" alone, as is technically possible for low-level models. Therefore, high-level models are heavily data driven or entirely data dependent (Janes and Yaffe, 2006; Thorne et al., 2007). The reliance of high-level models on biological measurements may be undesirable in theory. However, in practice, it allows high-level modeling to be more effective at revealing new relationships between molecules or cells, and in determining whether known pathways are supported by experiment. In this chapter, we present three different high-level approaches, in sections on Partial-least-squares Modeling of Signaling Networks, Bayesian Modeling of Transcriptional Networks, and Agent-based Modeling of Cellular Networks. Each approach is focused on a distinct biological problem, to give a sense of the breadth of questions that can be addressed by high-level modeling. To provide a common biological context, these models are applied to signaling, transcriptional and cell-fate regulation by the Hedgehog family of morphogens.

Morphogens and Shh Signal Transduction

The term "morphogen" refers to any signaling ligand that induces distinct cellular responses depending upon the concentration of the ligand. Morphogens have critical roles in development, overlapping concentration gradients of different morphogens specifying cell-fate patterning in the embryo (*see* Agent-based Modeling of Cellular Networks). Morphogens are also important in diseases such as cancer, in which aberrant reactivation of different morphogen signaling pathways can occur.

Sonic hedgehog (Shh) is one member of a family of lipophilic Hedgehog ligands that acts as a morphogen in many developing tissues,

INTRODUCTION

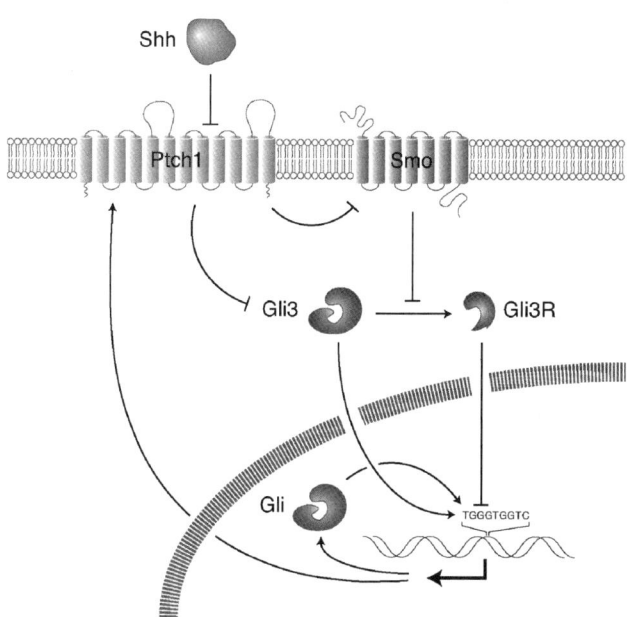

FIGURE 9.1 The Shh Signaling Pathway.
The network consists of five main signaling proteins: Shh, Ptch1, Smo, Gli3, Gli3R and Gli. See the main text for a description of the connections within the overall network.

including the neural tube and limb bud (Ingham and McMahon, 2001). Mature Shh is cholesterol modified and palmitoylated; therefore, Shh transport occurs across the cell membrane from a Shh "producing" cell to a Shh "receiving" cell (Jacob and Lum, 2007). Shh-receiving cells bind Shh through the 12-transmembrane Shh receptor, Patched (Ptch1) (Fig. 9.1). In the absence of Shh, Ptch1 prevents the seven-transmembrane protein, Smoothened (Smo), from inhibiting the proteolysis of the zinc-finger transcription factor, Gli3, into a cleaved form that is a transcriptional repressor (Gli3R). Shh binding to Ptch1 relieves the inhibition on Smo, causing uncleaved (active) Gli3 to accumulate and activate transcription after translocating to the nucleus (Fig. 9.1).

Gli transcription factors bind to the consensus DNA sequence, 5'-TGGGTGGTC-3' (Kinzler and Vogelstein, 1990), and Gli3-induced proteins provide important regulatory feedback to the Shh signaling network. Among the recognized targets of Gli3 are Gli1 and Gli2 (collectively referred to here as "Gli"), which bind to the same consensus as Gli3 and thus positively regulate their own transcription (Fig. 9.1). Gli3 also induces the expression of Ptch1, adding a negative-feedback circuit that dampens Gli3 activity. Besides reducing Gli3 concentrations through derepression of Gli3 proteolysis (Fig. 9.1), Ptch1 also downregulates total Gli3 protein via an unknown mechanism (Wang et al., 2000). Many other important questions remain (Jacob and Lum, 2007), including: (i) how quantitative activation of the Shh network converges on induction of Gli (*see* Partial-least-squares Modeling of Signaling Networks), (ii) how Gli induction causes the induction of specific target genes (*see* Bayesian Modeling of Transcriptional Networks), and (iii) how Shh-induced phenotypes collaborate with other morphogens to determine tissue patterns. All these topics can be explored with high-level modeling, as we will show below.

PARTIAL-LEAST-SQUARES MODELING OF SIGNALING NETWORKS

Introduction

A fundamental goal in nearly all systems models is prediction—prediction of molecular connections, cellular states and biological outcomes that have not already been tested by experiment. For low-levels models, it is possible to make predictions completely *in silico*, because these models are theoretically "complete" (Janes and Lauffenburger, 2006). High-level models, in contrast, omit or abstract many of the biochemical and biophysical events that underlie biological networks. Consequently, high-levels models often require data to make predictions, just as they require data during model construction (*see* High-level Modeling). Models of this kind that directly map measured (independent) variables on to predicted (dependent) variables are called regression models.

Partial least squares is an approach that was designed for modeling problems in which the number of variables exceeds the number of observations that constrain how these variables can contribute to a prediction. Such "underdetermined" regression models are degenerate, with an infinite number of solutions given the available data. Partial least squares emerged as a tool for underdetermined models from the field of spectroscopy (Geladi and Kowalski, 1986). Spectroscopy datasets often consist of hundreds of complex sample mixtures (observations), the spectra of which are measured at thousands of wavelengths (variables). Partial least squares has also found applications in sensory science and process control, in which several easily measured variables are used as indicators to predict complex responses (Martens and Martens, 2001).

Biological systems often collect information from many sources en route to reaching a specific outcome, and would therefore appear ideally suited for partial-least-squares modeling. Appropriate datasets have been lacking, however, because biologists typically design experiments that are univariate, to investigate the effect of one variable at a time. The recent growth in multiplex assays that can measure many biological variables simultaneously has changed this trend, and now multivariate biological datasets are emerging regularly (Albeck et al., 2006). Several large-scale studies of signaling networks have been specified as multivariate from the start (Janes et al., 2005; Natarajan et al., 2006), suggesting that techniques such as partial least squares will have integral roles in future systems-level experiments.

Theory and Computational Algorithms

Principal Components Analysis

Before delving into underdetermined regressions between multiple independent and dependent variables, it is important to introduce some basic ideas from linear algebra, concerning how data matrices are conceived. We start with a matrix (X) of m rows and n columns. Most datasets are organized such that the columns indicate a measured variable and the rows indicate an experimental observation of that variable. Ideally, a data matrix will not have missing elements, meaning that each variable was measured during every observation. (In practice, a small number of missing elements can be tolerated in the models described here.) We ordinarily inspect data matrices as a table of numbers; however, an alternative view is to think of each variable (matrix column) as a dimension in an n-dimensional data space (Janes and Yaffe, 2006). The matrix rows then specify the coordinates of an observation in the n-dimensional data space—how far an observation projects along the different dimensions. Conversely, the observations constrain how the n dimensions "point" relative to one another.

If $m = n$ and each row and column is linearly independent from all the others (that is, it cannot be expressed as a linear combination of the remaining rows or columns), then **X** has full rank. In a full-rank data space, all the variables are needed to describe where the observations project, and all the observations are needed to describe how the variables relate to one another. Full-rank data matrices are rare in data-driven applications. Usually, it is desirable to have more observations than variables ($m > n$). Extra observations provide added constraints (called degrees of freedom), which can be used to account for random errors in observed measurements. Degrees of freedom are essential for most estimation problems in classical statistics, such as determining whether two observations (or two variables) are significantly different from one another.

This section deals with the third type of data matrix, which has more variables than observations and thus is rank deficient ($m < n$). Such matrices are now common in biology, with the widespread use of oligonucleotide microarrays and the emerging applications of mass spectrometry and protein arrays (Albeck et al., 2006). For rank-deficient matrices, some of the dimensions in the data space are necessarily redundant, because at least $n-m$ variables can be expressed as linear combination of the others. This means that some dimensions must point in similar directions (Janes et al., 2005).

There are many techniques for dealing with rank-deficient matrices that can be useful, depending upon the application. For the models described here, our strategy is to identify a few latent dimensions, called principal components, that roughly capture where the variables point and how the observations project. A simple example of a latent dimension occurs if two or more variables are nearly collinear and thus point in a very similar direction. One can identify the common direction of the collinear variables, and then define a principal component that captures their joint behavior in a single dimension. Principal components are formally oriented in the direction of maximum variance for the entire dataset (i.e., the direction across which the observations change most dramatically). This ensures that each principal component will be more efficient than the original set of variables at describing the dataset. By further constraining principal components to be orthogonal to one another, it becomes possible to identify a series of latent dimensions that comprise a basis set for the data space (Janes et al., 2005).

Implementation of Principal Components Analysis

The problem of identifying these latent dimensions is posed as a factorization of the data matrix (**X**) into an iterative series of vector products between so-called scores vectors (**t**) and loadings vectors (**p**):

$$X \approx \begin{bmatrix} t_{11} \\ t_{21} \\ \vdots \\ t_{m1} \end{bmatrix} \begin{bmatrix} p_{11} & p_{12} & \cdots & p_{1n} \end{bmatrix} + \begin{bmatrix} t_{12} \\ t_{22} \\ \vdots \\ t_{m2} \end{bmatrix} \begin{bmatrix} p_{21} & p_{22} & \cdots & p_{2n} \end{bmatrix}$$

$$+ \ldots = t_1 p_1^T + t_2 p_2^T + \ldots$$

(9.1)

where ^{T} represents transpose. In this way, it is possible to describe the observed dataset completely by the product of all the scores vectors (**T**) and loadings vectors (**P**):

$$X = \begin{bmatrix} t_{11} & t_{12} & \cdots & t_{1\min(m,n)} \\ t_{21} & t_{22} & \cdots & t_{2\min(m,n)} \\ \vdots & \vdots & \ddots & \vdots \\ t_{m1} & t_{m2} & \cdots & t_{m\min(m,n)} \end{bmatrix}$$

$$\times \begin{bmatrix} p_{11} & p_{12} & \cdots & p_{1n} \\ p_{21} & p_{22} & \cdots & p_{2n} \\ \vdots & \vdots & \ddots & \vdots \\ p_{\min(m,n)1} & p_{\min(m,n)2} & \cdots & p_{\min(m,n)n} \end{bmatrix} = TP^T$$

(9.2)

Because there are many ways to factorize **X**, the score-loading factorization by itself does not have a unique solution and does not guarantee the identification of principal components. To do this, the first score-loading pair (which together identify the first principal component) must maximize the variance captured in **X**, which is achieved by searching for a loadings vector that fits the criterion:

$$p_1 = \underset{p_1^T p_1 = 1}{\arg\max} \mathrm{var}(Xp_1) \quad (9.3)$$

where arg max is maximum of the argument, and var is variance (loadings vectors are constrained to be orthonormal, so that they can serve as the latent variables of a basis set). This objective function is solved iteratively by: (i) starting with an observation from **X** as a first guess at a scores vector (**t**), (ii) projecting **t** onto **X** to get a first approximation of the loadings vector (**p**), (iii) normalizing **p** and then projecting it back onto **X** to get an updated scores vector (**t**$_{new}$), (iv) comparing **t** and **t**$_{new}$, and repeating steps (ii) to (iv) until **t** = **t**$_{new}$ (Geladi and Kowalski, 1986).

The subsequent score-loading pair and principal component are calculated iteratively by subtracting the variance captured by the first principal component and optimizing a second, orthogonal loadings vector based on the residual:

$$p_2 = \underset{p_2^T p_2 = 1,\, p_1^T p_2 = 0}{\arg\max} \mathrm{var}[(X - t_1 p_1^T) p_2] \quad (9.4)$$

Principal components can similarly be defined up to the rank of the data matrix:

$$p_i = \underset{p_i^T p_i = 1,\, p_i^T p_{j \neq i} = 0}{\arg\max} \mathrm{var}\left[\left(X - \sum_{k=1}^{\min(m,n)-1} t_k p_k^T\right) p_i\right] \quad (9.5)$$

Decomposing a data matrix into this series of latent variables is called "principal components analysis." Using all the principal components is simply a re-casting of the original data space. However, because principal components are defined to maximize the residual variance from the preceding component, one can typically approximate the data space with only a handful of the leading principal components. Principal components play a prominent role in partial-least-squares modeling for relating two rank-deficient datasets, as we will see below.

Partial Least Squares

Many aspects of partial least squares are extensions of principal components analysis but now applied to two data matrices, called an independent "block" (**X**) and a dependent block (**Y**). **X** and **Y** must have the name number of observations (rows), but can have different numbers of variables (columns). Whereas principal components analysis is essentially automatic in its decomposition of a single data matrix (Equation (9.5)), partial least squares specifies a hypothesized relationship between independent and dependent blocks: **Y** = f(**X**). Principal components must reduce the dimensionality of the overall data space and also be predictive of the latent variables in the dependent block. Consequently, the assignment of measured variables to independent or dependent blocks is a critical first step in constructing a successful partial-least-squares model. Poor organization of **X** and **Y** matrices will lead to a phenomenological model that stands little chance at uncovering new biological mechanisms (Janes and Yaffe, 2006). A generally safe strategy is to place all molecular "causes" (or possible causes) in the **X** block and all downstream "effects" in the **Y** block.

The identification of principal components through partial least squares occurs by simultaneous factorization of the independent and dependent blocks into their respective scores and loadings vectors:

$$X = TP^T$$
$$Y = UQ^T \quad (9.6)$$

where **T** and **P** are the matrices of scores and loadings vectors for the independent block (as in Equation (9.2)), and **U** and **Q** are the matrices of scores and loadings vectors for the dependent block. The simplest versions of partial least squares assume a linear relationship between the independent and dependent blocks. The regression for this relationship is specified through the scores vectors: $u_i = b_i t_i$ for the ith principal component, so that $Y = TBQ^T$. **B** then is a matrix of regression coefficients with row elements for each observation and column elements for each principal component. These regression coefficients allow prediction of new Y-block data based on the projection of the corresponding X-block data along the model-derived principal components.

Implementation of Partial Least Squares

The score-loading factorization is calculated iteratively using numerical algorithms that are very similar to those described for principal components analysis (Geladi and Kowalski, 1986). The critical difference between partial least squares and principal components analysis is that the loadings vectors are optimized to capture the covariance between the independent and dependent blocks:

$$p_i = \underset{\substack{p_i^T p_i = 1, p_i^T p_{j\neq i} = 0 \\ q_i^T q_i = 1, q_i^T q_{j\neq i} = 0}}{\operatorname{argmax}} \operatorname{cov}\left[\left(X - \sum_{k=1}^{\min(m,n)-1} t_k p_k^T\right)\right.$$

$$\left.\times p_i, \left(Y - \sum_{k=1}^{\min(m,n)-1} u_k q_k^T\right) q_i\right]$$

(9.7)

The decomposition of **X** and **Y** are computed as in principal components analysis (see above), except that X- and Y-block scores are swapped (**X** is projected on **u**, rather than **t**, and **Y** is projected on **t**, rather than **u**). This exchange of scores allows the covariance to be maximized, rather than the variance of the two individual blocks (Geladi and Kowalski, 1986). The result is a rotation in the scores and loadings vectors that will be less efficient at capturing the data in **X** compared with principal components analysis, but will be more accurate in predicting the data in **Y**. Other practical considerations for implementing partial least squares will be introduced when it is applied to the Shh signaling network (*see* Partial-least-squares Modeling of Shh Simulations, below).

Application to the Shh Signaling Network

A Low-level Model of Shh Signaling

The core Ptch1/Smo/Gli3 inhibitory cascade and the feedback circuits described in the section on Morphogens and Shh Signal Transduction constitute the currently understood network downstream of Shh (Fig. 9.1). The major proteins involved in Shh signaling have been identified and interconnected for some time, but most of the experimental evidence has been based on epistatic relationships identified through genetic studies (Lum and Beachy, 2004). Notably, there have yet to be described direct biochemical readouts of Ptch1, Smo or Gli3 that reflect activation of the Shh pathway. (Shh signaling is usually monitored at its endpoint by using an exogenous Gli reporter construct.) This precludes the collection of multivariate Shh datasets that would be directly amenable to partial least squares, because the only measurable variable in the network is the upregulation of Gli targets (the pathway output).

To circumvent these difficulties here, we turn to simulated data from a low-level model of Gli induction (Lai et al., 2004). This model codifies the network relationships described in Morphogens and Shh Signal Transduction, using rate equations and hyperbolic dose curves, but it abstracts the unknown mechanistic details. For example, in the model, the cleavage of Gli3 to Gli3R is proportional to Ptch1 and inversely proportional to Shh, but the exact state changes in Ptch1 and Smo that mediate the effect on Gli3 proteolysis are not specified. The model of Lai and colleagues incorporates both the positive feedback of Gli autoinduction and the negative feedback of Ptch1 induction by Gli3 via a sigmoidal model of transcriptional regulation (Keller, 1995). Adding these features to the Ptch1/Smo/Gli3 inhibitory cascade creates a highly non-linear system that can exhibit bistability and hysteresis similar to the decisive cell-state changes mediated by Shh *in vivo* (Lai et al., 2004).

The Shh model contains 12 parameters that were estimated from the literature or assigned on the basis of similar regulatory systems (Figs. 9.1 and 9.2A). The model parameters include: (i) the basal and inducible synthesis–degradation rates of Gli, Gli3 and Ptch1 (parameters 1, 2, 4 and 5); (ii) the rate and half-maximum constant (EC_{50}) for the cleavage of Gli3 to Gli3R (parameters 3 and 8); (iii) the ratio of affinities of Ptch1 for Shh relative to Ptch1 for Smo and of DNA binding sites for Gli relative to sites for Gli3 (parameters 6 and 11); (iv) three terms describing the transcriptional and translational pathways downstream of active Gli and active Gli3 (parameters 9, 10 and 12).

As is true for most low-level models, it is not immediately obvious which (if any) of these parameters constitutes a rate-limiting step for the Shh network. An additional complication is that the Shh model has essentially two outputs, Gli and Gli3, which share the ability to induce target genes but are under different regulatory constraints (Gli positively regulates its own concentrations, whereas Gli3 is inversely proportional to Ptch1). This arrangement is problematic for techniques such as sensitivity analysis, because Gli and Gli3 could be sensitive to different model parameters. Here, we will use partial least squares to perform a simple bivariate sensitivity analysis of the Shh model.

Partial-least-squares Modeling of Shh Simulations

To construct a sensitivity-based dataset that could be used with partial least squares, we ran simulations of the low-level Shh model using 24 different parameter sets. Each of the 12 parameters was individually changed to 10-fold above or below its published value (Lai et al., 2004); then, the network was stimulated with saturating Shh (10-fold above its affinity for Ptch1) and steady-state concentrations of Gli and Gli3 were recorded as the pathway outputs. On the basis of the results of these simulations (Fig. 9.2A; note that variables are shown as rows rather than columns for presentation purposes), the Shh model appears to be sensitive to only a subset of the parameters. Furthermore, there is an inverse relationship between steady-state Gli and Gli3 concentrations, with high levels of Gli often corresponding to low levels of Gli3, and *vice versa*. The overall dataset, with 24 observations and 12 variables × 2 outputs, lacks sufficient observations to be related by multiple linear regression and ordinary least squares. The regression is therefore well suited for partial least squares.

Before implementing partial least squares, it is important to preprocess the data matrix so that the variables can be fairly compared. In this example, each model parameter (variable) has different baseline values and units, and a model constructed without preprocessing will extract scores and loadings vectors that mostly reflect these differences, rather than how parameter changes affect the Shh model outputs. There are many important considerations when preprocessing a data matrix (Martens and Martens, 2001); here, we will "center" each variable about its mean and "scale" the mean-centered variable by the square root of its variance:

$$x_{i,scaled} = \frac{x_{i,raw} - \overline{x_{i,raw}}}{\sqrt{\mathrm{var}(x_{i,raw} - \overline{x_{i,raw}})}} \quad (9.8)$$

where x_i represents a column vector in the data matrix (variables in both the independent and dependent blocks are scaled). This preprocessing is equivalent to using the Z score of each parameter and model output.

The preprocessed dataset was factorized into scores and loadings vectors that captured the dependent block (steady-state Gli and Gli3; Fig. 9.2A). As seen in Figure 9.2B, the ability of the model to capture the observed changes in the **Y** block increases rapidly with the number of principal components. Using only two principal components, the model captures more than 95% of the variance of steady-state Gli and Gli3 across all parameter changes, with only a small increase (96% capture) after the addition of a third component.

Capturing the data in the **Y** block measures the degree of model fitting, but it does not indicate how stable the model is at predicting the outputs. To quantify the predictive ability of the model, a simple cross-validation is used, in which one observation is omitted from the dataset and the model is retrained. After recalculation of the principal components, the "leave-one-out" model attempts to predict the omitted observation by projecting it onto the derived loadings vectors, and the accuracy of this prediction is compared with the measured value. By repeating the cross-validation procedure through the entire dataset, one can gauge the overall stability of the model predictions.

Leave-one-out predictions of the cross-validation runs are commonly summarized by the root mean-squared error (RMSE) from the measured value. In Figure 9.2C, we see that the RMSE improves for both outputs when the number of principal components increases from one to two. Above two components, however, there is little to no improvement, and the RMSE actually begins to increase above three principal components, indicating that the model is overfit. Taken together, the diagnostics from Figures 9.2B and 9.2C suggest that a two-component model is best for the parameter dataset to predict Gli–Gli3 outputs.

The contribution of all Shh model parameters to Gli–Gli3 outputs can therefore be encompassed with a single partial-least-squares model that uses two principal components. To see how different parameters selectively affect Gli or Gli3, we can now inspect the loadings vectors for the two components in the independent and dependent blocks. In the independent block (Fig. 9.2D), the loadings quantify how much each parameter contributes to orienting the direction of the principal component. Similarly, in the dependent block (Fig. 9.2E), the loadings identify which principal components are important for pointing toward the Gli and Gli3 outputs. Starting with the dependent block, we see that the first principal component separates the divergent responses of Gli and Gli3, with Gli being positively weighted and Gli3 being negatively weighted. The second component then separates overall Gli–Gli3 responsiveness, isolating parameters that substantially affect the model outputs from those that do not.

Keeping in mind the role of the two principal components, we then can return to the loadings of the independent block to interpret the parameter sensitivities. Along the first component, we observe major contributions from the maximum rate of Gli synthesis (positive and thus toward Gli) and from the basal rate of Gli3 synthesis (negative and thus toward Gli3), with a smaller contribution from the Gli3→Gli3R conversion rate (toward Gli3). In the second component, major contributions are again seen from Gli and Gli3 synthesis rates, with a minor contribution from overall Gli transcriptional efficiency. Together, analysis of the partial-least-squares model supports the conclusion that steady-state Gli levels are most sensitive to the maximum rate of Gli synthesis, where as steady-state Gli3 levels are most sensitive to its basal rate of synthesis. The importance of the maximum rate of synthesis of Gli is consistent with a previous a

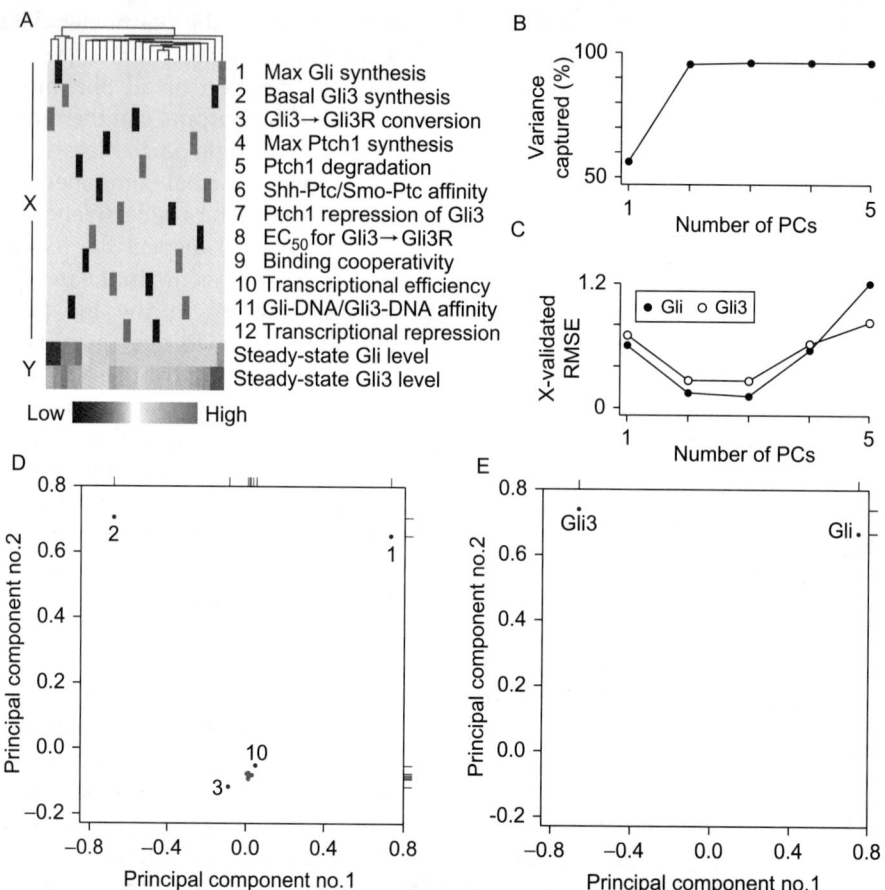

FIGURE 9.2 Sensitivity Analysis of a Low-level Model of the Shh Network, Based on Partial Least Squares.
(A) Training set for the partial-least-squares model. Simulated data were constructed by varying model parameters 10-fold above and below their published values (Lai et al., 2004) and then quantifying the steady-state levels of Gli and Gli3. After centering and scaling, the data were hierarchically clustered with a Pearson correlation distance metric and average linkage. The data matrix has been transposed and values log transformed for presentation purposes. (B) Change in variance captured with increasing number of principal components (PCs). Note that, after two components, the improvement in data capture is negligible. (C) Change in root mean-square error (RMSE) for cross-validated predictions of steady-state Gli and Gli3. Note that the RMSE increases dramatically after three components, indicating decreased model stability as a result of overfitting. (D) Loadings plot for the first two principal components of the independent block. The quantitative contribution of each model parameter to the individual loadings is shown as check marks on the top and right of the graph. Parameters with large contributions are shown in red, and the numbers refer to the parameters listed in Figure 9.2A. All other parameters are located around zero in both principal components, and are colored gray. (E) Loadings plot for the first two principal components of the dependent block. The quantitative contribution of each principal component to the prediction of Gli and Gli3 is shown as check marks on the top and right of the graph.

sensitivity analysis for steady-state Gli (Lai et al., 2004), whereas the role of basal Gli3 synthesis in steady-state Gli3 levels has not been reported. This straightforward example of partial least squares shows how complex datasets can often be reduced to simple linear combinations of measured variables that provide biological insight into the underlying molecular network.

BAYESIAN MODELING OF TRANSCRIPTIONAL NETWORKS

Introduction

High-throughput data such as gene expression arrays provide a wealth of biological information about the underlying transcriptional networks that govern cellular behavior. As an example, a single expression array provides quantitative measures of tens of thousands of genes in one fairly inexpensive experiment. Paradoxically, this bounty of quantitative biological data is problematic for many scientists, because it provides an overwhelming number of biological predictions. If we measure tens or hundreds of gene expression profiles of tens of thousands of genes, for example, we quickly accumulate millions of data points. These datasets are so large that they are difficult to visualize and are incompatible with many of the spreadsheet programs that are customarily used in the laboratory.

One solution to large datasets is to create high-level models that sort or structure the information in the data so that a human can interpret the result. Methods such as principal component analysis and partial least squares described in the section on Partial-least-squares Modeling of Signaling Networks provide an excellent method for gaining a coarse-grained view of the data. These preliminary methods reduce the dimensionality of the data, making the information more apparent. A complementary method for analyzing large datasets is to re-cast the data in terms of a network of causal interactions. For example, if a gene A regulates a target X, then an intuitive way to express this relationship is $A \rightarrow X$. Such causal maps are relatively common in biology texts and biological-pathway maps, and thus are readily accepted by the biological community.

Graphical models that describe causal interactions are well described by a class of probabilistic tools called Bayesian networks. Bayesian networks are a graphical statement of the conditional or causal relationships between variables. A key advantage of Bayesian networks is that these network structures can be learned directly from experimental data. This data-driven construction is in contrast to the manually constructed networks that one often sees in biology texts or curated reaction-network databases such as KEGG. In bioinformatics, Bayesian networks are finding wide use in interpreting gene expression data (Hartemink et al., 2001; Wang et al., 2007), proteomic data (Sachs et al., 2005; Woolf et al., 2005) and interaction data (Markowetz and Spang, 2007). Below, we will provide a simple example of how a Bayesian network is constructed and learned in the context of identifying new members in the Hedgehog network.

Theory and Computational Algorithms

The framework below describes how Bayesian networks are created, interpreted and learned. Bayesian networks have a significant history in the machine-learning community, with applications ranging from text mining to object recognition. The description below discusses only a fraction of the literature. For a more complete discussion on Bayesian networks, several textbooks are available (Jensen and Nielsen, 2007; Neapolitan, 2004).

Bayesian Networks

Bayesian networks are a graphical representation of a statement of conditional probability. As a simple example, consider a gene-regulatory network in which gene A regulates gene B, which in turn regulates gene C. Given this relationship, we could make the following statement of conditional probability:

$$P(A,B,C) = P(A)P(B \mid A)P(C \mid B) \quad (9.9)$$

This conditional probability statement says that the expression of gene A is independent of

B and C, but the expression of B depends on the value of A, and the expression of C depends on B. Graphically, this expression could be written as $A \to B \to C$.

A key feature of Bayesian networks is that they describe causal relationships. Biologically, such causal relationships are appealing, in that causal models bring us closer to a mechanistic understanding of the processes that govern cellular behavior. Unfortunately, for observational data alone (in which none of the variables have been directly externally manipulated), we cannot always uniquely identify causal relationships. Using the example above, the networks $A \to B \to C$ and $C \to B \to A$ both look the same in a Bayesian-network model, as they are both equivalent statements of conditional probability. This equivalency can be shown using Bayes' rule to rearrange the conditional probability statements describing the model, which shows that a finite set of alternative topologies describe an identical conditional probability assertion. These equivalence classes can be resolved either by setting an arrow direction on the basis of other knowledge about the network, or by using interventional data.

The conditional probability interpretation of Bayesian networks also requires that a Bayesian network be a directed acyclic graph (DAG). In a DAG, there can be no loops or cycles. Mathematically, this requirement arises directly from the conditional probability decomposition. Intuitively, the DAG requirement is needed to avoid circular reasoning. Biologically, however, loops and cycles are commonplace in regulatory networks. To allow these biological loops, a Bayesian network can be re-cast as dynamic, the values at some state, t_i, influencing states at some future time, t_{i+1}. In a dynamic Bayesian network, a variable can influence its future self or form loops in time without violating the DAG requirement. Dynamic Bayesian networks are finding wide use in computational biology for modeling time-series gene expression data (Perrin et al., 2003; Sugimoto and Iba, 2004), and whole-patient clinical models (Xiang et al., 2007).

Implementation: Network Scoring

Our central goal is to score a set of gene expression data as to how well it is described by a particular graphical structure. In general terms, this search can be cast as finding the network or model that is most likely, given the data. Using Bayes' rule we can rearrange the search to:

$$P(Model \mid Data) = \frac{P(Data \mid Model)P(Model)}{P(Data)}$$

(9.10)

Thus, if we limit our model space to those that fit the DAG criterion (i.e., Bayesian networks), the search can be re-stated as finding a model that maximizes P(Model | Data). The term P(Model) is the prior probability of the model, P(Data) is the prior probability of the data, and P(Data | Model) is the probability of the data, given a model. Each of these terms is discussed below.

To explain how P(Data | Model) is calculated, let us first introduce some notation. Assume a dataset, D, with m entries (rows). Each entry describes a state of n discrete-valued variables (columns). For any variable, i, let r_i equal the number of states (or the "arity") of the variable. Given a network model, each node represents a variable, and arrows represent apparently causal connections between nodes. Further, let each node (variable), i, have a list of parents called π_i, which can take on a total of q_i possible combinations of values. Finally, let N_{ijk} equal the total number of cases in the dataset in which variable i is in state k and the parent nodes are in state j. Similarly, let N_{ij} equal the number of cases in the dataset in which parents of the variable i are in state j. Given these terms, we can write a closed form expression for P(Data | Model):

$$P(Data \mid Model) = \prod_{i=1}^{n} \prod_{j=1}^{q_i} \frac{(r_i - 1)!}{(N_{ij} + r_i - 1)!} \prod_{k=1}^{r_i} N_{ijk}!$$

(9.11)

Intuitively, this expression describes the product of the probability of observing child nodes, i, in a particular state, k, given parents in some state, j (Cooper and Herskovits, 1992). This convenient closed-form expression is based on a multinomial model of discrete variables. Combinations of parents that are more informative for, or predictive of, the child values will have a higher probability.

Biologically, each node in the network is an experimentally accessible variable such as a gene expression value or cellular state. Arrows between nodes thus indicate apparent causal relationships uncovered within the data. It is important to note that arrows between nodes do not differentiate between positive, negative or more complicated interactions, but only indicate a directional relationship between variables.

Implementation: Discretization

To allow us to use the multinomial scoring function (Equation (9.11)) to calculate the probability of a model given data, the data need to be discretized into categorical states such as high, medium and low. Some types of data are already discretized and need no additional preprocessing—for example, a cellular differentiation state or a knockout cell line. Other variables, such as expression levels, need to be divided into a number of bins that are defined by the user. Common approaches for gene expression data are to divide the data into three equally sized bins as a first approximation of their states. Larger numbers of states (e.g. very high, high, medium, low, very low), or discretization schemes based on clustering, for example, have also been used, and discretization is an active area of research in Bayesian analysis (Steck and Jaakkola, 2004; Yu et al., 2004).

Implementation: Network Searching

Using the Bayesian scoring metric (Equation (9.11)), we can evaluate the likelihood of any topology, given experimental data. Search methods such as simulated annealing, greedy and genetic algorithms have all been used to search the combinatorial space of network solutions (Markowetz and Spang, 2007; Pe'er, 2005). These methods search for high-probability networks (given the available experimental data) by testing small changes to the network. Changes include the addition, reversal or removal of an arrow connecting two variables. In general, if the change to the network improves the fit of the network, then the change is accepted.

Application to Hedgehog Signaling

Here we describe a simple application of Bayesian networks to identify Shh pathway targets from gene expression data. Although the Shh pathway has been intensely studied, only a few of the genetic targets are known, because bona fide targets depend strongly on cellular context and sometimes exhibit only small changes in gene expression in response to Shh stimulation. Furthermore, because Shh is a morphogen, the targets of the pathway depend strongly on the exact activity of Shh, rather than a simple on–off relationship when Shh is present or absent. These complexities are difficult to address using standard statistical tools such as linear correlations, but can be addressed in a straightforward way using Bayesian networks as described below.

Data

Expression data describing the effects of various Shh mutations in mouse were used as the basis of the study and are described in more detail by others (Tenzen et al., 2006). The data consist of 44 Affymetrix U74v2 mouse arrays hybridized to cDNA samples from mouse embryos at three different developmental stages: 8 somites, 13 somites and E10.5. Triplicate 8- and

13-somite samples were taken from embryos with wild-type, Ptch1$^{-/-}$ or Smo$^{-/-}$ backgrounds. E10.5 embryos were divided into head (4x), trunk (3x), and limb (6x) fractions, in both wild-type and Shh$^{-/-}$ backgrounds. Together, these data survey a wide range of tissues and developmental stages that involve significant Hedgehog-related activity. Data were normalized and processed using standard techniques and gene values were discretized into three equally sized bins for Bayesian analysis.

Results

The gene expression data above were analyzed to identify genes responsive to changes in Shh and Ptch1, either by knockouts or by natural variations in the expression of these genes by other pathways. For profiles that are based on knockout data, we assumed that Shh or Ptch1 had an effective level of expression of zero in these cases. Topologically, we are searching for networks of the form shown in Figure 9.3A, in which Shh and Ptch1 influence some target gene, X.

After exhaustively scoring all possible target genes in the X position, the genes in Figure 9.3B were identified as the top-scoring target genes. Note that the scores are logarithmic transformations of the probability. Thus, the best-scoring network is the one with the most-positive value—Foxc2, with a log-probability score of

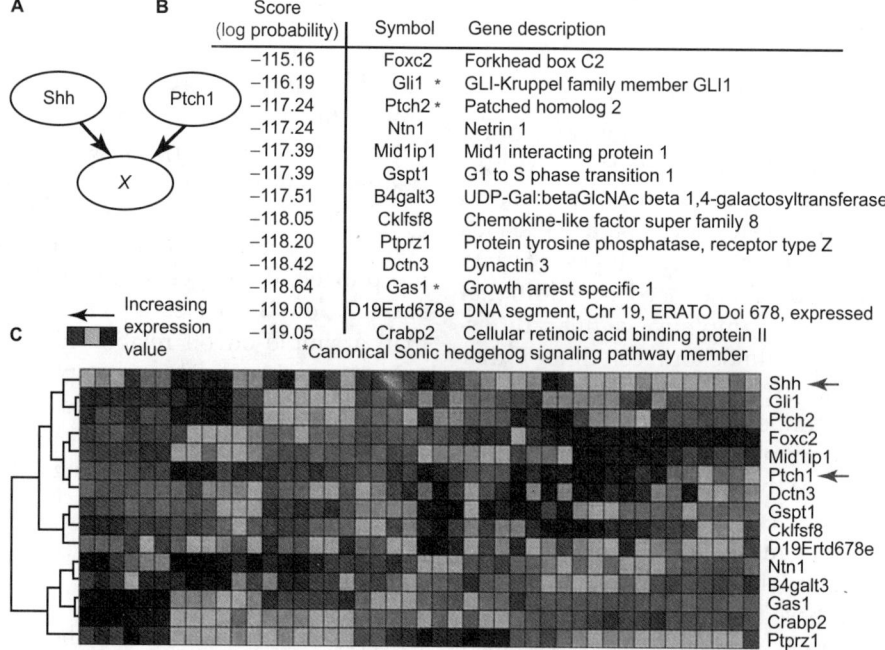

FIGURE 9.3 Bayesian-network Modeling of Hedgehog Target Genes.
(A) Small Bayesian network used to identify genes within the Hedgehog signaling pathway. The unknown genes are denoted as "X." (B) Sorted list of top-scoring targets for the Bayesian network in Figure 9.3A. Searching was done using PEBL (http://code.google.com/p/pebl-project/). (C) Two-dimensional hierarchical cluster of the gene expression profile data of both the regulators (Shh and Ptch1, highlighted with red arrows) and the targets. Note that the targets and regulators do not form close clusters, indicating that the Bayesian network identifies patterns distinct from more standard clustering approaches.

−115.16. In this case, many of the top-scoring networks have similar scores, meaning that these targets are all well described by the pattern of expression of Shh and Ptch1.

Many of the targets identified by this method are biologically reasonable. On the list of top targets, for example, Gli1 and Ptch1h2 are both canonical targets of Shh signaling (Dahmane et al., 1997; Marigo and Tabin, 1996; Marigo et al., 1996; Ruiz i Altaba, 1999). Growth arrest specific 1 (Gas1) is also a well known target of Shh signaling (Allen et al., 2007; Kang et al., 2007), and Foxc2 has been shown in be a downstream target of the Hedgehog pathway in combination with other developmental pathways (Jeong et al., 2004). Many, but not all, of the remaining targets have been associated with Shh signaling in other studies.

Hierarchical clustering of the top targets and the regulator genes Shh and Ptch1 shows the complexity of the relationships found using this Bayesian network structure (Fig. 9.3C). Instead of forming a simple cluster with either Shh or Ptch1, the top-scoring targets largely show different patterns of gene expression. The Bayesian network identifies these targets because they are well described by the combination of the expression values of Shh and Ptch1—not just one of the genes in isolation. In contrast, additive methods such as regression or naïve Bayesian networks assume that each regulator has a separable impact on the outcome—a requirement that is rarely satisfied by most biochemical pathways. Such complex, combinatorial regulation is expected in the Hedgehog pathway, because both Shh and Ptch1 are required for the pathway to function correctly (Fig. 9.1). These results demonstrate the power of small Bayesian networks in an exploratory analysis of large bodies of gene expression data. The problem of finding causal genetic regulatory targets is ubiquitous in molecular biology, but can be approached using high-level methods like those described here.

AGENT-BASED MODELING OF CELLULAR NETWORKS

Introduction

How do individual cells and their microenvironment give rise to larger-scale tissue phenomena? On the basis of prior knowledge of how cells respond to defined sets of environmental conditions, is it possible to predict outcomes when groups of cells interact dynamically in a spatially heterogeneous environment? Could such simulations suggest how the network is "wired" at the tissue level? Agent-based modeling (ABM) is uniquely suited to addressing these types of question, which are abundant in biology.

Agent-based modeling is a high-level modeling technique that simulates the behaviors of individual entities ("agents") as they interact with one another and with their environment in the context of a complex system. The behavior of each agent is governed by a "rule set," a series of if/then statements dictating an agent's decisions given the "state" described by factors such as its microenvironment and proximity to other agents. Agent states and behaviors are updated at each time increment, and thus population-level phenomena emerge from the collective behavior of individual agents.

The invention of ABM is attributed to John Louis von Neumann in the 1960's and has been used extensively in the fields of epidemiology (Burke et al., 2006), ecology (Grimm et al., 2005), financial forecasting (Terano, 2005) and behavioral and social sciences (Elliott and Kiel, 2004). More recently, this modeling technique has been applied to systems biology problems, including tumorigenesis (Zhang et al., 2007), angiogenesis (Peirce et al., 2004), embryo morphogenesis (Longo et al., 2004) and immune cell trafficking (Bailey et al., 2007; Tang et al., 2007). ABMs have been used to study many biological problems, but their predominant application has been in the study of multicell, tissue-level phenomena. For these applications, ABMs model biological cells as individual agents (Longo et al., 2004; Peirce et al., 2004). Each cell is endowed with the ability to exhibit biologically relevant behaviors, including migration, proliferation, differentiation and apoptosis. These outcomes are dictated by stimuli in the local environment, such as diffusible morphogens and growth factors, the extracellular matrix and cell–cell contacts. Typically, the rule set is derived empirically, relying heavily on accurate estimates of quantifiable behaviors derived from *in-vitro* assays.

The key motivation for using ABMs to study complex biological processes is that they allow the researcher to examine how single agents behave both individually and as an ensemble within a complex network. ABM graphical displays can be compared with microscopy images of the analogous experimental endpoint, which is particularly useful for ABM validation. Validated multicell ABMs can further provide individual cell tracking of the agents that gave rise to the final tissue-level pattern, suggesting lineage paths that would otherwise be difficult to examine experimentally. When intimately paired with experimental studies, ABMs are very effective at testing alternative or competing hypotheses about rule sets. Lastly, by disqualifying rule sets that do not match experiments, ABMs can also pinpoint gaps in our current understanding of how cellular networks interact within tissues.

Agent-based Theory and Computational Algorithms

Agents

Agents are the fundamental unit of an ABM. Each agent has a unique identity, the characteristics of which at any point in time are described by its state. States can be defined in an ABM by any combination of discrete numerical variables, which describe relative levels of stimuli, and Boolean variables, which simply describe whether a stimulus is present or absent. Example state descriptors include the time since last cell division (to capture the phase of the cell cycle), location in the tissue with respect to other cells, concentration of a certain protein being expressed, amount of protein being secreted, and the existence of a cell–cell contact with a neighboring agent. The first four examples would require a numerical state variable, whereas the last example would be defined by a true/false state. Because each agent has its own state that evolves with every time step, ABMs are able to accommodate the inherent spatial and temporal heterogeneities of biological tissues.

Rule Set

After a time step, agents are required to make behavioral decisions that are dictated by the ABM rule set. Rule sets take the agent state as an input and return defined or stochastic outputs that establish the agent behavior. Agent behaviors are often directly observable cell phenotypes, such as proliferation (generating a new agent in the ABM), migration (causing the agent to move across the simulation space), apoptosis (eliminating the agent) or expression of a marker protein (changing the agent's state). Changes in agent behaviors will cause changes in agent states that will affect the output behavior of the rule set. In this way, agents "interact" with one another and with their environment en route to tissue-level patterns.

Rules sets can be theoretically or empirically based, and can include both deterministic and stochastic rules. An example of a theoretically based rule is to use Fick's second law of diffusion to describe the diffusion of a growth factor (Peirce et al., 2004). An example of an empirically based rule is a dose–response curve describing cell migration speed as a function of morphogen concentration. Stochastic rules rely on probability distributions and are important when an agent state does not instruct a behavior explicitly but, rather, affects the likelihood of such a behavior occurring. Rules may be estimated from the literature or optimized from a training dataset, although it is generally better to quantify rules directly and empirically. Most tissues are heterotypic, and ABM rules are usually specific to a subset of agents that identify one particular cell type. In practice, rule sets can vary from as few as 10 rules to as many as 200 (Bailey et al., 2007; Grant et al., 2006).

Rule sets are the implicit hypothesis of an ABM. When ABMs are used for alternative hypothesis testing, "known" rules in the rule set are replaced with speculated rules. If an improved endpoint emerges in the ABM, one may conclude that the hypothetical rule set could be a possible explanation for the observed outcome. However, such an ABM result only supports the hypothetical rule and does not prove it, because other yet-to-be-tested rule sets could conceivably give the same outcome. Ideally, proof of such rules would then occur by directed experiments that map the relevant agent states to the behavior encoded by the hypothetical rule.

The composition, content and accuracy of a rule set has a profound impact on the output of an ABM. Slightly modifying a single rule can dramatically alter the output of even the simplest ABM. Therefore, in designing, constructing and implementing ABM rule sets, caution is urged to ensure that the rules are accurate, non-redundant, and necessary. The validity of a rule set can be checked by verifying ABM outputs against experimental data (Longo et al., 2004; Peirce et al., 2004; Simpson et al., 2007) and by performing a sensitivity analysis, in which rules are systematically removed or altered incrementally to determine the effect of their manipulation on the systems-level ABM output (Grant et al., 2006).

Simulation Space

Agents and rule sets must be implemented in a fixed region, and the simulation space defines the area in which agents are allowed to interact with one another. Most biological ABMs are implemented in a two-dimensional simulation space to lessen computing time and reduce model complexity for more rapid simulations. The entire simulation space is divided into a set of discrete pixels, in which agents typically occupy a single pixel at any given time. Pixels, like agents, can store spatial information about the system. For example, a pixel may store concentrations of diffusible factors such as chemokines or cytokines, or non-diffusible factors such as extracellular matrix proteins (Bailey et al., 2007; Peirce et al., 2004).

The edges of an ABM simulation space can have closed, open or periodic boundary conditions. With closed boundaries, neither agents nor diffusible stimuli can move past the boundaries, and the simulation area must therefore be sufficiently large relative to the area of agent interactions to avoid edge effects (Longo et al., 2004). Open conditions remove cells or protein from the simulation entirely after passing the boundaries (Bailey et al., 2007) and are appropriate when agents or agent states approach a background tissue level as they approach the simulation boundaries. Periodic simulation space has boundaries that wrap to the opposite side, so that an agent exiting the simulation through the left-hand border automatically re-enters from the right-hand border (Segovia-Juarez et al., 2004). Periodic boundary conditions are often used to simulate a portion of a larger tissue, such that agents exit and enter the simulation space with similar frequencies and there is no flux of agents out of the tissue.

Initial Conditions and Scaling

The positioning and state assignments for the agents at the start of an ABM simulation are specified through initial conditions. For tissue-level models, the initial conditions for agent position are frequently derived from microscopy images obtained at a starting time point (Bailey et al., 2007; Longo et al., 2004). This ensures that the initial cell numbers, positions and distributions in the simulation are realistic. If experimental observations are not destructive to the tissue, setting initial conditions in this way also enables direct comparison with the experimental system at later time-points for model validation. The initial states are set based on empirical data (histology, immunofluorescence, etc.) that describe baseline conditions for agent states.

Another important consideration when building an ABM is in selecting the spatial and temporal scales for the simulation. It is important to define a spatial scale, for example, that is small enough to be computationally tractable but large enough to study the tissue property of interest. The choice of time steps in an ABM is similarly important, because time steps are intimately linked to the rule sets that are evaluated at each step. ABM time steps can range from milliseconds to hours (Casal et al., 2005; Peirce et al., 2004), and the total simulation time can span years (Abbott et al., 2006). A good strategy is to pick a time step that matches the shortest time scale that is embedded in the rule set.

In this way, the ABM avoids oversampling or aliasing the rule set with too many or too few time steps.

Model Validation

The endpoint of most ABMs is a graphical output describing the spatial arrangements of agents and their final states. These patterns can subsequently be analyzed using image metrics that enable quantitative comparison with experimental data. A common pitfall in ABM validation is to choose patterns for validation that lie at the same level of abstraction as the empirical data upon which the model was based. For example, if an ABM's rule set is derived from tissue-level data, then making a prediction at the tissue level that identically matches the data from which the rules were derived only produces an intuitive output. A true tissue-level validation would require the ABM rule set to be assembled from *in-vitro* experiments, which then are validated at the tissue level by comparing the model results with those from *in-vivo* experiments. Validation could be

FIGURE 9.4 Agent-based Modeling of Neural Tube Domain Patterning.
(A) Schematic of a cross-section of the neural tube with dorsal–ventral axis, neuron subtypes and key anatomical features indicated. Blue regions indicate neural subdomains that organize in these locations during development. The five morphogens that are included in the ABM are indicated by shapes the widths of which correspond to concentration along the DV axis. (B) Screen-shot of the ABM, implemented using NetLogo software, indicating bone morphogenetic protein (BMP; green), retinoic acid (RA; pink), and Shh (red) diffusing from adjacent mesoderm. Gray neuroblasts in the neural tube are also shown. (C) Hypothesized feedback between morphogens. Fibroblast growth factor (FGF) signals are crucial in patterning of the most ventral domains, where they interact with Shh and RA (Lupo et al., 2006). It has been suggested that RA and FGF antagonize one another, whereas FGF represses Shh (Wilson and Maden, 2005). RA is suggested to inhibit Shh and, in the absence of RA, BMPs are downregulated (Wilson and Maden, 2005). RA induces neural differentiation in the intermediate domains and is responsible for downregulating FGF. Shh is responsible for inducing ventral neural cell types in a time- and concentration-dependent manner, predominantly via the inhibition of the GLI3 transcription factor. More ventral fates are specified in cells receiving both higher concentrations of Shh and longer durations of signal. Knockout of Shh causes the loss of ventral cell types (Ruiz i Altaba et al., 2003). Interestingly, double knockout of Shh and Gli3 partially recovers ventral cell fates, the only abnormality being in the floor plate and p3 domains. Therefore, specification of MN/p3 cells appears to be largely independent of Shh (Lupo et al., 2006). Shh inhibits BMP, and *vice versa*. BMPs are responsible for inducing dorsal neural cell types in a concentration-dependent manner, and their inhibition in the ventral region is essential for correct specification of ventral domains. BMP antagonists are expressed by the notochord and the mesoderm surrounding the neural tube (Wilson and Maden, 2005). Although Shh does not appear to influence dorsal patterning, there is a convincing amount of evidence to suggest that downregulation of BMPs influences ventral specification (Lupo et al., 2006). (D) ABM prediction of relative neuroblast

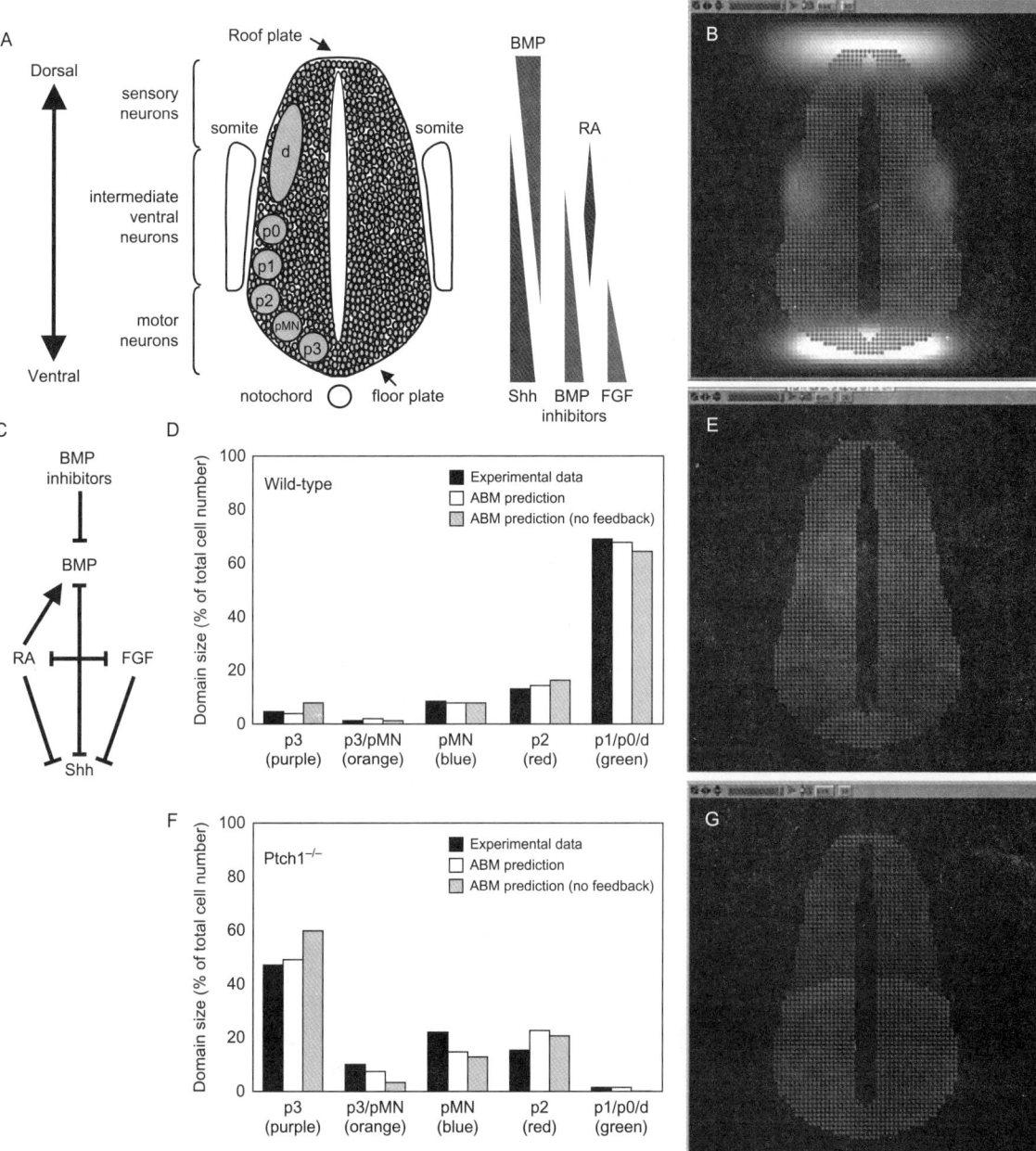

domain size in the wild-type, both with (white) and without (gray) feedback mechanisms included, as compared with experimental measurements by Jeong and McMahon (2005) (black). (E) ABM screen-shot of predicted wild-type domain patterning, with morphogen feedback mechanisms included. Neuroblast domains are colored according to those given on the X-axis labels in (D). (F) ABM prediction of relative neuroblast domain size in the Ptch1$^{-/-}$ mutant case compared with experimental measurements by Jeong and McMahon (2005). (G) ABM screen-shot of predicted Ptch1$^{-/-}$ mutant domain patterning with morphogen feedback mechanisms included.

similarly achieved by experimentally perturbing rule sets at the molecular level, and then using the ABM to predict the consequences of this perturbation at the tissue level.

Application to Multicell Morphogen-regulated Patterning

The neural tube is patterned in the dorsal–ventral (DV) axis from a very early stage in development, with a roof plate (dorsally: D), a floor plate (ventrally: V) and different types of neuroblasts, the precise position of which in the neural tube is essential for their correct development into different types of neurons (Wilson and Maden, 2005) (Fig. 9.4A). The underlying mesoderm of these structures modulates neural tube patterning via the production of different morphogens that specify distinct regions of the central nervous system (Fig. 9.4A). When neural tube morphogens are manipulated in transgenic knockout models or pathologically altered *in vivo*, profound patterning abnormalities ensue (Lupo et al., 2006). The effects of many morphogens have been studied alone or in combination by using transgenic and knockout embryos, but there remain unresolved questions regarding how they normally work together to direct correct neural tube patterning. Delineating how combinations of morphogens give rise to spatial patterns within developing tissues is a goal that is uniquely suited to an ABM approach. Here, we present a simplified model of DV neural tube patterning in a generic vertebrate, to examine how Shh might collaborate with other morphogens during development.

A number of morphogens are known to influence DV patterning, including fibroblast growth factor (FGF) produced by the caudal mesoderm, retinoic acid (RA) produced by the paraxial mesoderm (somites), Sonic hedgehog (Shh) produced by the notochord and floor plate, bone morphogenic protein (BMP) produced by the roof plate, and BMP antagonists, such as Noggin and Chordin, which sequester BMPs in the extracellular space (Piccolo et al., 1996) (Fig. 9.4A). Morphogens differ in the source of their production (Fig. 9.4B), and there is mounting evidence suggesting that these proteins directly inhibit each other's actions (Fig. 9.4C). Hypotheses from the literature regarding these interactions were input as part of the rule set in the ABM.

The ABM simulates the cells contained in a two-dimensional cross-section of the neural tube. At the start of the simulation (≈E8.5), five morphogens (Fig. 9.4A) diffuse from the surrounding mesoderm into the neural tube (Fig. 9.4B), according to an algorithm that approximates Fick's second law of diffusion in two dimensions (Peirce et al., 2004). For the sake of simplicity, the initial concentrations and diffusion coefficients of different morphogens were set equal to one another. Diffusion was allowed to proceed for 100 time steps, so that morphogens could diffuse throughout the entire neural tube. When two or more morphogens occupy the same pixel (e.g. an inhibitor, such as FGF, and one of its effectors, such as Shh), the inhibitor reduces the amount of effector in that pixel if the inhibitor exceeds a threshold level, according to the function:

$$\text{if INHIBITOR}_{(x,y)} > \text{INHIBITORthreshold} \\ \times [\text{set EFFECTOR}_{(x,y)}(\text{EFFECTOR}_{(x,y)} * 0.75)] \tag{9.12}$$

The threshold level for each inhibitor was set to 5% of its maximal concentration, which is relatively low and encourages the occurrence of inhibition. Inhibitory interactions result in a 25% reduction in the amount of the inhibited protein. The last step in the simulation is the correlation of morphogen concentration with DV patterning, which is accomplished through a simple transfer function that relates ventral differentiation to final Shh concentration, after the inhibition by other morphogens has occurred:

$$DV - \text{identity} = [Shh] \tag{9.13}$$

Thus, the ABM assumes that the concentration of Shh will be the ultimate driver of DV identity, specifying a neuron in the p3, MN, p2 or p1/p0/d domain.

First, the size of each neuroblast domain (i.e., total cell number) was fitted to published measurements (Jeong and McMahon, 2005) to capture the wild-type vertebrate case (Fig. 9.4D and E). Then, to investigate the possible role of morphogen cross-talk (Fig. 9.4C), the inhibitory interactions were removed from the rule set and the model was re-simulated. The results closely match to when cross-talk is included (compare gray and white bars), suggesting that the feedback rules in the wild-type state have minimal impact overall. This may be due to the manner in which feedback is implemented in the rule set (Equation (9.1)), or it may be a result of over-simplifying linkages between morphogens and cell patterning. Nevertheless, this result can be used as baseline for examining how sensitivity to cross-talk changes in the context of mutations in the Shh network.

To mimic Shh-network dysfunction, neural tube patterning was simulated in a Ptch1-deficient vertebrate (Fig. 9.4F and G). Ptch1 induces rapid endocytosis of Shh (Fig. 9.1) so, in this genetic background, there is an excess of Shh. We simulated Ptch1 deficiency by implementing a 20-fold increase in Shh concentration and increasing its diffusion time 7-fold. The predicted pattern of domain size emerges from this rule in combination with the morphogen feedback rules (Fig. 9.4F and G). For the Ptch1$^{-/-}$ mutant, the extent of ventral domains (p3-pMN; purple, orange and blue) are extended dorsally (upwards) relative to wild-type (compare Fig. 9.4E and G). Moreover, the quantitative prediction (white bars) approximates the summarized data (black bars) from Jeong and McMahon (2005). Also, there is now a more pronounced contribution from morphogen cross-talk in the Ptch1$^{-/-}$ case (Fig. 9.4F, gray bars). This simplified ABM implementation shows how feedback systems can exert non-uniform control on tissue function, becoming disproportionately important during disease.

References

Abbott, R.G., Forrest, S., Pienta, K.J., 2006. Simulating the hallmarks of cancer. Artif. Life 12, 617–634.

Albeck, J.G., MacBeath, G., White, F.M., Sorger, P.K., Lauffenburger, D.A., Gaudet, S., 2006. Collecting and organizing systematic sets of protein data. Nat. Rev. Mol. Cell Biol. 7, 803–812.

Allen, B.L., Tenzen, T., McMahon, A.P., 2007. The Hedgehog-binding proteins Gas1 and Cdo cooperate to positively regulate Shh signaling during mouse development. Genes. Dev. 21, 1244–1257.

Bailey, A.M., Thorne, B.C., Peirce, S.M., 2007. Multi-cell agent-based simulation of the microvasculature to study the dynamics of circulating inflammatory cell trafficking. Ann. Biomed. Eng. 35, 916–936.

Burke, D.S., Epstein, J.M., Cummings, D.A., et al., 2006. Individual-based computational modeling of smallpox epidemic control strategies. Acad. Emerg. Med. 13, 1142–1149.

Casal, A., Sumen, C., Reddy, T.E., Alber, M.S., Lee, P.P., 2005. Agent-based modeling of the context dependency in T cell recognition. J. Theor. Biol. 236, 376–391.

Cooper, G.F., Herskovits, E., 1992. A Bayesian method for the induction of probabilistic networks from data. Mach. Learn. 9, 309–347.

Dahmane, N., Lee, J., Robins, P., Heller, P., Ruiz i Altaba, A., 1997. Activation of the transcription factor Gli1 and the Sonic hedgehog signalling pathway in skin tumours. Nature 389, 876–881.

Elliott, E., Kiel, L.D., 2004. Agent-based modeling in the social and behavioral sciences. Nonlinear Dynamics Psychol. Life Sci. 8, 121–130.

Geladi, P., Kowalski, B.R., 1986. Partial least-squares regression—a tutorial. Anal. Chim. Acta. 185, 1–17.

Grant, M.R., Mostov, K.E., Tlsty, T.D., Hunt, C.A., 2006. Simulating properties of in vitro epithelial cell morphogenesis. *PLoS Comput. Biol.* 2.

Grimm, V., Revilla, E., Berger, U., et al., 2005. Pattern-oriented modeling of agent-based complex systems: lessons from ecology. Science 310, 987–991.

Hartemink, A.J., Gifford, D.K., Jaakkola, T.S., Young, R.A., 2001. Using graphical models and genomic expression data to statistically validate models of genetic regulatory networks. *Pac. Symp. Biocomput.* ?:422–433.

Ingham, P.W., McMahon, A.P., 2001. Hedgehog signaling in animal development: paradigms and principles. Genes Dev. 15, 3059–3087.

Jacob, L., Lum, L., 2007. Deconstructing the hedgehog pathway in development and disease. Science 318, 66–68.

Janes, K.A., Albeck, J.G., Gaudet, S., Sorger, P.K., Lauffenburger, D.A., Yaffe, M.B., 2005. A systems model of signaling identifies a molecular basis set for cytokine-induced apoptosis. Science 310, 1646–1653.

Janes, K.A., Lauffenburger, D.A., 2006. A biological approach to computational models of proteomic networks. Curr. Opin. Chem. Biol. 10, 73–80.

Janes, K.A., Yaffe, M.B., 2006. Data-driven modelling of signal-transduction networks. Nat. Rev. Mol. Cell Biol. 7, 820–828.

Jensen, F.V., Nielsen, T.D., 2007. Bayesian Networks and Decision Graphs, 2nd ed. Springer, New York, USA.

Jeong, J., Mao, J., Tenzen, T., Kottmann, A.H., McMahon, A.P., 2004. Hedgehog signaling in the neural crest cells regulates the patterning and growth of facial primordia. Genes Dev. 18, 937–951.

Jeong, J., McMahon, A.P., 2005. Growth and pattern of the mammalian neural tube are governed by partially overlapping feedback activities of the hedgehog antagonists patched 1 and Hhip1. Development 132, 143–154.

Kang, J.S., Zhang, W., Krauss, R.S., 2007. Hedgehog signaling: cooking with Gas1. Sci. STKE pe50.

Keller, A.D., 1995. Model genetic circuits encoding autoregulatory transcription factors. J. Theor. Biol. 172, 169–185.

Kinzler, K.W., Vogelstein, B., 1990. The GLI gene encodes a nuclear protein which binds specific sequences in the human genome. Mol. Cell Biol. 10, 634–642.

Lai, K., Robertson, M.J., Schaffer, D.V., 2004. The sonic hedgehog signaling system as a bistable genetic switch. Biophys. J. 86, 2748–2757.

Longo, D., Peirce, S.M., Skalak, T.C., et al., 2004. Multicellular computer simulation of morphogenesis: blastocoel roof thinning and matrix assembly in Xenopus laevis. Dev. Biol. 271, 210–222.

Lum, L., Beachy, P.A., 2004. The Hedgehog response network: sensors, switches, and routers. Science 304, 1755–1759.

Lupo, G., Harris, W.A., Lewis, K.E., 2006. Mechanisms of ventral patterning in the vertebrate nervous system. Nat. Rev. Neurosci. 7, 103–114.

Marigo, V., Scott, M.P., Johnson, R.L., Goodrich, L.V., Tabin, C.J., 1996. Conservation in hedgehog signaling: induction of a chicken patched homolog by Sonic hedgehog in the developing limb. Development 122, 1225–1233.

Marigo, V., Tabin, C.J., 1996. Regulation of patched by sonic hedgehog in the developing neural tube. Proc. Natl. Acad. Sci. USA 93, 9346–9351.

Markowetz, F., Spang, R., 2007. Inferring cellular networks—a review. BMC Bioinformatics 8 (suppl 6), S5.

Martens, H., Martens, M., 2001. Multivariate Analysis of Quality: An Introduction. John Wiley & Sons, Chichester, UK.

Natarajan, M., Lin, K.M., Hsueh, R.C., Sternweis, P.C., Ranganathan, R., 2006. A global analysis of cross-talk in a mammalian cellular signalling network. Nat. Cell Biol. 8, 571–580.

Neapolitan, R.E., 2004. Learning Bayesian networks. Pearson/Prentice Hall, Upper Saddle River, NJ, USA.

Pe'er, D., 2005. Bayesian network analysis of signaling networks: a primer. Sci. STKE pl4.

Peirce, S.M., Van Gieson, E.J., Skalak, T.C., 2004. Multicellular simulation predicts microvascular patterning and in silico tissue assembly. FASEB J. 18, 731–733.

Perrin, B.E., Ralaivola, L., Mazurie, A., Bottani, S., Mallet, J., d'Alche-Buc, F., 2003. Gene networks inference using dynamic Bayesian networks. Bioinformatics 19 (suppl 2), ii138–ii148.

Piccolo, S., Sasai, Y., Lu, B., De Robertis, E.M., 1996. Dorsoventral patterning in Xenopus: inhibition of ventral signals by direct binding of chordin to BMP-4. Cell 86, 589–598.

Ruiz i Altaba, A., 1999. Gli proteins encode context-dependent positive and negative functions: implications for development and disease. Development 126, 3205–3216.

Ruiz i Altaba, A., Nguyen, V., Palma, V., 2003. The emergent design of the neural tube: prepattern, SHH morphogen and GLI code. Curr. Opin. Genet. Dev. 13, 513–521.

Sachs, K., Perez, O., Pe'er, D., Lauffenburger, D.A., Nolan, G.P., 2005. Causal protein-signaling networks derived from multiparameter single-cell data. Science 308, 523–529.

Segovia-Juarez, J.L., Ganguli, S., Kirschner, D., 2004. Identifying control mechanisms of granuloma formation during M. tuberculosis infection using an agent-based model. J. Theor. Biol. 231, 357–376.

Simpson, M.J., Merrifield, A., Landman, K.A., Hughes, B.D., 2007. Simulating invasion with cellular automata: connecting cell-scale and population-scale properties. Phys. Rev. E Stat. Nonlin. Soft. Matter Phys. 76, 021918.

Steck, H., Jaakkola, T.S., 2004. Predictive discretization during model selection. In: Rasmussen, C.E., Buelthoff, H.H., Schoelkopf, B. (Eds.) Lecture Notes in Computer Science, Vol. 3175. Springer, Berlin, pp. 1–8.

Sugimoto, N., Iba, H., 2004. Inference of gene regulatory networks by means of dynamic differential Bayesian networks and nonparametric regression. Genome. Inform. 15, 121–130.

Tang, J., Ley, K.F., Hunt, C.A., 2007. Dynamics of in silico leukocyte rolling, activation, and adhesion. BMC Syst. Biol. 1, 14.

Tenzen, T., Allen, B.L., Cole, F., Kang, J.S., Krauss, R.S., McMahon, A.P., 2006. The cell surface membrane proteins Cdo and Boc are components and targets of the Hedgehog signaling pathway and feedback network in mice. Dev. Cell. 10, 647–656.

Terano, T., 2005. Agent-based Simulation. Springer, ?.

Thorne, B.C., Bailey, A.M., Peirce, S.M., 2007. Combining experiments with multi-cell agent-based modeling to study biological tissue patterning. Brief, Bioinform. 8, 245–257.

Wang, B., Fallon, J.F., Beachy, P.A., 2000. Hedgehog-regulated processing of Gli3 produces an anterior/posterior repressor gradient in the developing vertebrate limb. Cell 100, 423–434.

Wang, M., Chen, Z., Cloutier, S., 2007. A hybrid Bayesian network learning method for constructing gene networks. Comput. Biol Chem. 31, 361–372.

Wilson, L., Maden, M., 2005. The mechanisms of dorsoventral patterning in the vertebrate neural tube. Dev. Biol. 282, 1–13.

Woolf, P.J., Prudhomme, W., Daheron, L., Daley, G.Q., Lauffenburger, D.A., 2005. Bayesian analysis of signaling networks governing embryonic stem cell fate decisions. Bioinformatics 21, 41–53.

Xiang, Z., Minter, R.M., Bi, X., Woolf, P.J., He, Y., 2007. miniTUBA: medical inference by network integration of temporal data using Bayesian analysis. Bioinformatics 23, 2423–2432.

Yu, J., Smith, V.A., Wang, P.P., Hartemink, A.J., Jarvis, E.D., 2004. Advances to Bayesian network inference for generating causal networks from observational biological data. Bioinformatics 20, 3594–3603.

Zhang, L., Athale, C.A., Deisboeck, T.S., 2007. Development of a three-dimensional multiscale agent-based tumor model: simulating gene–protein interaction profiles, cell phenotypes and multicellular patterns in brain cancer. J. Theor. Biol. 244, 96–107.

CHAPTER 10

Systems Analysis for Systems Biology

Scott Hildebrandt, Neda Bagheri, Rudiyanto Gunawan, Henry Mirsky, Jason Shoemaker, Stephanie Taylor, Linda Petzold and Francis J. Doyle III

University of California, Santa Barbara

OUTLINE

Summary	249	Other Metrics for Systems Analysis	255
Definitions	250	**Applications**	**258**
Introduction	**250**	The Unfolded Protein Response	258
Sensitivity Analysis	**251**	Apoptotic Signaling Pathway	260
Review of Classical Sensitivity Analysis	251	Circadian Rhythm Gene Regulation in Fly, Mouse and Plants	262
Tool for Model Refinement	251	**Acknowledgements**	**270**
Tool for Design of Experiment	253		
Sensitivity Extensions: Stochastic Systems	253		

Summary

This chapter focuses on system's analysis tools and its application to the study of biological systems through mathematical modeling. The fundamental sensitivity analysis concept, or definition, is quite basic: perturbations in model parameters will affect model outputs. However, its implications, extensions and applications are profound and numerous in the field of systems biology. For example, sensitivity analysis results imply that certain parameters affect certain model outputs more or less than others, and may be used to guide model refinement and/or experimental design. The basic definition of sensitivity may be extended for application to specialized conditions that arise (although not exclusively) in biology, such as stochasticity and oscillatory behavior.

Examples of how these aforementioned sensitivity analysis implications and extensions have already been applied to biological systems are provided. The *Saccharomyces cerevisiae* unfolded protein response and the apoptotic signaling pathway are used to illustrate model refinement and experimental design guided by sensitivity analysis. The *Arabidopsis thaliana* circadian rhythm model is refined using an extension of the basic sensitivity analysis for oscillatory systems. The *Drosophila melanogaster* circadian rhythm is used for the further demonstration and development of the application of sensitivity analysis to the study of oscillatory systems. Finally, sensitivity analysis is used to explore a stochastic, oscillatory system: the mouse circadian rhythm.

Definitions

Chemical Master Equations (CMEs) Differential equations that represent the temporal evolution of state density functions and describe stochastic variations as Markov processes.
Circadian entrainment The process in which a circadian rhythm synchronizes its oscillations to match a cyclic external input.
D-optimal design Experimental design protocol that seeks to minimize parameter noise by maximizing the determinant of the Fisher Information Matrix.
Fisher Information Matrix (FIM) Scores parametric sensitivity based on Gaussian output measurement noise and output noise resulting from parametric / input perturbations.
Sensitivity analysis Specifically ascribes model output variation to its sources, such as certain parametric perturbations.
Stochasticity System property in which the system's current state is not wholly determined by its previous states, but exhibits random characteristics.

INTRODUCTION

As progress occurs in mathematical modeling of biological systems at the molecular, cellular and whole-organism levels, issues related to robustness of the models, in addition to the underlying biophysical network, have arisen. Of particular interest is the problem of pinpointing the areas of robustness ("insensitivity") and fragility ("sensitivity") within the biological networks. A recurring theme that has emerged over the past several years is that complex network architectures are *robust yet fragile* (Csete and Doyle, 2002). These tradeoffs are important both for model refinement through iterations with experiments and for unraveling design principles. Methods for approaching these issues have been developed in classical control and systems biology theory, including the use of *sensitivity* operators that relate system response to perturbations.

Parametric sensitivity has found widespread application in the analysis and design of both scientific and engineering systems (Varma et al., 1999). In the field of systems biology, sensitivity analysis has been used in a number of applications, including optimized design of synthetic circuits (Feng et al., 2004), design of experiments for optimal parameter estimation (Gadkar et al., 2005; Zak et al., 2003) and robustness analysis to provide insights into design principles (Stelling et al., 2004). The sensitivity operator describes the change in the system's outputs arising from variations in the parameters that affect the system dynamics. High sensitivity to a parameter suggests that the system's performance (e.g. growth, temperature, and so on) can drastically change with small variations in the parameter. Conversely, a small value of the sensitivity suggests that the system is not strongly affected by the parameter.

In this chapter, the tools from classical sensitivity analysis are outlined, and described with application to the unraveling of design principles

SENSITIVITY ANALYSIS

Review of Classical Sensitivity Analysis

Sensitivity analysis investigates the changes in a system's behavior in response to infinitesimal parametric perturbations. If the system dynamics are governed by a set of real ordinary differential equations of the form:

$$\frac{d\mathbf{y}}{dt} = \mathbf{f}(t, \mathbf{y}(t), \mathbf{p}) \quad (10.1)$$

a perturbation in some parameter p_j will cause a change in the state values $\mathbf{y}$. This phenomenon is quantified by sensitivity coefficients—the first-order partial derivatives of $\mathbf{y}$ with respect to $\mathbf{p}$:

$$S_{ij}(t) = \frac{\partial y_i}{\partial p_j}(t) \quad (10.2)$$

where y_i is the ith state and p_j is the jth parameter (Varma et al., 1999). It is straightforward to compute the values of S by coupling the system equations with the sensitivity differential equations:

$$\dot{\mathbf{S}} = \left(\frac{\partial \mathbf{f}}{\partial \mathbf{y}}\right)\mathbf{S}(t) + \frac{\partial \mathbf{f}}{\partial \mathbf{p}}, \quad \mathbf{S}(0) = 0 \quad (10.3)$$

This captures dynamical sensitivities; the sensitivities themselves change with time, much like the evolution of the states themselves. To reduce the data in $\mathbf{S}$ to a sensitivity score for each parameter, we use the Fisher Information Matrix (FIM). The theoretical underpinnings of the FIM relate information content to measurements with Gaussian noise. In this context, it is not information content in a noisy system, but the overall effect of a potential parametric perturbation that is measured by the FIM. Given the assumption that parametric perturbations will cause locally linear effects, the diagonal elements of the FIM provide a sensitivity score for each parameter. To compute the FIM, we sum the sensitivity coefficients and a covariance matrix for each state x_i at each time step t_k:

$$\mathbf{FIM} = \sum_{i=1}^{N_y} \mathbf{S}_{i*}^T \mathbf{V}_i^{-1} \mathbf{S}_{i*}, \quad \mathbf{V}_i = \begin{bmatrix} \sigma_i^2(t_1) & 0 & 0 \\ 0 & \ddots & 0 \\ 0 & 0 & \sigma_i^2(t_{Nt}) \end{bmatrix} \quad (10.4)$$

where the diagonal elements of $\mathbf{V}_i$ are $\sigma_i(t_k) = \text{relative\_scale}_i \cdot y_i(t_k) + \text{absolute\_min}_i$

In practice, it is useful to supply the same relative scaling factor for each state and a very small absolute minimum value. To produce the sensitivity score r_j for each parameter p_j, we normalize the diagonal of the FIM by the parameter values:

$$r_j = \sqrt{(\mathbf{D} \times \mathbf{FIM} \times \mathbf{D})_{jj}}, \quad \mathbf{D} = \begin{bmatrix} p_1 & 0 & 0 \\ 0 & \ddots & 0 \\ 0 & 0 & p_{Np} \end{bmatrix} \quad (10.5)$$

The parameters can be rank ordered; the system is most sensitive to the parameter with the largest sensitivity score.

Tool for Model Refinement

Sensitivity analysis results may be used in refining a mathematical model to improve its performance and/or reduce its dimensionality (number of equations). In the case of improving model performance (e.g. to achieve a better match with experimental data) sensitivity analysis identifies components most influential in determining overall model behavior. These components—indicated by parameters with large-magnitude sensitivity values—serve as focal points for initiating behavior modification.

The key to improving model performance using sensitivity analysis lies in the ability to define the property(ies) that best encapsulate(s) "improved model performance." For example, if one desires to use sensitivity analysis to achieve a certain steady-state concentration of protein, one must consider the steady-state sensitivities for that protein. The most descriptive sensitivities may not be as straightforward when dynamical data are being considered. Depending on the desired behavior, one or more of the following trajectory characteristics may be relevant: the final time point value, timing and/or value of a characteristic peak, mean value, period, phase difference as compared with another state. In addition, the sensitivities of the property(ies) must be considered. When more than one property is under consideration, the individual property sensitivities may be summed—*after* they have been property-scaled—to provide combined sensitivity measures, because of the assumption of model linearity within the parameter range of sensitivity calculation.

From the combined sensitivity measures (for correct comparison, they should also be parameter-scaled), one selects parameter sensitivities of relatively large magnitude, based on one's judgment, to guide the model refinement. When modification of model structure is desired, the selected parameters indicate points at which structure modifications most effectively modulate system behavior; the modifications should be carried out using one's familiarity with the biological system. When it is desired to modify parameter values, the values of the selected parameters should be altered, and the sensitivity results will guide these alterations in two ways. First, the directionality of the sensitivity values will prescribe directionality for the alterations: negative sensitivity values indicate a negative correlation between property and parameter value, and positive sensitivities indicate a positive one. Secondly, for strongly linear systems, sensitivities will prescribe the magnitude of the alterations, as small property changes resulting from small parameter changes during sensitivity calculation may be extended to larger spans of parameter space. That is, $S = (\partial y / \partial p) \approx (\Delta y / \Delta p)$ may be used to predict the change in parameter value required to produce the desired change in property value. Note that combined property- and parameter-scaled sensitivities must be decomposed and unscaled for performing these predictions. Even for non-linear systems, these predictions may provide insightful starting values.

When sensitivity analysis is used to reduce a model, small-magnitude sensitivities become of interest. Parameters responsible for these values signal points in the model structure with no great influence on the property at hand (when reducing, one typically considers overall system behavior sensitivity, obtained by summing all state-scaled state sensitivities; again, sensitivities should be parameter-scaled for comparison). Guided by one's familiarity with the scope and focus of the model, one may reduce it at these low-sensitivity points and expect negligible effects on model behavior, while keeping in mind one important caveat: removing system components may introduce perturbations too large for sensitivity analysis to provide an accurate prediction of the consequent output effects, again depending upon model linearity. In such cases, one may use an optimization approach, such as that proposed by Zhu and Petzold (1999), in which components are chosen for removal, so that the solution of the reduced model is closest to that of the full-size model.

Tool for Design of Experiment

Hypothesis Generation and Discrimination

Arguably, the most powerful application of mathematical models in biology is hypothesis generation and discrimination, and the use of models is becoming more common (Bagci et al., 2006; Blumenfeld et al., 2006). In large, complex systems such as those in biology, system complexity generally overwhelms experimental intuition. Models allow experimenters to generate testable hypotheses to differentiate complex behaviors in cellular networks via *in-silico* experimentation.

Several characteristics of differentiating models may be probed during hypothesis validation. Exploring time trajectories is often the first test when distinguishing two competing scenarios, but the value of these results is generally limited by experimental capacity in biology. Thus other model characteristics are often explored that may be more easily validated, such as steady-state characteristics (bifurcation diagrams) and sensitivity curves. An example of hypothesis generation and discrimination is provided later in the section on Applications (Hypothesis Discrimination).

Experiment Optimization

The quality of the data produced during experimentation is strongly correlated with the conditions in which the experiment is performed. Regardless of the analysis, poor data may lead to poor results, often incurring unnecessary financial and time losses, as it may be necessary to repeat procedures. Given a model system, the FIM provides a means of optimizing the quality of data by establishing the set of conditions in which the accuracy of parameter estimation is maximized—or, equally, the variability of the estimates is minimized.

Two important features in considering the quality of data during experimental design are measurement variability (i.e., measurement error) and the dependence of the measurements on changes in experimental factors (i.e., manipulated inputs, known disturbances, and so on). The FIM quantifies both of these characteristics. The "size" of the FIM is inversely proportional to the measurement noise, and directly proportional to sensitivity of the system. The condition required to use the FIM for experiment optimization is given by the Cramer–Rao inequality (Cover and Thomas, 1991), which states:

$$| \mathbf{V}_p | \geq | \mathbf{FIM}^{-1} | \qquad (10.6)$$

where $|\mathbf{V}_p|$ and $|\mathbf{FIM}^{-1}|$ are suitable norms for the matrices. Thus parameter variation due to noise in the measurements can be minimized by maximizing the "magnitude" of the FIM. There are many ways to describe the magnitude of a matrix. Here, D-optimal design, which maximizes the determinant of the FIM, is used, but several FIM-based criteria exist and have been applied to biological systems. Faller et al. (2003) used D-optimal design, along with several other design techniques, on a mitogen-activated protein kinase pathway, revealing that richer input dynamics increase parameter accuracy. Furthermore, D-optimal design has been integrated into an iterative technique of model identification and applied to an apoptosis model (Gadkar et al., 2005; Gunawan et al., 2006).

Sensitivity Extensions: Stochastic Systems

A cell can be likened to a microscopic chemical plant, in which different cellular components (mRNAs, proteins) are produced, transformed and consumed (or degraded) to accomplish cellular functions. However, unlike a typical chemical plant, cellular processes such as gene transcription and protein translation, involve very low concentrations of molecules (of the order of nanomolar) (McAdams and Arkin, 1999). Such low concentration means that these processes can only occur intermittently, as discrete and random events. This intrinsic stochastic behavior gives rise to variations in cellular phenotype, even in clonal cell population, which have been shown in both prokaryotes (Elowitz et al., 2002) and eukaryotes (Colman-Lerner et al., 2005). Thus, to understand the functional behavior of a biological network, the intrinsic variations in cellular processes should be explicitly taken into consideration in the system modeling and analysis.

For the reason mentioned above, discrete stochastic modeling through the use of chemical master equations (CMEs) has recently gained a lot of attention in the computational biology community (Arkin et al., 1998; Forger and Peskin, 2005; Weinberger et al., 2005). A CME describes the cellular stochastic variations as a Markov process, and is a very high-dimensional differential equation system representing the temporal evolution of the state density function under the assumption of a well mixed volume. At the thermodynamic limit (large number of molecules), the average of the density function described by a CME will effectively reduce to the reaction-rate differential equations (Gillespie and Mangel, 1981). Such stochastic descriptions of cellular behavior have been successful in explaining the phenotypic variations seen in experiments and providing biological insights such as microbial survivability (Wolf et al., 2005) and human immunodeficiency virus latency (Weinberger et al., 2005). Furthermore, the stochastic variations can induce system behaviors, such as bistability (Samoilov et al., 2005) and oscillation (Bratsun et al., 2005), that are different from the dynamics predicted by a deterministic (continuous) model. Indeed, a previous study indicated that ignoring the underlying stochastic behavior may lead to incorrect analysis of the system behavior (Gunawan et al., 2005). This study extended the sensitivity analysis to the case of CMEs, which is summarized below.

In a CME, the system states (such as protein and mRNA levels) are assumed to be random variables described by a joint probability distribution. This probability distribution changes as different cellular processes occur in a cell. As motivated above, because of the low molecular counts, each process has a likelihood of occurrence defined by the propensity function, a_j. Here, the quantity $a_j \Delta t$ gives the probability that the jth process will take place within the time window of Δt. Accounting for all the processes that can happen in a given system, the CME describes the evolution of the state joint probability distribution as a function time according to (Gillespie, 1977):

$$\frac{df(\mathbf{x},t;\mathbf{x}_0,t_0)}{dt} = \sum_{j=1}^{n} a_j(\mathbf{x} - \mathbf{v}_j, \mathbf{p}) f(\mathbf{x} - \mathbf{v}_j, t; \mathbf{x}_0, t_0) - a_j(\mathbf{x}, \mathbf{p}) f(\mathbf{x}, t; \mathbf{x}_0, t_0)$$

(10.7)

where $f(\mathbf{x}, t; \mathbf{x}_0, t_0)$ is the joint distribution function of the states $\mathbf{x}$ at time t with the initial condition $\mathbf{x}_0$ at time t_0, $\mathbf{v}_j$ is the vector of stoichiometric change of the state if the jth process occurs, $\mathbf{p}$ is the parameter vector, and n is the total number of processes in the system. An analytical solution to the CME is generally unavailable because of the enormous number of ordinary differential equations produced. However, a numerical solution based upon a Monte Carlo approach is achievable through the stochastic simulation algorithm (SSA) (Gillespie, 1976). Given a set of reaction propensities, the SSA derives the joint probability for the index of the next reaction and the time to this reaction, and is therefore able to simulate the CME to produce realizations of each state. A detailed introduction to the CME, SSA and the relationship between stochastic and deterministic descriptions of a system can be found in Gillespie and Petzold (2006).

The concept of sensitivity described in the previous sections does not directly translate to a CME, because taking the derivative of random variables is not well-defined. Nevertheless, there are at least two approaches to quantify sensitivities in the context of a joint probability distribution (Gunawan et al., 2005). The first is to measure the stochastic sensitivity (i.e., the sensitivity of a CME) using the joint distribution function according to:

$$\hat{S}_j = \frac{df(\mathbf{x},t;\mathbf{x}_0,t_0)}{dp_j} \quad (10.8)$$

The second approach uses the FIM, but without the normality (Gaussian) simplification. In this case, the FIM is expressed in terms of the score function of a probability distribution:

$$\tilde{S}_j = \frac{d\log f(\mathbf{x},t;\mathbf{x}_0,t_0)}{dp_j} \quad (10.9)$$

which can also be interpreted as a stochastic sensitivity measure. Here, each parameter sensitivity is correlated to the ability of that parameter to propagate noise (evident as a shift in probability distribution) to miscellaneous states. With a realized SSA, one may construct a probability distribution of values for any chemical species. One may then modify an SSA by individually multiplying any reaction propensity by lognormal random noise with a mean of one (lognormal noise is used to ensure that the reaction propensity remains positive and a mean of one is used so that the average reaction propensity across time remains unaltered). If this noise is multiplied to an insensitive parameter and probability distributions of states are constructed from the realized SSA, the probability distribution for each state will be essentially identical to that constructed from the SSA lacking extraneous noise. However, if the noise is multiplied to a sensitive parameter, the probability distribution for each state will be shifted substantially from nominal.

From information theory (Cover and Thomas, 1991), the FIM is simply the variance of the score function, that is:

$$FIM = E[\tilde{\mathbf{S}}\tilde{\mathbf{S}}^T] \quad (10.10)$$

where $\tilde{\mathbf{S}}$ is the score sensitivity matrix (i.e., $\tilde{\mathbf{S}} = [\tilde{\mathbf{S}}_1 \ \tilde{\mathbf{S}}_2 \ \cdots \ \tilde{\mathbf{S}}_p]$). This formulation also indicates that the FIM is related to the magnitude (squares) of the sensitivities. Under the assumption that the joint probability density function follows a (multivariate) normal distribution, the FIM reduces to the more familiar form as given in the previous section.

The application of these stochastic sensitivity measures to a gene toggle switch model (Gardner et al., 2000) revealed the importance of explicit noise consideration in describing cellular behavior. In particular, comparison of deterministic and stochastic analyses indicated differences in the key parameters, to which the switching behavior is highly sensitive. A previous study (Gunawan et al., 2005) found a bias caused by the molecular noise, such that the gene toggle can switch at a lower inducer concentration than that predicted by a (deterministic) differential equation model. Here, the underlying cause of the difference is the existence of several steady states in the toggle switch. In a deterministic model, the predicted behavior can only assume one of the steady states, whereas, in a stochastic model, the probability of each steady state is non-zero. In other words, there is always a non-zero likelihood that the system will assume any of the steady states. Such differences may lead to incorrect results when model sensitivity information is being used in systems biology for the purposes of: (i) gaining insights to a biological system, (ii) engineering / design of biological behavior (synthetic biology), and (iii) parameter identification of a biological model.

Other Metrics for Systems Analysis

As previously mentioned, sensitivity analysis may be applied to a variety of dynamic properties,

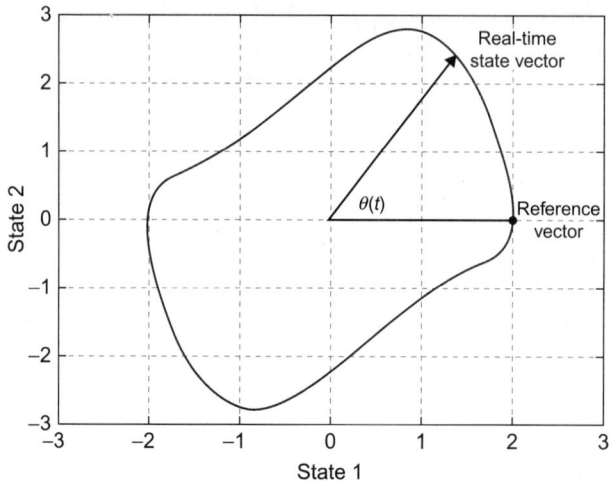

FIGURE 10.1 Limit Cycle Behavior of the Van Der Pol Oscillator. The behavior is mapped such that the origin lies within the enclosed shape. An arbitrary static reference points to the maximum state 1 value. Time-dependent phase measures are defined as the angular difference between the real-time state vector and the reference vector.

and certain measures of property sensitivity are more appropriate for certain systems under certain sets of conditions. For biological oscillators, classic measures include state-, period- and/or amplitude-based sensitivities. However, these oscillators have the ability to synchronize, or entrain, their phase to that of a forcing signal, without affecting the steady-state amplitude or period behavior. Consequently, a set of phase-based sensitivity metrics that take this technicality into account has been defined for the investigation of performance particular to oscillatory systems: period sensitivity, raw phase sensitivity, corrected phase sensitivity and relative phase sensitivity.

Consider a set of non-linear ordinary differential equations that describe a general oscillatory system:

$$\dot{\mathbf{y}} = \mathbf{f}(\mathbf{y}(t), \mathbf{p}), \mathbf{y}(t) \in \mathbb{R}^{Ny}, \mathbf{p} \in \mathbb{R}^{Np}$$
$$\mathbf{y}(t_0) = \mathbf{y}(0), \quad (10.11)$$
$$\mathbf{y}(t + \tau) = \mathbf{y}(t).$$

State dynamics are defined by the Ny time-varying states, and Np parameters. The system's input is defined as one of the Np parameters; the output is defined by an attribute of the system's phase as a measure of radians, $\theta(t,\mathbf{p})$, or time, $\phi(t,\mathbf{p})$.

The system's angular phase is defined by the radian difference between the real-time vector and a predetermined reference vector, $\mathbf{r}$, as projected on the system's limit cycle (Fig. 10.1). Phase measures may be calculated via the cosine rule:

$$\cos(\theta(t, \mathbf{p})) = \frac{\mathbf{y}(t, \mathbf{p})^T \cdot \mathbf{r}}{\| \mathbf{y}(t, \mathbf{p}) \| \cdot \| \mathbf{r} \|}. \quad (10.12)$$

Angular phase dynamics are recorded for independent parametric perturbations, where /tilde/ is used to denote results associated with a finite magnitude perturbation, δ, affecting the jth element of the parameter vector. $\hat{\mathbf{e}}_j$ reflects a unit vector in jth dimension.

$$\tilde{\mathbf{p}} = \mathbf{p} + \delta \cdot \hat{\mathbf{e}}_j. \quad (10.13)$$

Period sensitivity may be defined as the accumulation of the change in phase over an entire cycle. As a result, direct evaluation of phase

SENSITIVITY ANALYSIS

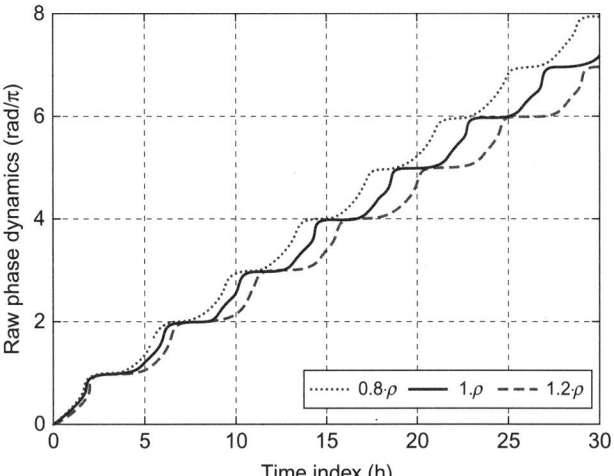

FIGURE 10.2 Raw Phase Trajectories.
The trajectories are plotted against time for ±20% perturbations of the van der Pol model's parameter, ρ. Period sensitivity measures are calculated by evaluating these time-dependent phase measures at a 2π interval and comparing the corresponding time indices. Raw phase sensitivity is determined by evaluating these measures at specific times and comparing their corresponding angular values.

trajectories at a 2π interval, L, yields phase-based period sensitivity:

$$S_j^\tau = \frac{1}{L} \cdot \frac{\tilde{k} - k}{\delta \cdot p_j}\bigg|_{\theta(k,p)=\theta(\tilde{k},\tilde{p})=2\pi \cdot L},$$
$$j \in [1, \mathbf{N}p], \quad L \in [1, \infty] \quad (10.14)$$

where the difference between the perturbed $2\pi L$-radian crossing time, $\tilde{k}$, and the nominal time, k, reflects a numerical approximation of periodic performance that is normalized with respect to the parametric perturbation (Fig. 10.2). The difference between radian measures reflects raw phase sensitivity, as it characterizes a perturbation-induced phase change with respect to the jth parameter, t_k hours after the perturbation:

$$S_j^\theta(t_k) = \frac{\theta(t, \tilde{\mathbf{p}}) - \theta(t, \mathbf{p})}{\delta \cdot p_j}\bigg|_{t=t_k}, j \in [1, \mathbf{N}p]$$

(10.15)

Phase sensitivity grows unbounded in time as a result of the non-uniform expansion of the periodic system. To correct for this response, which is attributed to the coupling of period and phase, each raw phase trajectory is normalized with respect to the perturbation-induced period, $\tilde{\tau}$. Scaling the time by $\tilde{\tau}$ decouples the system's phase from its period. Thus corrected phase trajectories begin and end at the same relative time points (0 and 100% of their respective cycles) (Fig. 10.3). This sensitivity measure characterizes the linear scaling of raw phase measures as a time-dependent performance quantity that identifies specific points of the cycle most susceptible to parametric uncertainty:

$$S_j^{\hat{\theta}}(t) = \frac{\theta(t/\tilde{\tau}, \tilde{\mathbf{p}}) - \theta(t/\tau, \mathbf{p})}{\delta \cdot p_j}, j \in [1, \mathbf{N}p]$$

(10.16)

Apart from an angular measure, phase also defines the time difference between the occurrences of two distinct events. Relative phase

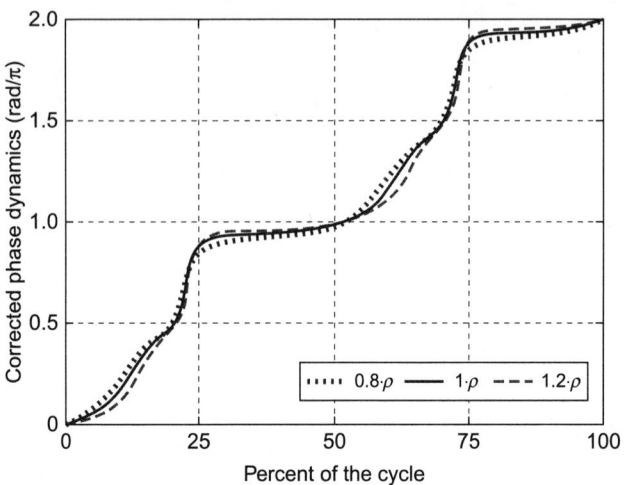

FIGURE 10.3 Corrected Phase Sensitivity.
Corrected phase sensitivity decouples phase and period dynamics by scaling each trajectory with respect to the perturbation-induced period: 7.72 h for 0.8ρ, 8.35 h for ρ and 9.02 h for 1.2ρ. Normalized phase dynamics provide corrected phase sensitivity measures by comparing phase angles as a function of the scaled time.

sensitivity investigates this time interval, $\phi(\mathbf{y}(t), \mathbf{p})$, by relating how individual system components change with respect to one another upon a parametric perturbation:

$$S_j^\phi = \frac{\phi(\mathbf{y}(t), \tilde{\mathbf{p}}) - \phi(\mathbf{y}(t), \mathbf{p})}{\delta \cdot p_j}, \; j \in [1, \mathbf{N}p] \quad (10.17)$$

Sensitivity metrics provide unique values that define system performance; the greater the magnitude, the more susceptible the system is to an isolated parametric perturbation. The methods described in this section are general, and may be applied to oscillators that exhibit stable-limit cycle behavior and monotonic phase dynamics.

APPLICATIONS

The Unfolded Protein Response

As a first exemplary application in biological modeling, sensitivity analysis is used to identify behavioral differences between two activation regulation models for the *Saccharomyces cerevisiae* unfolded protein response (UPR), to prescribe a model invalidation experiment to eliminate one of them. The UPR is triggered in all eukaryotes by increased unfolded protein loads on the secretory pathway within the endoplasmic reticulum, resulting from a variety of stressors including heat shock, chemical treatment and heterologous protein expression. It modulates the production of chaperones and foldases, which encourage and expedite correct protein folding to reduce unfolded protein levels. The *S. cerevisiae* UPR has been traditionally modeled as a negative feedback loop centered on the molecular chaperone, BiP (Kimata et al., 2003; Okamura et al., 2000; Welihinda and Kaufman, 1996). When BiP levels are insufficient to cope with current unfolded protein levels, unfolded protein sequesters it from Ire1p, a transmembrane kinase, and only BiP-free Ire1p may activate and initiate increased chaperone (including BiP) and foldase production—that is, the UPR.

APPLICATIONS

TABLE 10.1 Mean Unfolded Protein Response (UPR) Sensitivity to the BiP–Heterologous Unfolded Protein (Het. UP) Binding Rate for the Traditional and Newer UPR Activation Regulation Models

UPR Actviation Model	State- and Parameter- Scaled Sensitivity	Absolute Sensitivity Difference (New − Old)	Relative Sensitivity Difference	Mean UPR			
				Nominal Parameters	0.1 × BiP– Het.UP Binding	0.001 × BiP– Het.UP Binding	0.00001 × BiP– Het.UP Binding
Old	0.00246871	−0.2345367	1.01063787	641	627	288	149
New	−0.232068			669	1430	1803	1804

Subsequent experimental data have shown that Ire1p has potential for binding unfolded protein (Credle et al., 2005) and activates independent of BiP binding (Kimata et al., 2004). A competing UPR activation model was constructed to reflect the idea that unfolded protein may directly regulate UPR activation, whereas BiP only modulates it (Hildebrandt et al., 2007). When implemented mathematically, both models similarly reproduce experimental data, so a method was needed to systematically and comprehensively probe them for other behavioral differences. This method included performing sensitivity analysis on the two models and comparing the results to identify parameter modifications that effect the greatest behavioral inconsistencies between them.

In detail, a particular state (specifically, a green fluorescent protein marker) was said best to represent UPR behavior, and its sensitivities were calculated for each model for simulations in which the UPR was induced by heterologous unfolded protein expression. Mean sensitivities were scaled by both mean-state and parameter values, so that they could be compared across the models. Comparison involves a two-step process that considers sensitivity, magnitude and direction. First, the absolute difference between two sensitivities is taken by subtracting one sensitivity value from the other. If the magnitude of the absolute difference is heuristically large enough, a relative difference may be calculated:

$$\frac{|\hat{S}_{model1} - \hat{S}_{model2}|}{\max(|\hat{S}_{model1}|, |\hat{S}_{model2}|)} \quad (10.18)$$

where $\hat{S}_{modeln}$ denotes a state- and parameter-scaled sensitivity value for model n. The definition for the minimum significant relative difference is also heuristic, but a value of 0.99 indicates sensitivities two orders of magnitude apart.

Results from UPR sensitivity comparisons showed the greatest disparity between the BiP-heterologous unfolded protein binding rate sensitivities for the two models. In addition, the UPR of the traditional model was positively, and that of the newer model was negatively, correlated to this parameter. From these results, an experiment may be designed to invalidate one of the models: mutate the BiP binding sites on the heterologous unfolded protein to slow binding and observe whether the UPR decreases, according to the traditional model, or increases, according to the newer model, as shown in Table 10.1.

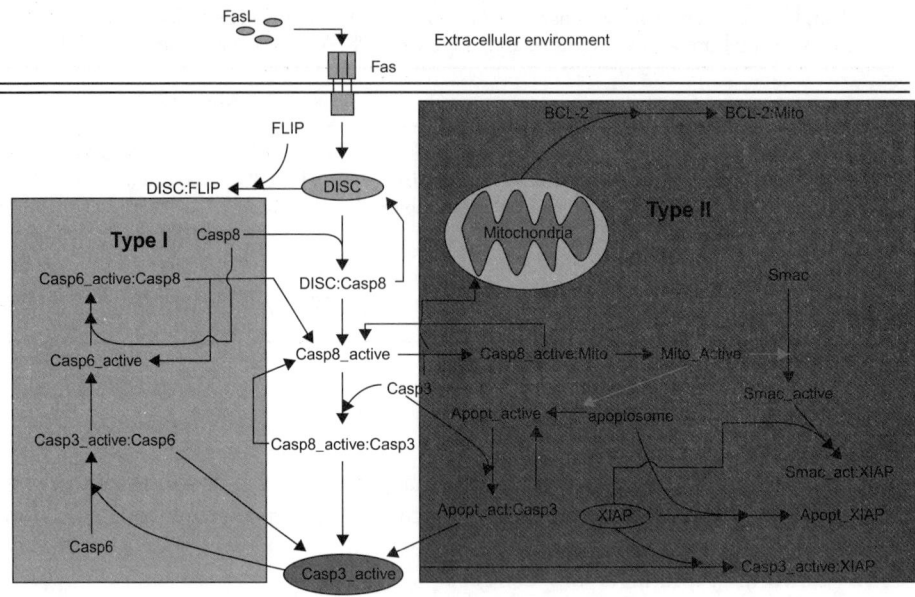

FIGURE 10.4 The Fas Apoptosis Model Proposed by Hua et al. (2006).

Apoptotic Signaling Pathway

As another example, the Fas apoptosis model, developed by Hua et al. (2006), is utilized to illustrate the value of sensitivity analysis in model-based experimental design. Apoptosis—programmed cell death—is critical in the immune response and the development and maintenance of multicellular organisms (Screpanti et al., 2005). Fas apoptosis (Fig. 10.4) is especially significant during the immune response as the apoptosis initiator, Fas ligand (FasL), is expressed on activated T cells and natural killer (NK) cells (Matter et al., 2006). FasL binding to its receptor, Fas, initiates a series of events that includes the formation of the death-inducing complex, transduction of the death signal via the activation of caspase 8 and concludes with the production of the executioner caspase, caspase 3. The death signal is amplified by one of two pathways. In type I dominant cells, positive feedback from the interaction of caspase 8 and caspase 6 allows for an "all-or-nothing" apoptotic response. In type II cells, the signal is amplified via mitochondrial interactions.

Hypothesis Discrimination

Consider two competing hypotheses. In Hypothesis I, type II behavior has been mapped and is considered to be solely responsible for the apoptotic behavior seen in the cellular population; Hypothesis II states that, in addition to type II signaling, caspase 3 production has a positive effect on caspase 8 activation. The model for Hypothesis I is the Hua et al. (2006) model with type I signaling removed. To develop a model for Hypothesis II, an enzymatic Michaelis–Menten kinetic reaction in which caspase 3 further activates caspase 8 production was added, and the parameters were fitted to experimental values when FasL was at its natural concentrations of 10 nM. In this example, the "experimental" system is the original Hua et al. model.

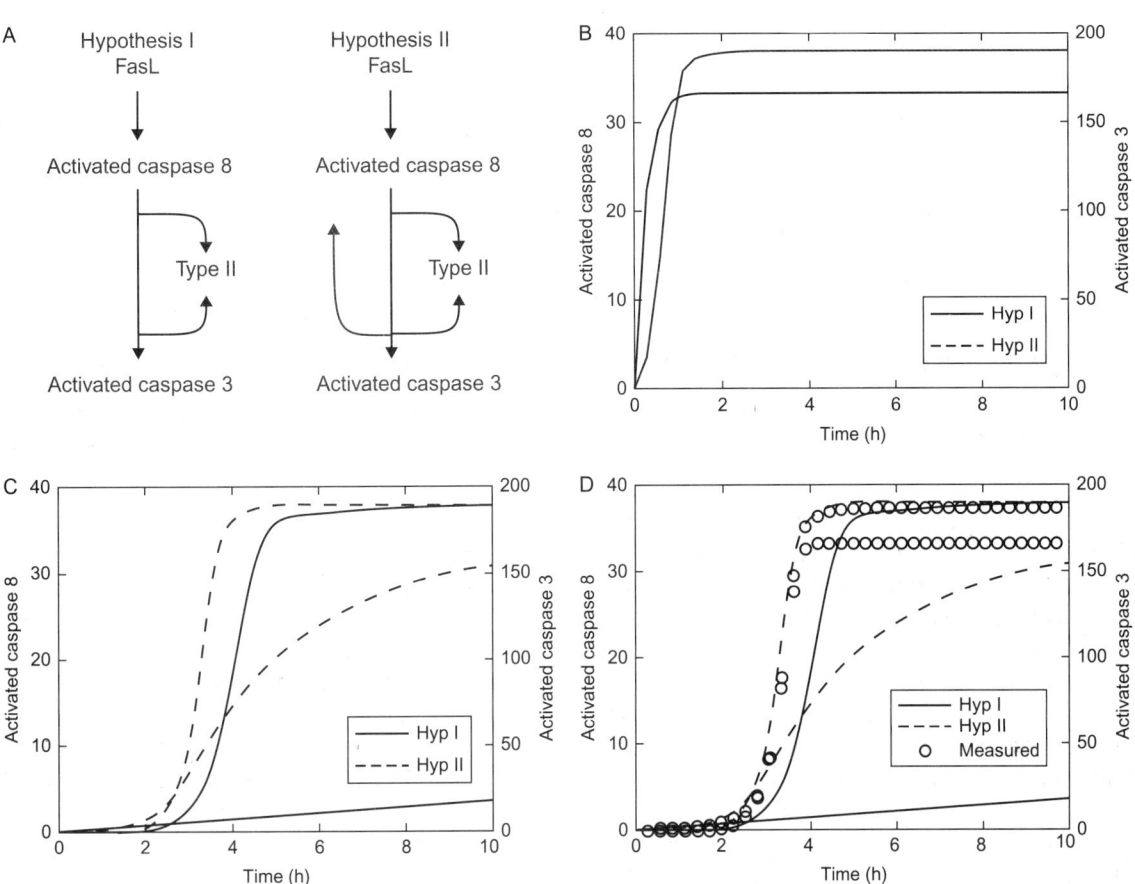

FIGURE 10.5 Hypotheses I and II.
(A) Schematic for Hypothesis I and Hypothesis II. (B–D) The activated caspase 3 (blue lines) and activated caspase 8 (black lines) response curves for both hypotheses. Hypothesis I is represented by a solid line, Hypothesis II by a dashed line. (B) Response curves in conditions of exposure to high FasL levels. (C) Response curves for both hypotheses in conditions of exposure to low FasL levels. (D) Comparing the predicted behaviors of both hypotheses with experimental data obtained with low FasL concentrations.

Once the models had been developed, the manipulatable experimental variables were explored to determine the conditions that maximize the difference between the model predictions. Figure 10.5 shows the predictions for each model in conditions of exposure to high and at low concentrations of FasL when activated caspase 3 and activated caspase 8 are the measurable variables. Measurement of activated caspase 3 alone would not discriminate between the competing hypotheses. With exposure to high levels of FasL, both activated caspase 3 and caspase 8 predictions are mapped identically by both models. With exposure to low levels, some slight variation between the two activated caspase 3 predictions is visible, but it is unlikely that this slight variation would be verifiable, especially given the inherent noise of biological systems. In contrast, activated caspase 8 concentrations predicted by each hypothesis in

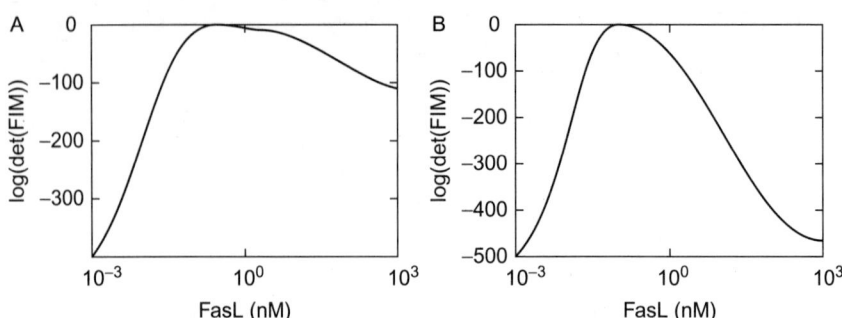

FIGURE 10.6 Applying D-optimal Criteria to the Fas Apoptosis System when the FasL Concentration is a Manipulatable Variable.
(A) The log of the determinant of the FIM [log(det(FIM))] when all states are measurable. (B) The log of the determinant of the FIM when caspases 3 and 8 are measurable.

response to exposure to low levels of FasL show characteristically distinct dynamics: Hypothesis I shows a slow, linear increase in the amount of activated caspase 8, whereas Hypothesis II shows a more rapid, sigmoidal response, clearly distinct from the behavior predicted in Hypothesis I. In Figure 10.5D, the experimental data are plotted against the two predictions for low level FasL exposure and, clearly, Hypothesis II is similar to the experimental data in shape and output gain. Thus Hypothesis I has been invalidated, and Hypothesis II should be further developed.

Experimental Optimization

D-optimal design was applied to the Hua et al. (2006) apoptosis model to identify the optimal conditions that guarantee the greatest accuracy during data collection. First, it was assumed that all states (protein concentrations, gene expressions, and so on) are measurable, and then this result was restricted to a more realistic scenario in which only caspase 3 and caspase 8 concentrations are measurable. For both situations, the concentration of FasL is the manipulatable, environmental variable. Figure 10.6 illustrates how the quality of the information from the experimental measurements varies with initial FasL concentrations. Using complete measurements, the experiment should be conducted using 0.37 nM FasL. Considering only caspase 3 and caspase 8 as measurable, 0.10 nM FasL is the optimal experimental condition. Most importantly, though, note the rapidity with which data quality decreases as a function of initial FasL concentration, particularly in the case when only caspase 3 and 8 are measurable. Small deviations from the optimal greatly depreciate the information content of the collected data.

Circadian Rhythm Gene Regulation in Fly, Mouse and Plants

Across the major kingdoms, organisms possess vital physiological behaviors that follow daily rhythms. Those rhythms are controlled by an endogenous oscillator—the circadian clock, from the Latin *circa* (about) and *dies* (day). The clock responds to environmental cues, adjusting its time-keeping to ensure processes and behaviors are correctly phased with the day. The 24 hour light / dark cycle is the primary entraining signal. Circadian clocks have been studied in bacteria, fungi, plants, flies and mammals. Although clock structure is not identical in these organisms, the core mechanism is conserved; in the gene regulatory network of certain cells, there is a negative feedback loop interlocked with a positive feedback loop. These final sections convey the roles that sensitivity analysis has assumed in studying the circadian clock in a few organisms.

Arabidopsis thaliana

Several genes have been implicated as clock components in the model plant, *Arabidopsis thaliana*; they encode the transcription factors LATE ELONGATED HYPOCOTYL (LHY), CIRCADIAN CLOCK ASSOCIATED 1 (CCA1), and the pseudoresponse regulators TIMING OF CAB (TOC1), PRR7 and PRR9 (Alabadi et al., 2001; Farre et al., 2005). Experimentation has revealed interactions between them, some of which are believed to be indirect. To simulate the proposed system, the first generation of mathematical models were developed (Locke et al., 2005a, 2005b; Zeilinger et al., 2006). They incorporated some or all of the putative clock components, the last two including hypothetical components (X and Y) to serve as intermediaries for the indirect interactions. Mass action and Hill kinetics were used in collections of autonomous ordinary differential equations demonstrating stable periodic (limit cycle) behavior. Because there were inadequate biochemical data to supply values for the kinetic parameters, an optimization procedure was used to find parameters that minimized the difference between model behavior and experimental data.

Model fidelity to plant behavior was assessed using both *in-silico* (numerical) experiments and sensitivity analysis. One would expect robustness to appear in parameters associated with the intrinsic operation of the clock; therefore perturbations caused by environmentally-induced kinetic variance (e.g. temperature fluctuations) would not appreciably affect clock performance. Conversely, one would expect the clock to be sensitive to parameters governing required environmental input. Unexpected sensitivity in a non-input parameter could then indicate a flaw in modeling: either additional regulators are absent, or the interactions are captured incorrectly.

The early models were tested for the robustness of rhythms despite small finite perturbations. They were shown to maintain periodic behavior with acceptable variation in period and amplitude despite 5% perturbations in parameters (Locke et al., 2005a, 2005b).

Zeilinger et al. (2006) used the FIM-based rankings to determine which processes were the most sensitive. Transcription of hypothetical component X was a sensitive process. Because X was modeled as a regulator of LHY and CCA1, Zeilinger and colleagues concluded that experimental energy must be expended to determine more about the regulation of LHY and CCA1. To show that these results pertained to the model structure, rather than the specific parameter set, a more comprehensive sensitivity analysis proposed by Stelling et al. (2004) was performed. Using a Monte Carlo method to explore parameter space, sensitivity rankings were evaluated at each point. The rankings were conserved with small variance across parameter sets (Fig. 10.7); this confirmed the conclusion that the model structure caused transcription of X to be sensitive.

Fly

In studies of the circadian rhythm of the fruit fly (*Drosophila melanogaster*), phase-based sensitivity metrics have been applied to the free-running 10-state mathematical model (Leloup and Golbeter, 1998). In this system, oscillations derive from two coupled negative feedback loops involving *period* and *timeless* genes and protein dynamics. The phase-based performance of states 1 (*per* mRNA) and 10 (nuclear PER/TIM complex) were highlighted for this study. The corresponding limit cycle was shifted such that the enclosed shape encompassed the origin. A reference vector that points to the maximum mRNA concentration was defined. Angular phase measurements were recorded for dynamics reflecting isolated

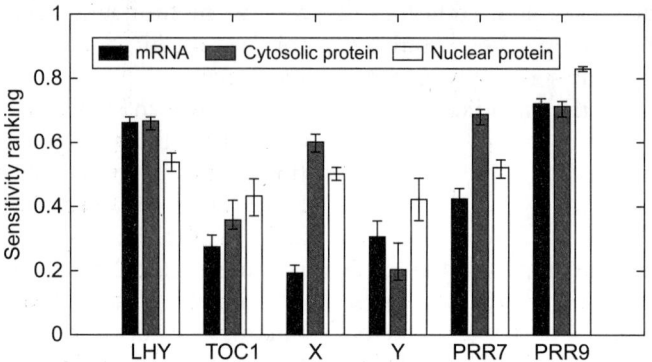

FIGURE 10.7 Sensitivity Rankings of the Monte Carlo Multidimensional Analysis for the PRR7-PRR9-Y' Model Proposed by Zeilinger et al. (2006).
Sensitivity rankings range from 0 (very sensitive) to 1 (not sensitive). Parameters are grouped by gene and then by component (mRNA, cytosolic protein and nuclear protein). Error bars denote standard deviations of the grouped rankings in the applied Monte Carlo search of 10 000 parameter sets. Adapted from Zeilinger et al. (2006), with permission.

parameter perturbations of ±10% for each of the 37 parameters. Angle measurements were unwrapped and evaluated at 18 hours, yielding raw phase sensitivity measures. These same trajectories were evaluated at $2\pi L$, providing phase-based period sensitivity measures. The perturbation-induced period was determined in each simulation and used to scale the corresponding the time index. Scaled phase data were used to measure corrected phase sensitivity.

For consistency, relative phase describes the timing between peak *per* mRNA (state 1) and nuclear PER/TIM complex (state 10) concentrations. The shrinking or expanding of this time interval was recorded for the same set of isolated parametric perturbations and used to generate relative phase sensitivity results.

Each performance measure provided unique sensitivity values that were rank-ordered from least to most sensitive. Parameters that greatly affect system performance have larger absolute sensitivity values and were assigned higher integer ranks. Table 10.2 lists each metric along with five of the 37 system parameters that greatly affect its performance and five that least affect performance. Similarity among the metrics rank distributions suggests a conservation of sensitivity, whereas differences highlight the definition of performance of an individual metric. One means of comparing sensitivity measures is through correlation diagrams: strongly correlated rank distributions suggest similar performance characteristics with respect to parametric perturbations. Select correlation diagrams for a *Drosophila* model [Leloup, J.-C., Goldbeter, A., 1998] are shown in Figure 10.8. A consistent result among these diagrams is that model performance is more sensitive to biochemical processes involving transcription, translation, mRNA degradation and other global parameter rate as these parameter are found in the upper right quadrant; performance is less sensitive to (de)phosphorylation and similar local parameter rates as their corresponding data points reside in the lower left quadrant. More specifically, global parameters describe core cellular reactions that are non-specific to the circadian network. Local parameters describe processes that are specific to the network and not shared with other cellular circuits (Stelling et al., 2004).

A more complete description of the Drosophila model [Leloup, J.-C., Goldbeter, A., 1998] parametric sensitivity distributions with respect to parameter function and type is depicted in

TABLE 10.2 Sensitivity Metrics Provide Unique Performance Measures with Respect to Isolated Parametric Perturbations Parameters assigned large sensitivity values greatly affect corresponding output dynamics. The five most and least sensitive parameters for each metric are defined below. Similarity among metrics suggests a conservation of sensitivity that is highlighted in Figures 10.8 and 10.9.

	Sensitivity rank	Raw Phase		Period		Corrected Phase		Relative Phase	
		Parameter index	Absolute sensitivity	Parameter index	Absolute sensitivity	Parameter index	Absolute sensitivity	Parameter index	Absolute sensitivity
Least sensitive	1	1	5.69E-20	27	0.071744	10	0.001105	19	0.055422
	2	7	6.61E-20	10	0.071744	27	0.001105	10	0.056982
	3	24	6.61E-20	31	0.080751	31	0.001985	27	0.056982
	4	28	9.09E-20	14	0.080751	14	0.001985	14	0.060061
	5	32	1.54E-19	9	0.212093	24	0.002958	31	0.060061
Most sensitive	33	21	1.9916E-15	33	11.394597	21	2.825322	33	10.772674
	34	3	2.1449E-15	18	11.394597	2	3.239289	18	10.772674
	35	5	1.4388E-13	35	20.159789	35	3.251999	35	19.983786
	36	36	1.4394E-13	37	45.158422	5	5.043859	37	42.969703
	37	37	1.4408E-13	5	59.543394	37	7.626592	5	53.597704

Figure 10.9, where parameters are grouped on eh basis of biochemical function (upper subplot) and type (lower subplot). Relative sensitivity ranks are denoted by the shading of each cell: dark shading indicates a lower average sensitivity rank among the function/group, whereas lighter shading indicates a greater average sensitivity. The vertical height of each shaded section reflects the number of parameters in each function/group relative to the total number of parameters. Figure 10.9 includes data from state-based sensitivity analysis (discussed in the section on Sensitivity Analysis (Review of Classical Sensitivity Analysis)) that further validates the conservation of sensitivity, as global parameters consistently influence performance more than local parameters. These metrics have been used to assess the performance of different circadian networks (namely, mammalian models) and provided similar results: although performance is a function of the defined output measure, there exists a conservation of sensitivity among parameter function and type.

Fly—Entrained

Circadian entrainment refers to the process in which a circadian rhythm synchronizes its oscillations to match a cyclic external input such as sunlight. This is arguably the most important function of circadian rhythms—that is, to tell the time of the day analogous to a (biological) clock. In fact, the circadian-ness of these rhythms evolves to achieve a robust entrainment, which

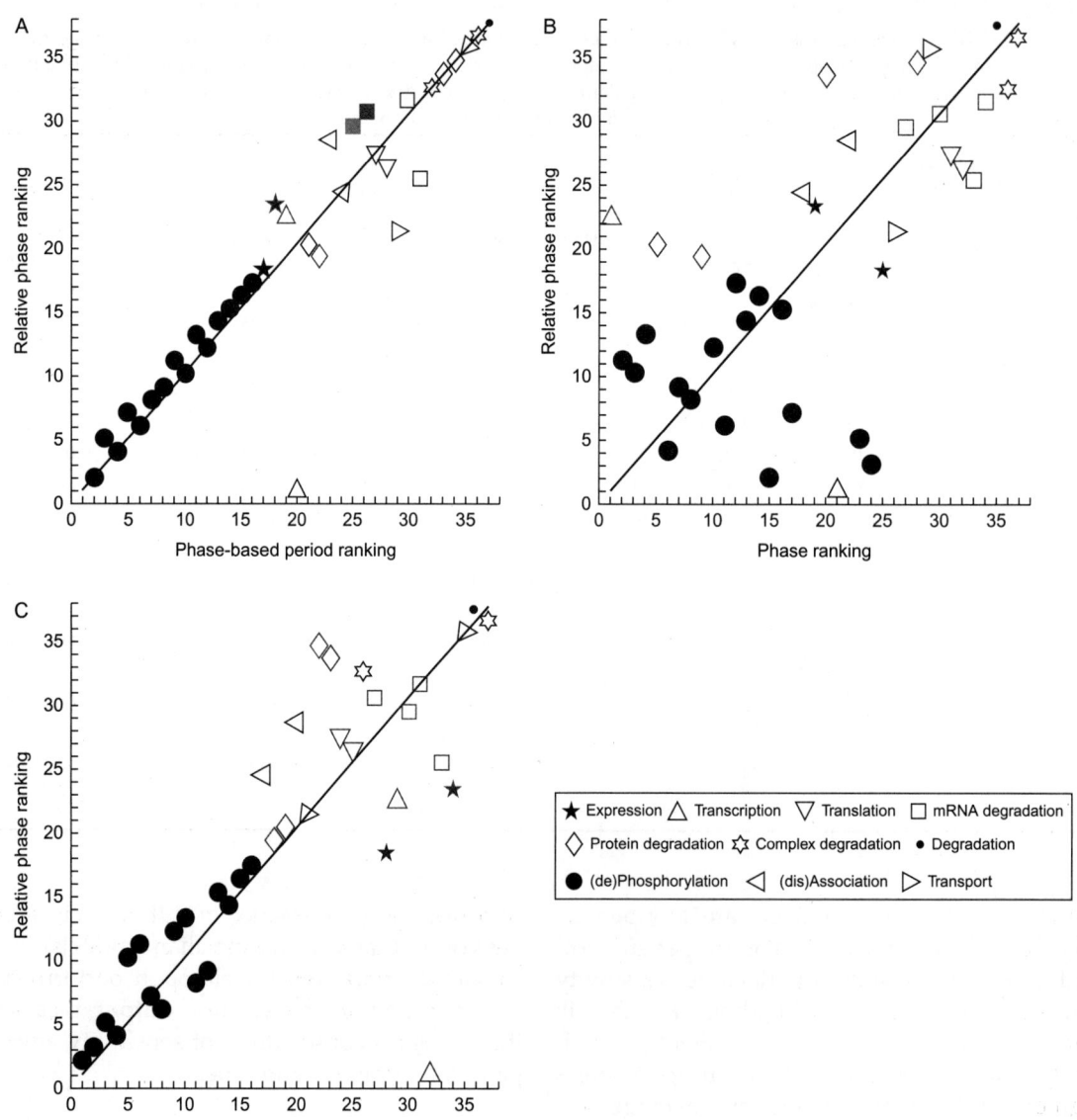

FIGURE 10.8 Comparing Sensitivity Measures Through Correlation Diagrams.
Sensitivity measures for a *Drosophila* model [Leloup, J.-C., Goldbeter, A., 1998] are rank ordered from least to greatest absolute value and assigned integer numbers reflecting their relative sensitivity. Resulting rank distributions are plotted against each other to investigate correlation: (A) period versus relative phase sensitivity, (B) raw phase versus relative phase sensitivity and (C) corrected phase versus relative phase sensitivity. Parameter function is denoted by the shape of the data point and the parameter type is described by the shading: white-filled shapes reflect global parameters; gray-filled shapes reflect mixed parameters; black-filled shapes reflect local parameters. *per*-related dynamics are outlined in red and *tim*-related dynamics in green. The conservation of sensitivity is noted by the consistency in the lower left (least sensitive) quadrants compared with the upper right (most sensitive) quadrant: black-filled circular shapes are consistently less sensitive than white-filled data points.

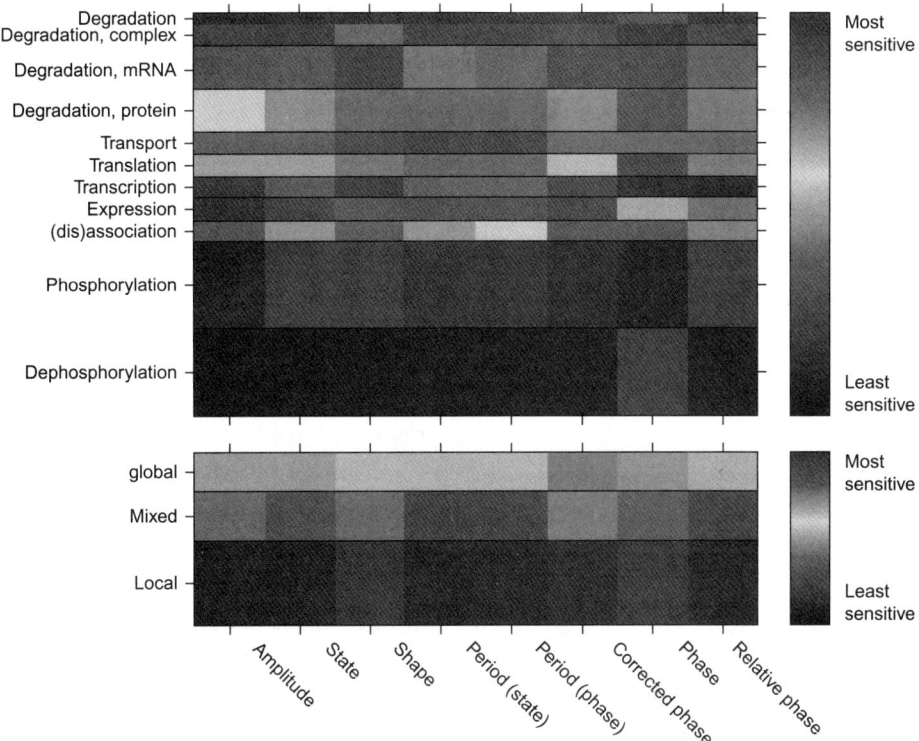

FIGURE 10.9 Average Sensitivity Rank of Parameters.
The average sensitivity rank among parameters of the same function (top subplot) and type (bottom subplot) is denoted by the color shading of each cell: the lighter the shading the higher the sensitivity rank. The average sensitivity of each group is mostly consistent across varying performance metrics, including state-based sensitivity analysis.

is defined by a stable phase angle between the entraining agent, called the *zeitgeber* (time-giver), and the daily cycles of the organism (Pittendrigh and Daan, 1976). There are two signatures of circadian entrainment: the first is period matching with a stable (unique) phase angle, and the second is the preservation of this phase angle upon removal of the zeitgeber (Johnson et al., 2003). The first characteristic allows circadian rhythms to control the physiological functions of organisms to anticipate daily cycles and to adapt to seasonal changes. The second implies that the zeitgeber carries along the internal circadian phase, as opposed to a synchronization of behavior without circadian rhythm interactions, known as *masking* ((Mrosovsky, 1999). The molecular aspect as to how a zeitgeber, most importantly light, affects the circadian rhythm regulation has been identified for many organisms, such as fly (Myers et al., 1996) and mouse (Dunlap, 1999). Despite the existence of a large amount of data, the underlying principle of circadian entrainment remains unclear.

Entrainment is inherently a phase behavior, and thus its analysis requires a measure of phase, as was described in the previous section. However, circadian entrainment is not an autonomous system, as the rhythm is entrained to a cyclic input. In this case, the phase analysis based on isochrons is not applicable, because all points that converge to the entrained limit cycle will have the same phase, by definition of entrainment.

One approach to the study of entrainment is to quantify the phase using extrema of the oscillations, such as the maximum and/or minimum concentrations of mRNAs and proteins. For example, in *Drosophila*, the peak level of PER mRNA appears to track dusk (Qiu and Hardin, 1996). This section summarizes the development of a novel sensitivity analysis of entrained oscillatory systems (Gunawan and Doyle, 2006).

Suppose that the entrained system is described by a set of ordinary differential equations:

$$\frac{d\mathbf{y}}{dt} = g(\mathbf{y}, \mathbf{p}, u) \quad (10.19)$$

where $\mathbf{y}$ and $\mathbf{p}$ are the state and parameter vectors, respectively, g is a vector of non-linear functions, and u is the cyclic input (e.g. zeitgeber). An extremum of the ith state is defined by:

$$g_i(\mathbf{y}_e(t_e), \mathbf{p}, u) = 0 \quad (10.20)$$

where $\mathbf{y}_e$ is the state vector at the extremum at time t_e. Taking the derivative of the above equation with respect to the parameter p_j, and followed by a simplification, gives the parametric sensitivity of the time of extremum t_e:

$$\frac{\partial t_e}{\partial p_j} = \frac{\partial \Psi}{\partial p_j} = -\left.\frac{\frac{\partial g_i^T}{\partial \mathbf{y}}\frac{\partial \mathbf{y}}{\partial p_j} + \frac{\partial g_i}{\partial p_j}}{\frac{\partial g_i^T}{\partial \mathbf{y}} g}\right|_{t=t_e} \quad (10.21)$$

where Ψ is the entrained phase angle as defined by the extremum of the ith state. This sensitivity analysis can be applied to investigate the robustness of entrainment to variations in the circadian periodicity and the length of day (seasonal tracking). Here, the two appropriate performance metrics are given by:

$$\pi_1 = \frac{d\Psi}{dT} \quad (10.22)$$

for periodicity and

$$\pi_2 = \frac{d\Psi}{dT_{day}} \quad (10.23)$$

for length of day variation. The variable T in the first metric actually denotes the zeitgeber period, instead of the circadian period. This is done to emulate a T-cycle experiment, in which the phase angles are measured for different zeitgeber periods T. In the second metric, T_{day} denotes the length of day, as expected.

The aforementioned sensitivity analysis was previously applied to elucidate the robustness of circadian entrainment using a *Drosophila* model (Gunawan and Doyle, 2006). *In-silico* T-cycle experiments and seasonal day length change studies were performed to highlight the roles of circadian period and phase in attaining a robust phase angle. The study was simulated under two competing hypotheses for circadian entrainment: complete (constant light during day) and skeleton (two light pulses in a cycle) photoperiods. The analysis indicated a trade-off between the contributions of period and phase modulations. In this case, the circadian period τ largely determined the phase angle when τ approximated the zeitgeber period T—that is, when the ratio τ/T nears one. In contrast, the phase modulation appeared to have greater control of the phase angle away from $\tau/T = 1$. This finding gave support for and extended previous single light pulse experiments to the case of photoperiodic entrainment. Furthermore, comparison of parameter sensitivity analysis between the complete and skeleton photoperiods gave indications of experiments to validate these competing hypotheses of entrainment.

Mouse

In studies of mammalian circadian rhythms, sensitivity analysis was performed on the Forger and Peskin (2003) mouse circadian clock

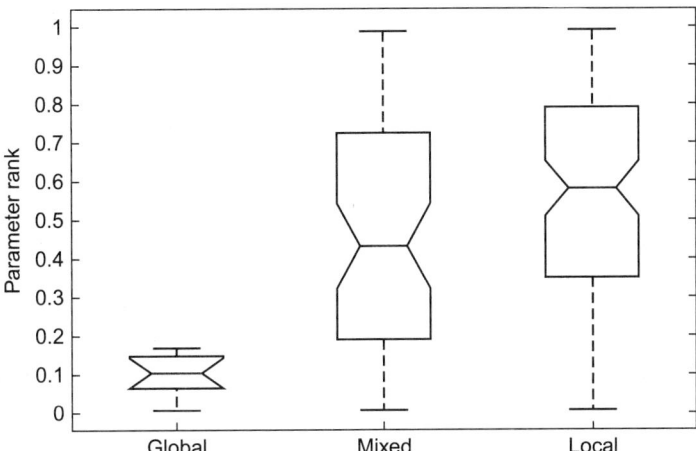

FIGURE 10.10 Normalized Parameter Sensitivity Ranks for the Global, Local, and Mixed Parameter Groups for the Forger and Peskin (2003) Mouse Circadian Clock.
The P value for the difference between global and local sets is 4.21×10^{-6}. A rank of 0 indicates maximum sensitivity of the model to a perturbation in that parameter. A rank of 1 indicates maximum insensitivity of the model to a perturbation in that parameter. Global parameters are those such as translation that are shared by many cellular systems, whereas local parameters are those such as clock protein phosphorylation that are clock specific. Mixed parameters have characteristics of both.

model to assess points of fragility and points of robustness. The software used was BioSens, part of BioSPICE. BioSens uses the FIM to develop an ordered list: the parameter that, when perturbed, has the greatest effect on the clock is listed first, followed by the parameter that, when perturbed, has the second-greatest effect on the clock, and so on through the list of all parameters. The position of each parameter in the generated list was then scaled such that the most sensitive parameter was given a value of 0 and the least sensitive parameter was given a value of 1. Parameters were sorted hierarchically into global, local and mixed classes (Stelling et al., 2004). Box plots were created for each class and the P values separating each class from the others determined (Fig. 10.10). The P value between the global and local set is 4.21×10^{-6}; this statistic and the figure clearly indicate the separation between these classes: the clock is sensitive to perturbations in global parameters and insensitive to perturbations in local parameters. The conclusion is biologically sensible, as a robust clock can be maintained if the global (i.e., non-clock-specific) parameters are fragile (but controlled by cellular machinery outside the clock) whereas the local (i.e., clock-specific) parameters are robust.

The Forger and Peskin model is also available in stochastic form (Forger and Peskin, 2005). One hundred 500-hour realizations of its SSA were made, with data sampled every 0.1 hour. The first 250 hours of each realization was discarded. For each chemical species in the circadian system, the 250 000 data points (100 realizations × 250 hours/realization × 10 data points/hour) were used to construct a probability distribution. Two parameters were then selected to independently receive extraneous noise. The first parameter, dcPtnpCn, is an insensitive, local parameter representing the rate at which kinase binds to the clock protein PER2 in its nuclear, singly phosphorylated state. The second parameter, tlPt, is a sensitive, global parameter representing the rate at which PER2 is translated from its corresponding mRNA. Lognormal noise with a mean of 1 was multiplied to the reaction governed by dcPtnpCn,

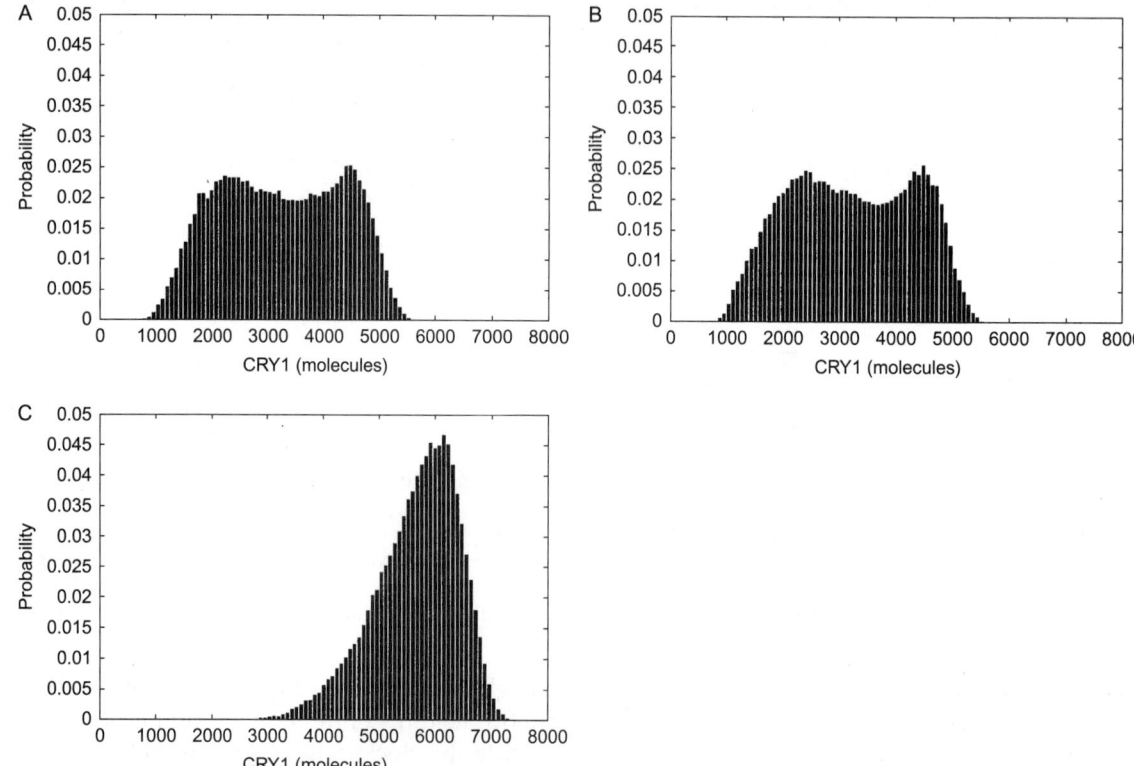

FIGURE 10.11 Comparisons of CRY2 Distribution Resulting from Simulation of the Forger and Peskin (2005) Stochastic Mouse Circadian Clock.
(A) No extraneous noise, (B) extraneous lognormal noise (mean = 1, standard deviation = 6) on dcPtnpCn, and (C) extraneous lognormal noise (mean = 1, standard deviation = 6) on tlPt. The data for each plot are derived from 100 realizations of a 500-hour simulation sampled every 0.1 hour. The first 250 hours of each simulation were discarded and therefore not included in the data.

and the SSA was realized and the data constructed as for the nominal case. The experiment was then repeated for the reaction governed by tlPt. Figure 10.11 shows the probability distributions for the clock protein CRY1 (the most abundant protein in the clock) for the nominal case (with no extraneous noise) and for the cases in which extraneous noise has been multiplied to dcPtnpCn and tlPt. Note that the probability distributions for the nominal case and for the case in which noise has been multiplied to dcPtnpCn are essentially identical, whereas the probability distribution for the case in which noise has been multiplied to tlPt is substantially modified. Similar behavior is observed for other states. Extraneous noise, therefore, is observed to propagate through the clock network when introduced into a sensitive parameter, but not when introduced into an insensitive parameter.

ACKNOWLEDGEMENTS

The authors would like to acknowledge the following sources of funding for the work presented in this chapter. Unfolded protein response: National Institutes of Health under grants R01

GM65507 and R01 GM75297; apoptotic signaling pathway: the National Science Foundation's IGERT Program under grant DGE02-21715 and the Institute for Collaborative Biotechnologies; *Arabidopsis thaliana* circadian rhythm: the National Science Foundation's IGERT Program under grant DGE02-21715, the Institute for Collaborative Biotechnologies through US Army Research Office Grant DAAD19-03-D-0004, and NSF/NIGMS grant GM078993; fruit fly (*Drosophila melanogaster*) circadian rhythm: the National Science Foundation's IGERT Program under grant DGE02-21715, the Institute for Collaborative Biotechnologies through US Army Research Office Grant DAAD19-03-D-0004, DARPA BioSPICE Program, and the Research Participation Program between the US DOE and AFRL/HEP; mouse circadian rhythm: the Institute for Collaborative Biotechnologies through US Army Research Office Grant DAAD19-03-D-0004.

References

Alabadi, D., Oyama, T., Yanovsky, M.J., Harmon, F.G., Mas, P., Kay, S.A., 2001. Reciprocal regulation between TOC1 and LHY/CCA1 within the Arabidopsis circadian clock. Science 293, 880–883.

Arkin, A.P., Ross, J., McAdams, H.H., 1998. Stochastic kinetic analysis of developmental pathway bifurcation in Phage lamda-infected *Escherichia coli* cells. Genet 149, 1633–1648.

Bagci, E.Z., Vodovotz, Y., Billiar, T.R., Ermentrout, G.B., Bahar, I., 2006. Bistability in apoptosis: roles of bax, bcl-2, and mitochondrial permeability transition pores. Biophys. J. 90, 1546–1559.

Blumenfeld, B., Preminger, S., Sagi, D., Tsodyks, M., 2006. Dynamics of memory representations in networks with novelty-facilitated synaptic plasticity. Neuron. 52, 383–394.

Bratsun, D., Volfson, D., Tsimring, L.S., Hasty, J., 2005. Delay-induced stochastic oscillations in gene regulation. Proc. Natl. Acad. Sci. USA 102, 14593–14598.

Colman-Lerner, A., Gordon, A., Serra, E., et al., 2005. Regulated cell-to-cell variation in a cell-fate decision system. Nature 437, 699–706.

Cover, T.M., Thomas, J.A., 1991. Elements of Information Theory. John Wiley & Sons, Inc., New York, NY.

Credle, J.J., Finer-Moore, J.S., Papa, F.R., Stroud, R.M., Walter, P., 2005. On the mechanism of sensing unfolded protein in the endoplasmic reticulum. Proc. Natl. Acad. Sci. USA 102, 18773–18784.

Csete, M.E., Doyle, J.C., 2002. Reverse engineering of biological complexity. Science 295, 1664–1669.

Dunlap, J.C., 1999. Molecular bases for circadian clocks. Cell 96, 271–290.

Elowitz, M.B., Levine, A.J., Siggia, E.D., Swain, P.S., 2002. Stochastic gene expression in a single cell. Science 297, 1183–1186.

Faller, D., Klingmüller, U., Timmer, J., 2003. Simulation methods for optimal experimental design in systems biology. Simulation 79, 717–725.

Farre, E. M., Harmer, S.L., Harmon F.G., Yanovsky, M.J., Kay, S.A., 2005. Overlapping and distinct roles of PRR7 and PRR9 in the Arabidopsis circadian clock. Curr. Biol. 15, 47–54.

Feng, X.-J., Hooshangi, S., Chen, D., Li, G., Weiss, R., Rabitz, H., 2004. Optimizing genetic circuits by global sensitivity analysis. Biophys. J. 87, 2195–2202.

Forger, D.B., Peskin, C.S., 2003. A detailed predictive model of the mammalian circadian clock. Proc. Natl. Acad. Sci. USA 100, 14806–14811.

Forger, D.B., Peskin, C.S., 2005. Stochastic simulation of the mammalian circadian clock. Proc. Natl. Acad. Sci. USA 102, 321–324.

Gadkar, K.G., Gunawan, R., Doyle III, F.J., 2005. Iterative approach to model identification of biological networks. BMC Bioinformatics 6, 155–174.

Gardner, T.S., Cantor, C.R., Collins, J.J., 2000. Construction of a genetic toggle switch in Escherichia coli. Nature 403, 339–342.

Gillespie, D.T., 1976. Exact stochastic simulation of coupled chemical reactions. J. Comput. Phys. 22, 403–434.

Gillespie, D.T., 1977. Exact stochastic simulation of coupled chemical reactions. J. Phys. Chem. 81, 2340–2361.

Gillespie, D.T., Mangel, M., 1981. Conditioned averages in chemical kinetics. J. Chem. Phys. 75, 704–709.

Gillespie, D.T., Petzold, L., 2006. Numerical simulation for biochemical kinetics. In: Szallasi, Z., Periwal, V., Stelling, J. (Eds.) System Modeling in Cellular Biology: from Concepts to Nuts and Bolts. MIT Press, Cambridge, pp. 331–353.

Gunawan, R., Cao, Y., Petzold, L., Doyle III, F.J., 2005. Sensitivity analysis of discrete stochastic systems. Biophys. J. 88, 2530–2540.

Gunawan, R., Doyle III, F.J., 2006. Phase sensitivity analysis of circadian rhythm entrainment. J. Biol. Rhythms. 22, 180–194.

Gunawan, R., Gadkar, K.G., Doyle III, F.J., 2006. Methods to identify cellular architecture and dynamics from experimental data. In: Szallasi, Z., Periwal, V., Stelling, J. (Eds.) System Modeling in Cellular Biology: from Concepts to Nuts and Bolts. MIT Press, Cambridge, pp. 221–242.

Hildebrandt, S., Raden, D., Robinson, A.S., Doyle III, F.J., 2008. A top-down approach to mechanistic biological modeling: application to the single-chain folding pathway. Bio Phys J. 95, 3535–3558.

Hua, F., Hautaniemi, S., Yokoo, R., Lauffenburger, D.A., 2006. Integrated mechanistic and data-driven modelling for multivariate analysis of signalling pathways. J. R. Soc. Interface 3, 515–526.

Johnson, C.H., Elliott, J.A., Foster, R., 2003. Entrainment of circadian programs. Chronobiol. Int. 20, 741–774.

Kimata, Y., Kimata, Y.I., Shimizu, Y., et al., 2003. Genetic evidence for a role of BiP/Kar2 that regulates Ire1 in response to accumulation of unfolded proteins. Mol. Biol. Cell 14, 2559–2569.

Kimata, Y., Oikawa, D., Shimizu, Y., Ishiwata-Kimata, Y., Kohno, K., 2004. A role for BiP as an adjustor for the endoplasmic reticulum stress-sensing protein Ire1. J. Biol. Chem. 167, 445–456.

Leloup, J.-C., Goldbeter, A., 1998. A model for circadian rhythms in Drosophila incorporating the formation of a complex between the PER and TIM proteins. J. Biol. Rhythms. 13, 70–87.

Locke, J.C.W., Millar, A.J., Turner, M.S., 2005a. Modelling genetic networks with noisy and varied experimental data: the circadian clock in Arabidopsis thaliana. J. Theor. Biol. 234, 383–393.

Locke, J.C.W., Southern, M.M., Kozma-Bognár, L., et al., 2005b. Extension of a genetic network model by iterative experimentation and mathematical analysis. Mol. Syst. Biol. 1, 0013.

Matter, C.M., Chadjichristos, C.E., Meier, P., et al., 2006. Role of endogenous Fas (CD95/Apo-1) ligand in balloon-induced apoptosis, inflammation, and neointima formation. Circulation 113, 1879–1887.

McAdams, H.H., Arkin, A., 1999. It's a noisy business! Genetic regulation at the nanomolar scale. Trends. Genet. 15, 65–69.

Mrosovsky, N., 1999. Masking: history, definitions, and measurement. Chronobiol. Int. 16, 415–429.

Myers, M.P., Wager-Smith, K., Rothenfluh-Hilfiker, A., Young, M.W., 1996. Light-induced degradation of TIMELESS and entrainment of the Drosophila circadian clock. Science 271, 1736–1740.

Okamura, K., Kimata, Y., Higashio, H., Tsuru, A., Kohno, K., 2000. Dissociation of Kar2p/BiP from an ER sensory molecule, Ire1p, triggers the unfolded protein response in yeast. Biochem. Biophys. Res. Commun. 275, 445–450.

Pittendrigh, C.S., Daan, S., 1976. A functional analysis of circadian pacemakers in nocturnal rodents. IV Entrainment: pacemaker as clock. J. Comp. Physiol. 106, 291–331.

Qiu, J., Hardin, P.E., 1996. *per* mRNA cycling is locked to lights-off under photoperiodic conditions that support circadian feedback loop function. Mol. Cell. Biol. 16, 4182–4188.

Samoilov, M., Plyasunov, S., Arkin, A.P., 2005. Stochastic amplification and signaling in enzymatic futile cycles through noise-induced bistability with oscillations. Proc. Natl. Acad. Sci. USA 102, 2310–2315.

Screpanti, V., Wallin, R. P. A., Grandien, A., Ljunggren, H. 2005. Impact of FASL-induced apoptosis in the elimination of tumor cells by NK cells. Mol. Immunol. 42,495–499.

Stelling, J., Gilles, E.D., Doyle III, F.J., 2004. Robustness properties of circadian clock architectures. Proc. Natl. Acad. Sci. USA 101, 13210–13215.

Varma, A., Morbidelli, M., Wu, H., 1999. ?Title of chapter/article?. In: Varma, A. (Ed.), Parametric Sensitivity in Chemical Systems. Cambridge University Press, Cambridge, pp. 10–11.

Weinberger, L.S., Burnett, J.C., Toettcher, J.E., Arkin, A. P., Schaffer, D.V., 2005. Stochastic gene expression in a lentiviral positive-feedback loop: HIV-1 Tat fluctuations drive phenotypic diversity. Cell 122, 169–182.

Welihinda, A.A., Kaufman, R.J., 1996. The unfolded protein response pathway in Saccharomyces cerevisiae. Oligomerization and trans-phosphorylation of Ire1p (Ern1p) are required for kinase activation. J. Biol. Chem. 271, 18181–18187.

Wolf, D.M., Vazirani, V.V., Arkin, A.P., 2005. Diversity in times of adversity: probabilistic strategies in microbial survival games. J. Theor. Biol. 234, 227–253.

Zak, D.E., Gonye, G.E., Schwaber, J.S., Doyle III, F.J., 2003. Importance of input perturbations and stochastic gene expression in the reverse engineering of genetic regulatory networks: insights from an identifiability analysis of an in silico network. Genome. Res. 13, 2396–2405.

Zeilinger, M.N., Farre, E.M., Taylor, S.R., Kay, S.A., Doyle III, F.J., 2006. A novel computational model of the circadian clock in Arabidopsis that incorporates PRR7 and PRR9. Mol. Syst. Biol. 2, 58.

Zhu, W., Petzold, L., 1999. Model reduction for chemical kinetics: an optimization approach. AIChE J. 45, 869–886.

CHAPTER

11

The Virtual Cell Project

Leslie M. Loew, James C. Schaff, Boris M. Slepchenko and Ion I. Moraru

R. D. Berlin Center for Cell Analysis and Modeling, Farmington

OUTLINE

Summary	273	Web-based Deployment and Client–Server Architecture	285
Introduction	274	Conclusion and Future Prospects	285
The Virtual Cell Database	275	Acknowledgement	287
Modeling Process in the Virtual Cell–Biomodel Interface	278		
Numerical Algorithms in Virtual Cell	282		

Summary

Elaborate biochemical reaction networks control the activity of cells and their responses to environmental stimuli. The challenge of understanding the behavior of such networks can be guided by the predictions generated from kinetic models. However, cells and their subcellular organelles have complex structures that provide a framework for the dynamic spatial distribution of signaling molecules. How this cellular architecture shapes and controls the response of cells to their environment must be incorporated in any attempt to understand a cellular process. The Virtual Cell is a computational modeling software environment that has been designed to address this need. It facilitates the organization of experimental data into quantitative hypotheses and the generation of predictions from them. A key feature of the Virtual Cell is that it permits the incorporation of experimental microscope images within full 3-dimensional spatial models of signal transduction networks. Reaction, diffusion, advection, membrane transport and electrophysiology are the biophysical mechanisms that are supported by the Virtual Cell. A variety of solvers are provided for ordinary differential equations and non-spatial stochastic simulations. The finite volume method is used for partial differential equation (i.e., spatial) models. A layered software architecture with a database backbone facilitates the reuse of models and model components. The database also permits collaborative model sharing and publication. This review presents the current design and structure of the Virtual Cell problem-solving environment.

INTRODUCTION

Traditionally, cell biology has been a descriptive science, but new experimental and computational tools are changing the face of modern cell biological research. Quantitative approaches can provide data spanning scales from single molecule turnover to cell–cell communication. Acquisition of such data is enabled primarily through outstanding advances in optical microscopy, but also from techniques such as patch clamp electrophysiology. In essence, the microscope can replace the test tube, allowing the elucidation of complex biochemical processes *in vivo* in living cells. These would include biochemical reaction rates, electrophysiological data on membrane transport dynamics, diffusion of cellular species within cellular compartments and the mechanical properties of cellular structures. To organize these heterogeneous data then requires the construction of models that can predict the overall behavior of the biological system. If the model correctly predicts the biological endpoint, one can hypothesize that the elements within the model are sufficient; furthermore, it is often possible to discern which of these elements are the most critical. This can then be tested by further experiments designed to specifically perturb or remove these elements (e.g. via RNA interference). However, it is never possible to be sure that a model is fully correct, as there may always be an as yet unperformed, or even not yet conceived, experiment that could disprove it. So it is perhaps actually more useful when the model is unable to predict the observed biology. This requires that the elements of the model are either incorrect or incomplete, and would lead the investigator to the design of new experiments to solve the problem. In other words, the cycle of experiment–model–experiment, is just a reformulation of the classical scientific method, in which the term "model" can be considered to be synonymous with the term "hypothesis."

To organize and make predictions from quantitative data, mathematical models that can produce simulations of the biology are required. Despite the clear benefits of the use of modeling as an adjunct to experiment, the difficulties associated with the formulation of mathematical models and the generation of simulations from them has impeded the adoption of this disciplined and quantitative approach to research in cell biology. Because biologists rarely have sufficient training in the mathematics and physics required to build quantitative models, modeling has been largely the purview of theoreticians who have the appropriate training but little experience in the laboratory. This disconnection to the laboratory has limited the impact of mathematical modeling in cell biology and, in some quarters, has even given modeling a poor reputation. The *Virtual Cell* (VCell) project aims to address this problem by providing a computational modeling framework that is accessible to cell biologists. It does this by abstracting and automating the mathematical and physical operations involved in constructing models and generating simulations from them. VCell is a modular computational framework that permits construction of models, application of numerical solvers to perform simulations, and analysis of simulation results.

VCell enables users to create and run simulations of biochemical networks, membrane transport and electrophysiology. These can be formulated as compartmental ordinary differential equation models and numerically solved with a choice of ordinary differential equation solvers. In addition, biochemical systems within small compartments, in which the number of molecules involved is small, can be treated discretely with simulations that use stochastic solvers. However, a key feature of VCell is that it permits the incorporation of realistic experimental geometries within full 3-dimensional (3D) spatial models. Thus the effects of diffusion and flow can be explicitly incorporated into models, and simulations provide solutions to the corresponding partial differential equations (PDEs). An intuitive JAVA interface includes options for database access, geometry definition (including directly from microscope images), specification of compartment topology, species definition and assignment, chemical reaction input, membrane transport mechanisms (including voltage dependence), initial conditions, boundary conditions, simulation solver choices and computational mesh. At the same time, the VCell provides a mathematical interface that allows theoreticians to examine and elaborate models through purely mathematical formulations. It allows for the direct entry of mathematical equations that describe a model, through a declarative language (Virtual Cell Mathematics Description Language, VCMDL). The mathematics is then automatically translated into C++ programming code that can than be sent to the numerics solvers. Thus modelers are relieved of the drudgery of writing *ad-hoc* code for every new modeling task. Furthermore, a VCMDL description of a model can be produced directly and automatically from a model that has been created within the biological interface. This dual interface has the additional benefit of encouraging communication and collaboration between the experimental and modeling communities.

This review is intended to summarize the current design and structure of the VCell problem-solving environment. Additional details on the algorithms within VCell can be found in several papers and some earlier reviews (Choi et al., 1999; Novak et al., 2007; Schaff et al., 1997, 2000, 2001; Slepchenko et al., 2000, 2003). Here, we will describe the physics and math supported by VCell, the numerical methods available for simulating the various classes of supported models, the layered workflow for assembling a BioModel, some of the visualization and analysis features of VCell, the rationale of our web-deployment strategy, and the functionality of the VCell database.

THE VIRTUAL CELL DATABASE

Models and geometries are maintained in an access-controlled central database. There are three database browsers, collected as three tabs within a "Database Manager" window, that provide a Windows Explorer file type of interface, one for each of the focused workspaces in VCell (BioModel Workspace, MathModel Workspace, Geometry Workspace). These database browsers allow interactive browsing of objects in the database and viewing of their corresponding descriptive metadata. Permissions to share a model with designated users or with the entire user community (i.e., making a model "Public") are set within the database browsers. A shared or public model can be opened by a user just like one of their own models, but altering the model or running new simulations requires that the user save a copy of the model under their own username. There is a Model Comparator Tool that compares any two models on the basis of their XML representation, and the resulting difference is displayed graphically in a hierarchical way.

VCell provides mechanisms to link to external resources to facilitate the sharing of models across various computational cell biology and systems biology tools. This is achieved by supporting the two prevalent XML languages that cover these fields: SBML (http://www.sbml.org/) and CellML (http://www.cellml.org/). The VCell team has been involved in developing both of these languages, including work on the development of SBML from its inception (Hucka et al., 2003). Exporting or importing CellML or SBML documents within VCell is simply achieved through appropriate menu items under the File menu. This facilitates the exchange of VCell model data between complementary software systems, as more than 100 different tools now support these two languages at varying levels. However, neither of these languages currently supports spatial modeling, and they have limited support for the abstractions used in VCell for membrane transport. Also, SBML does not support electrophysiological phenomena. So there was a need to develop an XML dialect that could completely capture a VCell model and, accordingly, Virtual Cell Markup Language (VCML) was developed to meet this need. In addition to allowing ready transfer and documentation of VCell models outside our central database, VCML is also used internally for efficient transport of model elements between software modules, and serves as a file format permitting a user to save a full copy of a model outside the central database for archival purposes. Other export utilities that are provided in the software are a translator into Matlab scripts and a pdf report generator in a format that contains all the model details in a human-readable format.

VCell offers access to external databases as a means to strengthen the utility of our own internal database and to provide additional modeling resources and data to users. To define a molecular species unambiguously, we have provided the ability to bind to a dictionary of species (controlled vocabulary) derived from (KEGG) (their Compound database for small molecules, metabolites, lipids, and so on and their Enzyme database for enzymes) and SwissProt (for proteins). This is illustrated in Figure 11.1, which shows the two steps in defining and binding a new species in VCell. In the top dialog box, a new species in the cytosol compartment is being created and is named IP3. Clicking "Add DB Link" brings up the second dialog box that allows the user to search the KEGG or SwissProt databases for the appropriate species definition ("Dictionary" is chosen). It also allows the user to search their own models ("My Models") or other public VCell models ("All Models") for molecules that have already been bound. In this case, the user has entered "inositol" in the Search Filter and from the list of resultant search hits has highlighted the appropriate entry for the inositol-trisphosphate species with which they wish to associate "IP3." VCell can also directly import and export models into Biomodels.net, a growing repository of SBML-encoded models (http://biomodels.net/) (Le Novere et al., 2006). This is somewhat limited by the level of compliance that a VCell model has with the SBML standard, as discussed above; however, currently about 50% of the models in Biomodels.net can be imported into VCell and all non-spatial and non-electrical VCell models can be exported to Biomodels.net. VCell also supports the MIRIAM (minimum information requested in the annotation of biochemical models) standard for model curation and annotation. In particular, VCML supports MIRIAM-compliant annotations in ? ? ? (RDF) format, and a user interface for viewing, adding, editing and deleting MIRIAM annotations is available in VCell.

VCell also permits automated searches for reactions within both the VCell database and the KEGG database of enzymatic reactions (http://www.genome.jp/kegg/reaction/) (Kanehisa et al., 2008) to facilitate building up a reaction network and defining and binding new species. This is illustrated in Figure 11.2, for a search that adds a reaction from the VCell database. It is built on a model for the turnover of the lipid, phosphatidylinositol-4,5-bisphosphate (PIP2) (Xu et al., 2003), where binding between the lipid PIP2 in the membrane and PH (representing the fluorescent label, PHδ1-GFP) is added to a reaction scheme in the Virtual Cell Reaction Editor. By right clicking within the reaction editor to reveal

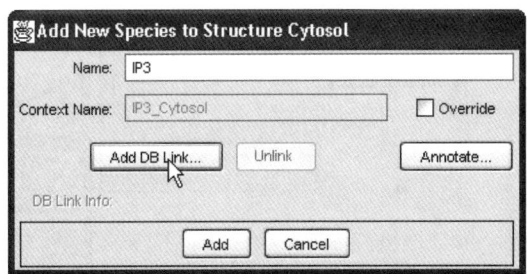
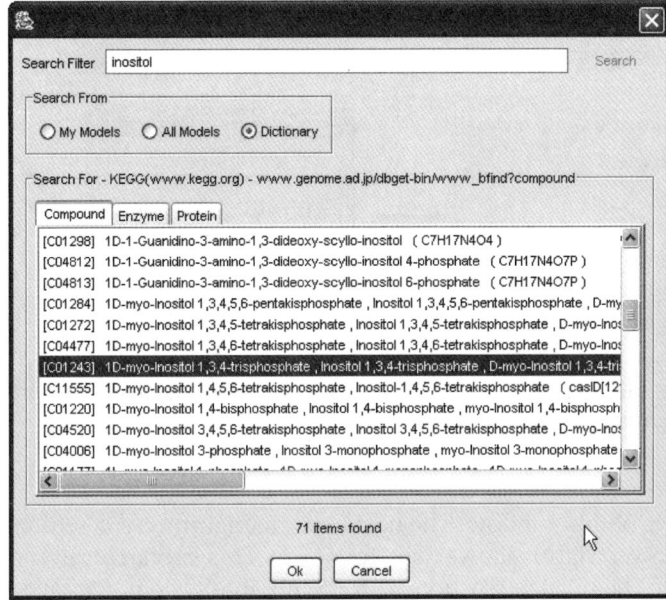

FIGURE 11.1 Defining and Binding a New Species in VCell. Top: New Species dialog box in which the species "IP3" is being created. Bottom: Searching for a species definition in the KEGG Compound database to bind "IP3."

the pop-up menu shown in the upper left, the "Add Searchable Reaction" wizard is launched. The first pane of the wizard (upper right) permits the user to choose whether to search from among User (i.e., the VCell database of models) or KEGG reactions. When choosing "User," only reactions within models that are accessible to the user will be searched (i.e., public models, those owned by the user under their username or those that have been explicitly shared with the user by a collaborator). The user is also asked to create a search filter—in this case they have chosen the string "PIP2" as an element that will be found within a reaction. Clicking Next brings up results of a search within the VCell database of all reactions in which PIP2 appears (Fig. 11.2, middle right). Clicking one of these in the upper pane of this window reveals, in the lower left pane, all the models in which this reaction occurs—in this case, two models under the username "hillelab", corresponding to two papers published by the laboratory of Bertil Hille (Horowitz et al., 2005; Suh et al., 2004); choosing the second of these reveals the corresponding parameters and their

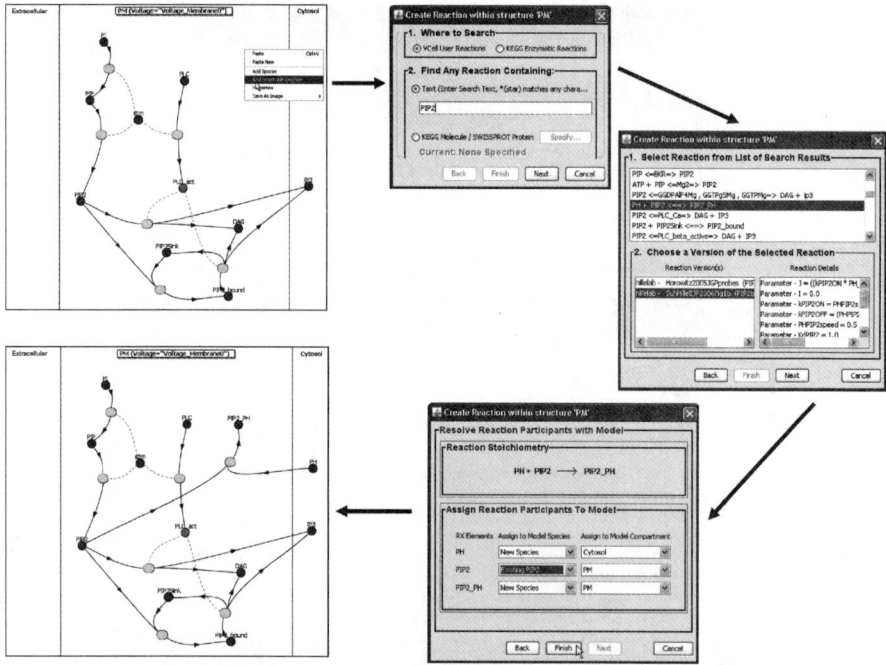

FIGURE 11.2 Automatic Import of Reactions into the Virtual Cell Reaction Editor from the VCell Database. For a detailed explanation, refer to the text.

values in the right pane of this window. The next window (Fig. 11.2, lower right) allows one to associate the species in the hillelab reaction with any existing species in the target reaction network; completing the wizard automatically adds the new reaction to the original pathway shown in the final reaction editor window on the lower left. An identical process is followed for searching and inserting reactions from KEGG.

MODELING PROCESS IN THE VIRTUAL CELL–BIOMODEL INTERFACE

The modeling process in the VCell–BioModel interface is facilitated by a conceptual decomposition into a hierarchical layered workflow. Figure 11.3 summarizes the way in which this modeling process is structured within the interface. This hierarchical layered structure starts with the system *Physiology* that describes the molecular species and mechanisms (reactions and fluxes) localized to cellular structures. Cellular structures are created by specifying the topological arrangement of membranes and membrane-bounded compartments. Biochemical reactions are defined within volumetric compartments of the cell as well as in membranes; molecular fluxes and electrical currents are defined across membranes. The reaction rate or flux rate is determined as an explicit function of the local environment (e.g. concentrations, surface densities, membrane potential) and one or more kinetic parameters (e.g. k_{on} and k_{off}). Mass action and Michaelis–Menten rate laws are available automatically, but user-defined general kinetic expressions are also readily entered. Membrane transport kinetics can be specified

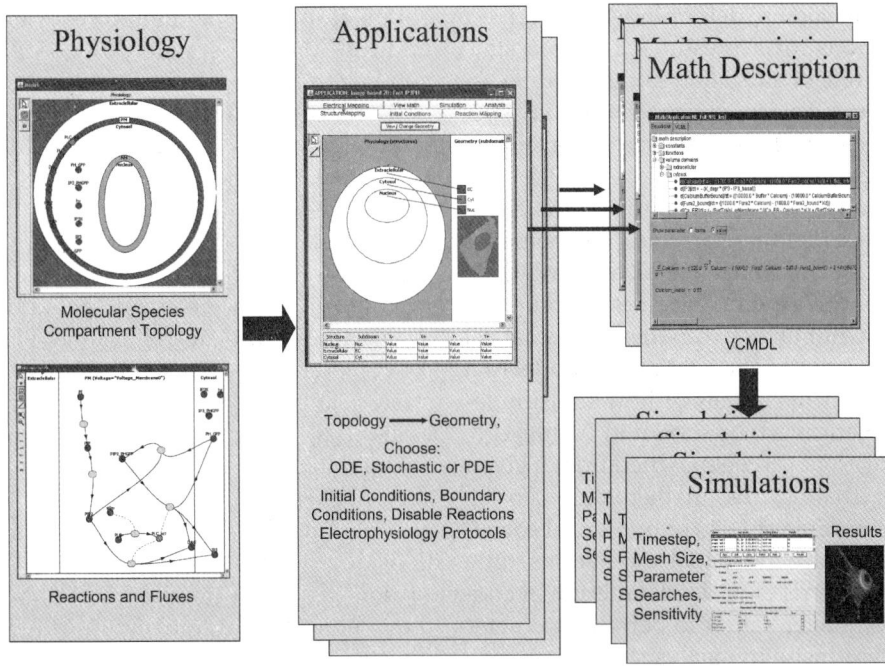

FIGURE 11.3 The Modeling Process Within the VCell–BioModel Workspace.
Each component of the overall model is labeled over a screen snapshot of the corresponding section of the user interface. A model entered through the MathModel workspace would have the geometry directly linked to the Math Description, but could still spawn several simulations. ODE, ordinary differential equation; PDE, partial differential equation; VCMDL, Virtual Cell Mathematics Description Language.

with expressions for molecular flux or, for ions, the electric current. The transport kinetics can be described in terms of standard electrophysiological formulas (e.g. Goldman–Hodgkin–Katz permeability or Nernst conductance) or as user-defined molecular flux or current.

The Physiology describes the overall mechanistic process under study; however, it can spawn several *Applications* that pose concrete experimentally testable problems. The three classes of Applications that can be generated from the Physiology require three kinds of mathematical solvers: non-spatial deterministic models require the solution of ordinary differential equations in which the geometrical features of each compartment are approximated in terms of their volumes and the surface areas of their membranes; non-spatial stochastic models explicitly solve for reaction probabilities and are used when the number of molecules in the model are too small to be treated as continuous concentration variables; deterministic spatial models treat diffusion and flow within a geometry, in which the user associates the compartments in the Physiology with structures within an image and the resultant reaction–diffusion equations require a PDE solver. VCell currently does not support stochastic spatial problems (MCELL is a modeling system that specializes in such problems; see Stiles and Bartol, 2001). In addition, within an Application, the user specifies boundary conditions, default initial concentrations and parameter values, and whether any of the reactions are sufficiently fast to permit a pseudo-steady-state approximation. Also at the Application level, individual reactions can be disabled as an aid in determining the correct initial conditions for a prestimulus stable state or to test the role of a reaction in the overall system behavior; likewise, concentrations of specific molecules can be clamped as in a virtual knockout experiment.

An Application of a Physiology is sufficient to completely describe the governing mathematics of the model and, as noted above, a VCMDL file is generated at this point. VCell is designed to maintain a separation between this mathematical description, generated via either a BioModel or a MathModel, and the details of how the simulations are implemented. As shown in Figure 11.3, several simulations can be spawned from a given Application; that is, the mathematics can be solved with multiple choices of numerical solver, time step, mesh size for spatial simulations, time duration and overrides of the default initial conditions or parameter values to permit parameter scans. A local sensitivity analysis service is also available at the simulation level to aid in parameter estimation and to determine which features of the model are most critical in determining its overall behavior. A particular simulation specification is, in turn, sufficient to describe the software requirements for numerically calculating solutions and VCell thus automatically generates and runs the appropriate C++ code to produce simulation results.

The VCell software displays spatial and non-spatial simulation solutions for the variables over time. For non-spatial models, data from several species can be displayed on the same plot of variable vs. time, as illustrated in Figure 11.4, which also illustrates how the same Physiology can spawn both deterministic and stochastic Applications. The model behind Figure 11.4 is a simple enzyme (E)-catalyzed reaction of substrate S to product P, in which the enzyme–substrate (ES) complex is explicitly included as an intermediate. In addition to the trajectories shown in Figure 11.4, the stochastic data viewer also permits the display of probability distributions at any time point after the automatic generation of several trajectories. All the data from these non-spatial simulations can be exported directly into spreadsheet format for additional analysis. The spatial data viewer displays a single plane section of a 3D data set, and can sample the solution along an arbitrary curve (piecewise linear or Bezier spline) or at a set of points. Membranes are displayed as curves superimposed on the volume mesh, and membrane

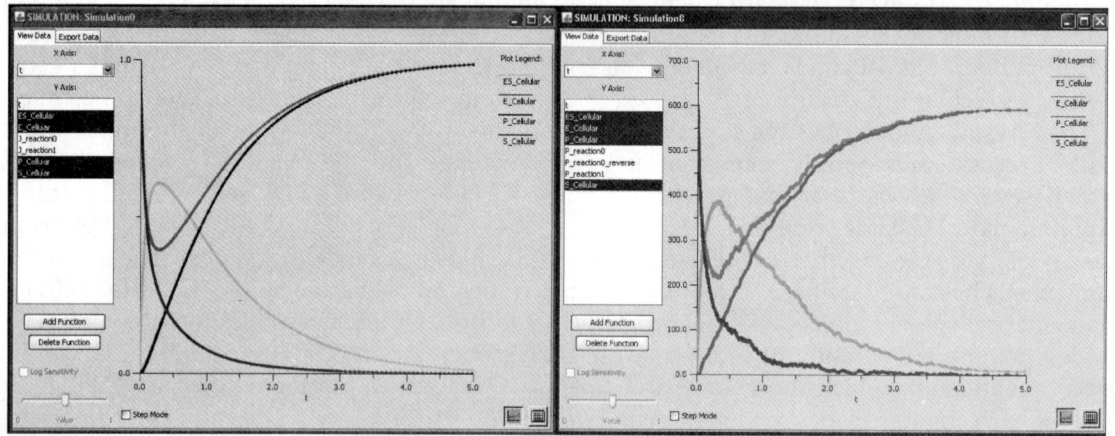

FIGURE 11.4 VCell Simulation Results.
Results from deterministic (left) and stochastic (right) Applications for a simple enzyme reaction.

variables are displayed along these curves. A 3D surface viewer and kymograph display are especially valuable for 3D datasets. Some of these visualization tools are displayed in Figure 11.5, which shows some screen-shots of a 3D spatial simulation of nucleocytoplasmic transport (Smith et al., 2002). A completely integrated data export service provides for data retrieval in a number of formats (e.g. comma-separated value, gif images, Apple QuickTime movies, animated gif movies) and data reduction schemes (subset of variables, time, and space including data sampling at selected points and along selected curves). Because the model can be mapped to a geometry acquired directly from the microscope, many of the same image analysis tools that are used to analyze experiments can be applied directly to simulation results.

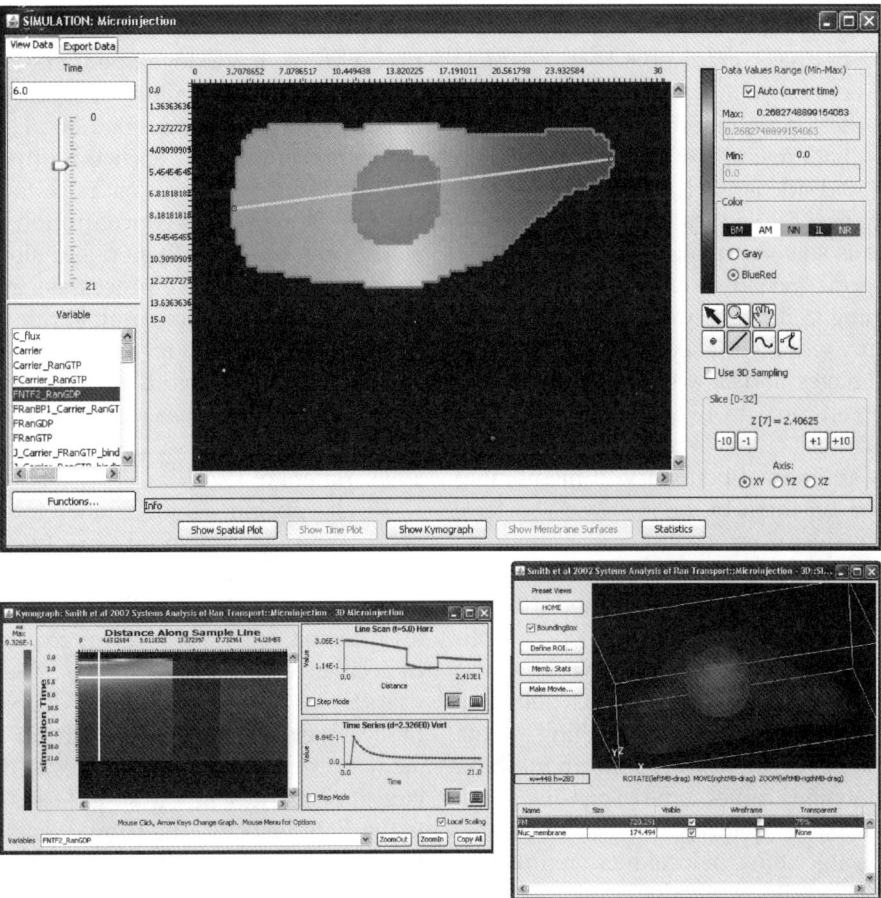

FIGURE 11.5 Simulation Results from a Spatial Application.
The top window shows a single X–Y plane through the 3D geometry, chosen at a Z position of 2.4 μm, displaying the distribution of the species FNTF2_RanGDP at the 6 s time-point. The line drawn with the line tool along the axis of the cell is used to generate a kymograph (i.e., time–space plot) as show in the lower left; cross-hairs can be positioned anywhere in the kymograph to display individual plots of the variable against distance and time. The lower right window shows a screenshot of the surface viewer for displaying the distribution of variables on membranes.

NUMERICAL ALGORITHMS IN VIRTUAL CELL

A physics framework for modeling spatiotemporal intracellular dynamics of molecular species is based on mass conservation. The dynamics are usually determined by kinetics of biochemical reactions and, in the presence of concentration gradients, by diffusive fluxes. Mathematically, the system is described by a set of PDEs of a reaction–diffusion type:

$$\partial_t[X] = \text{div}(D_X \text{grad}[X]) + \sum v_X \quad (11.1)$$

where $[X]$ is the concentration of a molecular species X, D_X is its diffusion coefficient and the sum in the right-hand side is taken over all the reaction rates v_X that affect the species X. In VCell, the system of PDEs is solved numerically on structured orthogonal grids (Schaff et al., 1997, 2001). This type of meshing facilitates sampling of cell geometry, particularly when it is taken from experimental microscope images, and allows one to move easily from one-dimensional to two- and three-dimensional applications. One issue with orthogonal grids is that an internal boundary (a membrane) is represented on them by a "staircase" surface, which may result in erroneous cross-membrane fluxes. To circumvent this problem, we have developed a "flux correction" method (Novak et al., 2007; Schaff et al., 2001) based on an optimal approximation for local normal vectors. The method ensures convergence to exact solutions and is equivalent to effective smoothing of the staircase. Another problem with uniform meshing is that computations can become expensive in the presence of disparate spatial scales. To address this issue, various algorithms of local mesh refinement (Berger, 1987; Colella et al., 2007) are currently being explored.

Spatial discretization of PDEs in VCell is achieved using a finite-volume scheme (Ferziger and Peric, 2002; Patankar, 1980). The method preserves exact mass conservation, even when numerical errors are large; this is important in biological applications. Time discretization is semi-implicit: we utilize a first-order backward Euler method with an explicit treatment of the reaction terms and membrane jump conditions. The resulting sparse linear algebraic system is solved iteratively using a preconditioned conjugate gradient method with an incomplete LU preconditioner (Saad, 2003). The explicit treatment of reactions and membrane fluxes leaves an opportunity for numerical instability if the corresponding time scales are vastly different ("stiff" systems). To partially alleviate the problem, we have developed an algorithm that performs an automatic pseudo-steady-state approximation (Slepchenko et al., 2000). The algorithm is invoked each time the user labels some of the reactions as infinitely fast. The method then updates concentrations in two substeps: first, due to diffusion and slow reactions, and then due to fast processes, in which the minimal set of non-linear algebraic equations is solved to equilibrate fast reactions. We are also currently testing various unconditionally stable numerical schemes based on the idea of operator splitting (Sportisse, 2000; Strang, 1968; Sun, 1996; Yanenko, 1971).

VCell capabilities for spatial modeling have been recently enhanced in two significant ways. First, in addition to diffusive fluxes, it is now possible to model directed flows that may arise in the cell as a result of forces exerted by molecular motors (Slepchenko et al., 2007) or due to polymerization and depolymerization of cytoskeletal structures, such as filamentous actin. In the presence of such flows, the total species flux is $\mathbf{j}_X = -D_X \text{grad}[X] + \mathbf{v}[X]$, where $\mathbf{v}$ is the flow velocity. The components of this vector field, which can be functions of time and spatial coordinates, are introduced by the user through the VCell mathematical user interface. The governing equations, sometimes termed as reaction–diffusion (*advection*) equations, have the form $\partial_t[X] = \text{div}(D_X \text{grad}[X] - \mathbf{v}[X]) + \sum v_X$. The current VCell implementation assigns a separate velocity field for each molecular species and, similarly to diffusion, the advection term is discretized using a finite volume method. For this, concentrations at the facets of control volumes, located half-way between the mesh points in VCell grids, must be evaluated. This is done using a hybrid scheme (Ferziger and Peric, 2002; Patankar, 1980), which is equivalent to the central difference scheme at low local Peclet numbers—that is, $v_x \Delta x / D < 2$—and to the upwind scheme with zero diffusion at high local Peclet numbers. It therefore preserves the accuracy of the central difference scheme when diffusive fluxes are significant, and the stability of the upwind scheme when the diffusive fluxes could be ignored. With the advection term, the linear system is no longer symmetric and requires a more general linear solver applicable to non-symmetric matrices—the generalized minimal residuals method (GMRES) (Saad, 2003).

The other addition to VCell spatial modeling tools is an algorithm for modeling lateral diffusion in cellular membranes coupled to reaction–diffusion processes in the cell volume (Novak et al., 2007). Diffusion on curved surfaces is described by a Laplace–Beltrami operator (Rosenberg, 1997), spatial discretization of which is a non-trivial task (Sbalzarini et al., 2006; Schwartz et al., 2005), particularly on pixilated surfaces. We have developed a method in which the Laplace–Beltrami operator is approximated locally by the Laplacian on the tangential plane. A local subset of the membrane mesh points, projected onto the tangential plane, forms an unstructured grid, to which Delaunay triangulation is applied. The resulting Voronoi cells are well suited for the finite-volume spatial discretization. Because the one-to-one correspondence between the membrane elements and the adjacent control volumes is preserved, coupling between diffusion on the surface and diffusion in the embedding volume is implemented on the basis of built-in exact mass conservation. One recent application of this capability relates to *in-vivo* measurements of the rate with which Rac, a G-protein regulating actin cytoskeleton, dissociates from the cell membrane (Moissoglu et al., 2006).

VCell has been used successfully for simulating electrophysiological experiments with non-neuronal cells (Horowitz et al., 2005; Suh et al., 2004). Because spatial equilibration of electric charges in this type of cells is fast on the time scale of interest, the membrane potential ϕ is approximated as a function of time only. The dynamics of ϕ are governed by conservation of charge: the total cross-membrane electric current is the sum of the capacitative current and the "direct" current associated with cross-membrane fluxes of ions and charged molecules:

$$I = C_m \frac{d\phi}{dt} + \sum I_X \qquad (11.2)$$

where I is the total outward cross-membrane electric current, C_m is the membrane capacitance, and the sum of direct currents is taken over all charged species X crossing the membrane. Note that, in VCell applications, the dynamics of membrane potential, described by Equation (11.2), can be coupled with spatially resolved dynamics of electrically charged species, such as calcium ion, governed by Equation (11.1). Indeed, in this case, the membrane flux density $j_{n,X}$ that constitutes the jump conditions for Equation (11.1) can be a function of ϕ and also determines the current I_X,

$$I_X = z_X F \int_{\partial \Omega_m} j_{n,X} dS,$$ where z_X is the valence of the species X, F is the Faraday constant, and $j_{n,X}$ is integrated over the entire membrane $d\Omega_m$. In mathematical terms, the problem in this case involves a coupled system of PDEs and integro-differential equations. Note that, in general, there might be several charged membranes electrically connected through currents. In this case, VCell automatically generates appropriate Kirchoff's current and voltage equations on the basis of a given topology of the system. A general formulation for the case of a spatially

resolved potential was proposed by Choi et al. (1999). In the quasi-one-dimensional case (neurons), this formulation reduces to equations of Cable Theory (Jack et al., 1975) that provide a mathematical basis for the popular software packages GENESIS and NEURON (Bower and Beeman, 1998; Hines and Carnevale, 1997).

The most recent VCell release supports non-spatial (compartmental) stochastic simulations. The implemented algorithm is based on the Gibson–Bruck Next Reaction method (Gibson and Bruck, 2000), an optimized version of one of the Gillespie algorithms (Gillespie, 1976***). These algorithms, sometimes called "exact stochastic simulators" to underscore the fact that they simulate events as they randomly occur and do not use fixed time step integration, are Monte Carlo techniques for solving a master equation that describes the Markov stochastic process in a "well stirred biochemical reactor"(Gardiner, 2004):

$$\frac{dP(n_1,...,n_k;t)}{dt} = \sum_{i=1}^{m}[a_i(n_1-v_{1i},...,n_k-v_{ki})$$
$$P(n_1-v_{1i},...,n_k-v_{ki};t)$$
$$-a_i(n_1,...,n_k)P(n_1,...,n_k;t)] \quad (11.3)$$

In Equation (11.3), n_i is the number of molecules of type i, $n_i \in (0,1,...,N_i)$, k is the number of molecular species in the system, m is the number of reactions, v_{ij} is the stoichiometry matrix, and the conditional probability rates $a_i(n_1,...,n_k)$ should be inferred from the corresponding reaction rates. One problem with deriving stochastic propensities from deterministic reaction rates is that the unambiguous interpretation of these in terms of Poisson stochastic processes is possible only for the mass-action kinetics and, even in this case, the reversible reactions should be decoupled into two separate processes. To address this issue, an analyzer tool has been developed in VCell that automatically determines whether the stochastic interpretation of reaction kinetics in the model is straightforward. In the case of ambiguity, the tool informs the user which mechanisms seem to be a combination of individual Poisson processes (for example, if they are passive fluxes) and which have to be recast into the mass-action type.

Exact stochastic simulators may be ineffective for systems that involve significantly different time scales (stiff systems). More efficient *approximate* stochastic algorithms can be utilized in the case $\min(N_i) >> \max(v_{ij})$ where noticeable change in the numbers of copies occurs only after multiple reaction firings (Gillespie, 2001). In this case, the variables $n_i(t)$ are advanced in time with a constant suitable time increment Δt:

$$n_i(t+\Delta t) = n_i(t) + \sum_{j=1}^{m} v_{ij} a_j(n_1(t),...,n_k(t))\Delta t$$
$$+ \sum_{j=1}^{m} \xi_j(0,1) v_{ij}(a_j(n_1(t),..., \quad (11.4)$$
$$n_k(t))\Delta t)^{1/2}, \quad i=1,...,k,$$

where $\xi_j(0,1)$ are uncorrelated normal random variables with the zero mean and unit variance (Gillespie, 2000). Equation (11.4) is a Langevin-type equation with the amplitude of the "fluctuating force" determined by reaction propensities (Gardiner, 2004) and is also known in the mathematical literature as a stochastic differential equation, or the Ito equation (Higham, 2001). A number of recently proposed hybrid algorithms (Haseltine and Rawlings, 2002; Rao and Arkin, 2003; Salis and Kaznessis, 2005; Salis et al., 2006) are being tested in VCell 4.5 (VCell alpha). In these methods, certain criteria are used to dynamically decouple the system into fast and slow subsystems. The fast subsystem is then simulated by solving Equation (11.4), whereas the slow subsystem is solved with an exact stochastic simulator. These methods allow the user to make a reasonable compromise between accuracy and efficiency by setting parameters for the fast–slow separation that would be appropriate for a particular application.

WEB-BASED DEPLOYMENT AND CLIENT–SERVER ARCHITECTURE

Biomedical computing software deployment strategies vary widely from complex stand-alone applications to simple web-based form page interfaces. We have chosen a client–server architecture with a web-based client deployment, web-based connectivity and centralized server-side infrastructure. This particular implementation of the distributed architecture of the VCell framework has been critical for scalability, interoperability, flexibility, continuous enhancement and multi-user support. However, it is important to emphasize that the current modular design of the VCell framework makes it very easy to construct many alternate implementations, ranging from fully packaged local installations to grid-based solutions. The current design is built on a few horizontal services (User Session Manager, Messaging, Authentication) and vertically integrated application services (Solvers, Object Persistence, Simulation Data Retrieval). Typical concerns for the viability of any application include: reliability, scalability, maintainability/extensibility and interoperability with third-party services and applications. There were six main considerations that influenced the choice of deployment strategy:

- *Portability*: the software should be compatible with Mac, Windows and Linux.
- *Resource requirements*: the users should be able to use the software without the need for additional software (compilers, libraries) or specialized hardware (high-performance computers, clusters).
- *Availability*: users need continuous access, with persistence of data and ability of the application to run uninterrupted for many days.
- *Maintenance*: we should be able to continuously update the software while maintaining backwards compatibility (automatically translating existing models in the database to new software formats).
- *Interoperability*: we should be able to add capabilities by linking to other software and services, also maintaining backwards compatibility.
- *Database functionality*: users should be able to share models and model components with other users while retaining control of access to their intellectual property.

Figure 11.6 shows an overview of the VCell framework in which individual components and services were grouped according to deployment considerations. This includes a client application that runs on individual users' computers and five server-side modules that run on computers at the R. D. Berlin Center for Cell Analysis and Modeling in Connecticut: a web portal (not shown), a main messaging server, a database service, a storage unit and compute nodes. There is no *a priori* reason for any of these modules to reside on separate computers, and the entire framework (including the client) could be deployed on a single workstation. The two main reasons to adopt a client–server design were (i) the desire to have a multi-user environment that can facilitate collaboration and model reuse, and (ii) the resource requirement issue stated above, which is particularly important in the case of our primary target audience, cell biologists, who typically have limited access to sophisticated and high-performance computer hardware and software.

CONCLUSION AND FUTURE PROSPECTS

This brief description of the current status of VCell can serve as an introduction to the functionality and operation of the software. We also hope it provides a view of the philosophy and rationale of the design of this software. We have been guided by the goals of providing a system that is both comprehensive and accessible, for the emerging field of computational

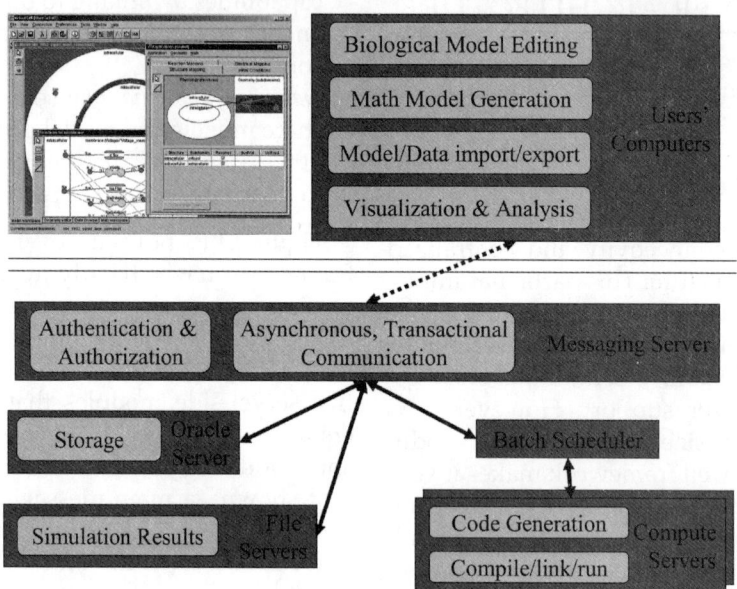

FIGURE 11.6 Current VCell Deployment Scheme.
Servers below the double line comprise the NRCAM computer cluster at University of Connecticut Health Center.

cell biology. We have placed emphasis on the re-usability of models and model components through both the hierarchical layered strategy for building models and the functionality of the VCell database system. The availability of both biologically and mathematically oriented interfaces, along with the centralized web-accessible model repository, facilitates interdisciplinary collaboration.

With regard to the impact that VCell is having at this juncture, our website (vcell.org) provides full bibliographies, a partial listing of papers that have been published in which VCell was used, in addition to sample applications, a User Guide and Tutorials. Table 11.1 shows the current (February 2008) level of VCell usage. Public models and simulations are available to anyone who logs on to VCell, as specified by their creators; the number of simulations is larger than the number of models, because models typically have several simulations associated with them. The figure for users who ran simulations probably is most representative of investigators who are actually using VCell productively, whereas the figure for total users reflects those who have been curious enough to register and explore the software or use the database to examine public models.

The range of cell biological problems that are encompassed by VCell is large, and we believe that it presents an extraordinarily palette of modeling opportunities to our user community.

TABLE 11.1 Impact of VCell (February 2008)

Total registered VCell users	11 082
Users who ran simulations	1737
Currently stored models	23 805
Currently stored simulations	112 974
Publicly available models	531
Publicly available simulations	1887

However, the physics and chemistry that control the operation of a cell are too rich to be satisfied by any one tool, even one as comprehensive as VCell. For example VCell does not have the ability to spatially model discrete events or the mechanical properties of cells. There are also features for analyzing models, such as bifurcation analysis, that are not covered in the current incarnation of VCell. We anticipate that community efforts such as CellML and SBML will help to fill these needs by permitting VCell models to be directly entered into other software tools (and *vice versa*). A new plug-in architecture and open source migration of the VCell codebase will further expand the range of functionality by allowing external developers to contribute directly. Finally, we are beginning to repackage the VCell software and algorithms into lightweight applications that are targeted to more specialized needs, such as tools for analyzing quantitative microscopy data.

ACKNOWLEDGEMENT

The Virtual Cell would not be possible without the dedicated work of an outstanding team of software developers and scientists. Current members of the VCell team include Frank Morgan, Fei Gao, Anuradha Lakshminaryana, Li Ye, Yung-sze Choi, Diana Resasco, Igor Novak, John Carson and Ann Cowan. The Virtual Cell project is supported through National Institutes of Health grant P41RR013186 from the National Center for Research Resources and, partially, through grant U54RR022232 that supports a NIH Technology Center for Networks and Pathways.

References

Berger, M.J., 1987. On conservation at grid interfaces. SIAM J. Numer. Anal. 24, 967–984.

Bower, J.M., Beeman, D., 1998. The Book of GENESIS: Exploring Realistic Neural Models with the General Neural Simulation System. Springer Verlag, New York.

Choi, Y.-S., Resasco, D., Schaff, J.C., Slepchenko, B.M., 1999. Electrodiffusion of ions inside living cells. IMA J. Appl. Math. 62, 207–226.

Colella, P., Graves, D.T., Ligocki, T.J., et al., 2007. Chombo Software Package for AMR Applications Design Document. Applied Numerical Algorithms Group, NERSC Division, http://seesar.lbl.gov/anag/chombo/ChomboDesign-2.0.pdf.

Ferziger, J.H., Peric, M., 2002. Computational Methods for Fluid Dynamics. Springer, Berlin.

Gardiner, C., 2004. Handbook of Stochastic Methods for Physics, Chemistry and the Natural Sciences. Springer-Verlag, New York.

Gibson, M.A., Bruck, J., 2000. Efficient exact stochastic simulation of chemical system with many species and many channels. J. Phys. Chem. A 104, 1876–1889.

Gillespie, D.T., 2000. The chemical Langevin equation. J. Chem. Phys. 113, 297–306.

Gillespie, D.T., 2001. Approximate accelerated stochastic simulation of chemically reacting systems. J. Chem. Phys. 115, 1716–1733.

Haseltine, E.L., Rawlings, J.B., 2002. Approximate simulation of coupled fast and slow reactions for stochastic chemical kinetics. J. Chem. Phys. 117, 6959–6969.

Higham, D.J., 2001. An algorithmic introduction to numerical simulation of stochastic differential equations. SIAM Review 43, 525–546.

Hines, M.L., Carnevale, N.T., 1997. The neural simulation environment. Neural Comput 9, 1179–1209.

Horowitz, L.F., Hirdes, W., Suh, B.-C., Hilgemann, D.W., Mackie, K., Hille, B., 2005. Phospholipase C in living cells: activation, inhibition, Ca2+ requirement, and regulation of M current. J. Gen. Physiol. 126, 243–262.

Hucka, M., Finney, A., Sauro, H.M., et al., 2003. The systems biology markup language (SBML): a medium for representation and exchange of biochemical network models. Bioinformatics 19, 524–531.

Jack, J., Noble, D., Tsien, R., 1975. Electric Current Flow in Excitable Cells. University Press, Oxford.

Kanehisa, M., Araki, M., Goto, S., et al., 2008. KEGG for linking genomes to life and the environment. Nucl. Acids Res. 36, D480–D484.

Le Novere, N., Bornstein, B., Broicher, A., et al., 2006. BioModels Database: a free, centralized database of curated, published, quantitative kinetic models of biochemical and cellular systems. Nucleic Acids Res. 34, D689–D691.

Moissoglu, K., Slepchenko, B.M., Meller, N., Horwitz, A.F., Schwartz, M.A., 2006. In vivo dynamics of Rac-membrane interactions. Mol. Biol. Cell 17, 2770–2779.

Novak, I.L., Gao, F., Choi, Y.-S., Resasco, D., Schaff, J.C., Slepchenko, B.M., 2007. Diffusion on a curved surface coupled to diffusion in the volume: application to cell biology. J. Comput. Phys. 226, 1271–1290.

Patankar, S.V., 1980. Numerical Heat Transfer and Fluid Flow. Taylor & Francis, ?Town.

Rao, C.V., Arkin, A.P., 2003. Stochastic chemical kinetics and the quasi-steady-state assumption: application to the Gillespie algorithm. J. Chem. Phys. 118, 4999–5010.

Rosenberg, S., 1997. The Laplacian on a Riemannian Manifold. University Press, Cambridge.

Saad, Y., 2003. Iterative Methods for Sparse Linear Systems. SIAM, Philadelphia, PA.

Salis, H., Kaznessis, Y., 2005. Accurate hybrid stochastic simulation of a system of coupled chemical or biochemical reactions. J. Chem. Phys. 122, 054103.

Salis, H., Sotiropoulos, V., Kaznessis, Y., 2006. Multiscale Hy3S: hybrid stochastic simulation for supercomputers. BMC Bioinformatics 7, 93.

Sbalzarini, I.F., Hayer, A., Helenius, A., Koumoutsakos, P., 2006. Simulations of (an)isotropic diffusion on curved biological surface. Biophys. J. 90, 878–885.

Schaff, J.C., Fink, C.C., Slepchenko, B.M., Carson, J.H., Loew, L.M., 1997. A general computational framework for modeling cellular structure and function. Biophys. J. 73, 1135–1146.

Schaff, J.C., Slepchenko, B.M., Choi, Y.-S., Wagner, J., Resasco, D., Loew, L.M., 2001. Analysis of nonlinear dynamics on arbitrary geometries with the Virtual Cell. Chaos 11, 115–131.

Schaff, J.C., Slepchenko, B.M., Loew, L.M., 2000. Physiological modeling with the Virtual Cell framework. In: Johnson, M. (Ed.), Methods in Enzymology, Vol. 321. Academic Press, San Diego, pp. 1–23.

Schwartz, P., Adalsteinsson, D., Colella, P., Arkin, A.P., Onsum, M., 2005. Numerical computation of diffusion on a surface. PNAS 102, 11151–11156.

Slepchenko, B.M., Schaff, J.C., Choi, Y.S., 2000. Numerical approach to fast reaction-diffusion systems: application to buffered calcium waves in bistable models. J. Comput. Phys. 162, 186–218.

Slepchenko, B.M., Schaff, J.C., Macara, I.G., Loew, L.M., 2003. Quantitative cell biology with the *Virtual Cell*. Trends Cell Biol 13, 570–576.

Slepchenko, B.M., Semenova, I., Zaliapin, I., Rodionov, V., 2007. Switching of membrane organelles between cytoskeletal transport systems is determined by regulation of the microtubule-based transport. J. Cell Biol. 179, 635–641.

Smith, A.E., Slepchenko, B.M., Schaff, J.C., Loew, L.M., Macara, I.G., 2002. Systems analysis of Ran transport. Science 295, 488–491.

Sportisse, B., 2000. An analysis of operating splitting techniques in the stiff case. J. Comput. Phys. 161, 140–168.

Stiles, J.R., Bartol, T.M., 2001. Monte Carlo methods for simulating realistic synaptic microphysiology using MCell. In: De Schutter, E. (Ed.), Computational Neuroscience: Realistic Modeling for Experimentalists. CRC Press, Boca Raton, pp. 87–127.

Strang, G., 1968. On the construction and comparison of difference schemes. SIAM J. Numer. Anal. 8, 506–517.

Suh, B.C., Horowitz, L.F., Hirdes, W., Mackie, K., Hille, B., 2004. Regulation of KCNQ2/KCNQ3 current by G protein cycling: the kinetics of receptor-mediated signaling by Gq. J. Gen. Physiol. 123, 663–683.

Sun, P., 1996. A pseudo-non-time-splitting method in air quality modeling. J. Comput. Phys. 127, 152–157.

Xu, C., Watras, J., Loew, L.M., 2003. Kinetic analysis of receptor-activated phosphoinositide turnover. J. Cell Biol. 161, 779–791.

Yanenko, N.N., 1971. The Method of Fractional Steps. Springer, New York.

CHAPTER

12

Software Tools for Systems Biology

Herbert M. Sauro and Frank T. Bergmann
University of Washington, Seattle

OUTLINE

Summary	289	Other Tools of Interest	299
Definitions	290	Commercial Tools	301
Introduction	**290**	Dedicated Libraries	301
The Problem	291	**Dedicated Tools for Stochastic Simulation**	**303**
The Need for Software	292	**Standards**	**305**
Functionality	292	CellML	305
A Brief Survey of Commonly Used Tools	**293**	SBML	305
COPASI	294	Other Related Standards	306
Jarnac	295	Other Ontologies	307
JSIM	295	Human-readable Formats	307
MathSBML	295	**Databases**	**308**
PySCeS	296	**Test Suites**	**309**
SBToolbox²	296	**Future Prospects**	**309**
Systems Biology Workbench	296	Re-usable Software Libraries	310
VCell	297	**Acknowledgements**	**310**
Visual Editors	297		
CellML-based Applications	298		

Summary

Probably one of the most characteristic features of a living system is its continual propensity to change as it juggles the demands of survival with the need to replicate. Internally, these changes are manifest by changes in metabolite, protein and gene activities. Such changes have become increasingly obvious to experimentalists with the advent of quantitative high-throughput technologies. Given the complexity of cellular networks, it is no surprise that researchers have also turned to computer simulation and the development of more theory-based approaches to augment and assist in the development of a fully quantitative understanding of cellular dynamics. In this chapter, we highlight some of the software tools and emerging standards for representing, simulating and analyzing cellular networks. The chapter will not be concerned with tools for managing high-throughput data or analyzing genome-scale data using bioinformatic approaches.

Definitions

API Application Programming Interface
CellML Cell Markup Language
MCA Metabolic control analysis
ODE Ordinary differential equation
PDE Partial differential equation
SBML Systems Biology Markup Language
SBW Systems Biology Workbench
SOSLib SBML ODE Solver Library
VCell Virtual Cell
XML Extensible Markup Language

INTRODUCTION

The use of simulation and theoretical studies in cellular and molecular biology has a long, if uneven, tradition spanning more than 70 years (Wright, 1934). With the recent advent of high-throughput technologies, interest in using more quantitative approaches to enhance our understanding of cellular dynamics has increased dramatically (Geva-Zatorsky et al., 2006; Kholodenko, 2006; Neves and Iyengar, 2002; Tyson et al., 2001). As part of this trend, there has been a significant increase in the availability of computer software to help us model, simulate and analyze dynamic models of cellular processes. In this chapter, we will briefly survey the available simulation software for systems biology. In addition, we will briefly discuss model databases, model exchange standards, ontologies and computational approaches that are relevant to the study of dynamics in biochemical networks. We will not be concerned with software tools for managing high-throughput data or analyzing genome-scale data using bioinformatic approaches.

Simulating biochemical networks has a long history dating back to at least the 1940s (Chance, 1943). The earliest simulations relied on building either mechanical or electrical analogs of biochemical networks. It was only in the late 1950s, with the advent of digital computers and the development of specialized software tools (Garfinkel, 1968), that the ability to simulate biochemical networks became more widely available. In the intervening years up to 1980, a handful of other software applications were developed (Burns, 1969, 1971; Park and Wright, 1973) to help the small community of modelers. In more recent years, particularly since the early 1990s, there has been a significant increase in interest in modeling biochemical processes, and a wide range of tools is now available to the budding systems biologist. Many tools have been developed by practicing scientists and are therefore available free (often in the form of open source), whereas others are commercial, such as SimBiology from MathWorks (http://www.mathworks.com/, 2006).

Given the recent explosion in interest in quantitative biology (Alon, 2006; Klipp et al., 2005), the number and variety of tools and approaches has likewise increased. In order to make the coverage more manageable, we will restrict our discussion to software that is aimed at modeling systems based on differential equations or stochastic chemical kinetics. We will not, therefore, be concerned with software for modeling Boolean models, agent-based models or models that use process calculi. For a discussion of these models and related software, the reader is referred to reviews by Fisher and Henzinger (2007) and Degenring et al. (2004).

We will, moreover, largely confine ourselves to dynamic models, which means that we will not discuss at any length the software that is designed to study the structural properties of networks, other than in a few notable cases. In particular, software used to build and compute flux balance models (Fell and Small, 1986; Kauffman et al., 2003; Lee et al., 2006; Palsson, 2007) or software for building isotopomer models (Schwender, 2008; Wiechert, 2001) will not be covered in detail, even though such analyses are crucial to the metabolic engineering community.

Finally, we will also not discuss tools that specialize in simulating spatial models or neurophysiology systems. More information on the former topic is to be found in articles by Ander et al. (2004), Broderick et al. (2005), Coggan et al. (2005), Hattne et al. (2005), Lemerle et al. (2005), Sanford et al. (2006) and Tomita et al. (1999). Details of simulating neural systems are given by Bhalla (2002), Bower and Beeman (1998), Carnevale and Hines (2006) and Hines (1993). Although this may appear to be a long list of exclusions, we are still left with more than 100 tools that focus on simulating non-spatial, deterministic or stochastic models.

The Problem

The software discussed in this chapter is concerned with analyzing two particular types of problem. One is the classical problem of solving systems of differential equations that describe the deterministic evolution of molecular species concentrations in time. These systems are generally written in the form:

$$\frac{d\mathbf{x}}{dt} = N\, v(x(p), p) \quad (12.1)$$

where $\mathbf{x}$ is the vector of species concentrations, $\mathbf{N}$ is the stoichiometry matrix, $\mathbf{v}$ is the rate vector and $\mathbf{p}$ is the vector of parameters. Often, the system of equations is overdetermined because of the presence of conserved moieties (Reich and Selkov, 1981), and the equation is then re-expressed in the form:

$$x_d = L_0 x_i + T$$
$$\frac{d\mathbf{xi}}{dt} = N_R v(x(p), p) \quad (12.2)$$

where $\mathbf{x}_i$ is the vector of independent species, $\mathbf{x}_d$ is the vector of dependent species, $\mathbf{T}$ is the vector of conserved mass totals, $\mathbf{N}_R$ is the reduced stoichiometry matrix and $\mathbf{L}_0$ is part of the Link matrix (Reder, 1988; Sauro and Ingalls, 2004). If the system of Equation (12.1) is overdetermined, then it is highly advisable to eliminate the redundant equations. There are a number of reasons for this, the most obvious being the reduction in the size of the model that accompanies the elimination. A more important reason is that the Jacobian matrix, a fundamental quantity in dynamical theory, is singular (Vallabhajosyula et al., 2006) in an overdetermined system. This in turn makes many important numerical methods unstable. Many simulators fail to carry out this important stage.

The second problem of interest is the realization of the master equation (Wilkinson, 2006). This equation describes the time evolution of the concentration probabilities. However, because we need one time evolution equation for every particle state in the system, the system of equations becomes unwieldy very rapidly as the size of the system increases. Instead, modelers use the exact stochastic simulation algorithm (SSA) and it variants, developed by Gillespie (1976). This approach, in which j indicates which reaction will fire and at what time in the future (τ), is summarized by Equation (12.3):

$$p(\tau, j \mid x, t) = a_j(x) e^{-a_0(x)\tau} \quad (12.3)$$

where t is the current time, τ is the time to the next reaction, $\mathbf{x}$ is the species vector, a_j is the propensity function of reaction j and a_o is the sum of all propensity functions. On its own, the SSA only generates a single trajectory or realization. In order to glean statistics on the model dynamics, many repeated runs must be made using this equation. As with the deterministic case, the system is overdetermined, and it is possible to reduce the work load by solving explicitly for the independent species only.

A third approach to modeling, which is intermediate between those represented by Equations (12.1) and (12.3), is to use the Langevin equation, which is a stochastic differential equation (Cyganowski et al., 2001). A stochastic differential equation can be constructed by appending a noise term to the deterministic formulation of Equation (12.1); however, very few tools currently provide facilities to solve stochastic differential equations, which is unfortunate (Adalsteinsson et al., 2004; Chickarmane et al., 2007).

Further information on modeling intracellular noise can be found in the excellent review by Rao et al. (2002).

The Need for Software

The first question one might ask is why develop specialized software to model biochemical networks? Given the availability of both generic commercial and freely available tools for numerical analysis, one might ask if there is such a need. There are probably at least two reasons why researchers develop their own specialized tools for modeling biochemical systems. The first is that specialized tools reduce the errors that occur when transcribing a reaction scheme (that is, a biological representation) into the mathematical formalism ready for simulation. Deriving the math equations by hand is often a source of error (especially in published papers), particularly in large models. The second important reason is that developing software offers an opportunity to codify and develop new numerical algorithms or new theoretical approaches that are specific to problems found in systems biology. Such examples include incorporating metabolic control analysis (MCA) (Kacser and Burns, 1973; Savageau, 1972) into software (which is the reason why one of us developed simulation software in the first place) or developing more efficient methods for network analysis (Vallabhajosyula et al., 2006). Although it is possible to carry many analyses in tools such as Matlab, Mathematica or SciLab, the process tends to be more tedious and error prone and certain analyses are unavailable to the user without the application of considerable effort.

Functionality

Given the long history of provision of software in modeling biochemical networks, we believe there is a minimum level of functionality that any newly developed or existing tool should have. Foremost is the ability to convert a biological description—that is, a set of biochemical reactions and corresponding rate laws—into a set of differential equations. The input format for the model can be in the form of the Systems Biology Markup Language (SBML) (Hucka et al., 2003) or Cell Markup Language (CellML) (Hedley et al., 2001) (described later, in the section on Standards), or it can be in the form of a human-readable text format that can be more easily edited and, if necessary, converted later into SBML or CellML for export. Tools such as the Systems Biology Workbench (SBW, discussed in the section A Brief Survey of Commonly Used Tools) provide facilities for converting SBML to simple human-readable text files that can be edited and loaded into the simulation tool.

Once a model has been converted into a set of appropriate differential equations, the solutions can be easily generated from widely available numerical integration routines. The US

Department of Energy, in particular, has developed a very useful series of sophisticated libraries, including SUNDIALS (Hindmarsh et al., 2005) and ODEPACK (Hindmarsh, 1983). These libraries are quite straight forward to incorporate into software, and can be used to solve even some of the most complex problems.

Together with generating a solution, some means of saving simulation results is obviously needed, and in a format that can be loaded by widely available tools such as GNUPLOT (Williams and Kelley, 1998) or Excel (microsoft.com). The final minimum requirement is some way in which to modify parameters and initial conditions to allow a user to repeat runs, although such functionality could simply involve editing the model in a text file and re-running the model.

What was just described is essentially the functionality of some of the earliest simulators dating back to the 1950s. Clearly, any simulator developed today should exceed these requirements.

Beyond the minimum requirements, there are a whole host of other desirable capabilities, including: model reduction by way of conservation laws, steady-state determination, sensitivity analysis (via MCA if possible), frequency analysis, bifurcation discovery and analysis, structural analysis and, finally, optimization and parameter fitting. In addition to these, other capabilities would also be desirable, such as access to a model database (particularly the BioModels Database (Le Novère, 2006), described in the later section on Databases), the availability of a variety of model editors (visual, text and GUI), and some way to generate camera-ready copy of network diagrams for publication purposes.

A BRIEF SURVEY OF COMMONLY USED TOOLS

In the past 10 years or so, numerous software applications have been written to support modeling of biochemical processes. The variety of software is huge, even within the restricted scope of this discussion. Almost every computer language has been used, at one time or another, to build simulation software. Some applications work on single operating platforms, others work across several platforms; some are trivial to install, whereas others require considerable persuasive efforts to make them work. There is also a wide variety of user interfaces, such as graphical user interfaces incorporating menus, buttons, lists, etc., network design interfaces that allow users to draw a pathway on the screen, and text-based scripts that enable users to control and define a computer model very precisely. Finally, application capabilities vary enormously: some attempt to be broad, offering many different capabilities; others choose to specialize in one particular area. Some of the tools are extensible—that is, new functionality can be added by a user either through scripting languages or by writing small plug-in applications. Most have some form of reference documentation, including tutorials to help users get started.

A visit to the software guide at the SBML.org web site will reveal more than 100 different tools for modeling or working with biochemical networks. The majority of these have been developed in the past eight years or so. However, although there appears to be a large number of offerings, many are not actively developed and have become orphaned software. In this chapter, we will focus only on those tools that are actively developed and have an excellent chance of being supported in the future.

We will focus initially on some tools we use ourselves. We sometimes use these tools because our software may lack certain features we need. More often, we also use them to compare simulation results.

Before continuing, however, we would also like to mention three legacy simulators which have influenced the development of most modern applications: GEPASI (Mendes, 1993), METAMOD (Hofmeyr and van der Merwe,

1986) and SCAMP (Sauro, 1993; Sauro and Fell, 1991). All three were developed in the 1980s, and in some cases continue to be used.

All the tools we will describe can import SBML and all, with the exception of JSIM, can export SBML; however, JSIM can also import CellML. Both SBML and CellML are established model exchange standards which we will discuss in more detail in a later section. All the tools we will describe are currently maintained and have an active user community. Most of the tools run on several platforms (Windows, Linux, Mac) and most, with the exception of one or two, are open source, although under varying licenses.

Given that we are also developers of simulation tools, it would be unfair for us to provide a detailed comparison of the different applications; instead, we refer interested readers to recent independent reviews by Alves et al. (2006), Manninen et al. (2006) and Vacheva and Eils (2006) and to two comparison web sites, one maintained by the VCell group at http://ntcnp.org/twiki/bin/view/VCell/SBMLFeatureToolMatrix, and the other by our own group at http://www.sys-bio.org/sbwWiki/compare. The feature matrix at the VCell site is a user-contributed table that lists the capabilities of each tool. In contrast, the comparison site at sys-bio.org does not attempt to make statements about particular capabilities, but instead runs each registered tool through every model in the BioModels Database (more than 170 models) and compares the results. From such results, a developer or user can judge the capabilities of a particular software tool without any bias from us.

Although not on the list, we should mention the use of Matlab as an excellent numerical and data analysis application in systems biology. Matlab is an application that we ourselves have frequently used for complex data analysis. MathWorks also supplies a specialized tool box called SimBiology, which offers many useful capabilities.

All these tools that we will now describe are capable of basic simulation—that is, solving differential equations or simulating a stochastic model; what makes them stand out is what they provide in addition to this basic functionality.

COPASI

Pedro Mendes wrote one of the earliest PC simulators, which he called GEPASI (Mendes, 1993). COPASI (Hoops et al., 2006) is essentially a rewrite of GEPASI that comes in two versions: a graphical user interface and a command-line version. The latter version is designed for batch jobs in which a graphical user interface is unnecessary, and in which runs can be carried out without human supervision. COPASI uses its own file format to store models; however, like all the tools discussed here, it can import and export SBML. One of its undoubted strengths is optimization and parameter fitting, which it inherited from its predecessor. It has an unique ability to optimize on a great variety of different criteria including metrics such as Eigen values, transient times, etc. This makes COPASI extremely flexible for optimization problems. Installation is very simple and entails using a one-click installer. Although the source code to COPASI is available and can be freely used for research purposes in academia, because of the way in which the development of COPASI was funded, there are restrictions on commercial use.

The graphical user interface is based on a menu/dialog approach, much like its immediate predecessor, GEPASI. COPASI has capabilities to simulate both deterministic and stochastic models, and includes a wide range of analyses. It correctly takes into account conservation laws, and has very good support for metabolic control analysis, amongst other things. COPASI is, without doubt, one of the better simulators available. Although the user interface is graphical, it does, because of its particular design, require some effort to master, but with the availability of the COPASI source code, there is the opportunity to provide alternative user interfaces. Finally, there is a version that has an SBW interface that allows SBW-enabled tools access to the functionality of COPASI.

Jarnac

Jarnac (Sauro, 2000) is a rapid prototyping script-based tool that was developed as a successor to SCAMP (Sauro and Fell, 1991). It is distributed as part of the SBW, which makes installation a one-click affair. Jarnac was developed in the late 1990s before the advent of portable GUI toolkits, which explains why it only runs under Windows, although it runs well under Wine (Windows emulator), thus permitting it to run under Linux. Visually, Jarnac has two main windows, a console where commands can be issued and results returned, and an editor where control scripts and models can be developed. The application also has a plotting window, which is used when graphing commands are issued.

Jarnac implements two languages: a biochemical descriptive language that allows users to enter models as reaction schemes (similar to a SCAMP script), and a second language, the model control language, which is a full-featured scripting language that can be used to manipulate and analyze a model. The main advantage of Jarnac over other tools is that models can be very rapidly built and modeled. From our experience with using many simulation tools over the years, Jarnac probably offers the fastest development time of any tool for model building. Models can also be imported or exported as SBML. Like COPASI and PySCeS, Jarnac offers many analysis capabilities, including extensive support for metabolic control analysis, structural analysis of networks and stochastic simulation. It has no explicit support for parameter fitting, but this is easily remedied by transferring a model directly to a tool such as COPASI via SBW.

JSIM

JSIM (Raymond et al., 2003) is a Java-based simulation system for building quantitative numeric models and analyzing them with respect to experimental reference data. JSIM can either be used from a web browser or downloaded to a desktop machine. The primary focus of JSIM is physiology and biomedicine; however, its computational abilities are quite general and applicable to a wide range of scientific domains. JSIM models may intermix ordinary differential equations (ODEs), partial differential equations (PDEs), implicit equations, integrals, summations, discrete events and procedural code as appropriate. One of the strengths of JSIM that makes it stand out from other simulators is its careful attention to dimensional analysis. Users can thus specify units for all terms in a model, and JSIM will then carry out an automatic check to ensure that the specified units are consistent with the model. In addition, JSIM can automatically insert conversion factors for compatible physical units. JSIM is one of the few modeling programs that can import both SBML and CellML formats.

The modeling language used by JSIM is mathematically orientated, and thus may not be suited to all users; however, the authors also define a more biologically orientated language called BCL, which allows users to specify models in a more biologically orientated manner.

MathSBML

MathSBML (Shapiro et al., 2004) is an open source package for working with SBML models in Mathematica. It provides facilities for reading SBML models, converting them to systems of ordinary differential equations for simulation and plotting in Mathematica, and translating the models to other formats. MathSBML is one of the few simulators to support differential/algebraic equations that may present themselves in models. For Mathematica users, MathSBML is a good choice.

PySCeS

PySCeS (Olivier et al., 2005) is probably the best Python-based simulator currently available. Although users interact with PySCeS via Python scripts, many of the underlying numerical capabilities are provided by well established C/C++ or FORTRAN-based numerical libraries. It was written by a team well seasoned in biochemical modeling, and as a result the software is reliable and comprehensive. As a portable free scripting tool for systems biology, PySCeS is currently one of the best. The only major element missing is parameter optimization, but such functionality can be added through additional Python scripting. As with COPASI and Jarnac, PySCeS correctly handles conservation laws and has very extensive support for metabolic control analysis, including extensive structural analysis capabilities. PySCeS is also one of the few tools to have some limited support for bifurcation analysis. Installation on Windows is very straightforward, with a single-click install. Although the current version of PySCeS is mainly concerned with deterministic simulations, there are plans to add stochastic capabilities in collaboration with the University of Newcastle, UK. There are a number of other Python-based simulators, including sloppyCell (Myers et al., 2007), Scrumpy (Poolman, 2006), ByoDyn (http://cbbl.imim.es:8080/ByoDyn) and PyLESS (http://sysbio.molgen.mpg.de/pyless/), which specializes in model reduction. PySCeS, however, is the most mature and comprehensive of these.

SBToolbox[2]

SBToolbox[2] is a very extensive Matlab tool box developed by Schmidt and Jirstrand (2006). The tool box has a wide range of capabilities. One of it unique features is the ability to interact with XPPAUT (Ermentrout, 2002) by generating the XPP files and launching XPPAUT. For a Matlab user, the SBToolbox[2] is a particularly useful tool to have available.

Systems Biology Workbench

The SBW (Bergmann et al., 2006; Sauro et al., 2003), unlike other tools described in this chapter, is not a simulation resource itself; it is instead an open source framework for connecting heterogeneous software applications. SBW is made up of two kinds of component:

- *Modules*: these are the applications that a user would use. There is available a broad collection of model editing, model simulation and model analysis tools.
- *Framework*: the software framework that allows developers to cross programming language boundaries and connect application modules to form new applications.

Modules in SBW can be written in a wide variety of languages, including C/C++, Java, .NET, Delphi, Matlab, Python and Perl. Each module will expose application programming interfaces that allow other application modules access to their functionality.

One of the core modules in SBW is the simulation module, roadRunner. roadRunner is implemented using the C# programming language and exploits the ability of .NET to generate model code on the fly, and subsequent compilation and optimization by the .NET framework. This approach leads to the generation of very fast simulation times. Numerical analysis is provided by the CVODE (Hindmarsh et al., 2005) integrator and the NLEQ library (http://www.zib.de/Numerik/numsoft/NewtonLib/)

for steady-state computations. roadRunner is available on the Windows platforms through the .NET framework and on POSIX systems through the mono project (http://www.mono-project.com). It relies on several SBW modules for the reading of SBML and for conservation analysis, resulting in a smaller set of ODEs to solve, but also the ability to generate non-singular Jacobian matrices, which is required for steady-state evaluation and other analyses. In addition to simulation and steady state evaluation, roadRunner also incorporates a full set of routines to compute sensitivities (i.e., MCA), frequency analysis, various structural metrics from the stoichiometry matrix and a basic continuation algorithm based on arc length (Kubicek, 1976; Kubicek and Marek, 1983). roadRunner is also the back-end simulator for the on-line simulation tools at sys-bio.org.

VCell

The Virtual Cell (VCell; see Chapter 11) (Moraru et al., 2002; Schaff et al., 1997; Slepchenko et al., 2003) is a client–server-based tool that specializes in three-dimensional cell simulations. It is unique in that it provides a framework for modeling, not only biochemical networks, but also electrophysiological and transport phenomena, while at the same time considering the subcellular localization of the molecules that take part in them. This localization can take the form of a three-dimensional arbitrarily shaped cell, in which the molecular species might be heterogeneously distributed. In addition, the geometry of the cell, including the locations and shapes of subcellular organelles, can be imported directly from microscope images. VCell is written in Java, but has numerical analysis carried out by C/C++ and FORTRAN-coded software to improve performance. Currently, modeling must be carried out using the client–server model, which necessitates a connection to the internet. In addition, models are generally stored on the VCell remote server rather than on the client's desktop. This operating model is not always agreeable to users, and as a result the VCell team are reorganizing the software so that it can also be run as a standalone application on a researcher's machine. Recently, the VCell team has incorporated the BioNetGen (Blinov et al., 2004) network generator, which allows models to be specified in a rule-based manner. VCell is also one of the few tools that can both import and export SBML and CellML. This feature could, in principle, be used to translate between SBML and CellML models.

Visual Editors

Tools that allow users to draw pathways on a screen and turn them into simulatable models seem to be fairly rare. We confine our attention here to tools that are specifically designed to assist in simulation, rather than pathway annotation. Examples of the latter include the Edinburgh Pathway Editor (Sorokin et al., 2006), Cytoscape (Shannon et al., 2003), BioUML (Kolpakov, 2004) and BioTapestry (Longabaugh et al., 2005); many others exist. We mention the latter tools specifically because they have some simulation capability, but their strengths lie elsewhere. A very complete review of non-simulation-based network viewers can be found in Suderman and Hallett (2007).

Probably one of the first visual editors to be written for simulation was a Mac-based tool called KineCyte (Cook and Atkins, 1997; Cook et al., 2001), and around the same time JDesigner (Bergmann et al., 2006) was developed by Sauro for the Windows platform. Other tools include applications such as SimWiz (Rost and Kummer, 2004), CADLive (Kurata et al., 2007) and Cellware (Dhar et al., 2004); unfortunately, Cellware does not appear to be under development any longer. The three main visual design tools still supported and geared towards simulation are JDesigner, ProMoT (Ginkel et al., 2003) and CellDesigner (Kitano et al., 2005).

JDesigner (Sauro et al., 2003; Bergmann et al., 2006) is open source (BSD license) and runs under Windows. It requires SBW to enable simulation capabilities. With SBW, models can be constructed using JDesigner and seamlessly transferred to other tools such as COPASI or any other SBW-enabled tool. Unlike CellDesigner, JDesigner takes a minimal approach to representing networks. CellDesigner has 12 node types (plus variants) and six different transition types. JDesigner, in contrast, has one node type, one generic reaction type and two regulatory types. All networks can be constructed from these four basic types. This minimal approach reflects the fact that the underlying models are the same regardless of the molecules or reaction types. Thus protein network models and metabolic models are indistinguishable at the mathematical level. Although JDesigner has only a limited number of types, nodes, reactions and membranes can be modified visually to change colors, shapes, etc. Moreover, nodes can be decorated with covalent sites and multimeric structures. JDesigner uses fully adjustable multibezier arcs to generate reactions and regulatory arcs, and has a variety of export formats that allow camera-ready copy to be generated for publications. Models are stored in native SBML, with specific open access annotations to store the visual information.

CellDesigner

CellDesigner (Kitano et al., 2005), developed by Akira Funahashi in the Kitano group, is a popular close-source, but cross-platform, Java-based tool. Like JDesigner, it needs external support to enable simulation, which can include SBW or SOSLib (Machné et al., 2006) (*see* Dedicated Libraries, SOSLib, below). One of the main strengths of CellDesigner is its visually appealing graphical representation, which has made CellDesigner a popular tool. Its other strength, although still under development, is the availability of a plug-in architecture that, in principle, will allow other third-party programmers to develop add-ons to the tool (Dräger et al., 2008). One potential drawback of CellDesigner is that the format that the tool uses to store the models is undocumented, so that only CellDesigner is capable of reading and writing the models. Only one other tool, the visual layout tool in SBW, can read CellDesigner models, and that was accomplished by reverse-engineering the CellDesigner format. With the advent of the Systems Biology Graphical Notation, it is hoped that tool writers will move towards a community-agreed and open format for representing biochemical networks. (More details are given in the section on Standards (Graphical Layout)).

Commercial Visual Design Tools

There are also some commercial pathway editors, including Cell Illustrator (http://www.cellillustrator.com), SimBiology from MathWorks and an interesting contribution from Gene Network Sciences (http://www.gnsbiotech.com/), which utilize a visual language called DCL (Diagrammatic Cell Language), which unfortunately was patented and thereby sealed its future; regardless, it seems no longer to be available.

CellML-based Applications

Although SBML is by and large one of the more popular exchange formats, CellML is also an important standard (particularly among cell physiologists), in which models combine biochemical network models with transport and electrophysiological behavior. For this reason, most applications developed with CellML import and export capabilities tend to be geared towards physiological modeling and often do not support SBML. Hybrid applications such as VCell and JSIM try to support both formats—with varying degrees of success, as the formats are not generally compatible.

We have already mentioned JSIM as an application that can import CellML models. In addition to JSIM, there are a number of prominent simulators in this category. The most important of these include Andre's CellML Tools, COR (Garny et al., 2003), PCEnv and VCell (Slepchenko et al., 2003). All these tools can import and export CellML.

Andre's CellML tools include a series of utilities to browse CellML models and carry out basic simulations. COR, another important CellML-based tool, is a Windows application developed by Alan Garny at Oxford University in the UK, and was probably the first simulator to support CellML. COR uses an interesting scripting language to describe a model, which means users do not need to know the intricacies of CellML. The language incorporates facilities to allow a user to specify units, much like the facilities found in JSIM. COR also supports high-speed simulation capabilities through runtime compilation. Installation is very simple, and uses a one-click installer.

PCEnv is a tool that is being development by the CellML team at Auckland. It incorporates a basic simulator permitting users to generate time-course simulations, change parameters and generate new models. Model generation is GUI-based, in which a user builds a tree representing the various components of the model. In addition to the GUI interface, there is also a JavaScript interface, which offers some control over the output and simulation. Installation is very simple and uses a one-click installer. Tools such as COR and PCEnv are under very active development, and it is hoped that in the future they will offer many of the facilities that are currently available in other systems biology simulation tools.

Other Tools of Interest

We list here some other tools that we have not mentioned but which are notable for one reason or another. Not all of these tools appear to be being actively developed, but they may experience continued development in the future. Most, if not all, of these tools support SBML import and export. All these tools are worth looking at, some implement particular functions very well. In the descriptions, only a brief hint is given concerning their capabilities, and the reader is strongly urged to investigate them further if some particular functionality is of interest.

BioNetGen: BioNetGen (Blinov et al., 2004) is a tool for automatically generating mathematical models of biological systems from user-specified rules for biomolecular interactions, particularly signaling pathways. Rules are specified in a script-based language from which the reaction scheme is generated and, subsequently, the mathematical model. There are not many tools that operate on a rule-based approach (*cf.* little b, http://www.littleb.org/), but all of them take a particular and fairly radical view of biology that assumes that all interactions are potentially significant, of which there may be many thousands in a given model, depending on the specified rules.

Cellerator/xCellerator: This is part of the SIGMOID project (Cheng et al., 2005) at Caltech and Irvine, although its origins are earlier. It is a Mathematica-based tool designed to facilitate biological modeling via automated equation generation. Two notable features of this tool include the ability to embed arrow-based chemical notation directly into Mathematica scripts- and support for multicellular models. Model analysis is fairly basic, confined largely to generating time-course simulations. The other Mathematica tool, MathSBML (Shapiro et al., 2004) has much more extensive analysis capabilities.

E-Cell: The E-Cell (Tomita et al., 1999) simulation environment is an object-oriented software suite for modeling, simulation and analysis of large-scale complex systems such as biological cells. It has been in development since 1996 and can, in the latest version, be accessed via Python. For some reason, E-Cell has never gained the popularity that perhaps is should have. Early versions suffered from a user interface that was difficult to use, which most probably slowed its acceptance by the community; furthermore, model interchange support has been weak, which also hampered acceptance of E-Cell by the wider community.

JigCell: JigCell (Vass et al., 2004) is a modeling tool developed by the Tyson group, who are well known for their cell cycle models (Tyson et al., 2002). Many tools are deigned by programmers rather than modelers, but JigCell is one of those few tools that was written specifically by a well established modeling group to fit models to data and test the models against numerous experimental results. The system works in a similar way to regression testing in software design, in which the computational model is repeatedly tested as the model evolves or new experimental data are made available. This enables the generation of robust and more reliable models. As part of this goal, JigCell also supports parameter estimation and the ability to maintain an ensemble of models. The unique functionality provided by JigCell reflects the fact that the authors are modelers, rather than just software developers.

ProMoT: ProMoT (Ginkel et al., 2003) stands for "process modeling tool" and originated from the process engineering community, but has since evolved to encompass biochemical modeling. Currently, it runs well only on Linux, but plans have been made to make a Windows version. It is notable for its ability to model differential algebraic equations and is one of the few tools to provide visual support for dealing with model libraries, modules and hierarchical models.

Oscill8: Oscill8 (http://oscill8.sf.net/) is a bifurcation analysis tool developed by Emery Conrad of the Tyson group. It runs well on the Windows platform and takes XPP scripts as input. Oscill8 represents one of the few bifurcation packages with a modern GUI interface. SBW supplies a special SBML-to-XPP translator that is designed to work with Oscill8. Although the XPPAUT site also provides an SBML-to-XPP translator, this is unsuitable for many biochemical models because it doesn't take conservation laws into consideration in the models, which renders the Jacobian singular and thereby unsuitable for the AUTO numerical algorithms.

PottersWheel: This is a very comprehensive parameter-fitting tool (Maiwald and Timmer, 2008) that works well with the SBToolBox^2 (Schmidt and Jirstrand, 2006), but can also be used alone. In a number of cases it betters the capabilities of COPASI, particularly in the area of generating non-linear confidence limits on parameter fits and analyzing the resulting fit. The experimental data input formats are also very flexible. The tool provides, out of the box, a number of optimization algorithms, including Genetic and simulated annealing approaches. For a Matlab user interested in doing parameter fitting properly, this tool is a serious contender, especially as the built-in optimization methods in Matlab itself are not sufficiently robust for fitting biochemical models. A further advantage of this tool is that is comes with copious documentation. PottersWheel combined with the SBToolbox^2 is a powerful mix.

R Packages: There is currently limited support for dynamic modeling in R, but this is changing. Given the growing interest in using R in biological research, it would not be surprising if further work is done in this area. Currently, the two tools that are of interest include the SBMLR package by Tomas Radivoyevitch and a more modern version by Michael Lawrence, called RSBML. Modeling is, however, in all cases limited to simple time-course simulations. Both packages use the ODEPACK library for integrating the ODEs, which arguably is superior to CVODE from SUNDIALS, thanks to the ability of ODEPACK to switch integration modes during the integration.

SBMLPET: SBMLPET (Zi and Klipp, 2006) is a SBML-based Parameter Estimation Tool. Of interest is that the tool not only supports event handling in SBML, but also uses the stochastic ranking evolution strategy (SRES) (Runarsson and Yao, 2005) for fitting, which is arguably one of the best fitting strategies to use (Moles et al., 2003).

SBMLToolbox: This is a Matlab tool box developed by the Caltech SBML team (Keating et al., 2006). Its primary function is to load and save SBML in to Matlab data structures. It uses the built-in Matlab functions to carry out simulations. Its importance lies in its careful adherence to the SBML specifications. Other Matlab-related tools add functionality to this toolbox.

sloppyCell: This is a Python-based tool developed at Cornell (Myers et al., 2007). It has some significant capabilities in parameter fitting, related to estimating confidence limits in fitted models. For a Python-based tool that supports parameter fitting, this is probably the most mature, although the supplied optimization methods are limited in scope (Levenberg, 1944; Marquardt, 1963; Nelder and Mead, 1965). It does support ensemble model fitting, which is very useful and is probably its main *raison d'être*. It does not, however, compare to PySCeS in other areas. If additional fitting methods—for example an SRES (Runarsson and Yao, 2005)—were included, a combination of sloppyCell and PySCeS would be extremely powerful.

XPPAUT: Although XPP (Ermentrout, 2002) is not a tool that was written specifically for the systems biology community, its great utility is its extensive support for bifurcation analysis, a largely neglected field in the software development community, particularly in systems biology. XPP gains its computational capabilities from a well established software library called AUTO (Doedel, 1981). Although it is possible to use AUTO on its own, XPP adds a user interface to make it easier to use. Although very capable, the user interface of XPP is, however, not very modern by current standards, and does take a little getting used to. Running XPP on Windows is awkward, and XPP is really meant to be run on the Linux/Unix platform. For an easier tool, but perhaps with more limited capability, Oscill8 is a good choice for the Windows user.

For Python users, there is an interesting tool called PyDSTool (Myers et al., 2007) (inspired by the original DSTool of Back et al., 1992) although users must derive the differential equations themselves, and installation is by no means trivial. However, it may be possible to modify the tool for the systems biology community.

Commercial Tools

There is a small but growing list of commercial titles available in the market. The most prominent of these include Berkeley Madonna, Jacobian, SimBiology from MathWorks, and Terranode. We should also mention SimPheny from Genomatica even though it is not a dynamic simulation package, but because it is a well established tool for flux balance analysis. Klamt et al. (2007) describe a non-commercial flux balance tool; note, however, that this tool requires a commercial copy of Matlab to operate. With the exception of Berkeley Madonna, all these tools can export SBML; however, COPASI can export Berkeley Madonna files. The one real issue with commercial tools is the lack of transparency with regard to the numerical algorithms they utilize and the impossibility of changing the methods when necessary. MathWorks, to its credit, has documentation on the methods used, but the code itself is not visible to the researcher. This is a significant problem for a research-based community, less so perhaps for a commercially-funded project. It is, of course, a difficult issue to reconcile for commercial vendors, because the underlying numerical methods are often the source of value in the product.

Dedicated Libraries

Up to now, we have focused on describing end-user applications with which a user would download an installer and in a very short time be ready to start defining a model and running a simulation. As mentioned previously, there are a huge number of such tools available, although sadly many are started but left unfinished. In addition, many tools re-invent basic functionality over and over again, wasting considerable human intellect and time. In this section we would like to describe a small but growing list of software libraries dedicated to dynamic simulation in systems biology and targeted at developers of new software. These libraries are cross-platform and, most significantly, cross-language solutions to common computational and data management problems in systems biology. They enable developers to create new applications from existing well tested and documented solutions, and enable developers to focus on novel functionality rather than spending most of their effort on re-inventing well understood themes. Furthermore, from a historical perspective, good, well tested software libraries tend to survive the turmoils of funding cycles and researcher turnover, whereas end-user applications tend not to.

libSBML

libSBML (Bornstein et al., 2008) is a very useful software library, provided by the SBML team, which can be used to read and write SBML. The success of SBML over competing standards can be ascribed in part to libSBML. The software library is based around a C/C++ core, with wrappers provided for many programming languages. Furthermore, the library is available for Windows and POSIX operating systems in which a C and C++ based Application Programming Interface (API) is exposed and thus can be linked to virtually any other computer language with relative ease. With an abundance of documentation and examples, software developers can readily use libSBML for their SBML support.

By using libSBML, a developer can focus on how to interpret computational models, rather than concerning themselves with the mechanics of reading and writing SBML. At the time this chapter was written, libSBML had released version 3. This version had new features, including the ability to validate the model, such as unit consistency checking, or checks on whether the model assignment expressions are overdetermined. libSBML also provides support for MIRIAM-compatible annotations (Le Novère et al., 2005). libSBML is a very well developed library that sets a high standard for the development of other software libraries in the systems biology community.

SOSLib

The SBML ODE Solver Library (Machné et al., 2006), or SOSLib, is a simulation library that can be linked against any application using the C programming language. At the core, SOSLib uses the SUNDIALS suite (Hindmarsh et al., 2005) and libSBML. Like most SBML-capable simulators, it does not deal with models using delayed differential equations and algebraic equations. Conversely, SOSLib is one of the few simulators that can handle events reasonably well. Supporting SBML events has proved to be a difficult undertaking for many developers, because of the numerical difficulties that they generate. Very few ODE integrators support event detection, and as a result only very few simulators (such as SOSLib and roadRunner) are capable of correctly handling them.

SOSLib can be run in two modes. In the interpreted mode, SOSLib will use the abstract syntax trees of libSBML to evaluate the kinetic laws and other equations. The use of the abstract syntax tree also permits SOSLib to invoke symbolic evaluation when computing the elements of the Jacobian matrix—a technique also utilized by SCAMP (Sauro, 1993; Sauro and Fell, 1991). In the second mode, the right-hand side of every ODE is compiled, using either GCC on POSIX environments or tcc (http://fabrice.bellard.free.fr/tcc/) on Windows. This allows SOSLib to generate fast simulation times. However, SOSLib has one significant drawback, namely its inability to remove dependent variables from the model. If this deficiency could be corrected, SOSLib would be a library of much greater use to the community.

libStructural

The libStructural library is a software library for conservation and structural analysis of stoichiometric networks and is written in C/C++ for cross-platform portability (http://sys-bio.org/libStructural).

One of the initial steps in a simulation (deterministic or stochastic) is to consider the stoichiometric structure of a model. This is carried out for a number of reasons: first it allows model reduction to take place and permits faster simulation times, and secondly it allows users to study the structural characteristics of the model, such as flux and moiety conservation. The flux constraints can be further used to establish linear programming models for flux balance analysis (Fell and Small, 1986; Palsson, 2007) and also as an aid to constructing the isotopomer dynamic models used in isotopic measurements of fluxes (Schwender, 2008; Wiechert, 2001). The library provides more than 60 API calls, which give information on various stoichiometric properties such as the kernel, link, dependent and independent flux, and species matrices. In addition, the library exposes some useful functionality from the LAPACK library (Anderson et al., 1999). The library can also be built against libSBML, so that models in standard SBML can be analyzed; otherwise, the library accepts raw stoichiometry matrices. The library is fully documented and has been tested against the very large models from the Palsson group (Price et al., 2003) and more than 20 smaller test models.

DEDICATED TOOLS FOR STOCHASTIC SIMULATION

Stochastic simulation has received much attention in the last 10–20 years, owing to the realization that continuous models are not always an appropriate description of what is, at the molecular level, a fundamentally discrete process. The development of practical algorithms for stochastic simulation owes its origin to a series of classical papers published by Gillespie in the 1970s. Gillespie's approach yielded an algorithm that was extremely straightforward to implement in software, but was largely unknown until the early 1990s in biology. Two of the first studies to utilize Gillespie's approach in biology were those by Kraus et al. (1992) and Moniz-Barreto and Fell (1993). However, it was probably the study by Arkin et al. (1998) that convinced many of the importance of stochastic dynamics in biology. In the intervening years, there has been an explosion in interest in stochastic dynamics, attracting researchers from many diverse fields (Curti et al., 2003; Ullah and Wolkenhauer, 2007; Wilkinson, 2006).

Together with modeling efforts there have been developments in software, particularly in relation to making the basic Gillespie method more efficient. An excellent and highly readable review of the current state of numerical methods is given by Gillespie (2007). Here, we will briefly review some of the software available for stochastic simulation. We will not consider hybrid methods that combine discrete with continuous modeling, as the methods are still under development (details are given by Salis et al., 2006); however, a brief review is given by Ullah and Wolkenhauer (2007). We will also not consider here spatial stochastic modeling tools such as MCell (Stiles and Bartol, 2001).

Unlike deterministic models in which a single run provides all the information on the trajectory, the Gillespie method only generates one of a very large number of possible realizations. Ideally, stochastic simulators should support ensemble simulations, so that statistics can be collected on the behavior of the model. Many simulators do not provide for this facility and presumably expect the user to manually make the necessary repeats (which, ideally, should run into tens of thousands of runs). Only a few simulators support ensemble runs (e.g. COPASI), but only one software tool, Gillespie-GUI (Vallabhajosyula and Sauro, 2007), computes a wide range of statistics for analyzing stochastic models.

As with models based on differential equations, there is a test suite available that allows developers of stochastic simulators to evaluate their efforts (see Test Suites, below). The test suite was developed and is maintained by the Wilkinson group at Newcastle, UK (Evans et al., 2008). An example of how the test suite can be used is given by Vallabhajosyula and Sauro (2007).

As for software, there are a number of tools that support stochastic simulation, many of which include the tools we have described in previous sections—for example, COPASI and Jarnac. SBW also incorporates a number of stochastic solvers, including a high-speed solver written using .NET. Other more specific tools that focus exclusively on stochastic simulation include BioNetS (Adalsteinsson et al., 2004), which is a Mac-based tool (a version with a Java front end also exists for Windows and Linux) that incorporates a number of stochastic related solvers, including Gillespie and a capability to solve Langevin equations. This latter ability is rare, and makes BioNetS a very useful tool for this kind of work.

Two other well known applications are Dizzy and StochSim. Dizzy (Ramsey et al., 2005) is a Java-based application that was developed by Stephen Ramsey at the Institute of Systems Biology in Seattle; it incorporates a number of stochastic methods. It is capable of reading SBML level 1 and has an SBW programmatic interface. StochSim (Le Novère and Shimizu, 2001) was developed in the 1990s at Cambridge University, UK by Carl Firth in Bray's group, and subsequently developed further by Le Novère and Shimizu. It uses a method slightly different from the Gillespie approach that, according to the authors, scales better when a system contains molecules that can exist in several states. In addition, later versions have provision for spatial simulation in two dimensions. One significant difference is that StochSim uses a fixed time-step the size of which will determine the accuracy of the algorithm. In contrast, the Gillespie SSA method uses an exact approach in which the step size is computed as part of the algorithm itself. However, subsequent variants of SSA such as tau-leaping are also approximate, and for detailed statistical analysis of stochastic runs such approximate methods should probably be avoided.

Other examples of stochastic simulators include CytoSim, written in Java, from the Microsoft Trento group (Sedwards and Mazza, 2007), and ESS from the University of Tennessee (Cox et al., 2003). CytoSim incorporates an interesting and easy to learn script language for describing biochemical networks. ESS and its descendants are notable for implementing what is probably the world's fastest stochastic simulation software.

Finally, there currently exists one software library, StochKit, that is dedicated to implementing a wide variety of Gillespie-based approaches (Li et al., 2008) and is being developed by the Petzold group in Santa Barbara, USA. StochKit is a C++-based library and therefore can, in principle, be linked easily only to other C++ applications; a mundane but more useful C-based API would make the library much more portable to other software languages. StochKit also currently lacks many of the advanced analysis methods that a stochastic solver would need for practical use. Moreover, support for Windows appears to be very limited, which makes the library essentially a Linux-based tool. StochKit has made a promising start, but has some way to go before it reaches the usability and portability of libraries such as SUNDIALS (Hindmarsh et al., 2005) or ODEPACK Hindmarsh (1983). The Tennessee group that developed ESS (Cox et al., 2003) is developing a very-high-performance C-based solution that will incorporate many advanced features, such as support for discrete events and ensemble simulations. There are, in addition, dedicated hardware solutions to stochastic simulation that involve the use of field-programmable gate arrays and other technology to build what could potentially be very-high-speed simulation engines (McCollum et al., 2003; Peterson and Lancaster, 2002; Yoshimi et al., 2004).

STANDARDS

With the surge in the number of incompatible simulation tools since the year 2000, it was realized by at least two communities that some form of standardization for model exchange was necessary. CellML and SBML are the two standards that emerged. CellML is primarily a notation for representing biochemical models in a strict mathematical form; as a result it is, in principle, completely general. In contrast, SBML uses a biologically inspired notation to represent networks from which a mathematical model can be generated. Each has its strengths and weaknesses, but SBML has a simpler structure than CellML and as a result there is more software support for SBML. Most software tools at the present time support import and export of SBML. Both standards have very active communities, intracellular models being primarily the domain of SBML and physiological models for CellML.

CellML

CellML (Hedley et al., 2001; Lloyd et al., 2004) represents cellular models using a mathematical description. In addition, CellML represents entities using a component-based approach in which relationships between components are represented by connections. The literal translation of the mathematics, however, goes much further; in fact the representation that CellML uses is very reminiscent of the way an engineer might wire up an analog computer to solve the equations (although without specifying the integrators). As a result, CellML is very general and, in principle, could probably represent any system that has a mathematical description. However, the generality and explicit nature of CellML also results in increased complexity, especially for software developers.

Another key aspect of CellML is its provision for metadata support. The metadata can be used to provide a context for a model, such as the author's name, when it was created and what additional documents are available for its description. CellML uses standard XML-based metadata containers such as Resource Description Framework (RDF) and, within RDF, the Dublin Core. CellML metadata support, such as BioPAX (Luciano and Stevens, 2007: http://www.biopax.org), is the means by which biological information can be introduced into a CellML model.

The CellML team has amassed a very large suite (hundreds) of models (Lloyd et al., 2008: www.cellml.org/models/) that provides many real examples of CellML syntax. This is an extremely useful resource for the community.

SBML

Whereas CellML attempts to be highly comprehensive, SBML was designed to meet the immediate needs of the modeling community, and is therefore more focused on a particular problem set. One result of this is that the standard is simpler than CellML, although more recent revisions have added new functionality, so that the difference in complexity between CellML and SBML is becoming less significant. Like CellML, SBML is based on XML; however, unlike CellML, it takes a different approach to representing cellular models. The way in which SBML represents models closely maps the way that existing modeling packages represent models. Whereas CellML represents models mathematically, SBML represent models as a list of chemical transformations. As every process in a biological cell can ultimately be broken down into one or more chemical transformations, this was a natural representation to use. However, SBML does not have generalized elements such as components and connections; rather, it uses specific elements to represent spatial compartments, molecular species and chemical transformations. In addition to these, SBML also has provision for rules that can be used to represent constraints, derived values and general math that for one reason or another cannot be transformed into a chemical scheme.

SBML, like any standard, evolves with time (Finney and Hucka, 2003). Major revisions of the standard are captured in levels, whereas minor modifications and clarifications are captured in versions. An example of a major change within the standard would be the use of MathML in level 2 of SBML, whereas level 1 encoded infix strings to denote reaction rates and rules. In contrast, a minor change would, for example, be the introduction of semantic annotation (in form of SBO terms and MIRIAM annotations), that can be added to SBML Level 2 Version 2 documents, whereas this was not possible in a supported fashion in earlier versions (see Systems Biology Ontology, below). At the time this chapter was being written, SBML level 3 was still in development. With level 3, the standard will develop in an extensible manner. This means there will be a set of core features that must be supported and around which additional features, such as spatial modeling, can be included.

There has been little effort to develop methods to interconvert between SBML and CellML; however, Schilstra in the UK developed a tool called CellML2SBML (Schilstra et al., 2006), which allows users to convert CellML-based models into SBML. It is also possible to use tools such as VCell to interconvert between these two standards.

Other Related Standards

Graphical Layout

Graphical modeling applications (Bergmann et al., 2006) routinely enhance computational models by layout annotations. Recently, the SBML community has decided on a common standard on how to embed the layout information within SBML. The layout extension (Gauges et al., 2006) allows a model to store the size and dimension of all model elements, along with textual annotations and reactions. Originally the intention was to embed the layout extension in a model annotation for level 2 versions of SBML, but with the expected level 3 the layout extension will be added to the SBML as a first-class construct. LibSBML has been modified to provide access to all elements of the layout extension. In addition, several reference implementations exist (Bergmann et al., 2006; Deckard et al., 2006).

Whereas the layout extension is concerned with representing simple elements, the Systems Biology Graphical Notation (SBGN) (http://sbgn.org) aims to standardize the visual language of computational models unambiguously. This standard is still in development and, strictly speaking, independent of the SBML effort. Experience in other fields such as electrical engineering has demonstrated the essential need for standardizing the visual notation for representing models in diagrammatic form.

MIRIAM

Model definition languages such as SBML and CellML target the exchange of models. They aim to pass on the quantitative computational models from one software tool to another. However, these description formats do not concern themselves with semantic annotations. Both SBML and CellML have launched efforts to remedy this problem. Both communities agreed on the Minimum Information Requested In the Annotation of biochemical Models (MIRIAM) (Le Novère et al., 2005). These annotations aim to add further confidence in quantitative biochemical models, making it easier and more precise to search for particular biochemical models, enabling researchers to identify biological phenomena captured by a biochemical model and, perhaps most importantly, facilitating model re-use and model composition.

In order to call a model MIRIAM compliant, the model has to be encoded in a standard format, such as SBML. Furthermore, it needs to be tied to a reference description, describing the properties and results that can be obtained from the model. Parameters of the computational model have to be provided, so that the model can be loaded into a simulation environment in which the results can be reproduced. Other information that has to be provided is a name for the model, the creator of the model, the date and time of the last modification and a statement about the terms of distribution.

Systems Biology Ontology

In order to assign meaning to model constituents, an ontology specific to Systems Biology has been developed: the Systems Biology Ontology (SBO) (http://www.ebi.ac.uk/sbo/). The ontology consists of five controlled vocabularies and two relationships: is-part-of and is-a. Qualifying model participants—say as enzyme, macromolecule, metabolite or small species such as an ion—will make it easier to generate meaning from the model. It will make the generation of standard visual notations such as SBGN possible. Moreover, it presents a solution as to how to interpret the model computationally, as the SBO allows tagging a model as continuous, discrete or logical. One could even go a step further, making kinetic interactions in a model obsolete, by just referencing that the rate law is one specified by an ontology identifier (e.g. tagging a reaction as following Henri–Michaelis–Menten enzyme kinetics and specifying the parameters). The SBO is community driven, and new terms or modifications to the existing ontology can be requested by the community.

Other Ontologies

The most recent developments in the CellML— and particularly the SBML—communities revolve around the creation of ontologies and refining the exchange semantics. Apart from classifying model constituents with an appropriate ontology, one of the current areas of interest is describing the dynamical behavior of a model. Terminology for the Description of Dynamics (TEDDY) (http://www.ebi.ac.uk/compneursrv/teddy/) provides a rich ontology to describe and quantify the kind of behavior that a computational model is able to exhibit (e.g. the characteristics of a model could describe bifurcation behavior in which the functionality of a model could be described as featuring oscillations or switch behavior). However, knowing that a model exhibits interesting behavior is not enough; more information is needed in order to recreate that behavior. The Minimum Information About a Simulation Experiment (MIASE) (http://www.ebi.ac.uk/compneursrv/miase/) project focuses in this problem. MIASE will help to describe the simulation algorithms and the simulation tool used, along with all needed parameter settings. In order to do so it will use the Kinetic Simulation Algorithm Ontology (KiSAO) that relates simulation algorithms and methods to each other. As these ontologies are still currently under development, it will be interesting to see how they progress and are taken up by the community.

Lastly, we should mention Biological Pathway Exchange (BioPAX) (Luciano and Stevens, 2007). BioPAX is an XML-based format that will act as a bridge between different pathway databases and data. In relation to modeling software, BioPAX may offer a means to embed rich annotation data into an SBML or CellML model. Some of this capability is being addressed, to a limited extent, by the new ontologies being developed at EBI in Cambridge, UK. However, given its role to allow a common exchange of biological data between pathway databases, BioPAX may offer a useful complementary way to bind data to computational models.

Human-readable Formats

SBML and CellML are examples of formats that use XML to represent information. One advantage to using XML is that there is much software available to assist in reading and manipulating XML-based data. However, XML is not suited for human consumption, but is designed strictly to be read by computer software. In order for humans to build and read models, human-readable formats are required; often these are text-based, but sometimes they are graphical. In relation to text-based formats, there has been a long tradition of using human-readable formats for representing biochemical models, starting with BIOSSIM (Garfinkel et al., 1970). Other examples of early human-readable formats include, for example, work by Burns (1971) and Park and Wright (1973). In more recent years, simulators such as SCAMP (Sauro and Fell, 1991) and METAMOD (Hofmeyr and van der Merwe, 1986) also introduced human-readable formats to define models. Both software tools were developed in later years, into Jarnac and PySCeS, respectively.

Other formats of interest include composable languages developed by McCollum at the University of Miami, Sauro and Bergmann at the University of Washington (Bergmann and Sauro, 2006) and Pederson at the University of Edinburgh (Pedersen and Plotkin, 2008). Blinov, Faeder, Goldstein and Hlavacek developed BioNetGen (Blinov et al., 2004), which is a rule-based format for representing systems with multiple states; CytoSim, which we have mentioned previously, incorporates an interesting human-readable language for representing biochemical systems. The SBML community (Wilkinson, 2007) has also developed a human-readable script called SBMLshorthand. This notation maps directly on to SBML, but is much easier to handwrite than SBML (as are all these human-readable formats). The shorthand is also much less verbose and uses infix to represent expressions, rather than MathML. Finally, we should mention a lisp-based language called little b (http://www.littleb.org/) that is being developed at Harvard University. The aim of little b is to allow biologists to build models quickly and easily from shared parts.

DATABASES

Along with the standardization of model representation, there has been an obvious desire to create model repositories where models published in journals can be stored and retrieved. There are, at the present time, five repositories, with varying degrees of quality and usability. Probably the most promising is the UK-based, searchable, BioModels Database, which at July 2008 held more than 170 fully curated and working models that can be downloaded in standard SBML and other formats. BioModels also has the great benefit of providing programmatic access to its database via web services, which allows any software program to access the database seamlessly across the internet. Models stored in the BioModels Database are curated, meaning that models will reproduce the original intention of the author. In addition, the models are annotated, so that model components can be referenced from other database sources.

Another large database has been assembled by the CellML community (Lloyd et al., 2008). It has more than 300 models stored in CellML format. From their site it is possible, in principle, to convert the CellML into standard C code for compilation in to a working model.

The JSIM group at the University of Washington has a large database of physiological models (http://nsr.bioeng.washington.edu/Models/) stored in the mathematical language used by the JSIM simulation application. These models can only be read by JSIM, and currently there is no simple way to translate these to any of the common exchange formats; however, this is likely to change in the future.

Another small but very useful database is the JWS online database developed by Olivier and Snoep (2004), which has almost 80 fully working models. JWS allows export in both SBML and the script format PySCeS, which can be easily translated to other formats such as Jarnac script. JWS is arguably one of the first databases of models, although physiological models such as those supported by JSIM have been available for longer. Many of, if not all, the models on JWS have also been imported to the BioModels Database and *vice versa*.

The database DOQCS (http://doqcs.ncbs.res.in/) focuses on signaling networks and contains more than 200 models. However, models in DOQCS can only be downloaded in GENESIS format (Bhalla, 2002), which limits the portability to other frameworks. Recently, the DOQCS database has been merged with the BioModels Database.

Finally, there is a major database called Sigmoid, sponsored by the National Institutes of Health (Cheng et al., 2005), which currently has about 20 models. The focus of the Sigmoid project, however, appears to be infrastructure rather than curation, which explains the limited number of models available. Access to the database is limited to the model explorer tool SME (www.sigmoid.org), thus access from other applications may not be possible. In addition, models can only be accessed from the web interface using the Cellerator format, which limits portability to other frameworks. Work on Sigmoid is continuing, and no doubt changes will occur in the future to make it more open.

TEST SUITES

An important need in the simulation community is some means to compare and test simulation codes. Currently, there are available a number of test suites expressed in SBML. One is provided by Andrew Finney (http://sbml.org/wiki/Semantic_Test_Suite) and includes various tests for deterministic models; another, by Evans et al. (2008), represents a stochastic test suite. Currently, the deterministic test suite is undergoing a redesign, because it has significant issues related to numerical stability. The stochastic test suite has recently gone through a second iteration and is an extremely useful resource. Another suite of models that can be used for testing is the BioModels Database of models. Although test results are not available, it is possible to use the database models for comparison purposes, as has been done by Bergmann and Sauro (2008: http://www.sysbio.org/sbwWiki/compare). The comparison site gives detailed side-by-side information as to how different simulators solve a given SBML model. Overall agreement between the simulation packages appears to be high.

The CellML team in Auckland are in the process of developing a test suite for CellML, which should aid considerably in testing CellML-compliant applications.

FUTURE PROSPECTS

In surveying the development of software in systems biology, we see a vibrant and sometimes innovative community with a very wide range of tools to satisfy all manner of users. There are still some areas that are lacking, most notably bifurcation analysis and model composition. There are some very notable tools for bifurcation analysis, but they have been written more for general use than specifically for systems biology (Oscill8 being a notable exception). User interface design is still somewhat primitive in these bifurcation tools, and there is much opportunity for innovation in this area, particularly with respect to interactive bifurcation analysis. The second area that is lacking is model composition (*cf.* ProMoT). As models become more commonplace, there is a growing desire to be able to take models and combine them easily. Currently, this is not possible without considerable effort. Model composition is not a simple problem to solve, however, as there are many issues to consider, including unit consistency and interface protocols. Nevertheless, the benefits would be significant, and with the rise of synthetic biology there is even more reason to develop the idea.

Re-usable Software Libraries

One of the issues that has plagued software development in systems biology is chronic reinvention. Many tools, particularly those listed at SBML.org, carry out similar functions at their core (solving ODEs, computing steady states, sensitivities, etc.). The fact that each tool re-implements the same functionality is arguably a waste of resources, and it would be of great benefit to the community if some of the core functionality could be released in the form of re-usable software libraries. There are many benefits to such an approach, including improved testing, documentation, maintainability and extensibility. Unless there are strong reasons to do so, very few developers now write their own stiff ODE solver or SBML reader. There are already some useful libraries in the community, such as libSBML, SUNDIALS, ODEPACK, LAPACK. These libraries are successful for a number of reasons: they are well documented, open and, most importantly, they are written in languages (C and FORTRAN) that make it easy to interface them to other programming languages. Libraries that are written in other languages, such as Java or C++, or in which a C interface is not exposed, tend to be less successful. We have seen some efforts to develop additional libraries, most notably SOSLib and StochKit, but these are still under development, and lack some critical functionality (SOSLib lacks the ability to remove dependent species) or ease of integration (in the case of StochKit). These issues will no doubt be resolved in the future, and will then allow developers to focus on other areas of interest such as user interface design and the development of new approaches to analysis.

ACKNOWLEDGEMENTS

We would like to acknowledge the generous support from a number of funding agencies, including the US Department of Energy GTL program and the NIH (1R01GM08107001). We would also like to acknowledge the many useful discussions we have had over the years with our colleagues in the software and computational systems biology community, in particular we wish to acknowledge the contributions of Athel Cornish-Bowden, David Fell, Jannie Hofmeyr, Mike Hucka and Pedro Mendes.

References

Adalsteinsson, D., McMillen, D., Elston, T.C., 2004. Biochemical network stochastic simulator (bionets): software for stochastic modeling of biochemical networks. BMC Bioinformatics 5, 24.

Alon, U., 2006. An Introduction to Systems Biology: Design Principles of Biological Circuits. Chapman & Hall/Crc Mathematical and Computational Biology Series. Chapman & Hall/CRC, Boca Raton, FL.

Alves, R., Antunes, F., Salvador, A., 2006. Tools for kinetic modeling of biochemical networks. Nat. Biotechnol. 24, 667–672.

Ander, M., Beltrao, P., Di Ventura, B., et al., 2004. SmartCell, a framework to simulate cellular processes that combines stochastic approximation with diffusion and localisation: analysis of simple networks. Syst. Biol. (Stevenage) 1, 129–138.

Anderson, E., McKenney, A., Sorensen, D., et al., 1999. LAPACK Users' Guide. Society for Industrial and Applied Mathematics Philadelphia, PA, USA.

Arkin, A., Ross, J., McAdams, H.H., 1998. Stochastic kinetic analysis of developmental pathway bifurcation in phage lambda-infected Escherichia coli cells. Genetics 149, 1633–1648.

Back, A., Guckenheimer, J., Myers, M., Wicklin, F., Worfolk, P., 1992. DsTool: computer assisted exploration of dynamical systems. Notices Am. Math. Soc. 39, 303–309.

Bergmann, F.T., Sauro, H.M., 2006. Human Readable Model Definition Language. Available from http://sys-bio.org/sbwWiki

Bergmann, F., Sauro, H., 2008. Comparing Simulation Results of SBML Capable Simulators. Bioinformatics 24, 1963–1965.

Bergmann, F.T., Vallabhajosyula, R.R., Sauro, H.M., 2006. Computational tools for modeling protein networks. Current Proteomics 3, 181–197.

REFERENCES

Bhalla, U.S., 2002. Use of Kinetikit and GENESIS for modeling signaling pathways. Methods Enzymol. 345, 3–23.

Blinov, M.L., Faeder, J.R., Goldstein, B., Hlavacek, W.S., 2004. BioNetGen: software for rule-based modeling of signal transduction based on the interactions of molecular domains. Bioinformatics 20, 3289–3291.

Bornstein, B., Keating, S., Jouraku, A., Hucka, M., 2008. LibSBML: an API library for SBML. Bioinformatics 24, 880–881.

Bower, J., Beeman, D., 1998. The Book of GENESIS: Exploring Realistic Neural Models with the GEneral NEural SImulation System. Springer-Verlag New York Inc., New York.

Broderick, G., Ru'aini, M., Chan, E., Ellison, M.J., 2005. A life-like virtual cell membrane using discrete automata. In. Silico. Biol. 5, 163–178.

Burns, J., 1969. Steady states of general multi-enzyme networks and their associated properties. Computational approaches. FEBS Lett. 2 (suppl 1), S30–S33.

Burns, J.A., 1971. Studies on Complex Enzyme Systems [PhD thesis]. University of Edinburgh, Edinburgh. Available from http://www.sys-bio.org/BurnsThesis.

Carnevale, N., Hines, M., 2006. The NEURON Book. Cambridge University Press, Cambridge.

Chance, B., 1943. The kinetics of the enzyme–substrate compound of peroxidase. J. Biol. Chem. 151, 553–577.

Cheng, J., Scharenbroich, L., Baldi, P., Mjolsness, E., 2005. Sigmoid: a software infrastructure for pathway bioinformatics and systems biology. IEEE Intell. Syst. 20, 68–75.

Chickarmane, V., R., A., Sauro, H.M., Nadim, A., 2007. A model for p53 dynamics triggered by DNA damage. SIAM J. Applied Dynamical Syst. 6, 61–78.

Coggan, J.S., Bartol, T.M., Esquenazi, E., et al., 2005. Evidence for ectopic neurotransmission at a neuronal synapse. Science 309, 446–451.

Cook, D.L., Atkins, W.M., 1997. Enhanced detoxification due to distributive catalysis and toxic thresholds: a kinetic analysis. Biochemistry 36, 10801–10806.

Cook, D.L., Farley, J.F., Tapscott, S.J., 2001. A basis for a visual language for describing, archiving and analyzing functional models of complex biological systems. Genome Biol. 2:RESEARCH0012.

Cox, C., Peterson, G., Allen, M., et al., 2003. Analysis of noise in quorum sensing. OMICS 7, 317–334.

Curti, M., Degano, P., Baldari, C.T., 2003. Causal picalculus for biochemical modelling. In: CMSB '03: Proceedings of the First International Workshop on Computational Methods in Systems Biology. Springer-Verlag, London, UK, pp. 21–33.

Cyganowski, S., Kloeden, P., Ombach, J., 2001. From Elementary Probability to Stochastic Differential Equations with MAPLE." Springer-Verleg, Heidelberg, Berlin, London.

Deckard, A., Bergmann, F.T., Sauro, H.M., 2006. Supporting the SBML layout extension. Bioinformatics 22, 2966–2967.

Degenring, D., Röhl, M., Uhrmacher, A.M., 2004. Discrete event, multi-level simulation of metabolite channeling. Bio. Systems. 75, 29–41.

Dhar, P., Meng, T.C., Somani, S., et al., 2004. Cellware—a multi-algorithmic software for computational systems biology. Bioinformatics 20, 1319–1321.

Doedel, E.J., 1981. Auto: a Program for the Automatic Bifurcation Analysis of Autonomous Systems. In: Proceedings of the 10th Manitoba Conference on Numerical Mathematical Computing, Allston, J.V. (Ed.), University of Manitoba, Winnipeg, Canada. [Congressus Numeratium, 30:265–284].

Dräger, A., Hassis, N., Supper, J., Schröder, A., Zell, A., 2008. SBMLsqueezer a CellDesigner plug-in to generate kinetic rate equations for biochemical networks. BMC Syst. Biol. 2, 39.

Ermentrout, B., 2002. Simulating, Analyzing, and Animating Dynamical Systems: A Guide to XPPAUT for Researchers and Students, 1st ed. Society for Industrial Mathematics, Philadelphia.

Evans, T.W., Gillespie, C.S., Wilkinson, D.J., 2008. The SBML discrete stochastic models test suite. Bioinformatics 24, 285–286.

Fell, D.A., Small, J.R., 1986. Fat synthesis in adipose tissue: an examination of stoichiometric constraints. Biochem. J. 238, 781–786.

Finney, A., Hucka, M., 2003. Systems biology markup language: level 2 and beyond. Biochem. Soc. Trans. 31, 1472–1473.

Fisher, J., Henzinger, T.A., 2007. Executable cell biology. Nat. Biotechnol. 25, 1239–1249.

Garfinkel, D., 1968. A machine-independent language for the simulation of complex chemical and biochemical systems. Comput. Biomed. Res. 2, 31–44.

Garfinkel, D., Garfinkel, L., Pring, M., Green, S.B., Chance, B., 1970. Computer applications to biochemical kinetics. Annu. Rev. Biochem. 39, 473–498.

Garny, A., Kohl, P., Noble., D., 2003. Cellular open resource (COR): a public CellML based environment for modeling biological function. Int. J. Bifurcat. Chaos. 12, 3579–3590.

Gauges, R., Kummer, U., Sahle, S., Wegner, K., 2006. A model diagram layout extension for SBML. Bioinformatics 22, 1879–1885.

Geva-Zatorsky, N., Rosenfeld, N., Itzkovitz, S., et al., 2006. Oscillations and variability in the p53 system. Mol. Syst. Biol. 2, 2006.0033.

Gillespie, D.T., 1976. A general method for numerically simulating the stochastic time evolution of coupled chemical reactions. J. Comp. Phys. 22, 403–434.

Gillespie, D.T., 2007. Stochastic simulation of chemical kinetics. Annu. Rev. Phys. Chem. 58, 35–55.

Ginkel, M., Kremling, A., Nutsch, T., Rehner, R., Gilles, E.D., 2003. Modular modeling of cellular systems with ProMoT/Diva. Bioinformatics 19, 1169–1176.

Hattne, J., Fange, D., Elf, J., 2005. Stochastic reaction-diffusion simulation with MesoRD. Bioinformatics 21, 2923–2924.

Hedley, W.J., Melanie, N.R., Bullivant, D., et al., 2001. CellML specification. Available from http://www.cellml.org

Hindmarsh, A.C., 1983. ODEPACK, a systematized collection of ODE solvers in scientific computing. In: Stepleman, R. (Ed.), Scientific Computing. North-Holland, Amsterdam, pp. 55–64.

Hindmarsh, A.C., Brown, P.N., Grant, K.E., et al., 2005. SUNDIAL S: suite of nonlinear and differential/algebraic equation solvers. ACM Trans. Math. Software 31, 363–396.

Hines, M., 1993. NEURON—a program for simulation of nerve equations. In: Eeckman, F. (Ed.), Neural Systems: Analysis and Modelling. Kluwer Academic Publishers, Amsterdam, pp. 127–136.

Hofmeyr, J.-H.S., van der Merwe, K.J., 1986. Metamod: software for steady-state modelling and control analysis of metabolic pathways on the BBC microcomputer. Comp. Appl. Biosci. 2, 243–249.

Hoops, S., Sahle, S., Gauges, R., et al., 2006. COPASI—a complex pathway simulator. Bioinformatics 22, 3067–3074.

Hucka, M., Finney, A., Sauro, H.M., et al., 2003. The Systems Biology Markup Language (SBML): a medium for representation and exchange of biochemical network models. Bioinformatics 19, 524–531.

Kacser, H., Burns, J.A., 1973. The control of flux. In: Davies, (Ed.), Rate Control of Biological Processes. Symposia of the Society for Experimental Biology, Vol. 27. Cambridge University Press, Cambridge, pp. 65–104.

Kauffman, K.J., Prakash, P., Edwards, J.S., 2003. Advances in flux balance analysis. Curr. Opin. Biotechnol. 14, 491–496.

Keating, S.M., Bornstein, B.J., Finney, A., Hucka, M., 2006. SBMLtoolbox: an SBML toolbox for Matlab users. Bioinformatics 22, 1275–1277.

Kholodenko, B.N., 2006. Cell-signalling dynamics in time and space. Nat. Rev. Mol. Cell Biol. 7, 165–176.

Kitano, H., Funahashi, A., Matsuoka, Y., Oda, K., 2005. Using process diagrams for the graphical representation of biological networks. Nat. Biotechnol. 23, 961–966.

Klamt, S., Saez-Rodriguez, J., Gilles, E.D., 2007. Structural and functional analysis of cellular networks with cellnetanalyzer. BMC Syst. Biol. 1, 2-2.

Klipp, E., Herwig, R., Kowald, A., Wierling, C., Lehrach, H., 2005. Systems Biology in Practice. Wiley-VCH Verlag, Weinheim.

Kolpakov, F., 2004. BioUML—open-source extensible workbench for systems biology. In: Proceedings of the Fourth International Conference on Bioinformatics of Genome Regulation and Structure. Vol. 2. 25–30 July 2004, Novosibirsk, Russia, pp. 77–80.

Kraus, M., Lais, P., Wolf, B., 1992. Structured biological modelling: a method for the analysis and simulation of biological systems applied to oscillatory intracellular calcium waves. Bio. Systems 27, 145–169.

Kubicek, M., 1976. Algorithm 502 dependence of solution of nonlinear systems on a parameter. ACM Trans Math. Software 2, 98–107.

Kubicek, M., Marek, M., 1983. Computational Methods in Bifurcation Theory and Dissipative Structures. Springer Series in Computational Physics, Springer-Verlag, Berlin/Heidelberg.

Kurata, H., Inoue, K., Maeda, K., Masaki, K., Shimokawa, Y., Zhao, Q., 2007. Extended CADLIVE: a novel graphical notation for design of biochemical network maps and computational pathway analysis. Nucl. Acids Res. 35, e134.

Lee, J.M., Gianchandani, E.P., Papin, J.A., 2006. Flux balance analysis in the era of metabolomics. Brief. Bioinform. 7, 140–150.

Lemerle, C., Di Ventura, B., Serrano, L., 2005. Space as the final frontier in stochastic simulations of biological systems. FEBS Lett. 579, 1789–1794.

Le Novère, N., 2006. Model storage, exchange and integration. BMC Neurosci. 7 (suppl 1), S11.

Le Novère, N., Shimizu, T.S., 2001. Stochsim: modelling of stochastic biomolecular processes. Bioinformatics 17, 575–576.

Le Novère, N., Finney, A., Hucka, M., et al., 2005. Minimum information requested in the annotation of biochemical models (MIRIAM). Nat. Biotechnol. 23, 1509–1515.

Levenberg, K., 1944. A method for the solution of certain nonlinear problems in least squares. Q. Appl. Math. 2, 164–168.

Li, H., Cao, Y., Petzold, L., Gillespie, D., 2008. Algorithms and software for stochastic simulation of biochemical reacting systems. Biotechnol. Prog. 24, 56–61.

Lloyd, C.M., Halstead, M.D., Nielsen, P.F., 2004. CellML: its future, present and past. Prog. Biophys. Mol. Biol. 85, 433–450.

Lloyd, C.M., Lawson, J.R., Hunter, P.J., Nielsen, P.F., 2008. The CellML Model Repository. Bioinformatics 24, 2122–2123.

Longabaugh, W., Davidson, E., Bolouri, H., 2005. Computational representation of developmental genetic regulatory networks. Dev. Biol. 283, 1–16.

Luciano, J.S., Stevens, R.D., 2007. e-Science and biological pathway semantics. BMC Bioinformatics 8 (suppl 3), S3.

Machné, R., Finney, A., Müller, S., Lu, J., Widder, S., Flamm, C., 2006. The SBML ODE Solver Library: a native API for symbolic and fast numerical analysis of reaction networks. Bioinformatics 22, 1406–1407.

Maiwald, T., Timmer, J., 2008. Dynamical modeling and multi-experiment fitting with PottersWheel. Bioinformatics 24, 2037–2043 10.1093/bioinformatics/btn350.

Manninen, T., Makiraatikka, E., Ylipaa, A., Pettinen, A., Leinonen, K., Linne, M.L., 2006. Discrete stochastic simulation of cell signaling: comparison of computational tools. Conf. Proc. IEEE Eng. Med. Biol. Soc. 1, 2013–2016.

Marquardt, D., 1963. An algorithm for least-squares estimation of nonlinear parameters. J. Soc. Ind. Appl. Math. 11, 431–441.

McCollum, J., Lancaster, J., Bouldin, D., Peterson, G., 2003. Hardware acceleration of pseudo-random number generation for simulation applications. In System Theory, 2003. Proceedings of the 35th Southeastern Symposium on, Piscataway, NJ, USA pp. 299–303.

Mendes, P., 1993. GEPASI: a software package for modelling the dynamics, steady states and control of biochemical and other systems. Comput. Applic. Biosci. 9, 563–571.

Moles, C.G., Mendes, P., Banga, J.R., 2003. Parameter estimation in biochemical pathways: a comparison of global optimization methods. Genome. Res. 13, 2467–2474.

Moniz-Barreto, P., Fell, D.A., 1993. Simulation of dioxygen free radical reactions. Biochem. Soc. Trans. 21, 256.

Moraru, I., Schaff, J.C., Slepchenko, B.M., Lowe, L.M., 2002. The Virtual Cell: an integrated modeling environment for experimental and computational cell biology. Ann. NY Acad. Sci. 971, 595–596.

Myers, C.R., Gutenkunst, R.N., Sethna, J.P., 2007. Python unleashed on systems biology. Comput. Sci. Eng. 9, 34–37.

Nelder, J., Mead, R., 1965. A simplex method for function minimization. Comput. J. 7, 308–313.

Neves, S., Iyengar, R., 2002. Modeling of signaling networks. BioEssays 24, 1110–1117.

Olivier, B., Snoep, J., 2004. Web-based kinetic modelling using JWS Online. Bioinformatics 20, 2143–2144.

Olivier, B.G., Rohwer, J.M., Hofmeyr, J.H., 2005. Modelling cellular systems with PySCeS. Bioinformatics 21, 560–561.

Palsson, B.O., 2007. Systems Biology: Properties of Reconstructed Networks. Cambridge University Press, Cambridge.

Park, D.J.M., Wright, B.E., 1973. METASIM, a general purpose metabolic simulator for studying cellular transformations. Comput. Programs Biomed. 3, 10–26.

Pedersen, M., Plotkin, G., 2008. A language for biochemical systems. In: Danos, V. Schachter, V. (Eds.), Computational Methods in Systems Biology. Springer, Berlin/Heidelberg, pp. 63–82. Available from http://homepages.inf.ed.ac.uk/s0677975/papers/lbs.pdf.

Peterson, G.D., Lancaster, J.M., 2002. Stochastic simulation of biological cellular processes using VHDL-AMS. Behavioral Modeling and Simulation, 2002. In "Proceedings of the 2002 IEEE International Workshop on Behavioral Modeling and Simulation," Piscataway, NJ, USA pp. 118–122.

Poolman, M.G., 2006. Scrumpy: metabolic modelling with python. IEE Proc. Syst. Biol. 153, 375–378.

Price, N.D., Papin, J.A., Schilling, C.H., Palsson, B.O., 2003. Genome-scale microbial in silico models: the constraints-based approach. Trends Biotechnol. 21, 162–169.

Ramsey, S., Orrell, D., Bolouri, H., 2005. Dizzy: stochastic simulation of large-scale genetic regulatory networks. J. Bioinform. Comput. Biol. 3, 415–436.

Rao, R., Wolf, D.M., Arkin, A.P., 2002. Control, exploitation and tolerance of intracellular noise. Nature 420, 231–237.

Raymond, G.M., Butterworth, E., Bassingthwaighte, J.B., 2003. JSIM: free software package for teaching physiological modeling and research. Exper. Biol. 280, 102.

Reder, C., 1988. Metabolic control theory: a structural approach. J. Theor. Biol. 135, 175–201.

Reich, J.G., Selkov, E.E., 1981. Energy Metabolism of the Cell. Academic Press, London.

Rost, U., Kummer, U., 2004. Visualisation of biochemical network simulations with SimWiz. Syst. Biol. (Stevenage) 1, 184–189.

Runarsson, T., Yao, X., 2005. Search biases in constrained evolutionary optimization. IEEE Trans. Systems Man Cybernetics C 35, 233–243.

Salis, H., Sotiropoulos, V., Kaznessis, Y.N., 2006. Multiscale Hy3S: hybrid stochastic simulation for supercomputers. BMC Bioinformatics 7, 93.

Sanford, C., Yip, M.L., White, C., Parkinson, J., 2006. Cell++ − simulating biochemical pathways. Bioinformatics 22, 2918–2925.

Sauro, H.M., 1993. SCAMP: a general-purpose simulator and metabolic control analysis program. Comput. Appl. Biosci. 9, 441–450.

Sauro, H.M., 2000. Jarnac: a system for interactive metabolic analysis. In: Hofmeyr, J.-H.S., Rohwer, J.M., Snoep, J.L. (Eds.), Animating the Cellular Map: Proceedings of the 9th International Meeting on BioThermoKinetics. Stellenbosch University Press, Stellenbosch.

Sauro, H.M., Fell, D.A., 1991. Scamp: a metabolic simulator and control analysis program. Mathl. Comput. Modelling 15, 15–28.

Sauro, H.M., Ingalls, B., 2004. Conservation analysis in biochemical networks: computational issues for software writers. Biophys. Chem. 109, 1–15.

Sauro, H.M., Hucka, M., Finney, A., et al., 2003. Next generation simulation tools: the Systems Biology Workbench and BioSPICE integration. OMICS 7, 355–372.

Savageau, M.A., 1972. The behaviour of intact biochemical control systems. Curr. Topics Cell Reg. 6, 63–130.

Schaff, J., Fink, C.C., Slepchenko, B., Carson, J.H., Loew, L.M., 1997. A general computational framework for modeling cellular structure and function. Biophys. J. 73, 1135–1146.

Schilstra, M.J., Li, L., Matthews, J., Finney, A., Hucka, M., Le Novère, N., 2006. CellML2SBML: conversion of CellML into SBML. Bioinformatics 22, 1018–1020.

Schmidt, H., Jirstrand, M., 2006. Systems Biology Toolbox for Matlab: a computational platform for research in systems biology. Bioinformatics 22, 514–515.

Schwender, J., 2008. Metabolic flux analysis as a tool in metabolic engineering of plants. Curr. Opin. Biotechnol. 19, 131–137.

Sedwards, S., Mazza, T., 2007. CytoSim: a formal language model and stochastic simulator of membrane-enclosed biochemical processes. Bioinformatics 23, 2800–2802.

Shannon, P., Markiel, A., Ozier, O., et al., 2003. Cytoscape: a software environment for integrated models of biomolecular interaction networks. Genome. Res. 13, 2498–2504.

Shapiro, B.E., Hucka, M., Finney, A., Doyle, J., 2004. MathSBML: a package for manipulating SBML-based biological models. Bioinformatics 20, 2829–2831.

Slepchenko, B.M., Schaff, J., Macara, I.G., Loew, L.M., 2003. Quantitative cell biology with the Virtual Cell. Trends Cell Biol. 13, 570–576.

Sorokin, A., Paliy, K., Selkov, A., et al., 2006. The pathway editor: a tool for managing complex biological networks. IBM J. Res. Dev. 50, 561–573.

Stiles, J.R., Bartol, T.M., 2001. Monte Carlo methods for simulating realistic synaptic microphysiology using MCell. In: Schutter, E.D. (ed.), Computational Neuroscience: Realistic Modeling for Experimentalists. CRC Press, Springer-Verlag, Berlin, Heidelberg, Longdon, pp. 87–127.

Suderman, M., Hallett, M., 2007. Tools for visually exploring biological networks. Bioinformatics 23, 2651–2659.

Tomita, M., Hashimoto, K., Takahashi, K., et al., 1999. E-cell: software environment for whole-cell simulation. Bioinformatics 15, 72–84.

Tyson, J.J., Chen, K., Novak, B., 2001. Network dynamics and cell physiology. Nat. Rev. Mol. Cell Biol. 2, 908–916.

Tyson, J.J., Csikasz-Nagy, A., Novak, B., 2002. The dynamics of cell cycle regulation. BioEssays 24, 1095–1109.

Ullah, M., Wolkenhauer, O., 2007. Family tree of Markov models in systems biology. IET Syst. Biol. 1, 247–254.

Vacheva, I., Eils, R., 2006. Computational systems biology platforms. IT Info. Technol. 48, 140–147.

Vallabhajosyula, R.R., Sauro, H.M., 2007. Stochastic simulation GUI for biochemical networks. Bioinformatics 23, 1859–1861.

Vallabhajosyula, R.R., Chickarmane, V., Sauro, H.M., 2006. Conservation analysis of large biochemical networks. Bioinformatics 22, 346–353.

Vass, M., Allen, N., Shaffer, C.A., Ramakrishnan, N., Watson, L.T., Tyson, J.J., 2004. The JigCell model builder and run manager. Bioinformatics 20, 3680–3681.

Wiechert, W., 2001. 13C metabolic flux analysis. Metab. Eng. 3, 195–206.

Wilkinson, D.J., 2006. Stochastic Modelling for Systems Biology. Chapman and Hall, Boca Raton.

Wilkinson, D., 2007. SBML shorthand. Available from http://www.staff.ncl.ac.uk/d.j.wilkinson/software/sbml-sh/

Williams, T., Kelley, C., 1998. GNUPLOT: an interactive plotting program. Manual, version 3.

Wright, S., 1934. Physiological and evolutionary theories of dominance. Am. Nat. 68, 24–53.

Yoshimi, M., Osana, Y., Fukushima, T., Amano, H., 2004. Stochastic simulation for biochemical reactions on FPGA. In: The 14th International Conference on Field Programmable Logic and Applications. Vol. 3203. ?Publisher, Town?, pp. 105–114.

Zi, Z., Klipp, E., 2006. SBML-PET: a systems biology markup language-based parameter estimation tool. Bioinformatics 22, 2704–2705.

SECTION III

APPLICATIONS OF SYSTEMS BIOLOGY

CHAPTER 13

Physiome Mark-up Languages for Systems Biology: Model Modularization and Re-use

M.T. Cooling[1], E.J. Crampin[2] and P.J. Hunter[1]

[1]Auckland Bioengineeing Institute, University of Auckland
[2]Department of Engineering Science, University of Auckland

OUTLINE

Definitions	317	Implications of Modularity	324
Introduction	318	Incorporating Cellml Models into Tissue and Organ Models	325
Conceptual Modularization	319		
Component-based Implementation	321		

Much of the material presented in pages 319–327 has been previously presented in Cooling et al., 2008.

Definitions

Accounting chain/cycle A set of reactions that accounts for the mass of a particular molecular species. It may include conservation of mass, but may not (e.g. if species are removed from the model). Depending on the reactions, possible topologies of the graph of this reaction set include cycles and chains.

Component A distinct unit of a model implemented in some computer-readable format. When used specifically in the context of the model discussed in this chapter, components are CellML "components" as defined in the CellML specification (available at http://www.cellml.org). We distinguish between functional and messenger components.

Functional component A component that implements a functional module once messenger species are separated out into their own messenger components.

Messenger component A component that encapsulates the amount of a molecular species that is likely to be used as a messenger species, communicating between functional components.

Module A conceptual entity encompassing a biological function. In this discussion, a module forms an accounting chain or cycle for the molecular species deemed key to that biological function. Modules are implemented in computer-readable form by functional and messenger components.

INTRODUCTION

The study of human physiology deals with the integrative function of proteins, carbohydrates and lipids within the approximately 200 cell types and four basic tissue types (muscle, nerve, epithelium and connective tissue) of the organs that make up the 12 organ systems of the human body. A quantitative understanding of how proteins, carbohydrates and lipids contribute to cell and tissue function, in the 10^9 range of spatial scales from proteins (scale $\approx 1\,nm$) to the whole body ($\approx 1\,m$), is dependent on the development of mathematical models that describe biophysical mechanisms. Some of the common physiological mechanisms that depend on proteins are: membrane ion channel electrophysiology (including voltage-dependent ion channels, exchangers and ATP-dependent pumps), signal transduction networks (often linking membrane receptors to sites of protein phosphorylation in the cytosol), metabolic pathways and gene regulatory pathways. In some cases these models deal with so-called "lumped parameter" systems—in which spatial effects are averaged—and in other cases they represent the spatial variations in cell or tissue properties. In the first case, the models are typically based on systems of ordinary differential equations and algebraic equations; in the second, they typically rely on partial differential equations. In both cases, there is a need to develop computer languages for describing the structure and mathematical expression of the models, together with associated metadata that provide biological meaning to the mathematics by referencing bio-ontologies. The eXtensible Markup Language (XML) offers a suitable framework for such a language, and two XML languages, CellML (http://www.cellml.org) (Lloyd et al., 2004) and FieldML (http://www.fieldml.org), have been developed to deal with lumped parameter systems and spatially varying systems, respectively.

Some of the advantages in establishing such a framework are: (i) models developed by different groups can be combined using commonly agreed ontological terms within the metadata; (ii) models can be modularized and used in libraries to make it easier to create complex models by importing and combining simpler ones; (iii) ensuring consistency—for example of physical units—between models could perhaps be automated (Terkildsen et al., 2008). In addition, the development of smaller models that may easily be combined to form more complex models provides opportunities for analyzing models representing functional biological components in isolation, assisting in identifying and rectifying any inaccuracies before complex and time-consuming analysis of the model as a whole, and more readily identifying common patterns or motifs in subcellular systems. In this chapter, we discuss the use of modularity in constructing and reusing models of biological function, using CellML. It is appropriate to take advantage of biological modularity to construct models at particular temporal and spatial scales. Modules describing biological components at one scale can then be treated as "black boxes" that summarize lower-level detail while linking to the level of abstraction directly above (Hunter and Borg, 2003).

At the subcellular level, many valuable models of biological systems have been produced. Regrettably, many of these models are not readily available to the community for re-use, because of a lack of a sufficiently accurate description (Le Novere et al., 2005; Smith et al., 2007). Some researchers do make available computer code or otherwise executable component-based implementations for their models (Bhalla and Iyengar, 1999; Lukas, 2004), but the recombination of these components to form new modules often requires the editing of this code (whether textually, or visually in a graphical environment) in order to ensure that molecular species are linked appropriately for the biological system under investigation.

The concept of modularity is not unambiguously defined, however. Conceptually, modules are unlikely to be rigid structures, with species belonging to different modules at different times, depending on perspective (Hartwell et al., 1999) (an example of this is given below). This flexibility is not easily represented in computer code formulations, and can lead to conflicts when components from different researchers are being combined. Although some degree of "gluing" code is likely to be necessary, ideally, existing module implementations should not have to be modified in order for previously unanticipated connections to be made. It would be more efficient if module implementations could also be relied upon to act as "black boxes," without the need to understand how they are coded.

Below, we discuss modularity using CellML, illustrating these concepts with the example of an inositol triphosphate (IP3) signaling cascade model broken into distinct conceptual modules (Cooling et al., 2008). We discuss how component boundaries should be formed, and develop leading practice for such implementations, to aid future model construction via the aggregation of existing components with minimal code alterations.

CONCEPTUAL MODULARIZATION

We will illustrate modularization using a biological reaction schematic of an existing IP3 signaling pathway model (Cooling et al., 2007) as shown in Figure 13.1A.

We define a module as being a collection of molecular species both with relatively strong internal interactions and representing a particular biological function (Alon, 2007; Hartwell et al., 1999). Conceptually, we can divide the reaction schema into three functional modules, depicted in Figure 13.1B. The model is composed of the GPCR module (reactions R1-R6), a module that describes the interactions of PLCβ, $G_\alpha GTP$ and Ca^{2+} (reactions R8-R13) and a third conceptual module that describes the production and degradation of IP3 (shown by reactions R14-R16). In each case, the module is defined by a set of states of most pertinent molecular species for the function that the module performs, and the reactions describing the transitions between those states.

The GPCR module receives an extracellular signal (via a ligand) and transduces this across the plasma membrane to the inside of the cell via GPCR receptor activation. This module therefore represents an "accounting cycle" for receptors—it encompasses all the possible complexes (states) of that particular species, governed by differential equations measuring their concentrations derived from the reactions between those complexes. Accounting cycles may also be mass conservation cycles of the species of interest, as can be understood by considering the differential equations for the receptor and receptor complexes R, R_l, R_g and R_{lg}, the fluxes for which sum to zero, as shown in Table 13.1.

Similarly, the second module, in which the intracellular signal primes the key enzyme, PLCβ, exhibits a similar accounting property for that enzyme via reactions R8-R12. A module does not require a cycle for an accounting relationship to hold; an "accounting chain"(in which mass is accounted for, but the graph of the reactions in the relationship is not closed) is also possible. This is the case for the third module, which describes the production and degradation of the IP3 signal, which terminates in a sink state (i.e., mass is not conserved in that module).

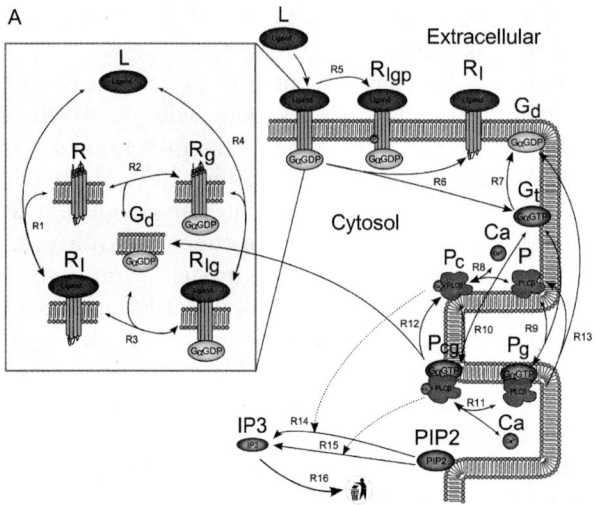
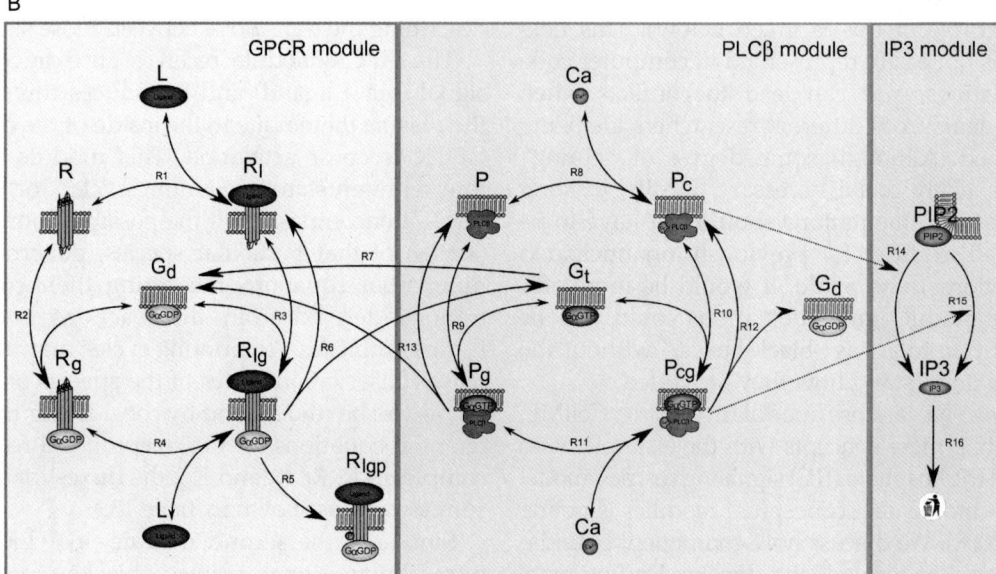

FIGURE 13.1. (A) Reaction scheme of the IP3 production system. The extracellular ligand (L) binds to receptors (R), whether precoupled with $G_\alpha GDP$ (G_d) or not. Fully activated receptors (R_{lg}) release $G_\alpha GTP$ (G_t) which, along with calcium (Ca), stimulates phospholipase Cβ (PLCβ) (P). In the unstimulated state, PLCβ-Ca^{2+} (P_c) hydrolyses phosphatidylinositol bisphosphate (PIP2) to produce IP3 via reaction R14. When stimulated, PLCβ-Ca^{2+}-G_αGTP (P_{cg}) hydrolyses PIP2 at a faster rate than reaction R14, via reaction R15. Free IP3 is degraded via reaction R16. (B) Conceptual model. Conceptually, the model is made up of three functional modules: the GPCR module, the PLCβ module, and the IP3 module. The G_αGDP, Ca^{2+}, and ligand species (G_d, Ca, and L, respectively) are represented twice for visual clarity.

Reproduced from Cooling et al. (2008) (Fig. 1), with permission.

TABLE 13.1 The Conservation Cycle for Receptors. Illustrated here by the reaction fluxes (J_i, where i denotes the reaction number) for the receptor complexes summing to zero, defining the accounting relationship for the G protein-coupled receptor (GPCR) module. Flux directions (signs) are chosen to reflect the dominant direction under stimulated, physiological conditions (Cooling et al., 2007).

	=						
$\frac{dR}{dt}$	=	$-J_1$	$-J_2$				
$\frac{dR_l}{dt}$	=	$+J_1$		$-J_3$			$+J_6$
$\frac{dR_g}{dt}$	=		$+J_2$		$-J_4$		
$\frac{dR_{ls}}{dt}$	=			$+J_3$	$+J_4$	$-J_5$	$-J_6$
$\frac{dR_{lgp}}{dt}$	=					$+J_5$	
Sum:	=	0	+0	+0	+0	+0	+0	=0

Modules defined in this manner are conceptual entities, and must be implemented as code before they can be readily manipulated by computer.

COMPONENT-BASED IMPLEMENTATION

To take advantage of modularization, models must adhere to standards and semantics that encourage their compatibility with one another. The model representation should also be independent of the solver algorithm and technology platform that act on it. A CellML representation fulfills these requirements, being a human- and machine-readable XML-based exchange format for mathematical models. Here we discuss representing the modules defined above using the current version of the CellML specification (version 1.1; available at http://www.cellml.org/specifications).

CellML models are partitioned into "components" that encapsulate internal variables and mathematical relationships. Communication between components is performed via CellML "connections," which map a given variable from one component onto another variable in a second component. Components may reside in separate files, connected by the "import" functionality of CellML. A conceptual module may be composed of one or more CellML components. This flexible approach facilitates the combination of modules designed by different researchers, while keeping the mathematical details of the module specification encapsulated in independently constructed components (Lloyd et al., 2004). In addition, a framework for integrating models for processes at different spatial and time scales, implemented as CellML components, already exists (Nickerson et al., 2006).

Implementing modules as CellML components requires forethought as to how they should be constructed in order to maximize their usability in future models. To aid re-use, we make a distinction between highly connected "messenger" components and non-messenger "functional" components. Diffusible molecules, such as the extracellular ligands, calcium and IP3, have greater potential to be consumed or produced by several modules than do localized species, and therefore should be only loosely coupled with other species. Membrane-bound molecules that are nonetheless messengers, such as G_α subunits (with attendant self-GTPase reaction R7), should be considered similarly. Hence, in this formulation, all messenger molecules (ligand, G_α subunits, calcium and IP3) are formed in separate components.

It is important that components hide information that is unnecessary to other components, but, in the CellML framework, these messenger components must expose the current concentrations of the messenger molecule species to allow these concentrations to be used in the calculation of kinetic rates inside other components. It is also necessary to allow for the connection of fluxes representing the gain or loss of messenger molecule species, as a result of reactions that use or produce these molecules in other components. These "sources" and "sinks" can be summed to a single flux, $J_{gain.species\_name}$, which each messenger molecule component exposes to be contributed to by other components in which the messenger molecule is produced or consumed. The summing of other source and sink fluxes from other components to this single flux is implemented in an "interface" component, which can be defined by the model builder who connects the components together. Through these mechanisms, components can both use and contribute to messenger molecule concentrations defined in separate messenger components, without requiring any changes to their own internal CellML code.

In this formulation, examples of functional components are those that preserve an accounting relationship for a non-messenger species of interest, such as in the GPCR and PLCβ modules described above. Once the messenger species have been isolated in separate components, the rest of the module can be directly translated into functional CellML components. This is shown as the "GPCR_Cycle" and "PLC_Cycle" components in Figure 13.2, which depicts the resultant partitioning of conceptual modules into CellML files and components, following these principles.

Figure 13.2 shows the contents of the main CellML file, which imports subsidiary files, each of which contains a model component and could have been developed independently by different researchers. The main file also contains the interface components and the component that holds the parameters defining the cell's geometry. In Figure 13.2, faded species represent those for which the differential equation is contained by other components. Fluxes involving such species are exposed by their containing component, as they will be summed to a $J_{gain.species\_name}$ variable in an interface component. There is no ligand or PIP2 interface component, as the concentrations of both species are fixed for this model. Two of the states of PLCβ, PLCβ-Ca^{2+}-G_αGTP and PLCβ-Ca^{2+}, are monitored by the PIP2 component (as P$β_c$ and P$β_{cg}$, respectively), which contains the reactions for the hydrolysis of PIP2 that they perform.

One potential conflict that may occur is that the same species could be considered the basis for different accounting relationships. If, for example, we allowed messenger molecules also to be the basis of an accounting relationship, it would be possible, in this case, to make the claim that the G_α component could therefore contain all the forms of that species—which would include several receptor-bound and PLCβ-bound forms. Such a component would form a conservation cycle for G_α subunits, as the fluxes for dG_d/dt, dR_g/dt, dR_{lg}/dt, dR_{lgp}/dt, dG_t/dt, dP_{cg}/dt and dP_g/dt (reactions R2-R13 inclusive) also sum to zero. This naturally reflects the conservation of this species in the system. To do so, however, would force the removal of those forms from their previously assigned components, because, whereas variable and parameter values can be shared between components, the differential equations that control the change of a variable over time can only belong to one. Therefore a choice must be made, in this case, whether to emphasize the accounting cycles of GPCR and PLCβ, or the accounting cycle of G_α. We assert that considering messenger molecules such as G_α as their own components, rather than embodying them in an accounting cycle or chain: (i) resolves this conflict, (ii) enables the translation of the GPCR functional module almost directly into a CellML component, keeping the semantic focus on the receptors as the basis of that functional unit, and (iii) allows easier connectivity with potential future components, as species likely to communicate between components (and therefore the nodes that communicate between the modules that those components represent) are decoupled, requiring additions only to interface

COMPONENT-BASED IMPLEMENTATION

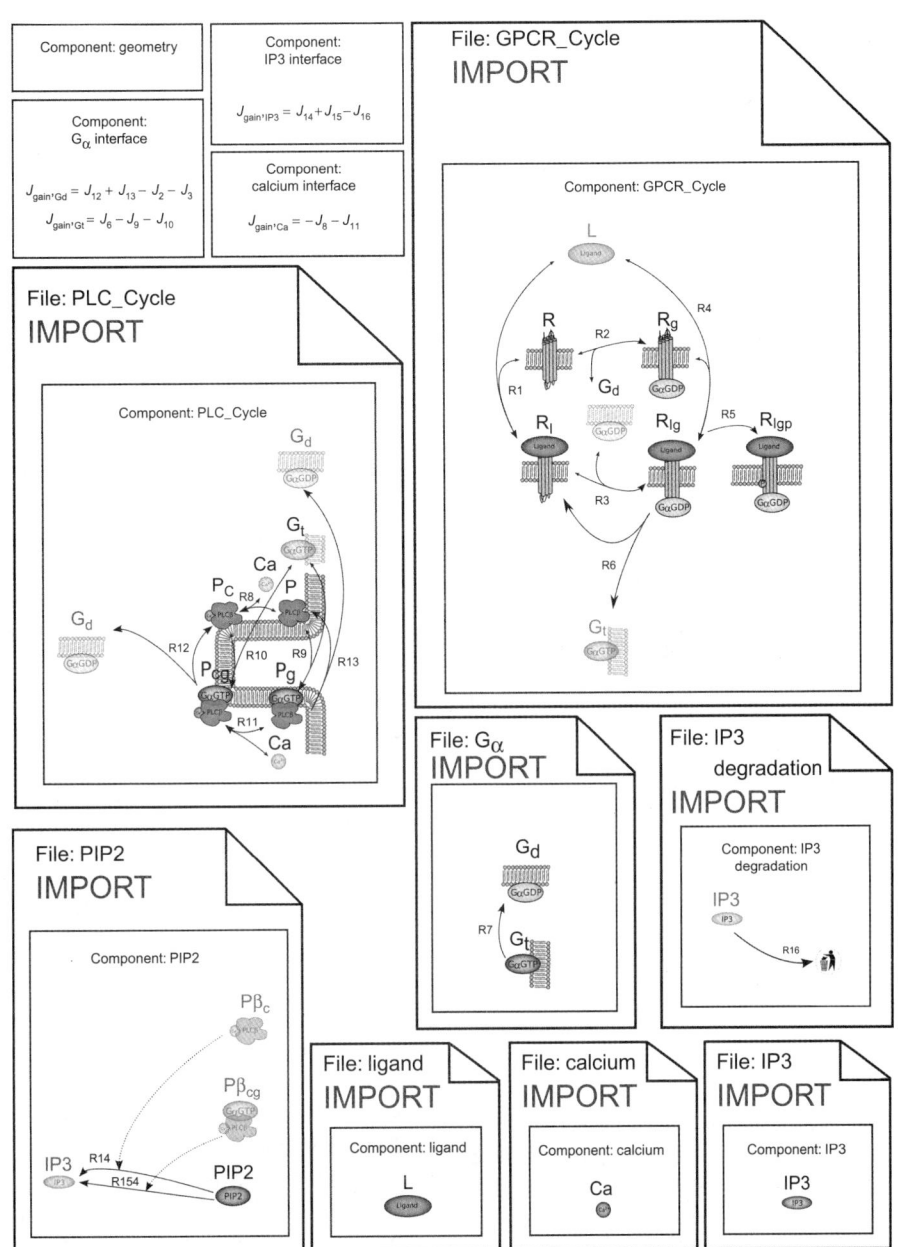

FIGURE 13.2. CellML File Schematic of the IP3 Model.
The contents of the main CellML file for the model. It contains the geometry component in order to define the cell, but imports signal transduction models from other files. Diffusive or mobile messengers are abstracted into their own components: "ligand," "calcium," "G_α," and "IP3." The functional components "GPCR_Cycle," "PLC_Cycle," "PIP2" and "IP3 degradation" are also imported. Components that link via fluxes from other components are connected through interface components. The complete CellML code for the model can be found on line (http://www.cellml.org/models, under the hyperlink for Cooling et al., 2008).
Modified from Cooling et al. (2008) (Fig. 2), with permission.

component code, and not changes to existing functional or messenger components.

When formulating components, it may be realized that one conceptual module may become two or more components once the distinction between messenger and non-messenger molecules is made. For example, the "IP3 Module" here becomes two components: (i) a PIP2 component centered on PIP2 and containing hydrolysis reactions forming the messenger IP3 (and diacylglycerol, which is not shown for the purposes of this model), and (ii) the IP3 component, which is a messenger and contains its own degradation reaction. The IP3 Module is, at the component level, a PIP2 hydrolysis component with an associated self-degrading messenger. The IP3 messenger molecule forms the communication carrier between the PIP2 component (and this model as a whole) and possible downstream components.

An important distinction can be drawn between the IP3 degradation reaction (R16) and the G_α subunit self-hydrolysis reaction (R7). For the former, the reaction is known to be a lumped description of the conversion of IP3 to either IP4 or IP2 (Cooling et al., 2007). This requires the interaction of other molecular species, such as kinases and phosphatases, with their associated metabolic pathways. This is a clue that we have a potential functional component for this step. It is conceivable that a modeler using these components might wish to expand the IP3 degradation abstraction by including one or more of these pathways. To facilitate this, we advocate placing such abstractions that rely on other pathways in their own component (component "IP3 degradation"), allowing the replacement of this reaction with a more detailed formulation without affecting the IP3 component itself or the rest of the model. By contrast, in the case of the G_α subunit self-hydrolysis, no other proteins or pathways are necessary for the reaction to occur, hence this process is unlikely to be expanded upon further, and can reside within the messenger component (component "G_α").

IMPLICATIONS OF MODULARITY

These components could be re-used to construct models for other pathways. For example, following appropriate reparameterization, the GPCR component could be used for any instance of a GPCR that produces G_αGTP— whether that product interacts with PLCβ or some other protein, in whatever pathway. Should, for some reason, a more detailed formulation for the GPCR be needed for the IP3 pathway, the GPCR component can be replaced with one containing a more detailed formulation, without affecting the other components. In addition, by formulating the components in which IP3 is in its own messenger component, we make it possible for components derived from additional functional modules to be added and read the IP3 signal and extend the pathway, without requiring code changes to the non-interface components in the existing model.

Aside from the distinctions between messenger and functional component discussed above, component boundaries may also be defined by physical or functional containment. For example, in a membrane that contains several types of ion channel, it seems logical that each ion channel should reside in its own component, these components being added to larger models should those channels be required. This is the case for many existing electrophysiological models (a range of electrophysiological examples coded in CellML are described in Nickerson and Hunter, 2006).

In signal transduction, more complex relationships are possible, including protein-to-protein interactions. For example, in this model PLCβ interacts with PIP2 to form IP3. This was implemented by forming the PIP2 component such that it expects to receive concentrations from PLCβ complexes from other components, and contains the kinetic rate constants for the hydrolysis of PIP2 by those specific enzymes. However, the expectation of a specific complex from another component represents a tighter coupling than is ideal. In some cell types, PIP2 is hydrolyzed by PLCγ complexes (van Leeuwen and Samelson, 1999), which give different kinetic parameters for those reactions. The PIP2 component could be generalized (in keeping with its role as a PIP2 hydrolysis component) by the addition of reactions using those alternative isoforms, which, when connected to the other components in the present model, would have enzyme concentrations of zero and hence be inactive. These additional reactions have not been shown, as they are not needed for this example.

Had the PIP2 and PLC_Cycle components been defined independently by different researchers, on the basis of their own modeling perspective alone, it is conceivable that both components could have been expected to have ownership of the differential equation for the PLCβ species. If both components were to be imported into the same model, the conflicts between two definitions of the same PLCβ species—and possibly the contingent reactions—would have to be resolved. The current CellML specification (version 1.1) does not provide a standardized way of handling this potential conflict, but work is under way to address these issues. Future plans for CellML include the binding of biologically relevant identifiers to CellML elements via metadata tags that use the CellML Bio Ontology currently being developed.

Two CellML variables or reactions with the same identifier will be semantically equivalent, regardless of their CellML representation, and it is envisaged that duplicates could be automatically determined via these identifiers during model construction. Once this functionality is available, it is likely that leading practice for CellML model design will include defining each species and reaction in its own component, which is then encapsulated into higher-level components to represent the physical or functional modules as defined above. This design enables the reformulation of higher-level components by the model builder at the time of composition of the model. Once duplicates had been detected, the resultant conflicts could be resolved by manually choosing one or the other, the components of which are then linked (at the CellML code level) automatically. Thus, for signal transduction, modules may still be combined without having to edit the code for the components that implement them; however, we envisage that a strictly black-box approach may not always be possible, as component contents would have to be understood well enough for the modeler to decide how such conflicts should be resolved. This technology would support, rather than replace, human intelligence in the model-building process.

INCORPORATING CELLML MODELS INTO TISSUE AND ORGAN MODELS

The challenge for the Physiome Project is to incorporate cellular-level models of protein pathways into tissue- and organ-level models of physiological function. We illustrate one example of such multi-scale modeling here, with the heart modeling work from the Auckland Bioengineering Institute. Figure 13.3 shows models used at spatial scales ranging from the 1 nm scale of proteins to the 1 m scale of the torso.

The cellular processes incorporated into the current generation of whole-heart cardiac models are shown in Table 13.2.

There are, of course, many other aspects of cellular function that could be included in a fully integrative heart model, depending on the particular physiological questions being asked of the model. At the tissue level, the physiological processes are: (i) myocardial electrical activation (Clayton and Panfilov, 2007), (ii) large-deformation wall mechanics (Nash and Hunter, 2000), (iii) ventricular fluid mechanics (Nordsletten et al., 2007) and (iv) coronary

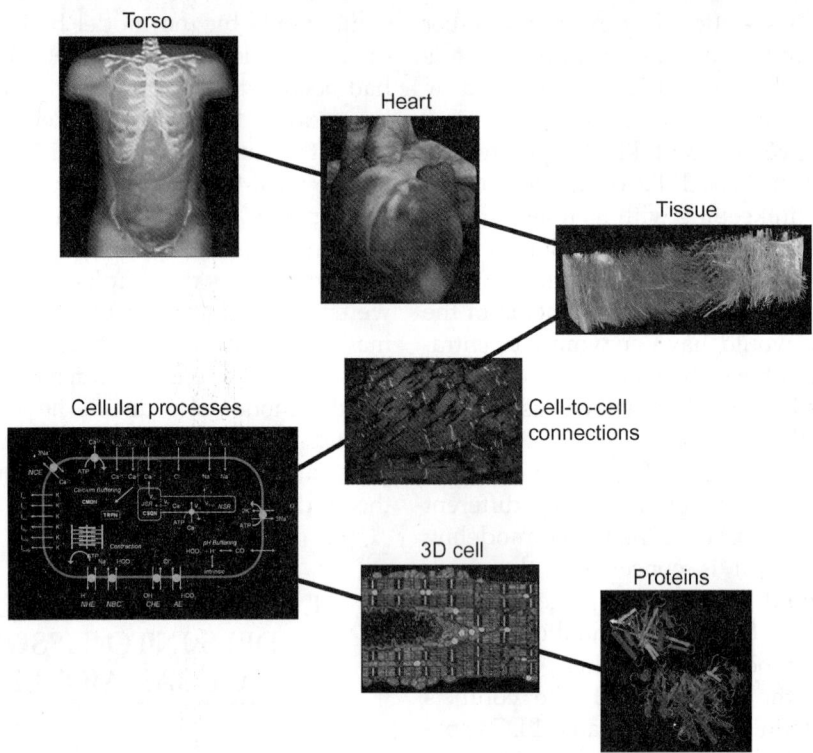

FIGURE 13.3. Multi-scale Modeling for the Heart.
CellML models defining subcellular processes are incorporated into whole-organ models that include the structure and material properties of the tissue.

Adapted from Austin et al. (2006), with permission.

TABLE 13.2 Whole-heart Cardiac Model Cellular Processes

(i)	Electrophysiology (ten Tusscher et al., 2004)	www.models.cellml.org/ workspace/tentusscher_ noble_noble_panfilov_2004
(ii)	Myofilament kinetics (Niederer et al., 2006)	www.models.cellml. org/workspace/niederer_ hunter_smith_2006
(iii)	Metabolic pathways (Beard, 2005)	www.models.cellml.org/ workspace/beard_2005
(iv)	β-adrenergic signaling (Saucerman and McCulloch, 2004)	www.models.cellml.org/ workspace/saucerman_ mcculloch_2004
(v)	IP3 signaling (Cooling et al., 2007)	www.models.cellml. org/workspace/cooling_ hunter_crampin_2007

Links to the CellML models are shown on the right.

flow and energetics (Smith et al., 2002). No single model yet includes all these physical processes—the computational cost is still too high—but several groups are close to achieving this goal (reviewed by Hunter et al., 2003). Several other organ system projects are at a similar stage of development —for example, the lungs (Burrowes et al., 2007), the musculoskeletal system (Fernandez et al., 2005) and the digestive system (Cheng et al., 2007).

An important goal for the tissue and organ models is to define a standard for encapsulating the spatial fields required to define the anatomical shape and tissue structure of organs (e.g. the fibrous-sheet structure of the heart), the spatial distribution of protein expression (e.g. the ion channel distributions in the heart) and the spatial fields that define boundary conditions and initial conditions for solution of the partial differential equations governing physical processes such as myocardial activation and ventricular mechanics. Finally, the time-varying dependent variable fields that result from the solution of these equations also need to be available in a standard format for visualizing in graphical display software. The standard being developed for all of these purposes is called FieldML. This currently evolving standard (version 1.0 is not yet released) deals primarily with fields defined via finite-element models. FieldML and CellML are complementary, and are designed to work together. For example, FieldML files representing the anatomy of the heart can reference the CellML files identifying the types of cell model at various material locations around the heart. These CellML files would identify which proteins vary spatially and point to the FieldML files that describe the spatially varying levels of expression for these proteins.

References

Alon, U., 2007. An Introduction to Systems Biology: Design Principles of Biological Circuits. Chapman and Hall/CRC, Boca Raton.

Austin, T.M., Hooks, D.A., Hunter, P.J., et al., 2006. Modeling cardiac electrical activity at the cell and tissue levels. Ann. NY Acad. Sci. 1080, 334–347.

Beard, D.A., 2005. A biophysical model of the mitochondrial respiratory system and oxidative phosphorylation. PLoS Comput. Biol. 1, e36.

Bhalla, U.S., Iyengar, R., 1999. Emergent properties of networks of biological signaling pathways. Science 283, 381–387.

Burrowes, K., Swan, A., Warren, N., Tawhai, M., 2008. Towards a virtual lung: multi-scale, multi-physics modelling of the pulmonary system. Phil. Trans. R. Soc. A 366, 3247–3263.

Cheng, L.K., Komuro, R., Austin, T., Buist, M., Pullan, A.J., 2007. Anatomically realistic multiscale models of normal and abnormal gastrointestinal electrical activity [invited paper]. World J. Gastroenterol. 13, 1378–1383.

Clayton, R.H., Panfilov, A.V., 2008. A guide to modelling cardiac electrical activity in anatomically detailed ventricles. Progr. Biophys. Mol. Biol. 96, 19–43.

Cooling, M., Hunter, P., Crampin, E.J., 2007. Modelling hypertrophic IP3 transients in the cardiac myocyte. Biophys. J. 93, 3421–3433.

Cooling, M.T., Hunter, P., Crampin, E.J., 2008. Modeling biological modularity with CellML. IET Syst. Biol. 2, 73–79.

Fernandez, J.W., Ho, A., Walt, S., Anderson, I., Hunter, P.J., 2005. A cerebral palsy assessment tool using anatomically based geometries and free-form deformation. Biomech. Model. Mechanobiol. 4, 39–56.

Hartwell, L.H., Hopfield, J.J., Leibler, S., Murray, A.W., 1999. From molecular to modular cell biology. Nature 402, C47–C52.

Hunter, P.J., Borg, T.K., 2003. Integration from proteins to organs: the Physiome Project. Nat. Rev. Mol. Cell Biol. 4, 237–243.

Hunter, P.J., Pullan, A.J., Smaill, B.H., 2003. Modeling total heart function. Annu. Rev. Biomed. Eng. 5, 147–177.

Le Novere, N., Finney, A., Hucka, M., et al., 2005. Minimum information requested in the annotation of biochemical models (MIRIAM). Nat. Biotechnol. 23, 1509–1515.

Lloyd, C.M., Halstead, M.D.B., Nielsen, P.F., 2004. CellML: its future, present and past. Progr. Biophys. Mol. Biol. 85, 433–450.

Lukas, T.J., 2004. A Signal transduction pathway model prototype I: from agonist to cellular endpoint. Biophys. J. 87, 1406–1416.

Nash, M.P., Hunter, P.J., 2000. Computational mechanics of the heart. J. Elast. 61, 113–141.

Nickerson, D.P., Hunter, P.J., 2006. The noble cardiac ventricular electrophysiology models in CellML. Progr. Biophys. Mol. Biol. 90, 346–359.

Nickerson, D.P., Nash, M.P., Nielsen, P.F., Smith, N., Hunter, P., 2006. Computational multiscale modeling in the IUPS Physiome Project: modeling cardiac electromechanics. IBM J. Res. Dev. 50, 617–630.

Niederer, S.A., Hunter, P.J., Smith, N.P., 2006. A quantitative analysis of cardiac myocyte relaxation: a simulation study. Biophys. J. 90, 1697–1722.

Nordsletten, D.A., Hunter, P.J., Smith, N.P., 2007. Conservative and non conservative arbitrary Lagrangian-Eulerian forms for ventricular flows. Int. J. Numer. Methods Fluids 56, 1457–1463 10.1002/fld.1647.

Saucerman, J.J., McCulloch, A.D., 2004. Mechanistic systems models of cell signaling networks: a case study of myocyte adrenergic regulation. Progr. Biophys. Mol. Biol. 85, 261–278.

Smith, N.P., Crampin, E.J., Niederer, S.A., Bassingthwaite, J.B., Beard, D.A., 2007. Computational biology of cardiac myocytes: proposed standards for the Physiome. J. Exp. Biol. 210, 1576–1583.

Smith, N.P., Pullan, A.J., Hunter, P.J., 2002. An anatomically based model of coronary blood flow and myocardial mechanics. SIAM J. Appl. Math. 62, 990–1018.

ten Tusscher, K.H.W.J., Noble, D., Noble, P.J., Panfilov, A.V., 2004. A model for human ventricular tissue. Am. J. Physiol. Heart Circ. Physiol. 286, H1573–H1589.

Terkildsen, J., Niederer, S.A., Crampin, E.J., Hunter, P.J., Smith, N.P., 2008. Using Physiome standards to couple cellular functions for cardiac excitation-contraction. Exp. Physiol. 93, 919–929.

van Leeuwen, J.E.M., Samelson, L.E., 1999. T cell antigen-receptor signal transduction. Curr. Opin. Immunol. 11, 242–248.

CHAPTER 14

Systems Approaches to Developmental Patterning

Claudiu A. Giurumescu and Anand R. Asthagiri
California Institute of Technology, Pasadena

OUTLINE

Introduction	329	Processing, Refining and Integrating Signals Downstream of Specification Cues	341
Specification Cues	330		
Short-range Specification	330	Conclusions	346
Long-range Specification and Morphogens	332	Acknowledgments	347

INTRODUCTION

Understanding the mechanisms that transform a fertilized egg into a multicellular organism is a deeply captivating fundamental question in biology. Insights into this question can have profound biomedical implications. Uncovering the regulatory mechanisms that control multicellular morphodynamics and tissue formation can offer design strategies for engineering synthetic environments to facilitate the formation of multicellular structures or for stimulating and accelerating natural biological processes that may promote tissue healing and regeneration. These design strategies can advance applications such as tissue engineering and regenerative medicine. Misguided strategies can have significant repercussions, as we now know that aberrations in developmental regulatory mechanisms provide some of the most potent driving forces for the structural and functional regression of tissues during cancer development (Hanahan and Weinberg, 2000).

Development begins with the partitioning of the fertilized egg into distinct groups of cells or "progenitor fields" that will go on to form future organs (Davidson, 1993). This early partitioning occurs through asymmetric divisions of the zygote. The cells within each progenitor field commit to expressing a distinct panel of genes, which lead them toward a unique developmental fate. The next round of specification cues further subdivides the progenitor field, with each subgroup now executing a distinct specification (i.e., gene expression) program. Thus development involves successive rounds of exposure to specification cues followed by commitment to the corresponding gene expression program. At each iteration, the gene expression program prompts cells to execute behaviors such as division, migration, death and extracellular matrix deposition and remodeling. These cell behaviors shape and functionalize developing tissues, and ultimately, the organism.

Tremendous advances are being made in uncovering molecular signals that drive developmental patterning, with particular emphasis on elucidating the specification cues and the network of biochemical reactions that process these cues to induce the appropriate gene expression program. Specification cues must encode spatial information, as groups of cells must be partitioned according to a precise three-dimensional geometry. Once the specification cue has been perceived, cells must then execute the downstream gene expression program in a *context-sensitive* manner. Context-sensitive cell response is essential, because the same specification cue is often used at different times and places to trigger distinct cell fate choices and patterns. These distinct outcomes arise partly because the response to a particular specification cue is often determined in the context of other concurrent signals. In addition, cellular response to a specification cue is contingent on the cell's developmental history.

In this chapter, we examine specification cues and the downstream context-dependent response that propels the development of multicellular organisms. We focus on the progress and the significant challenges in developing a systems-scale quantitative understanding of developmental signaling. Specific molecular networks and developmental systems are discussed, to provide illustrative examples.

SPECIFICATION CUES

Specification cues instruct cells to commit to a particular cell fate, typically by stimulating a specific gene expression program within the target cell. This gene expression program can have multiple effects. In some cases, it may trigger changes in cell behaviors such as cell division, polarization, directed cell migration or apoptosis. In addition, the gene expression changes could "prime" the cell to become competent (i.e., responsive) to the next round of specification cues or stimulate the production of new specification cues for patterning its neighbors. Regardless of the precise downstream response, a crucial feature of specification cues is that they induce a spatial pattern of cell fate choices. The spatial range of patterning has been used classically to group specification cues into two broad categories.

Short-range Specification

When adjacent cells commit to distinct cell fates, signaling proteins at sites of direct cell–cell contact often serve as the specification cues. This short-range mode of specification is conserved among invertebrates and vertebrates (Lai, 2004) with a prominent example involving the ligand, Delta, and the receptor, Notch. Upon binding Delta, several proteolytic events act on the transmembrane Notch protein, ultimately releasing the Notch intracellular domain (Kadesch, 2004). The cytoplasmic domain of Notch associates with the transcription factor Suppressor of Hairless (Su(H)), and regulates gene expression.

Different developmental scenarios utilize the Delta/Notch signaling pathway (Fig. 14.1). During gonad development in *Caenorhabditis elegans*, two neighboring equipotent cells diverge to become the anchor cell and the ventral uterine cell (Kimble and Simpson, 1997). Each cell initially is capable of assuming either fate, but a stochastic imbalance in Delta expression initiates the binary fate choice (Fig. 14.1A). The cell with the slightly higher Delta expression (referred to as the "sender") stimulates Notch signaling in its neighbor. Increased Notch signaling in the "receiver" cell is amplified by an intracellular positive-feedback loop that further increases Notch expression. Meanwhile, as Notch signaling impedes the synthesis of Delta, the receiver cell fails to present Delta to its neighbor, thereby depressing Notch activity in the neighbor. With relatively less Notch activity (and, therefore, better Delta production), the sender continues to produce Delta at a higher rate than its neighbor, which further strengthens Notch activity in the receiver. In this manner, an intercellular positive-feedback loop that is intrinsic to the Notch/Delta pathway reinforces and amplifies the initial random bias. In the final state, the pair of equipotent cells

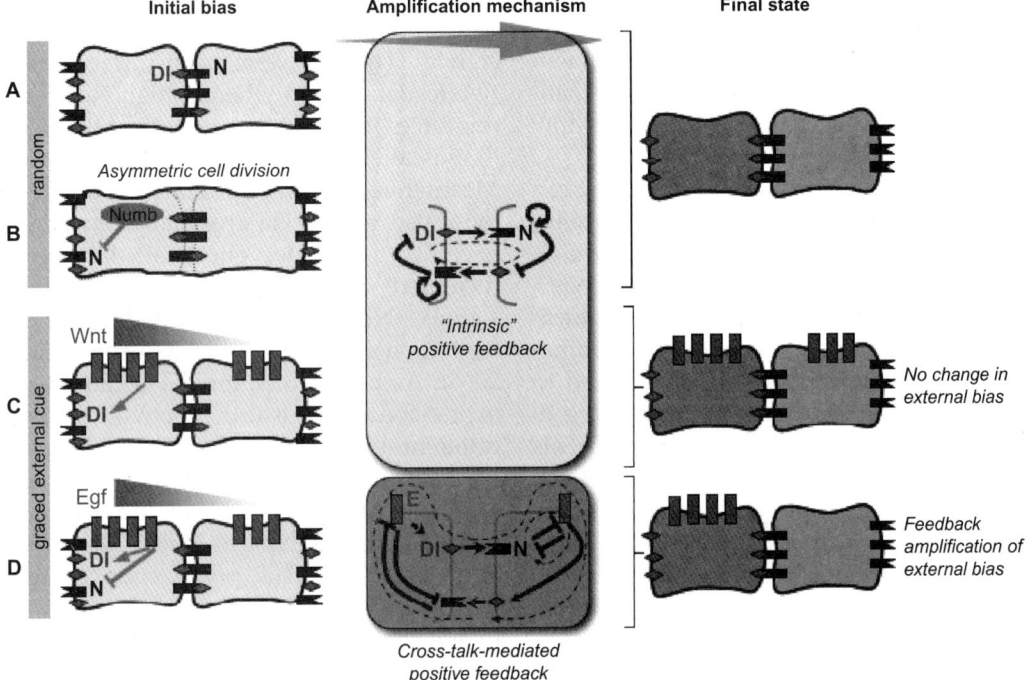

FIGURE 14.1 Different Modes of Delta/Notch Signaling in Short-range Specification.
(A) A stochastic imbalance in the production of Delta ligand (Dl) or Notch receptor (N) can generate an initial asymmetry. This initial bias is amplified by a positive-feedback loop that is intrinsic to the Notch/Delta pathway (yellow box). (B) Following asymmetric division, an imbalance in the amount of transcription factor (Numb) between the two daughter cells provides an initial stochastic bias that is amplified as in the first case. In both (A) and (B), the final state is the polarization of a single signal, Notch activity. (C) An external bias (Wnt gradient) initially polarizes Notch signaling, and differences are further amplified by the intrinsic Notch/Delta positive-feedback loop. This leads to polarization of Notch activity, while the graded Wnt signal remains unchanged. (D) An external bias (epidermal growth factor [EGF] gradient) introduces an initial bias in Delta/Notch signaling, which in turn is amplified via a positive-feedback loop that involves cross-talk between Notch and EGF signaling (green box). From the perspective of Notch signaling, this cross-talk circuit establishes positive-feedback loops that are similar to the classical intrinsic mechanism (compare dotted lines in the green box with the solid lines in the yellow box), with the important exception that all the critical steps are transduced through cross-talk with EGF signaling. This coupling results in the concomitant polarization of two signals (Notch activity and EGF signaling) in (D) as opposed to only the Notch signal as in (A), (B) and (C).

exhibits a large polarity in Notch signaling. The cell receiving high levels of Notch activity executes the ventral uterine fate; meanwhile, the absence of Notch activity in the sender cell drives it to the anchor cell fate.

In other systems, asymmetric cell division provides the initial random bias in the Delta/Notch pathway (Fig. 14.1B). For example, one of the daughter cells of the sensory organ precursor cells in *Drosophila* contains a higher level of the intracellular protein, Numb (Rhyu et al., 1994). Numb enhances Notch endocytosis and thereby attenuates Notch signaling. This initial random bias in Numb levels and Notch downregulation is then amplified by the aforementioned positive-feedback mechanism (Berdnik et al., 2002).

The initial bias for Delta/Notch signaling can also come from gradients in soluble extracellular factors (Fig. 14.1C, D). A gradient in the concentration of the morphogen, wingless (Wnt), biases Notch signaling during R3/R4 specification of photoreceptors in the *Drosophila* ommatidium. The presumptive R3 cell is exposed to a higher local concentration of Wnt, leading to an increase in Delta expression in this cell. This increased expression of Delta enhances Notch activity in its neighbor, the presumptive R4 cell. Notably, once the Wnt gradient has provided this initial bias, it seems to play a minimal role in subsequent amplification of Notch polarity, which is achieved through the classical intercellular positive-feedback pathway intrinsic to the Notch/Delta pathway. Furthermore, the polarization of Notch signaling does not feed back to affect Wnt-mediated signaling.

In contrast to the unidirectional effect of Wnt on Delta/Notch signaling in R3/R4 specification, an intriguing bidirectional coupling between a soluble factor and Delta/Notch guides the specification of vulval precursor cells in *C. elegans* (Fig. 14.1D). A gradient in the soluble factor LIN-3 (an epidermal growth factor [EGF]-like extracellular signal) provides the initial bias in Notch signaling. LIN-3 stimulates the expression of Delta-like ligands (Chen and Greenwald, 2004) and the downregulation of Notch (Shaye and Greenwald, 2002); thus the cell exposed to the lower local EGF concentration exhibits an initial relative bias favoring Notch activity. How this initial bias is amplified deviates from the classical Notch positive-feedback loop. Instead of regulatory pathways intrinsic to the Notch/Delta pathway, the feedback loops work through cross-talk between Notch and EGF (Fig. 14.1D, yellow box). Within each cell, Notch inhibits EGF-mediated signaling pathways, while EGF inhibits Notch activity. The net effect is an intracellular positive-feedback loop wherein high Notch activity reinforces itself but the strength of that feedback loop is affected by the local EGF concentration. Meanwhile, the intercellular positive-feedback loop also occurs via cross-talk between Notch and EGF. The net effect of this cross-talk-mediated positive-feedback loops is that two signals—Notch and EGF signaling—are polarized in neighboring cells (Giurumescu et al., 2006). As both Notch and EGF can affect gene expression programs, this network allows four different states (high EGF/high Notch, high EGF/low Notch, low EG/high Notch and low EGF/low Notch), rather than the two cell states encoded by the classical Notch/Delta pathway (Fig. 14.1A–C). This polarization of two signals may be particularly useful in this system, in which six cells acquire three distinct fates, in contrast to a binary fate choice based on the polarity of a single Notch signal.

Long-range Specification and Morphogens

Gradients in soluble factors play an even more prominent role in patterning cell fates over longer scales of distance. Classical models hypothesized that spatial gradients in soluble cues may encode positional information necessary to pattern large cell fields (Crick, 1970; Wolpert, 1969). Such soluble cues or morphogens were envisioned to induce two or more cell fate choices in a concentration-dependent manner (Fig. 14.2A) (Tabata and Takei, 2004). Direct evidence for the morphogen hypothesis came from the studies of activin during mesoderm induction in *Xenopus* embryos (Gurdon et al., 1994) and of Bicoid (Driever and Nusslein-Volhard, 1988) and decapentaplegic (Dpp) (Ferguson and Anderson, 1992; Nellen et al., 1996) during the anterior–posterior and dorsal–ventral patterning in *Drosophila* embryos. Since then, four major families of extracellular morphogens have been identified: fibroblast growth factor (FGF), hedgehog (Hh), wingless (Wg/Wnt) and transforming growth factor-β (TGFβ) (Anderson and Ingham, 2003). These factors are conserved evolutionarily and operate across both invertebrates (*Drosophila, C. elegans* and sea urchin) and vertebrates (*Xenopus*, zebrafish, mouse and chicken). It should be noted that morphogens need not be extracellular factors. The early *Drosophila* embryo contains no cell boundaries and is a multinuclear syncytium in which gradients in maternal gene products, such as Bicoid, impart anterior–posterior patterns in gene expression.

At the core, the formation of a morphogen gradient involves a source of morphogen, its transport across the field of target cells that will be patterned and a "sink" (i.e., a mechanism for its degradation). Extracellular morphogens are often secreted through proteolytic cleavage of transmembrane precursors (Hill and Sternberg, 1992; Lee et al., 2001). Morphogen release may be regulated through intracellular process, such as retention in the endoplasmic reticulum as in the case of the release of the Spitz morphogen during *Drosophila* eye development (Schlesinger et al., 2004).

In some cases, the source that secretes the morphogen is an individual cell, and the gradient may reach across only a short distance/few cells. A good example is the case of LIN-3 during *C. elegans* vulval development (Hill and Sternberg, 1992). Alternatively, an array of cells secretes Dpp during anterior–posterior patterning of the *Drosophila* wing (Lecuit et al., 1996). In this case, the gradient can span hundreds of cells, although short-range coverage is also possible, as in Hh-initiated anterior–posterior patterning in the *Drosophila* wing (Tabata and Kornberg, 1994). Precisely what factors

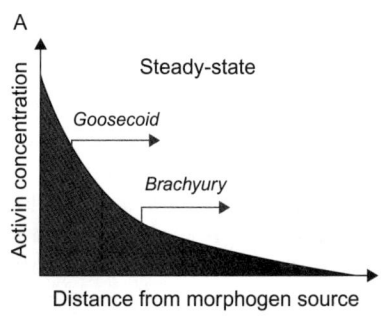
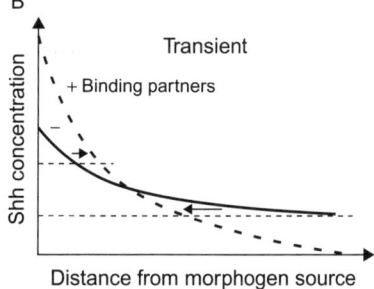

FIGURE 14.2 Spatial Patterning by Morphogens.
(A) Cells are exposed to a gradient in activin concentration. The local concentration of activin determines the gene expression response. The highest activin concentration promotes expression of *goosecoid*. At intermediate distances, a moderate concentration of activin induces the expression of *brachyury*. Cells farthest from the morphogen source receive the least amount of morphogen and do not express either gene. (B) The presence of reversible binding partners can slow down the evolution of the morphogen gradient, so that at an early time, the morphogen Sonic hedgehog (Shh) remains concentrated near the source. Far from the source, this has the expected effect of diminishing the working range of the morphogen. However, close to the source, the range of the morphogen is extended.

(A) Adapted from Giurumescu and Asthagiri (2008), with permission. Copyright 2008 American Chemical Society.

determine the spatial "reach" and quantitative form of a morphogen gradient is a critical issue and is discussed further below.

Meanwhile, the timing (initiation and duration) of secretion is also an important issue. If more than one source cell is involved, how are they synchronized? If the secreting group of cells is small, direct cell–cell communication may help to synchronize the secreting cells. Relay mechanisms may also be used to synchronize and extend the spatial reach of the morphogen. For example, a short-range gradient in Hh sets up a long-range gradient in Dpp morphogen patterns the *Drosophila* wing (Strigini and Cohen, 1999).

The secreted morphogen must be transported across the cell field to establish a gradient. Although diffusion-mediated transport is the most straightforward possibility, some mathematical models have suggested that passive diffusion may be too slow to establish a meaningful steady-state morphogen gradient (Kerszberg and Wolpert, 1998). For the parameter values studied in this model, the morphogen saturated the available cell surface receptors much more quickly than it could be transported. Thus diffusion-mediated transport produced only a traveling wave of morphogen-occupied receptors. At steady state, all available cell surface receptors would be bound to the morphogen, yielding uniform receptor signaling across the entire cell field.

Intriguing experimental observations further suggested a need to re-evaluate the role of diffusion. One such observation came from mosaic animals in which a patch of mutant cells were deficient in endocytosis, a process by which morphogen-bound receptors are internalized into the cell. A fraction of these internalized species are degraded; the remainder is recycled to the cell surface (for a review of receptor trafficking, see Lauffenburger and Linderman, 1993). In conditions in which a mutant patch of cells was deficient in receptor endocytosis, a transient depression or "shadow" in morphogen concentration was observed adjacent to the patch on the side opposite from the secreting morphogen source. This apparent inability of the morphogen to transport into and across mutant cell patches seemed to rule out diffusion and raised the possibility that morphogen transport may occur by an active, receptor-assisted process labeled "transcytosis" (Fig. 14.3) (Dubois et al., 2001; Entchev et al., 2000). In this process, morphogen-bound receptors are brought into the cell by endocytosis and then expelled back to the cell surface by exocytosis. These exocytosed morphogen–receptor complexes dissociate and release the morphogen back into the extracellular microenvironment. If transcytosis is isotropic (i.e., spatially non-biased exocytosis), this mode of morphogen transport can be characterized by an effective diffusion coefficient (Vincent and Dubois, 2002) and, unlike diffusion, would depend on receptor internalization, consistent with experimental observations.

These theoretical and experimental results brought into question the role of diffusion; however, new insights emerged from a systems-level re-examination of morphogen diffusion alongside key biochemical pathways such as receptor–morphogen trafficking and degradation (Lander et al., 2002). The interplay of four steps—morphogen synthesis, its diffusion, its degradation and its reversible binding to receptor—was shown to determine the shape of the steady-state gradient of morphogen-bound receptors. Consider a cell field being patterned as a closed system. Morphogen is injected into the system at one end. If there is no degradation, its concentration will simply build up over time, and at steady-state all receptors will be occupied. Interestingly, binding to receptors itself triggers intracellular trafficking and morphogen degradation (Entchev et al., 2000; Gonzalez-Gaitan, 2003). When this degradation operates at a rate that competes with morphogen synthesis, diffusion can yield a steady-state spatial gradient in morphogen-bound receptors. The steady-state gradient in bound

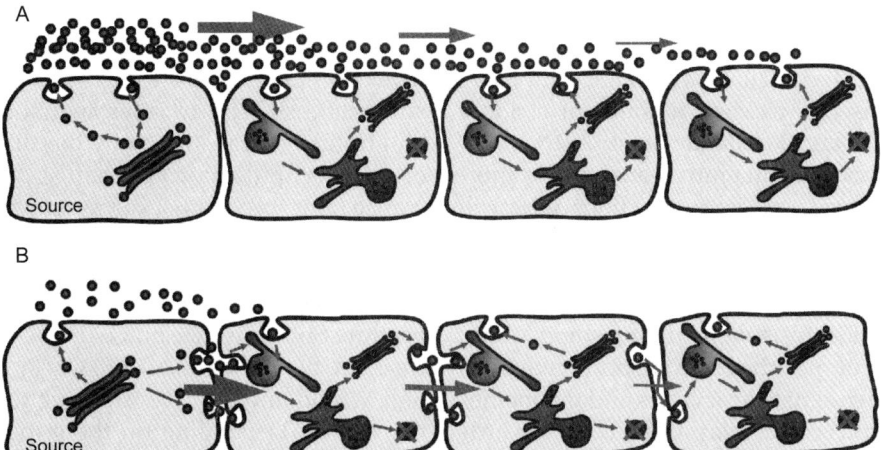

FIGURE 14.3 The Role of Receptor–Ligand Trafficking in Morphogen Transport.
Receptor–ligand trafficking plays a crucial role in establishing morphogen gradients, irrespective of whether morphogen transport occurs by (A) diffusion or (B) transcytosis. In both scenarios, morphogen is synthesized and released from the Golgi (green) of a source cell (left). In (A), the morphogen is transported by diffusion across the extracellular space. Receptors (not shown) on the surface of target cells bind the morphogen and mediate its internalization. A fraction of internalized ligand is recycled back into the microenvironment, but the remainder is degraded in lysosomes (blue). The rate of morphogen degradation influences the shape of the steady-state morphogen gradient. In contrast, in transcytosis (B), successive rounds of endocytosis and recycling of ligand mediates its transport across the cell field; in the absence of receptor–ligand trafficking, the morphogen is assumed to be immobile in the extracellular space.
Reprinted from Giurumescu and Asthagiri (2008), with permission. Copyright 2008 American Chemical Society.

morphogen also hinges on morphogen binding to its receptor. If the cell expresses a high level of receptors or the receptor binds rapidly to the morphogen, the cell surface receptors will be saturated with morphogen. An analysis of morphogen receptors, however, shows that their ligand affinity tends to be low, thereby avoiding saturation at typical physiological morphogen concentrations.

In fact, a closer look at physiological parameter values suggests that diffusion-mediated transport may be physically more plausible than transcytosis (Lander et al., 2002). Non-physiological rates for subcellular processes would be required to make the transcytosis model plausible. For example, to form mophogen gradients on typical developmental time scales, the morphogen would have to be transported across a single cell within 100 seconds. This time scale is achievable by diffusion; however, transcytosis would be too slow as it involves numerous relatively slow steps such as receptor association, internalization, directed transport through the cell, exocytosis and receptor dissociation.

In support of the transcytosis model, it remains a possibility that *in-vivo* rates of subcellular processes, such as internalization and exocytosis, may be optimized to facilitate transcytosis within developmental time scales (Vincent and Dubois, 2002). Furthermore, the diffusion/endocytosis model is not consistent with all experimental data (Kruse et al., 2004). Recall the experiment involving a mutant patch of cells that is defective in endocytosis. The patch casts a transient morphogen "shadow" next to the patch on the side opposite from the morphogen source. The diffusion/endocytosis model explains this shadow: because receptor degradation is blocked, receptor expression is predicted to increase well above normal levels in an endocytosis-defective patch. This increased receptor expression would sequester the morphogen and retard (but, would not completely halt) its transport, yielding a transient shadow effect (Kruse et al., 2004; Lander et al., 2002).

In summary, an integrative analysis of morphogen transport and its interactions with cell surface receptors demonstrates that diffusion is adequate for establishing morphogen gradients in developmentally relevant time scales and in an endocytosis-dependent fashion. Other mechanisms of morphogen transport have been proposed, including transcytosis and cytonemes or cytoplasmic projections from cells towards the source of the morphogen (Ramirez-Weber and Kornberg, 1999). It remains unclear how cells extend cytonemes in the absence of an additional positional cue. A role for convective transport in establishing morphogen gradients is also emerging, particularly in low-flow interstitial spaces. Under these low-flow conditions, convective transport may establish a gradient in vascular endothelial growth factor (VEGF), a chemotactic factor driving capillary formation (Helm et al., 2005).

The free diffusion of morphogen may also be affected by binding partners in the extracellular matrix or on the cell surface. Systems-level mathematical modeling has been used to dissect the effect of these binding partners on the formation of a Sonic hedgehog (Shh) morphogen gradient during vertebrate neural tube development (Saha and Schaffer, 2006). Sonic hedgehog (Shh) interacts with two cell surface molecules: its cell-surface receptor, Patched (Ptch), and a non-signaling membrane glycoprotein, Hip (Chuang and McMahon, 1999). Model analysis suggests that the signaling-deficient Shh–Hip complexes may act as a non-signaling endocytic sink for Shh, thereby shunting the morphogen from the extracellular space toward a degradation pathway. In this manner, Hip may limit the spatial range of Shh.

Meanwhile, Shh also binds extracellular matrix components, including heparan sulfate proteoglycans (HSPGs) (The et al., 1999) and vitronectin (Pons and Marti, 2000). Model analysis revealed that the transient gradient in Shh signaling can exhibit a broader spatial range when Shh transport is restricted by binding to HSPGs or vitronectin (Saha and Schaffer, 2006). At first glance, this prediction seems counterintuitive, because one would expect that sequestering Shh ought to constrain its transport. Indeed, transport-restricting mechanisms help to concentrate Shh near the source (Fig. 14.2B); in contrast, in the absence of HSPGs or vitronectin, Shh would move more effectively away from the source. Depending on the critical Shh concentration at which gene expression is turned on (or off), the effect of HSPG and vitronectin could be to enhance or diminish the spatial range of the Shh morphogen. Such predictions reveal that even seemingly innocuous changes in the mechanisms that govern morphogen transport can have significantly non-intuitive consequences, further stressing the importance of systems-level modeling and analysis of developmental regulatory networks.

In addition to binding immobile partners in the extracellular matrix or cell surface, morphogens may also encounter binding partners that are diffusing. A classical example involves the morphogen Dpp that establishes dorsal patterning of the *Drosophila* embryo (reviewed by O'Connor et al., 2006). A prior gradient in the transcription factor Dorsal along the dorsal–ventral axis leads to the expression of *short gastrulation* (*sog*) in the neurogenic ectoderm on the ventrolateral side of the embryo and the expression of the non-neurogenic genes *decapentaplegic* (*dpp*), *twisted gastrulation* (*tsg*) and *tolloid* (*tld*) in the dorsolateral part of the embryo. Sog, Dpp, Tsg and Tld are all secreted proteins (Francois et al., 1994; Marques et al., 1997; Mason et al., 1994). The Dpp receptor, Thickveins (Tkv), is uniformly distributed along the dorsal–ventral axis of the embryo. Release of Sog from its expression domain forms a gradient (Srinivasan et al., 2002) that drives the refinement of the uniform, low-concentration Dpp field to a narrow strip along the dorsal midline of the embryo that further patterns the dorsal side of the embryo. Interestingly, the mechanism of induction of asymmetry from Sog to Dpp does not involve Sog inhibition/degradation of Dpp in the lateral-most region. Indeed, such inhibition/degradation would be ineffectual towards creating a sharp concentration gradient at midline, as Dpp, at already low concentration, is unable to signal through its receptor. Instead, as Sog diffuses into the dorsolateral region, it forms, together with Tsg, a complex with Dpp. This complex sequesters Dpp and does not allow it to interact with its receptor. Under the driving force of the Sog concentration gradient, the Sog–Tsg–Dpp complex is transported towards the midline. Here, the protease Tld cleaves Sog in the Sog–Tsg–Dpp complex and releases Dpp, allowing binding to Tkv receptors and further signaling (Ashe and Levine, 1999; Shimmi and O'Connor, 2003; Shimmi et al., 2005).

The above examples of Shh and Dpp clearly demonstrate the rich network of mechanisms that regulate morphogen gradient formation. Mathematical models have proven critical to elucidate how these different mechanisms contribute to the dynamics of morphogen gradients (Bergmann et al., 2007; Mizutani et al., 2007; Saha and Schaffer, 2006). Furthermore, the rapid emergence of quantitative imaging techniques for measuring the dynamics of morphogen gradients *in vivo* has allowed systems-level predictions to be tested experimentally. Gradient dynamics have been directly observed *in vivo* using green fluorescent protein (GFP) fusion constructs. This approach has been used to study the formation of the Dpp and Wg gradients in *Drosophila* during the anterior–posterior patterning of wing discs and during embryonic development, respectively (Entchev et al., 2000; Pfeiffer et al., 2002; Teleman and Cohen, 2000). A similar strategy has been used to study Dpp and Bicoid gradients during dorsal–ventral and anterior–posterior patterning of the *Drosophila* embryo (Gregor et al., 2007b; Houchmandzadeh et al., 2002; Shimmi et al., 2005). In addition to testing how specific perturbations affect the dynamics and shape of the gradient, quantitative imaging has also enabled the estimation of parameters governing morphogen synthesis, diffusion and degradation (Gregor et al., 2007b; Kicheva et al., 2007).

In some cases, however, the morphogen gradient cannot be visualized directly because of technical difficulties in expressing GFP-fused morphogens or in using antibodies to detect low concentrations of morphogens. In these cases, an intracellular event activated by the morphogen, such as the expression of a gene target, may be used as an indirect marker. For example, during *C. elegans* vulval development, the presence of a gradient in an EGF-like soluble factor (LIN-3) has been confirmed by imaging the graded activation of a reporter of the mitogen-activated protein kinase (MAPK) pathway, *egl-17* (Yoo et al., 2004). Although this approach confirmed the existence of a spatial gradient in LIN-3, elucidating the precise quantitative form of this gradient remains encumbered by the lack of a direct sensor for LIN-3.

Working under similar constraints in another developmental system, Goentoro and colleagues (2006) used a model-based approach to infer the quantitative shape of the steady-state gradient in the morphogen, Gurken, in the *Drosophila* egg chamber. Because the Gurken morphogen gradient was not directly observable, they manipulated the level of expression of the Gurken receptor (epidermal growth factor receptor [EGFR]) and quantified the effect on the expression of the target gene, *pipe*. This quantitative dataset related the level of expression of EGFR to the spatial boundaries of *pipe* expression. To extract quantitative information about the Gurken gradient from these measurements, the quantitative dataset was fitted to a systems-scale model of Gurken gradient formation and signaling. This analysis uncovered the value of a key metric of gradient steepness: the ratio L/λ, where λ is the characteristic decay-length scale of the morphogen gradient and L is the length of the field of cells to be patterned (Houchmandzadeh et al., 2005; Lander et al., 2002). The steady-state Gurken gradient was characterized by an L/λ value of 2.7. This model-based estimation of L/λ provided a quantitative assessment of the shape of the Gurken gradient and revealed the sensitivity of downstream gene expression to the concentration of Gurken. For example, a mere threefold change in Gurken concentration induces a significant change in the gene expression program, revealing switch-like ultrasensitivity to Gurken concentration.

With systems-level insights emerging from mathematical modeling and quantitative imaging, it has become tractable to ask why development systems have adopted a particular set of mechanisms to form morphogen gradients. From an evolutionary perspective, what selective advantages does a particular set of mechanisms confer? Along these lines, three properties of morphogen gradients have drawn recent attention: its shape (graded versus steep), its robustness and its scalability.

The most basic requirement is that morphogen-shaping mechanisms produce a biologically useful morphogen gradient. One hypothesis is that a useful morphogen gradient should not be too shallow or too steep. Using the aforementioned metric of gradient steepness, a biologically useful gradient would have a steepness characterized by $L/\lambda = 1$, where the characteristic length scale of the morphogen gradient is approximately equal to the length of the cell field being patterned. Indeed, the Gurken gradient discussed above ($L/\lambda = 2.7$) seems to satisfy this requirement. Quantitative characterization of Bicoid localization in Drosophila embryos shows that the morphogen gradient is distributed across the patterning field, with $L/\lambda = 3.8$ (Houchmandzadeh et al., 2005), whereas the L/λ value for the Dpp gradient in the Drosophila wing disc is 2.5 (Kicheva et al., 2007).

Mathematical models provide insights into the interplay of mechanisms that yield a biologically useful gradient (Lander et al., 2002). In the context of an extracellular morphogen transported by diffusion and degraded by receptor endocytosis, biologically useful gradients are formed when the morphogen–receptor binding constant, k_{on}, is less than $O(10^5)$ M^{-1} s^{-1} and the degradation rate constant of endocytosed complexes, k_{deg}, is $O(10^{-4})$ s^{-1} (30). Larger values of k_{on} restrict the dynamic range of the number of morphogen–receptor complexes per cell, hence limiting the system to shallow gradients. Meanwhile, for smaller values of k_{deg}, morphogen synthesis outweighs degradation and leads to steady accumulation of morphogen and saturation of cell surface receptors.

It should be noted that, even for systems that achieve a seemingly optimal morphogen gradient characterized by $L/\lambda \approx 1$, this gradient ultimately must subdivide the cell field into distinct patterns of gene expression. Sharp borders in cell response must be established. In some cases, such borders are achieved by sharpening the signals that come downstream of a spatially graded morphogen concentration profile. Such signal processing downstream of morphogens is discussed in the next section.

Here we note that, in certain developmental contexts, mechanisms have evolved to encode sharp borders directly at the level of the morphogen gradient itself. As noted above, during Drosophila dorsal patterning, the bone morphogenetic protein (BMP) homologue Dpp becomes highly localized at the dorsal midline through Sog–Tsg–Tld-mediated shuttling (Shimmi et al., 2005). In addition, a second BMP (Scw), localized along the entire dorsoventral axis, is required for the correct midline localization of Dpp (Arora et al., 1994). It was recently shown that Dpp and Scw can exist as heterodimers (Shimmi et al., 2005) and homodimers. Sog associates more effectively with the heterodimer, forming a complex that is a better substrate for Tld-mediated

Sog cleavage. Thus the heterodimer is shuttled more effectively and concentrates to the midline. Meanwhile, the homodimeric Dpp remains more broadly distributed across the dorsal region. Interestingly, Dpp–Scw binds to a synergistic pair of receptors, yielding more potent downstream signaling. Meanwhile, the Dpp homodimer binds only one of these receptors and signals relatively more modestly. These two levels of signals trigger two different programs of gene expression: genes that require a lower level of signal are triggered by the Dpp homodimer, whereas those that require a higher threshold of signal are triggered by the Dpp–Scw heterodimer only in the dorsal midline. Thus, in this system, ligand dimers with distinct strength of interactions with transport facilitators (Sog, Tsg, Tld) and with the signaling apparatus (receptors) provide a sharp border of gene expression, distinguishing the dorsal midline from the dorsolateral regions.

Interestingly, the mechanisms responsible for sharpening the Dpp–Scw gradient may also confer robustness to changes in the level of expression of Sog, Tsg, Tld or Scw. Mutants heterozygous for these genes develop normally. Although $dpp^{+/-}$ heterozygous embryos do not develop, reduced Sog dosage in $dpp^{+/-}$; $sog^{+/-}$ embryos rescues the dpp haploinsufficiency (Eldar et al., 2002; Mizutani et al., 2005). However, there are limits to the ability of the system to buffer perturbations. Complete elimination of sog (Eldar et al., 2002; Francois et al., 1994), scw (Arora and Nusslein-Volhard, 1992; Shimmi et al., 2005), or tld (Arora and Nusslein-Volhard, 1992) will completely disrupt Dpp downstream signaling and gene expression, leading to ventralization of the embryo and abnormal development. Thus, as in engineered systems, robustness is achieved with respect to perturbations in specific parameters, but not others. In this case, interaction among the system components yields robustness. Eldar et al. (2002) identified several criteria: (i) cleavage of Sog by Tld requires Dpp binding, (ii) the complex involving Sog–Dpp must be diffusible, whereas Dpp by itself is not, (iii) Sog can capture Dpp when bound to receptors, and (iv) Dpp can only bind Sog–Tsg complexes. These criteria point to the criticality of Tld and Sog for the functioning of the system. Maintenance of a Sog gradient is necessary for transport of Dpp towards the dorsal midline as Sog–Dpp complexes. In turn, the Sog gradient is preserved by Tld through gene expression at the ventrolateral side and degradation at the dorsal side of Sog–Dpp complexes. In the absence of Tld, Sog would flood the dorsal side of the embryo and the potential difference of the Sog gradient would be only short lived. Furthermore, the differential affinity of Sog for Dpp–Scw rather than for Dpp or Scw homodimers, and the ability of Dpp–Scw to bind only Sog–Tsg, further refine Dpp transport and enhance the robustness of its gradient formation. Through a two-step mechanism, potential fluctuations in the amounts of Dpp, Scw, Sog or Tsg are buffered, reducing the variability in the quantities of Dpp–Scw and Sog–Tsg complexes. These more precise inputs then lead to further reduction in fluctuations in the amount of Dpp–Scw–Sog–Tsg, the complex transported to the midline for Tld cleavage (Shimmi et al., 2005).

In other systems like *Drosophila* embryonic patterning by Bicoid, in which synthesis, diffusion and degradation are presumably the only principal mechanisms of morphogen gradient formation, we would expect that this gradient may be more prone to high variability. However, recent measurements have shown that this is not the case (Gregor et al., 2007a). By quantifying the gradient in absolute concentrations of Bicoid across numerous *Drosophila* embryos, it was demonstrated that the amount of inter-embryo variability is ~10%, a value that is close to the physical limits of precision (Gregor et al., 2007a). Precisely what mechanisms confer this precision is unclear.

As with Dpp in dorsal patterning, the Bicoid gradient is not robust to all types of perturbation.

A change in the dosage of maternal Bicoid (the morphogen source) alters the Bicoid gradient (Gregor et al., 2007b). However, in other systems, the morphogen gradient is buffered against fluctuations in the source. Increases in the morphogen secretion rate are buffered by a feedback loop during anterior–posterior patterning of *Drosophila* wing (Eldar et al., 2003). Here, the Hh morphogen induces localized expression of its receptor, Ptch, which in turn sequesters and directs Hh to endocytic degradation. This negative feedback loop is a robust mechanism that limits the morphogen from reaching distant cells in the event of increased morphogen secretion. Such a feedback mechanism does not seem to exist in the Bicoid system, possibly because the maternal injection of Bicoid is itself well regulated and is not a significant source of fluctuations.

A particularly intriguing aspect of robustness of the Bicoid gradient is that it scales with embryo length (Gregor et al., 2005, 2007b). Embryo length (L) varies significantly between species in the *Drosophila* genus. Remarkably, the concentration of Bicoid at a particular scaled position (x/L) along the embryo varies only by 2% among these species (Gregor et al., 2005). The working hypothesis is that the morphogen degradation rate has adapted to changes in embryo length across species. While variations in compensating parameters may explain the scaling of Bicoid across different species, it is unclear what drives similar scaling across more the modest variations in embryo length observed within *Drosophila melanogaster* itself (Gregor et al., 2007b).

Recent work in *Xenopus* dorso–ventral patterning has offered new insights into the mechanisms providing robustness and scalability of morphogen gradients. *Xenopus* dorsal–ventral patterning uses a conserved set of molecules, the ligand Bmp, the BMP inhibitor Sog/Chordin (Chd), the modulator Tsg/xTsg and the protease Xlr. Similar to the mechanism in invertebrates, the Bmp is expressed along the entire dorsoventral axis, whereas Chd inhibitor is expressed locally on the dorsal side to drive the formation of a steep Bmp gradient. Unlike in *Drosophila*, in *Xenopus* the concentrations of Bmp morphogen are increased at the ventral midline, and an additional BMP-type ligand, Admp, is expressed at the dorsal midline, but its transcription levels are inhibited by BMP signaling. Using a computational model, Ben-Zvi et al. (2008) showed that, in the absence of Admp (in which case the model is equivalent to that previously presented for *Drosophila* dorsal–ventral patterning by Eldar et al., 2002), a correct Bmp morphogen gradient is formed that is robust to the dosage of Bmp, Chd, or Xlr, but is unable to provide correct scaling with changes in embryo dimensions along the dorsal–ventral axis. Introduction of Admp expression around the dorsal midline resulted in a model that was able to preserve robustness to dosage in network components, in addition to displaying correct scaling along the dorsal–ventral axis. Moreover, in this model the most likely mechanism of BMP (Bmp + Admp) gradient formation was inferred to be shuttling of BMP ligands by Chd to the ventral midline, provided that the following conditions were satisfied: (i) diffusion of BMP ligands is greatly enhanced by their binding to Chd, (ii) Chd degradation by Xlr requires its binding to BMP ligands, and (iii) Chd has greater affinity for Bmp than for Admp. We have seen how the shuttling mechanism naturally explains the robustness of the gradient to fluctuations in dosage of different network components—but how is scaling achieved? The key is Admp and its ability to be repressed by BMP signaling. The BMP morphogen gradient in this system is dynamic until Admp concentrations increase at the dorsal midline such that they surpass the level needed for BMP signaling to inhibit Admp expression. At this point, no more Admp is introduced into the system and the BMP gradient stabilizes according to the shuttling mechanism. Hence, if the size of the embryo is changed, this Admp "pumping" mechanism allows for scaling by changing the timing required for reaching the threshold Admp concentration around the dorsal midline.

It is abundantly clear that the dynamics of establishing morphogen gradients can involve a significant departure from simple diffusion with a source and sink. These additional regulatory mechanisms confer functional advantages, such as robustness and scalability. Interestingly, this remarkable level of regulatory complexity is found just at the level of presenting the specification cue(s) to the cell field, without even considering the remaining non-trivial challenge of translating these cues into appropriate cell responses.

PROCESSING, REFINING AND INTEGRATING SIGNALS DOWNSTREAM OF SPECIFICATION CUES

A first step in responding to specification cues involves cell surface receptors. In the context of morphogens, the classical view has been that the number of morphogen-bound receptors determines the extent of intracellular signaling and the gene expression program. Alternatively, the *ratio* of the number of bound to the number of unbound receptors may also dictate downstream signaling, as in the case of the morphogen, Hh (Casali and Struhl, 2004). The Hh receptor, Ptch, inhibits another transmembrane protein, Smo. Upon ligand binding, Hh-bound Ptch is no longer able to inhibit Smo. In this manner, Hh relieves Smo inhibition and enables Smo-mediated gene expression. Casali and Struhl showed that Hh-bound Ptch not only releases Smo to signal, but also impedes free Ptch from sequestering Smo. Thus the ratio of bound to unbound Ptch determines the degree of repression of Smo.

Beyond this initial sensing step, however, lies the challenge of decoding receptor signals into an appropriate dose-dependent cell response. This decoding must account for and be influenced by two key factors: (a) the cell's developmental history and (b) concomitant additional cues in the cellular microenvironment. The need for the cell response to be contingent on temporal and environmental context can be appreciated by the fact that a handful of common morphogens (e.g. Wnt, BMP, Hh) are used repeatedly to achieve cell patterning in distinct tissues and at different developmental time points. Thus a single one-to-one correspondence between specification cue and cell response cannot be applied ubiquitously to every developmental context.

Consistent with this idea, the spatial gradient in a single morphogen is inadequate to explain the final multicellular pattern in certain developmental contexts. Anterior–posterior segmentation of the Drosophila blastoderm occurs through the hierarchical activity of gap, pair-rule and segment-polarity genes (reviewed by Jaeger and Reinitz, 2006). The maternal protein gradients in Bicoid and Caudal are the direct inputs to the first layer of the hierarchy: the gap genes *hunchback* (*hb*), *kruppel* (*Kr*), *knirps* (*kni*) and *giant* (*gt*). The pattern of expression of gap genes segments the embryo along the anterior–posterior axis and serves as input to the subsequent layer, the pair-rule genes. However, Bicoid and Caudal alone cannot establish the sharp boundaries of gap-gene expression segments (Houchmandzadeh et al., 2002). Through a combination of gene-expression imaging followed by quantitation and mathematical modeling, Reinitz and colleagues showed that, in addition to the inputs Bicoid and Caudal, the gap genes require significant cross-regulation in order to be expressed in defined sharp segments (Jaeger et al., 2004a, 2004b).

Another example of cross-talk between specification cues occurs during vulval development in *C. elegans*. As described above, the cross-talk between Notch and EGF-like LIN-3 signaling pathways has a critical role in generating a sharp difference in the level of MAPK signal

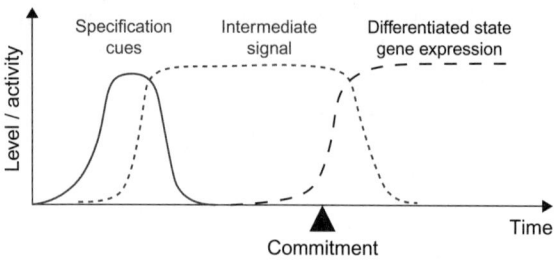

FIGURE 14.4 Transient Cues and Signals Drive Fate Commitment.
Specification cues (red) and intermediate signals (green) are re-used as development progresses even within the same spatial domain. Thus these components must be used transiently, but still produce a permanent differentiated state (blue).

Adapted from Giurumescu and Asthagiri (2008), with permission. Copyright 2008 American Chemical Society.

between neighboring cells. In the absence of this cross-talk, the gradient in the fate-inducing intracellular MAPK signal can at best mimic the likely shallow gradient in the extracellular specification cue, LIN-3.

Mitogen-activated protein kinases are involved broadly in signal processing and refinement downstream of morphogen gradients in numerous other developmental contexts. This signaling pathway exhibits certain quantitative properties that may be desirable in a developmental context. Foremost, the MAPK cascade can produce a switch-like output in response to a graded stimulus. This feature has clear utility in converting an analog signal (e.g. spatial gradient in morphogen) into a digital output (e.g. a fate choice). The cascade structure of the MAPK module contributes to this switch-like behavior. The major contribution, however, involves positive-feedback loops (Ferrell, 1999). For example, in *Xenopus* oocyte extracts, active MAPK triggers an upregulation of Mos, which is itself an upstream activator of the MAPK pathway. When this positive feedback is eliminated (by blocking the upregulation of Mos), the switch-like performance of the MAPK cascade is lost.

Increasing the gain of the positive feedback provides another feature of the MAPK pathway that is useful in the context of development: irreversibility (Fig. 14.4). For example, the MAPK pathway mediates irreversible maturation of the *Xenopus* oocyte following a transient exposure to progesterone (Xiong and Ferrell, 2003). This process involves two coupled positive-feedback loops: the first is found in the MAPK module (Mos, MEK, p42), and the second involves Cdc2, Cdc25 and Myt1. Active Cdc2 promotes accumulation of Mos and active MAPK inhibits Myt1, a negative regulator of Cdc2. As Cdc2/Cdc25 are implicated in cell cycle control (Yang et al., 1999), this positive reinforcement between modules seems to interlock the fate specification signal (via MAPK) and commitment to cell division (via Myt1) (Santos and Ferrell, 2008). The net effect is that the progesterone activates maturation and, even upon removal of the stimulus, the cell remains committed to that fate.

Such fate-locking is crucial in many developmental settings, because specification cues are often present for a sufficient time to elicit a cell response, but must be cleared from the system so that it may be re-used for subsequent developmental steps. Thus converting a transient stimulus to a longer-lasting, irreversible commitment signal is crucial. For example, in *C. elegans*, the anchor cell releases the morphogen LIN-3 and specifies the fate of vulval precursor cells (Hill and Sternberg, 1992); later, the descendants of vulval precursor cells release LIN-3 toward the anchor cell to induce vulval–uterine attachment (Sherwood and Sternberg, 2003). In *Drosophila*, the EGFR pathway functions in numerous processes during embryonic and post-embryonic development (reviewed by Shilo, 2003). EGFR signaling through the receptor, DER, occurs twice during patterning of neuroectoderm: (i) during gastrulation at stage 6, in two bands of lateral cells spanning the neuroectoderm anteroposteriorly, to specify the lateral neuroblasts, and (ii) at stage 10, in a single band of cells centered around the ventral midline, to specify medial neuroblasts (Gabay et al., 1997; Skeath, 1998).

It should be noted that even intermediate signals, such as MAPK, are not permanently dedicated to a single commitment step. They are re-used much like extracellular specification cues. MAPKs may be irreversibly activated on the time-scale of fate commitment, but will decay back to a basal level in order to be available for the next round of developmental patterning. Clearly, there must be other downstream mechanisms for locking-in fate choices. This requirement is a trivial one if the fate is cell division or death—choices that are obviously irreversibile. However, in cases in which fate execution involves the expression of specific genes, other positive-feedback loops at the level of gene regulation, histone acetylation and/or DNA methylation may work to maintain the gene expression program once the specification cue and intermediate signals have receded.

Converting an analog signal, such as a morphogen gradient, into an irreversible digital signal, such as MAPK, is great for making binary fate choices. However, cell fields are commonly divided into three or more distinct patterns of gene expression. Here again, integrating signals from several specification cues seems to be a common solution. Returning to the example of *C. elegans* vulval development, the cross-talk between the specification cues Notch and EGF-like LIN-3 establishes sharp distinctions in MAPK signaling and in Notch signaling. This enables, in principle, four distinct states: high/high, high/low, low/high and low/low levels of MAPK and Notch activity, with each state mapping to a distinct fate choice. Another example involves the aforementioned interplay between gradients in the transcription factors Bicoid and Caudal during anterior–posterior patterning of the *Drosophila* embryo.

These examples underscore the concept that different doses and combinations of transcription factors are used to trigger distinct gene expression responses. Precisely how the expression of specific genes may be sensitive to transcription factor dosage and permutations is starting to emerge. The calculus driving gene expression occurs at the *cis*-regulatory promoter regions upstream of the target gene. *Cis*-regulatory elements contain binding sites for several transcription factors—some activators, and others repressors, of gene expression. Combinatorial processing of these multiple inputs determines the net level of gene expression.

Uncovering how *cis*-regulatory elements integrate inputs from several concomitant transcription factors remains a key challenge. A paradigm for how this integration is accomplished comes from the quantitative analysis of the gene *endo-16*, an endoderm specification marker during the development of the sea-urchin embryo (Yuh and Davidson, 1996). Six modules, A, B, DC, E, F and G, located in a stretch of DNA 2300 base pairs upstream of the gene promoter, control the expression of *endo-16* (Fig. 14.5). Modules A, B and G activate gene expression, whereas the other elements have a repressive role (Yuh et al., 1998). The quantitative contributions of modules A and B to *endo-16* expression, working either alone or synergistically, have been measured, and a model has been constructed to relate the binding status of the different DNA regulatory sequences in these modules to the quantitative output of the module (Istrail and Davidson, 2005; Yuh et al., 2001).

These types of quantitative signal processing and integration that occur at *cis*-regulatory modules provide both a spatial and a temporal context. During early development, expression of *endo-16* is observed in the entire vegetal plate—that is, progeny of cells derived from the veg_2 blastomeres. This expression increases further as development progresses in the endoderm and future archenteron; meanwhile, *endo-16* expression decays back to a basal level in veg_2 progeny cells that are destined to be mesoderm. While these events are occurring among the progeny of veg_2 cells, expression of *endo-16* remains quiescent in micromeres or veg_1 progeny cells. In each of these spatial and temporal contexts, different transcription factors act on

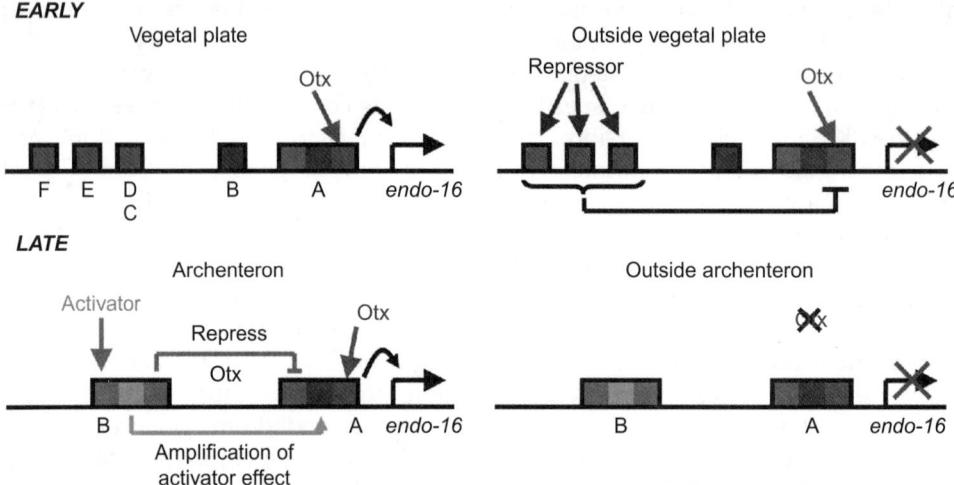

FIGURE 14.5 The Spatial and Temporal Regulation of *endo-16* by its *Cis*-regulatory Modules. Six modules (A, B, DC, E, F and G [not shown]) are found in the *cis*-regulatory region of *endo-16*. During early phases of sea-urchin development, the transcription factor, Otx, works through module A to stimulate expression of *endo-16* in the vegetal plate. Outside the vegetal plate, various repressors bind to modules DC, E and F and repress Otx-mediated expression of *endo-16*. In later stages, cells in the archenteron express an activator (Activator) that binds to module B and amplifies non-Otx-mediated transcription via module A. These events further increase the expression of *endo-16*.

Reprinted from Giurumescu and Asthagiri (2008), with permission. Copyright 2008 American Chemical Society.

the *cis*-regulatory modules of *endo-16*, thereby repressing and inducing its expression at different levels. These differences in the levels of expression of transcription factors are dictated in turn by *cis*-regulatory elements upstream of genes that encode these transcription factors. Thus the history of genes that were expressed in a particular cell encodes its temporal context, thereby priming the cell to respond appropriately to its current specification cues.

This cascade of gene expression events is not a simple linear pathway, but rather a gene regulatory network that operates over spatial and temporal dimensions. The genes and the associated *cis*-regulatory elements that comprise these genetic circuits have been elucidated for a wide range of developmental contexts, including endomesoderm specification in sea-urchin (Davidson et al., 2002), dorsoventral axis patterning in *Drosophila* (for reviews, see Levine and Davidson, 2005; Stathopoulos and Levine, 2005), vulva differentiation in *C. elegans* (Inoue et al., 2005), mesoderm specification in *Xenopus* (Koide et al., 2005), and anterior–posterior patterning and segmentation of the *Drosophila* embryo (Ochoa-Espinosa et al., 2005).

Assessing the quantitative calculations that occur at each *cis*-regulatory element nevertheless remains an important challenge. Approaches similar to the quantitative analysis of *endo-16* will need to be scaled up to cover a larger panel of *cis*-regulatory elements that belong to a common circuit. A significant advance along these lines was reported for the early stages of anterior–posterior patterning of the *Drosophila* embryo (Jaeger et al., 2004b, 2007). Quantitative measurements of the transcription factors and their target gene products were fitted to a mathematical model of the gene regulatory circuit. The parameter values

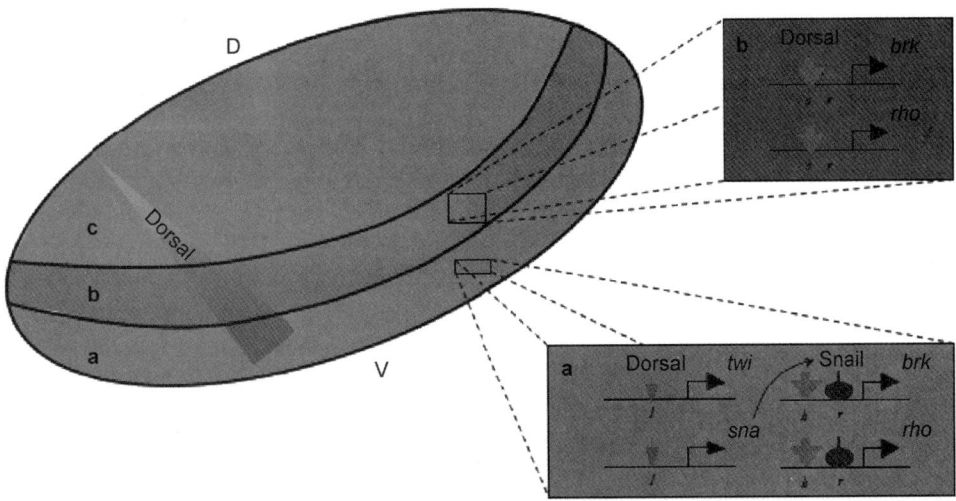

FIGURE 14.6 The Role of *Cis*-regulatory Sequences in Dorsal–ventral Patterning of the *Drosophila* Embryo.
Dorsal–ventral patterning involves the differential expression of specific genes in different regions (a, b and c) of the *Drosophila* embryo. A spatial gradient in the transcription factor, Dorsal, induces this gene expression pattern. Where the concentration of Dorsal is highest (region a, near the ventral [V] region), the target genes (*twi* and *sna*) with low (*l*)-affinity Dorsal binding sites in their *cis*-regulatory region are effectively expressed. These genes fail to be expressed in other regions in which the Dorsal concentration falls below a critical threshold needed to engage the low-affinity *cis*-regulatory regions. In contrast, optimal (*o*) Dorsal binding sites in the *cis*-regulatory regions of *rho* and *brk* permit their expression in region b. Importantly, the *cis*-regulatory region of *rho* and *brk* also contain binding sites (*r*) for the repressor Snail, thereby preventing *rho/brk* expression in the ventral-most region. Finally, the genes expressed in the dorsal-most region, c, are repressed by Dorsal in the ventral regions, a and b. As nuclear translocation of Dorsal does not occur in the dorsal-most nuclei, these genes are expressed in region c.
Adapted from Giurumescu and Asthagiri (2008), with permission. Copyright 2008 American Chemical Society.

uncovered by this approach provided quantitative characterization of the interactions between transcription factors and their gene targets. Moreover, this study delineated quantitatively when, where and to what extent individual transcription factors affected the expression of a particular target gene.

Quantitative characterization of the calculus that occurs at *cis*-regulatory regions presents the challenge of uncovering general principles that determine the quantitative functionality of these pivotal nodes in a gene circuit. Recent findings from the analysis of Dorsal-mediated gene expression during dorsal–ventral patterning of the *Drosophila* embryo offer intriguing insights (Stathopoulos and Levine, 2005) (Fig. 14.6). Target genes (e.g. *twist*, *snail*), the *cis*-regulatory elements of which contain low-affinity binding sites for Dorsal, are expressed strongly in the ventral-most region where concentrations of Dorsal are high. In contrast, target genes (e.g. *rho*), having *cis*-regulatory elements that contain high-affinity binding sites for Dorsal, are expressed toward the dorsal end where concentrations of Dorsal are low. Thus high-affinity sites are used to compensate for low Dorsal concentrations in order to achieve gene expression. In fact, across four divergent species of drosophilids, the overall strength of Dorsal binding sites on *cis*-regulatory elements (as measured by the number and affinity) correlates with the pattern of dorsoventral gene expression (Papatsenko and Levine, 2005).

These findings strongly suggest that the number and affinity of *cis*-regulatory binding regions determine the sensitivity of gene expression to the local concentration of transcription factor. Where the transcription factor concentration is low, genes with high-affinity transcription factor binding sites will be expressed. In contrast, genes with high-affinity transcription factor binding sites may be expressed even if the transcription factor concentration is low. However, this model still leaves open an important question: how do high-affinity binding sites remain unresponsive in regions in which the level of expression of transcription factor is high? For example, why is *rho* not effectively expressed in the ventral region? This additional selectivity is prescribed by repressor binding sites in the *cis*-regulatory region of *rho* (see Fig. 14.6 for details). Thus a combination of binding affinity, number of binding sites and repressors/activators antagonism determines the quantitative functionality of a *cis*-regulatory region.

These advances in uncovering quantitative aspects of gene regulatory networks that operate during narrow developmental windows in model organisms have inspired a bold new challenge: to elucidate the spatiotemporal gene regulatory network that transforms a fertilized egg into a multicellular organism. A first step is to build quantitative atlases of wild-type gene expression at cellular resolution, starting from the fertilized egg, throughout gastrulation and morphogenesis. Progress toward this goal has been made in *Drosophila* (Fowlkes et al., 2008), *C. elegans* (Dupuy et al., 2007; Hunt-Newbury et al., 2007; Murray et al., 2008), sea-urchin (Davidson et al., 2002; Howard-Ashby et al., 2006; Samanta et al., 2006) and the ascidian, *Ciona intestinalis* (Imai et al., 2006). Among these model organisms, *C. elegans* and *Ciona intestinalis* share the advantage of invariant cell lineages during development (Satoh, 1994; Sulston et al., 1983), which simplifies the acquisition of dynamic gene expression data at cellular resolution. Nevertheless, using a combination of quantitative imaging and image registration, the members of the Berkeley Drosophila Transcription Network Project have reported an atlas of the expression of 95 genes in the fruit fly at nuclear resolution and across six time domains of blastoderm development (Fowlkes et al., 2008; Keranen et al., 2006; Luengo Hendriks et al., 2006). With gene expression atlases to hand, genome-scale perturbation studies must be undertaken to uncover functional relationships between genes, thereby yielding the regulatory gene circuit that gives rise to the observed gene expression atlas.

CONCLUSIONS

Our understanding of the molecular signals that drive developmental patterning is growing at a phenomenal pace. Both the specification cues and the regulatory networks that translate these cues into cell responses are being uncovered in numerous model systems. Mathematical models have proven to be essential tools for analyzing the network of mechanisms that govern the spatiotemporal dynamics of specification cues, the cross-talk among cues and the gene expression program. The challenge, of course, is that none of these individual regulatory layers is solely sufficient to drive developmental patterning. Establishing a morphogen gradient does not guarantee a pattern of gene expression across a field of cells. Meanwhile, a gene regulatory network can adequately describe which genes are turned on or off in a particular cell, but genes do not cross cell borders! Models that integrate the numerous layers of regulatory mechanisms (specification cues, post-translational intracellular networks, gene regulatory networks) will be needed to provide an understanding of how development marches forward in space and time.

The promise of such an integrated model is that one could, in principle, "stitch" together successive rounds of specification, cross-talk and gene expression, so that the emergence of a multicellular organ, tissue or even the entire organism can be simulated. There is a key additional element that will be needed to meet this goal. While molecular signals and networks orchestrate development, it is the cells instructed by these signals that ultimately form the remarkable multicellular patterns and structures associated with development. In most cases, developmental signals (e.g. the expression of a particular gene) have been correlated to a specific cellular fate or behavior and, thus, serve as markers of cell response. A major challenge is to elucidate the mechanistic relation between these molecular developmental markers and cell responses. This insight will foster future mechanistic models (which undoubtedly must account for mechanics as well as biochemistry) that predict, not only the spatiotemporal evolution of developmental signals, but also the cellular rearrangements and turnover as development progresses.

ACKNOWLEDGMENTS

This work was supported by the Institute for Collaborative Biotechnologies Grant DAAD 19-03-D-0004 from the U.S. Army Research Office. C.A.G. was partially supported by the Center for Biological Circuit Design.

References

Anderson, K.V., Ingham, P.W., 2003. The transformation of the model organism: a decade of developmental genetics. Nat. Genet. 33 (Suppl), 285–293.

Arora, K., Nusslein-Volhard, C., 1992. Altered mitotic domains reveal fate map changes in Drosophila embryos mutant for zygotic dorsoventral patterning genes. Development 114, 1003–1024.

Arora, K., Levine, M.S., O'Connor, M.B., 1994. The screw gene encodes a ubiquitously expressed member of the TGF-beta family required for specification of dorsal cell fates in the Drosophila embryo. Genes. Dev. 8, 2588–2601.

Ashe, H.L., Levine, M., 1999. Local inhibition and long-range enhancement of Dpp signal transduction by Sog. Nature 398, 427–431.

Ben-Zvi, D., Shilo, B.Z., Fainsod, A., Barkai, N., 2008. Scaling of the BMP activation gradient in Xenopus embryos. Nature 453, 1205–1211.

Berdnik, D., Török, T., González-Gaitán, M., Knoblich, J.A., 2002. The endocytic protein alpha-Adaptin is required for numb-mediated asymmetric cell division in Drosophila. Dev. Cell. 3, 221–231.

Bergmann, S., Sandler, O., Sberro, H., et al., 2007. Pre-steady-state decoding of the Bicoid morphogen gradient. PLoS Biol. 5, e46.

Casali, A., Struhl, G., 2004. Reading the Hedgehog morphogen gradient by measuring the ratio of bound to unbound Patched protein. Nature 431, 76–180.

Chen, N., Greenwald, I., 2004. The lateral signal for LIN-12/Notch in C. elegans vulval development comprises redundant secreted and transmembrane DSL proteins. Dev. Cell. 6, 183–192.

Chuang, P.T., McMahon, A.P., 1999. Vertebrate Hedgehog signalling modulated by induction of a Hedgehog-binding protein. Nature 397, 617–621.

Crick, F., 1970. Diffusion in embryogenesis. Nature 225, 420–422.

Davidson, E.H., 1993. Later embryogenesis: regulatory circuitry in morphogenetic fields. Development 118, 665–690.

Davidson, E.H., Rast, J.P., Oliveri, P., et al., 2002. A genomic regulatory network for development. Science 295, 1669–1678.

Driever, W., Nusslein-Volhard, C., 1988. The bicoid protein determines position in the Drosophila embryo in a concentration-dependent manner. Cell 54, 95–104.

Dubois, L., Lecourtois, M., Alexandre, C., Hirst, E., Vincent, J.P., 2001. Regulated endocytic routing modulates wingless signaling in Drosophila embryos. Cell 105, 613–624.

Dupuy, D., Bertin, N., Hidalgo, C.A., et al., 2007. Genome-scale analysis of in vivo spatiotemporal promoter activity in Caenorhabditis elegans. Nat. Biotechnol. 25, 663–668.

Eldar, A., Dorfman, R., Weiss, D., Ashe, H., Shilo, B.Z., Barkai, N., 2002. Robustness of the BMP morphogen gradient in Drosophila embryonic patterning. Nature 419, 304–308.

Eldar, A., Rosin, D., Shilo, B.Z., Barkai, N., 2003. Self-enhanced ligand degradation underlies robustness of morphogen gradients. Dev. Cell. 5, 635–646.

Entchev, E.V., Schwabedissen, A., Gonzalez-Gaitan, M., 2000. Gradient formation of the TGF-beta homolog Dpp. Cell 103, 981–991.

Ferguson, E.L., Anderson, K.V., 1992. Decapentaplegic acts as a morphogen to organize dorsal-ventral pattern in the Drosophila embryo. Cell 71, 451–461.

Ferrell Jr., J.E., 1999. Building a cellular switch: more lessons from a good egg. Bioessays 21, 866–870.

Fowlkes, C.C., Hendriks, C.L., Keränen, S.V., et al., 2008. A quantitative spatiotemporal atlas of gene expression in the Drosophila blastoderm. Cell 133, 364–374.

Francois, V., Solloway, M., O'Neill, J.W., Emery, J., Bier, E., 1994. Dorsal-ventral patterning of the Drosophila embryo depends on a putative negative growth factor encoded by the short gastrulation gene. Genes. Dev. 8, 2602–2616.

Gabay, L., Seger, R., Shilo, B.Z., 1997. In situ activation pattern of Drosophila EGF receptor pathway during development. Science 277, 1103–1106.

Giurumescu, C.A., Asthagiri, A.R., 2008. Signal processing during developmental multicellular patterning. Biotechnol. Prog. 24, 80–88.

Giurumescu, C.A., Sternberg, P.W., Asthagiri, A.R., 2006. Intercellular coupling amplifies fate segregation during Caenorhabditis elegans vulval development. Proc. Natl. Acad. Sci. USA. 103, 1331–1336.

Goentoro, L.A., Reeves, G.T., Kowal, C.P., Martinelli, L., Schüpbach, T., Shvartsman, S.Y., 2006. Quantifying the Gurken morphogen gradient in Drosophila oogenesis. Dev. Cell. 11, 263–272.

Gonzalez-Gaitan, M., 2003. Endocytic trafficking during Drosophila development. Mech. Dev. 120, 1265–1282.

Gregor, T., Bialek, W., de Ruyter van Steveninck, R.R., Tank, D.W., ns Wieschaus, E.F., 2005. Diffusion and scaling during early embryonic pattern formation. Proc. Natl. Acad. Sci. USA. 102, 18403–18407.

Gregor, T., Tank, D.W., Wieschaus, E.F., Bialek, W., 2007a. Probing the limits to positional information. Cell 130, 153–164.

Gregor, T., Wieschaus, E.F., McGregor, A.P., Bialek, W., Tank, D.W., 2007b. Stability and nuclear dynamics of the bicoid morphogen gradient. Cell 130, 141–152.

Gurdon, J., Harger, B., Mitchell, P., Lemaire, A., 1994. Activin signalling and response to a morphogen gradient. Nature 371, 487–492.

Hanahan, D., Weinberg, R.A., 2000. The hallmarks of cancer. Cell 100, 57–70.

Helm, C.L., Fleury, M.E., Zisch, A.H., Boschetti, F., Swartz, M.A., 2005. Synergy between interstitial flow and VEGF directs capillary morphogenesis in vitro through a gradient amplification mechanism. Proc. Natl. Acad. Sci. USA. 102, 15779–15784.

Hill, R.J., Sternberg, P.W., 1992. The gene lin-3 encodes an inductive signal for vulval development in C. elegans. Nature 358, 470–476.

Houchmandzadeh, B., Wieschaus, E., Leibler, S., 2002. Establishment of developmental precision and proportions in the early Drosophila embryo. Nature 415, 798–802.

Houchmandzadeh, B., Wieschaus, E., Leibler, S., 2005. Precise domain specification in the developing Drosophila embryo. Phys. Rev. E Stat. Nonlin. Soft Matter Phys. 72, 061920.

Howard-Ashby, M., Materna, S.C., Brown, C.T., et al., 2006. High regulatory gene use in sea urchin embryogenesis: implications for bilaterian development and evolution. Dev. Biol. 300, 27–34.

Hunt-Newbury, R., Viveiros, R., Johnsen, R., et al., 2007. High-throughput in vivo analysis of gene expression in Caenorhabditis elegans. PLoS Biol. 5, e237.

Imai, K.S., Levine, M., Satoh, N., Satou, Y., 2006. Regulatory blueprint for a chordate embryo. Science 312, 1183–1187.

Inoue, T., Wang, M., Ririe, T.O., Fernandes, J.S., Sternberg, P.W., 2005. Transcriptional network underlying Caenorhabditis elegans vulval development. Proc. Natl. Acad. Sci. USA. 102, 4972–4977.

Istrail, S., Davidson, E.H., 2005. Logic functions of the genomic cis-regulatory code. Proc. Natl. Acad. Sci. USA. 102, 4954–4959.

Jaeger, J., Reinitz, J., 2006. On the dynamic nature of positional information. Bioessays 28, 1102–1111.

Jaeger, J., Blagov, M., Kosman, D., et al., 2004a. Dynamical analysis of regulatory interactions in the gap gene system of Drosophila melanogaster. Genetics 167, 1721–1737.

Jaeger, J., Surkova, S., Blagov, M., et al., 2004b. Dynamic control of positional information in the early Drosophila embryo. Nature 430, 368–371.

Jaeger, J., Sharp, D.H., Reinitz, J., 2007. Known maternal gradients are not sufficient for the establishment of gap domains in Drosophila melanogaster. Mech. Dev. 124, 108–128.

Kadesch, T., 2004. Notch signaling: the demise of elegant simplicity. Curr. Opin. Genet. Dev. 14, 506–512.

Keranen, S.V., Fowlkes, C.C., Luengo Hendriks, C.L., et al., 2006. Three-dimensional morphology and gene expression in the Drosophila blastoderm at cellular resolution II: dynamics. Genome. Biol. 7, R124.

Kerszberg, M., Wolpert, L., 1998. Mechanisms for positional signalling by morphogen transport: a theoretical study. J. Theor. Biol. 191, 103–114.

Kicheva, A., Pantazis, P., Bollenbach, T., et al., 2007. Kinetics of morphogen gradient formation. Science 315, 521–525.

Kimble, J., Simpson, P., 1997. The LIN-12/Notch signaling pathway and its regulation. Annu. Rev. Cell Dev. Biol. 13, 333–361.

Koide, T., Hayata, T., Cho, K.W., 2005. Xenopus as a model system to study transcriptional regulatory networks. Proc. Natl. Acad. Sci. USA. 102, 4943–4948.

Kruse, K., Pantazis, P., Bollenbach, T., Jülicher, F., González-Gaitán, M., 2004. Dpp gradient formation by dynamin-dependent endocytosis: receptor trafficking and the diffusion model. Development 131, 4843–4856.

Lai, E.C., 2004. Notch signaling: control of cell communication and cell fate. Development 131, 965–973.

Lander, A.D., Nie, Q., Wan, F.Y., 2002. Do morphogen gradients arise by diffusion?. Dev. Cell. 2, 785–796.

Lauffenburger, D.A., Linderman, J.J., 1993. Receptors: Models for Binding, Trafficking, and Signaling. Oxford University Press, New York p. 365.

Lecuit, T., Brook, W.J., Ng, M., Calleja, M., Sun, H., Cohen, S.M., 1996. Two distinct mechanisms for long-range patterning by Decapentaplegic in the Drosophila wing. Nature 381, 387–393.

Lee, J.R., Urban, S., Garvey, C.F., Freeman, M., 2001. Regulated intracellular ligand transport and proteolysis control EGF signal activation in Drosophila. Cell 107, 161–171.

Levine, M., Davidson, E.H., 2005. Gene regulatory networks for development. Proc. Natl. Acad. Sci. USA. 102, 4936–4942.

Luengo Hendriks, C.L., Keränen, S.V., Fowlkes, C.C., et al., 2006. Three-dimensional morphology and gene expression in the Drosophila blastoderm at cellular resolution I: data acquisition pipeline. Genome. Biol. 7, R123.

Marques, G., Musacchio, M., Shimell, M.J., Wünnenberg-Stapleton, K., Cho, K.W., O'Connor, M.B., 1997. Production of a DPP activity gradient in the early Drosophila embryo through the opposing actions of the SOG and TLD proteins. Cell 91, 417–426.

Mason, E.D., Konrad, K.D., Webb, C.D., Marsh, J.L., 1994. Dorsal midline fate in Drosophila embryos requires twisted gastrulation, a gene encoding a secreted protein related to human connective tissue growth factor. Genes. Dev. 8, 1489–1501.

Mizutani, C.M., Nie, Q., Wan, F.Y., et al., 2005. Formation of the BMP activity gradient in the Drosophila embryo. Dev. Cell. 8, 915–924.

Murray, J.I., Bao, Z., Boyle, T.J., et al., 2008. Automated analysis of embryonic gene expression with cellular resolution in C. elegans. Nat. Methods.

Nellen, D., Burke, R., Struhl, G., Basler, K., 1996. Direct and long-range action of a DPP morphogen gradient. Cell 85, 357–368.

O'Connor, M.B., Umulis, D., Othmer, H.G., Blair, S.S., 2006. Shaping BMP morphogen gradients in the Drosophila embryo and pupal wing. Development 133, 183–193.

Ochoa-Espinosa, A., Yucel, G., Kaplan, L., et al., 2005. The role of binding site cluster strength in Bicoid-dependent patterning in Drosophila. Proc. Natl. Acad. Sci. USA. 102, 4960–4965.

Papatsenko, D., Levine, M., 2005. Computational identification of regulatory DNAs underlying animal development. Nat. Methods 2, 529–534.

Pfeiffer, S., Ricardo, S., Manneville, J.B., Alexandre, C., Vincent, J.P., 2002. Producing cells retain and recycle Wingless in Drosophila embryos. Curr. Biol. 12, 957–962.

Pons, S., Marti, E., 2000. Sonic hedgehog synergizes with the extracellular matrix protein vitronectin to induce spinal motor neuron differentiation. Development 127, 333–342.

Ramirez-Weber, F.A., Kornberg, T.B., 1999. Cytonemes: cellular processes that project to the principal signaling center in Drosophila imaginal discs. Cell 97, 599–607.

Rhyu, M.S., Jan, L.Y., Jan, Y.N., 1994. Asymmetric distribution of numb protein during division of the sensory organ precursor cell confers distinct fates to daughter cells. Cell 76, 477–491.

Saha, K., Schaffer, D.V., 2006. Signal dynamics in Sonic hedgehog tissue patterning. Development 133, 889–900.

Samanta, M.P., Tongprasit, W., Istrail, S., et al., 2006. The transcriptome of the sea urchin embryo. Science 314, 960–962.

Santos, S.D., Ferrell, J.E., 2008. Systems biology: on the cell cycle and its switches. Nature 454, 288–289.

Satoh, N., 1994. Developmental Biology of Ascidians. Cambridge University Press, New York p. 251.

Schlesinger, A., Kiger, A., Perrimon, N., Shilo, B.Z., 2004. Small wing PLCgamma is required for ER retention of cleaved Spitz during eye development in Drosophila. Dev. Cell. 7, 535–545.

Shaye, D.D., Greenwald, I., 2002. Endocytosis-mediated downregulation of LIN-12/Notch upon Ras activation in Caenorhabditis elegans. Nature 420, 686–690.

Sherwood, D.R., Sternberg, P.W., 2003. Anchor cell invasion into the vulval epithelium in C. elegans. Dev. Cell. 5, 21–31.

Shilo, B.Z., 2003. Signaling by the Drosophila epidermal growth factor receptor pathway during development. Exp. Cell Res. 284, 140–149.

Shimmi, O., O'Connor, M.B., 2003. Physical properties of Tld, Sog, Tsg and Dpp protein interactions are predicted to help create a sharp boundary in Bmp signals during dorsoventral patterning of the Drosophila embryo. Development 130, 4673–4682.

Shimmi, O., Umulis, D., Othmer, H., O'Connor, M.B., 2005. Facilitated transport of a Dpp/Scw heterodimer by Sog/Tsg leads to robust patterning of the Drosophila blastoderm embryo. Cell 120, 873–886.

Skeath, J.B., 1998. The Drosophila EGF receptor controls the formation and specification of neuroblasts along the dorsal-ventral axis of the Drosophila embryo. Development 125, 3301–3312.

Srinivasan, S., Rashka, K.E., Bier, E., 2002. Creation of a Sog morphogen gradient in the Drosophila embryo. Dev. Cell. 2, 91–101.

Stathopoulos, A., Levine, M., 2005. Genomic regulatory networks and animal development. Dev. Cell. 9, 449–462.

Strigini, M., Cohen, S.M., 1999. Formation of morphogen gradients in the Drosophila wing. Semin. Cell Dev. Biol. 10, 335–344.

Sulston, J.E., Schierenberg, E., White, J.G., Thomson, J.N., 1983. The embryonic cell lineage of the nematode Caenorhabditis elegans. Dev. Biol. 100, 64–119.

Tabata, T., Kornberg, T.B., 1994. Hedgehog is a signaling protein with a key role in patterning Drosophila imaginal discs. Cell 76, 89–102.

Tabata, T., Takei, Y., 2004. Morphogens, their identification and regulation. Development 131, 703–712.

Teleman, A.A., Cohen, S.M., 2000. Dpp gradient formation in the Drosophila wing imaginal disc. Cell 103, 971–980.

The, I., Bellaiche, Y., Perrimon, N., 1999. Hedgehog movement is regulated through tout velu-dependent synthesis of a heparan sulfate proteoglycan. Mol. Cell. 4, 633–639.

Vincent, J.P., Dubois, L., 2002. Morphogen transport along epithelia, an integrated trafficking problem. Dev. Cell. 3, 615–623.

Wolpert, L., 1969. Positional information and the spatial pattern of cellular differentiation. J. Theor. Biol. 25, 1–47.

Xiong Jr., W., Ferrell, J.E., 2003. A positive-feedback-based bistable 'memory module' that governs a cell fate decision. Nature 426, 460–465.

Yang, J., Winkler, K., Yoshida, M., Kornbluth, S., 1999. Maintenance of G2 arrest in the Xenopus oocyte: a role for 14-3-3-mediated inhibition of Cdc25 nuclear import. EMBO J. 18, 2174–2183.

Yoo, A.S., Bais, C., Greenwald, I., 2004. Crosstalk between the EGFR and LIN-12/Notch pathways in C. elegans vulval development. Science 303, 663–666.

Yuh, C.H., Davidson, E.H., 1996. Modular cis-regulatory organization of Endo16, a gut-specific gene of the sea urchin embryo. Development 122, 1069–1082.

Yuh, C.H., Bolouri, H., Davidson, E.H., 1998. Genomic cis-regulatory logic: experimental and computational analysis of a sea urchin gene. Science 279, 1896–1902.

Yuh, C.H., Bolouri, H., Davidson, E.H., 2001. Cis-regulatory logic in the endo16 gene: switching from a specification to a differentiation mode of control. Development 128, 617–629.

CHAPTER

15

Applications of Immunologic Modeling to Drug Discovery and Development

Daniel L. Young, Saroja Ramanujan and Lisl K.M. Shoda

Entelos, Inc., Foster City

OUTLINE

Summary	352	Immune Cell–Cancer Interactions: Homogenous Single-compartment Models	361
Introduction	352		
Challenges to Drug Discovery and Development in Immune-related Diseases	352	Lymphocyte Trafficking and Tumor Infiltration: Spatial and Multicompartment Models	364
Systems Biology for Drug Discovery and Development	353	Future Work	367
Basic Immunology	354	**Allergic and Autoimmune Diseases**	**367**
Infectious Diseases	**355**	T Cell Vaccination	368
Challenges in Treating Infectious Diseases, Specifically HIV	355	Disease-specific Efficacy of Cytokine Blockade	369
Central Mathematical Model of HIV Infection	356	Evaluation and Prioritization of Drug Targets for Rheumatoid Arthritis	370
Insights into Viral Drug Resistance	358	**Conclusion**	**372**
Optimizing Treatment Administration	358	**Acknowledgements**	**373**
Cancer	**360**		

Summary

The study of immunological diseases is challenged by the diversity and complexity of immune responses to environmental and endogenous stresses. *In vitro* studies have revealed many important insights into immunologic function, but these reductionist approaches do not address many of the interactions integral to understanding dynamic, distributed disease processes. Conversely, although animal models embody integrated disease processes, they are not typically predictive of treatment responses in human patients. Furthermore, some of the mechanisms underlying animal responses can be difficult to study in the laboratory. In this chapter we review the use of mathematical modeling to enhance drug discovery and development for several diseases characterized by dysfunction of the immune system. Examples are drawn from infectious diseases, cancer and allergic and autoimmune diseases—each representative of advantages that immunological modeling brings to the challenges facing drug research in these areas. The chapter highlights insights that immunological modeling can provide throughout the pharmaceutical process, from early-stage drug discovery such as target prioritization, to development efforts aimed at optimizing treatment schedules and personalizing treatment approaches. The use of quantitative models can greatly facilitate the integration and interpretation of data, providing a framework that is much needed, given the current explosion in experimental data, including genomic and proteomic assays. Further, models allow the researcher to simulate biological processes and analyze the consequences of manipulating the underlying biology. Such model-driven analysis and simulation can yield novel insights and testable predictions to guide and improve rational drug research.

INTRODUCTION

Challenges to Drug Discovery and Development in Immune-related Diseases

The course of many human diseases is shaped by immune responses. A complex immunologic system composed of specialized tissues, cells and molecules has evolved to combat the multitude of pathogens encountered in everyday life and to support the maintenance of good health through the removal of dead or mutated cells. Infectious diseases and cancers progress because the immune response fails to clear pathogens or cancerous cells, respectively. As a result, many drug discovery and development efforts in these areas have focused on strategies to directly attack the invasive organisms or cells. Strategies that aim to enhance the immune response could, if successful, treat current disease and provide long-lasting protection against disease recurrence. In contrast to infectious diseases and cancers, allergic and autoimmune diseases occur as a result of a relatively robust immune response to normally innocuous environmental substances (e.g. pollen) or self-tissues (e.g. pancreatic beta cells). In these cases, efforts in drug discovery and development have focused on strategies to suppress the overactive immune response.

Several challenges impede the discovery and development of better treatments for these diseases. First, researchers are still discovering and characterizing fundamental components of the immune response, therefore our understanding of the immune system is akin to a puzzle with pieces missing or not in place. Secondly, specific immune components can serve different roles in different diseases; thus there is a need to understand the interactions occurring in a disease-specific context. Thirdly, insufficient knowledge and tools have limited our ability for selective modulation of the disease-specific immune response without affecting general immune status: for example, attempts to enhance an insufficient immune response carry the risk of immune overactivation and associated toxicity, whereas, conversely, attempts to suppress an immune response can increase the risk of opportunistic infection and compromise wound healing. Fourthly, patient-to-patient variability can limit the effectiveness of treatment strategies. Finally, although drug combination therapies are promising and sometimes effective, the ramifications of new combinations or regimens are difficult to predict and expensive to test. Mathematical modeling of immunologic responses can be used to address each of these challenges, providing researchers with a platform that explicitly defines the biology of interest, enabling systematic investigation and, ultimately, improved experimental design and decision making (Friedrich and Paterson, 2004).

Systems Biology for Drug Discovery and Development

Reductionist approaches that focus on the study of isolated elements of complex systems have flourished recently in the biological sciences as advances in experimental technologies have allowed scientists to explore intracellular and molecular interactions with ever greater detail and efficiency. Although reductionist science has undoubtedly increased our understanding of specific biological functions, the data describing such elemental relationships do not readily explain system-level behaviors that characterize the functions of cells, tissues and organisms. Emergent system-level behaviors of an organism ultimately account for health and disease.

Systems-level approaches have traditionally been used in disciplines such as telecommunications and aerospace, in the pre-emptive investigation of complex non-linear multicomponent networks for emergent behaviors otherwise difficult to anticipate (Von Bertalanffy, 1976). Scientific investigation of biology also has much to gain from quantitative approaches that enable theoretical analysis, modeling and predictive simulation of systems-level interactions. The renowned cyberneticist, Norbert Wiener, pioneered the application of mathematical modeling to the investigation of biological hypotheses (Wiener, 1948). Over time, biological modeling has gained acceptance, particularly in the pharmaceutical sciences, where targeted pharmacokinetic models focused specifically on the absorption and distribution properties of particular drugs have proven valuable in the design of clinical trials.

This chapter reviews several studies in which mathematical modeling has provided insights into the mechanisms and treatment of human immunological diseases. Because of their complexity, human immune responses are ideal candidates for study by systems biology approaches. The studies reviewed here include mathematical models that represent a range of biological complexity—from the spatial and temporal interaction of a few cell types to the interactions of several tissues, cells and molecules. In all cases, these models integrate disparate experimental data into a coherent quantitative framework supporting model validation and hypothesis testing. These systems-level models facilitate drug discovery and development in several ways, including the identification of drug targets and the *in-silico* evaluation of new compounds and treatment regimens (Table 15.1). Analyses of the results of simulations from these models have led to predictions of novel biomarkers of clinical response, in addition to insights

TABLE 15.1 Summary of Systems Biology Applications Reviewed in this Chapter

Applications of Systems Biology to Drug Discovery and Development	Applicable Immunologic Diseases Reviewed in this Chapter
Identifying and prioritizing immunotherapeutic targets	Cancer, RA
Optimizing treatment dose and schedule	Cancer, EAE, HIV, leukemia, RA
Understanding and reducing drug resistance	Cancer, HIV
Enhancing drug delivery	Cancer
Identifying biomarkers of patient response and phenotype	HIV
Assessing impact of treatment (non-)adherence	HIV
Improving personalized treatment approaches	HIV
Evaluating novel compounds and treatments	RA
Determining key drug mechanisms of action	RA

EAE, experimental autoimmune encephalomyelitis; HIV, human immunodeficiency virus; RA, rheumatoid arthritis.

into optimal treatment administration and individualization of patient care. Refinement of these systems-level approaches should continue to improve our understanding of complex immunological systems and enhance our ability to restore and preserve patient health.

Basic Immunology

For better understanding of how immunologic modeling is being applied to drug discovery and development, we first briefly describe some basic concepts and components in immunology. The immune system is characterized by innate and adaptive immunity, both of which contribute to the control of infections. However, whereas innate immune cells respond rapidly to an immunological stimulus but have limited ability to discriminate different stimuli, adaptive immune cells have an extensive repertoire permitting discrimination of different stimuli, but are slower to respond.

The innate immune response occurs when cells such as macrophages and dendritic cells are activated by pattern recognition receptors (PRRs). Resident populations of macrophages and dendritic cells are found at all body surfaces and in various tissues, and serve a surveillance function. The engagement of PRRs by common molecular elements that are found on several pathogens signals macrophages and/or dendritic cells to produce mediators that combat pathogens and recruit other immune cells to the tissue site. Other innate immune cells include natural killer (NK) cells, eosinophils, mast cells and basophils. When activated, these cells may potentiate the inflammation and combat the infection through production of mediators and cell contact mechanisms.

The innate immune response is a potent and critical aspect of immunity, but adaptive immunity generates a more targeted response, in addition to immunological memory. Dendritic cells, in particular, are important cells that bridge innate and adaptive immunity. Dendritic cell surveillance includes sampling the environment and processing acquired materials into small protein segments, called antigens, that are displayed on the dendritic cell surface. These antigens may be recognized by T lymphocytes—cells of the adaptive immune system. Each T lymphocyte expresses a T cell receptor (TCR) recognizing a particular antigen. On encountering its specific antigen presented by a dendritic cell, a T lymphocyte will become activated, proliferate and differentiate, ultimately leading to an antigen-specific immune response. Although dendritic cells primarily encounter antigen in peripheral tissues (e.g. skin), the initial interaction between naïve lymphocytes and antigen-bearing dendritic cells generally occurs in lymphoid tissues (e.g. lymph nodes, spleen), which are specialized to support the priming of an adaptive immune response. $CD4^+$ T lymphocytes (also known as helper T lymphocytes) are critical to the expansion of antigen-specific B lymphocytes that ultimately produce antibodies, and to the expansion of antigen-specific $CD8^+$ T lymphocytes (also known as cytotoxic lymphocytes [CTLs]). Both $CD4^+$ and $CD8^+$ T lymphocytes can exhibit effector activity. Activated $CD4^+$ T lymphocytes may destroy pathogens or cells through the production of pro-inflammatory cytokines or through contact with death-inducing cell surface molecules. Although $CD8^+$ T lymphocytes also produce pro-inflammatory cytokines, they recognize and are activated by their cognate antigen expressed on the target cells, providing a direct and antigen-guided form of killing. Antibodies produced by B cells bind antigens or cells expressing them, marking them for subsequent immune clearance. In addition to effector activity, T and B lymphocyte expansion generates memory cells. Memory T and B lymphocytes are long-lived and enable a faster, more potent recall immune response on secondary encounter with an immunological stimulus. Finally, regulatory T lymphocytes dampen or prevent antigen-specific immune responses, providing a counterbalance to inappropriate or uncontrolled immune responses. Together, the innate and adaptive immune responses are generally sufficient to maintain human health. However, failures in these responses are implicated in many diseases (e.g. infectious disease, cancer, allergy and autoimmunity).

INFECTIOUS DISEASES

Challenges in Treating Infectious Diseases, Specifically HIV

Several groups have applied modeling approaches to study the dynamics and immune responses associated with persistent infections, such as bacterial infections, hepatitis C virus (HCV), hepatitis B virus (HBV), and human immunodeficiency virus (HIV). These approaches have successfully integrated a wealth of experimental data within mathematical models to gain insights that can be experimentally validated and to guide future drug development and treatment decisions. To illustrate the value of these approaches, this section focuses specifically on several investigations of HIV.

HIV is a retrovirus transmitted as an enveloped RNA virus. Upon infection of the target cell, reverse transcriptase converts HIV RNA to DNA. Viral DNA is integrated into the DNA of the infected cell by a virally encoded integrase, allowing the viral genome to be transcribed. After infecting the target cell, either the virus becomes latent and the infected cell continues normal function, or the virus becomes active and replicates, causing a large number of infectious virions to be released from the infected cell. HIV infects primarily naïve and memory $CD4^+$ T lymphocytes, monocytes, macrophages and dendritic cells. Over time, infection leads to diminished $CD4^+$ T lymphocyte numbers by direct and indirect induction of infected cell death. Infected $CD4^+$ T lymphocytes are also killed by cytotoxic $CD8^+$ T lymphocytes specific for HIV antigens. The progressive loss of $CD4^+$ T cells, a hallmark of acquired immunodeficiency syndrome (AIDS), renders the infected individual unable to combat secondary infections and disease. HIV has been shown to establish latent infections in resting memory $CD4^+$ T lymphocytes, monocytes and macrophages (Chun et al., 1997). These leukocytes harbor the latent infectious HIV for decades, making complete eradication of the virus difficult and increasing the risk of viral rebound even after prolonged viral suppression.

Despite discovery of the HIV virus more than 25 years ago, numerous uncertainties remain regarding the best treatment options for managing this pandemic disease. As HIV is likely to remain one of the most common chronic infectious diseases for many decades, there continues to be an urgent need to apply laboratory, clinical and systems biology approaches to gain better understanding of the disease process. Current research is focused on several aspects of HIV infection, including methods to avoid or reduce drug resistance, to identify the best drug combinations for specific types of patient, and to optimize treatment regimens according to patient symptoms and treatment history.

Currently, three classes of antiretroviral drugs approved by the US Food and Drug Administration (FDA) target different stages of the viral lifecycle. Of these, the most commonly administered antiretroviral drug classes include the nucleoside/nucleotide or non-nucleoside reverse transcriptase inhibitors that block infection of target cells by free viral particles, and the protease inhibitors that cause infected cells to produce immature and therefore non-infectious virions. More recently developed, the third class of antiretroviral drugs acts by inhibiting viral entry into a cell. Highly active antiretroviral therapy (HAART)—the combined administration of one protease inhibitor and one or more reverse transcriptase inhibitors—has been very successful in suppressing HIV in treatment-naïve patients. Approximately 90% of treatment-naïve patients achieve significant virologic benefit (i.e., plasma HIV RNA concentrations maintained below the limit of detection) at or beyond 48 weeks of treatment (Gallant et al., 2006).

Despite the favorable responses seen in treatment-naïve patients, drug treatment fails in 40–60% of treatment-experienced patients during the first year of a new regimen (Struble et al., 2005). Moreover, certain classes of patient, such as children, pregnant women and the elderly, require individualized treatment regimens to achieve efficacy while limiting side-effects. Virologic failure (i.e., detectable concentrations of plasma HIV RNA) in patients may arise as a result of a variety of host and viral factors (Deeks, 2003), complicating treatment recommendations and trial design. To enhance patient outcomes, mathematical models of HIV have been used to investigate methods to improve the efficacy of treatment protocols, limit side-effects by reducing treatment durations, improve drug absorption properties and prevent the emergence of drug-resistant virus.

Central Mathematical Model of HIV Infection

For more than 15 years, mathematical models of HIV dynamics have been used to gain insights into the disease process and to investigate therapeutic approaches (reviewed by Perelson, 2002). Early insights into the turnover and lifespan of HIV were gained from mathematical models that represented fundamental features of the disease process (Perelson et al., 1996). The model (Fig. 15.1) adopted by many investigators represents the dynamics of both uninfected and productively infected target cells (T_u and T_i, respectively), and of infectious and non-infectious viral particles in the plasma (V_i and V_n, respectively) in the following non-linear system of ordinary differential equations:

$$\frac{dT_u}{dt} = \lambda - (1-\varepsilon)kV_iT_u - dT_u$$

$$\frac{dT_i}{dt} = (1-\varepsilon)kV_iT_u - \delta T_i$$

$$\frac{dV_i}{dt} = (1-\eta)N\delta T_i - cV_i$$

$$\frac{dV_n}{dt} = \eta N\delta T_i - cV_n \qquad (15.1)$$

where λ represents the rate of production of uninfected target cells (cells/day), k is the rate

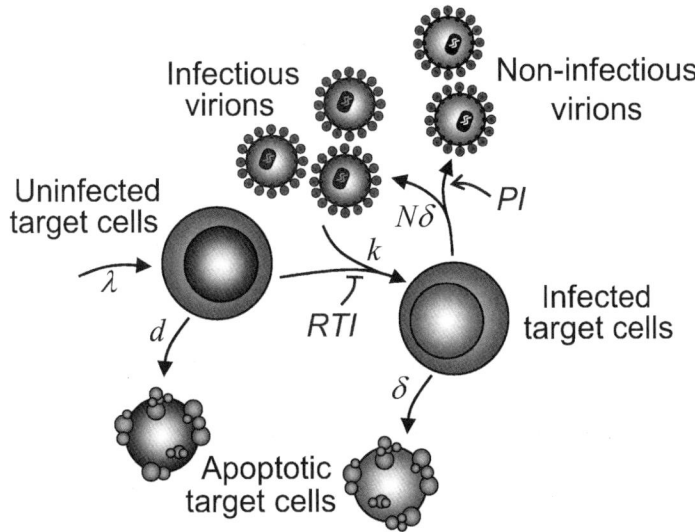

FIGURE 15.1 Biological Components Represented in a Mathematical Model of HIV Infection. Uninfected targets cells, produced at a constant rate by the host, are targeted by infectious virions at a rate that can be inhibited by reverse transcriptase inhibitor (RTI) treatment. Infected targets cells yield both infectious and non-infectious virions, the latter enhanced by protease inhibitors (PI). Both populations of target cells apoptose at different rates. (See text for details/definitions of model parameters and model behaviors).

constant for target cell infection per infectious virion (virion^{-1}days^{-1}), d and δ are the rate constants describing the loss of uninfected and infected target cells, respectively (both, days^{-1}), N is the number of new virions produced per infected cell during its lifespan (virions/cell), and c is the rate constant describing the clearance of virions from the plasma (days^{-1}). Pretreatment, reverse transcriptase inhibitor and protease inhibitor treatment conditions are modeled by the appropriate specification of the parameters ε ($0 < \varepsilon < 1$) and η ($0 < \eta < 1$). The pretreatment condition is represented by $\varepsilon = \eta = 0$, where the rate of target cell infection is maximal and all virions produced are assumed infectious. The effect of reverse transcriptase inhibitor or protease inhibitor treatment is represented by $\varepsilon > 0$ or $\eta > 0$, respectively, where complete block of target cell infection or complete inhibition of infectious virion production occurs when $\varepsilon = 1$ or $\eta = 1$. Sustained viral infection or viral clearance in the absence of treatment can be predicted by the basic reproductive ratio, Ro ($Ro = k\lambda N/dc$) (Nowak and Bangham, 1996). This ratio describes the number of newly infected cells resulting from one infected cell at the time of initial host infection. If $Ro < 1$, the virus is cleared; however, when $Ro > 1$, the virus will replicate and expand in number until a steady-state infection is reached, in which the rate of viral replication is balanced by the rate of viral loss.

Analysis of this mathematical model of HIV dynamics led to several important insights regarding treatment strategies. Perelson et al. (1996) estimated parameter values describing the disease process by using non-linear least-squares fitting utilizing human HIV viral load data from five infected individuals after administration of a protease inhibitor. Infected cells were estimated to have an average lifespan ($1/\delta$) of 2.2 ± 0.8 days, whereas plasma virions were estimated to have an average lifespan ($1/c$) of 0.3 ± 0.1 days. This estimated rate of viral clearance suggested that effective and non-effective treatments could be differentiated by measuring the plasma viral load after only a few days of treatment. These early indicators of treatment efficacy could be used to adjust treatment dose and/or regimen in a clinical trial and/or in the clinic.

Insights into Viral Drug Resistance

The emergence of resistant viruses resulting from genetic mutation is one of the major factors leading to the loss of treatment efficacy (Coffin, 1995). The expected emergence rate of viral resistance is dependent in part on the viral replication rate, the frequency of genetic mutations, and the ability of the virus to function despite the presence of multiple mutations. It was previously estimated that genetic mutation occurs at every base pair in the HIV genome every day in an infected individual (Coffin, 1995). From analysis of the model shown in Equation (15.1) and patient data, Perelson et al. (1996) estimated that the average rate of production of HIV was 10.3×10^9 virions per day, about 15 times greater than other estimates at the time of their investigation. To limit the emergence of drug resistance from mutation at this high rate of replication, and assuming that the virions continue to function despite mutations, these findings highlighted the need to treat HIV-infected patients with a combination of drugs from several antiretroviral classes and/or design novel drugs not affected by any single point mutation. Additional modeling studies have since demonstrated the capability of the virus to escape from the selective pressures associated with treatment and host immunity (reviewed by Nowak and May, 2000).

Poor adherence to treatment regimens is another factor believed to contribute to viral drug resistance. Several modeling studies have investigated the role of non-adherence in the treatment of patients infected with HIV. Using an impulse differential equation model in which the mutant viral strain is assumed to be susceptible only to high drug concentrations whereas the wild-type strain responds to both intermediate and high drug concentrations, it was predicted that drug resistance could arise in response to intermediate and high net exposures to drug, whereas the risk was lower at low net exposure to drug (Smith and Wahl, 2005). The findings of this study suggested that an optimal treatment response could be achieved with dosages and regimens that permit a sufficiently high drug exposure to eliminate both mutant and wild-type viral strains. Intermediate levels of drug exposure that could result from non-adherance present the greatest risk of resistance. Utilizing a model of wild-type and drug-resistant virus in combination with a pharmacokinetic model that included blood and cellular compartments, Rong et al. (2007) showed that intermediate, but not low or high, levels of adherence may result in the dominance of the drug-resistant virus several months after the initiation of treatment. Interestingly, not only is the level of adherence important, but the pattern of adherence also can influence treatment efficacy. Specifically, when the number of consecutive doses missed increases, but the total fraction of missed doses remains constant, the average drug efficacy is predicted to decline (Rong et al., 2007). These mathematical studies provide insights into the interplay between treatment adherence and drug resistance and could lead to new methods to detect patients at greatest risk for virologic failure, based on their viral load and host immune characteristics. Moreover, such insights can help guide the selection of candidate compounds and trial design by optimizing drug pharmacokinetics and treatment regimens to maximize net exposure to the drug.

Optimizing Treatment Administration

Long-term continuous HAART can lead to numerous adverse side-effects, making lifelong treatment with current antiretroviral drugs infeasible (Flexner, 2007). Accordingly, temporary breaks from continuous treatment, known as scheduled treatment interruptions (STIs), have been investigated in the clinic setting (Altfeld and Walker, 2001). Although they remain controversial because of the risk of viral rebound or the emergence of drug resistance, STIs also hold the promise of delaying disease progression by boosting HIV-specific immune responses. Accordingly, recent modeling efforts have focused on identifying patients likely to benefit from STIs and the optimal STI regimens for these patients.

To identify factors that could influence the clinical outcomes of STIs, a mathematical model was developed that includes cell and viral dynamics in the blood and representative lymphoid tissue (Bajaria et al., 2002, 2004). This model was validated by comparing the simulated outcomes of different STI protocols with the data from clinical studies. Subsequently, simulation results predicted that patients with a significant delay in viral return would be better candidates for STIs, supporting the hypothesis that measures of viral load and $CD4^+$ T lymphocyte counts during the first treatment interruption can reveal a patient's immune status, whereas the degree of viral suppression during treatment is not predictive of the effectiveness of an STI. Additional simulations predicted that greater than 40% inhibition of viral infection and production rates is required during a 1-month STI in order for the viral load to remain below the limit of detection. However, simulations also predicted that short-term viral suppression during an STI does not guarantee long-term clinical benefit (Bajaria et al., 2004). If confirmed in clinical studies, these modeling insights could be used to guide the selection of patients most likely to benefit from STI, according to their viral and $CD4^+$ T cell profiles.

In addition to reducing side-effects, STIs may also serve to boost HIV-specific immunity by boosting the sustained $CD8^+$ T cell memory response, possibly resulting in long-term suppression of HIV infection without continuous treatment (Wodarz and Nowak, 1999). For instance, STIs designed to induce a sustained $CD8^+$ T lymphocyte response could help control HIV infection during subsequent STIs by promoting infected cell lysis and preventing viral replication. Wodarz and Nowak (1999) used a mathematical model to study the $CD8^+$ T lymphocyte response. Simulation results predicted that treatment separated by a drug holiday induces an efficient memory $CD8^+$ T lymphocyte response that is long-lived in the absence of viral antigen. These modeling results confirmed earlier suggestions by other investigators regarding the possibility of inducing a sustained memory response against the virus (reviewed by Altfeld and Walker 2001). In confirmation of these modeling predictions, non-human primate studies (Lifson et al., 2000; Lori et al., 2001) demonstrated that sustained viral control can be achieved by a robust memory $CD8^+$ T cell response, and that STIs can help suppress viral rebound. Moreover, clinical studies have demonstrated that STIs applied during the acute phase of the disease can boost viral-specific immunity (Rosenberg et al., 2000). The mixed results reported to date in additional clinical studies of STIs may be attributable to differences in the disease stage at which treatment is initiated, heterogeneity of host immunity and differences in the duration of treatment interruption (Bajaria et al., 2004).

Significant host and viral heterogeneity argue for personalized treatment approaches to manage HIV infection. Successful personalization would be greatly facilitated by a systems-level approach that can quantitatively integrate several data sources to identify biomarkers for guiding treatment decisions. An elegant study by Wu et al. (2005) utilized a model of long-term HIV dynamics and considered uncertainties in drug potency, drug exposure/adherence and drug resistance to study patient and viral diversity. Individualized model parameters for each patient were estimated using a hierarchic Bayesian model allowing individual patient records to be combined optimally with population-level data. Interestingly, a large interindividual variation was found for dynamic parameter estimates describing patient and viral characteristics. The model allowed individualized patient assessments in order to determine if a given antiretroviral regimen would be able to suppress viral replication in that patient. Moreover, improved treatment regimens optimizing dosage and time of initiation could be recommended on the basis of the patient's baseline viral loads and $CD4^+$ T cell counts. This systematic, quantitative approach that captures the impact of patient-specific diversity on treatment outcomes could improve the administration of personalized care to patients with HIV.

CANCER

Cancers typically arise from mutations that disrupt control of differentiation, maturation and growth in host cells, yielding extensive proliferation and inadequate cell death. To sustain this imbalance and perpetuate growth, the tumor must evade the host immune system's cytotoxic control mechanisms. Unlike infection, in which the goal of the host immune system and of treatment is to eradicate a foreign invader, in cancer the goal is to control a self-derived aggressor. This situation poses a distinct challenge: how to recognize and attack the tumor cells without causing significant damage to other host cells. Various researchers have studied the interaction between the immune system and tumors, hoping to enhance immune function to achieve control or eradication of the tumor. These efforts have led to different approaches to cancer immunotherapy involving administration of cytokines (e.g. interleukin [IL]-2, IL-12, granulocyte macrophage-colony stimulating factor, tumor necrosis factor [TNF]α), vaccines based on antigens or dendritic cells, or other immune cells (T cells, NK cells), all designed to boost antitumor responses of the host. Phase I–III clinical trials are in progress in various types of cancer, including prostate, breast, colon, ovarian, melanoma, leukemia and lymphoma (*see* Internet Resources). However, as yet, no therapy has advanced to the market and, only recently, application for approval of a dendritic-cell-based vaccination for prostate cancer treatment (Provenge®) was rejected by the FDA. As with any novel approach, many challenges to clinical success and approval exist, including regimen determination, scale-up from rodent models and biomarker identification. Approaches based on mathematical modeling may prove valuable in guiding these efforts via quantitative integration and interrogation of therapeutic impact, ultimately enabling clinical researchers, pharmaceutical companies and healthcare organizations to optimize therapeutic strategies to maximize efficacy in heterogeneous populations of patients.

Most commonly, models of tumor immunology have examined tumor, immune cell and cytokine interactions assuming a well mixed single compartment, using ordinary differential equation (ODE) formulations. Other modeling approaches have considered immune cell delivery to and infiltration and control of solid tumors using multicompartment ODE, partial differential equation (PDE), and cellular automata models. Finally, a growing literature has focused specifically on cancers of immune cells themselves, specifically leukemias and lymphomas. In this section, we discuss illustrative examples of the first two approaches to modeling immune cell–tumor interactions, focusing on the general approach and the nature of the insight they can offer into therapeutic avenues in oncology. Because much of the modeling work in leukemia has focused on stem cell dynamics and differentiation, as opposed to immunologic interactions, we refer the reader to a recent review of modeling in chronic myelogenous leukemia by Roeder and Glauche (2007).

Immune Cell–Cancer Interactions: Homogenous Single-compartment Models

The majority of mathematical modeling efforts in tumor immunology have focused on characterizing the relationship between the immune system and the tumor, using ODEs to track cell populations and assuming homogenous distribution in a single "well mixed" tissue compartment. Simplistically, the tumor–immune interaction models includ: (i) tumor growth, (ii) generation (recruitment or activation) of immune effectors by the tumor cells, typically as a result of indirect mechanisms driven by antigens on the latter, (iii) expansion of the effector population by cytokines such as IL-2 and (iv) the killing of cancer cells by the immune effectors (Fig. 15.2).

These mechanisms are illustrated, for example, in a much cited model of minimal tumor–immune interaction developed by Kirschner and Panetta (1998). The model represents the dynamics of cancer cells (C), cytotoxic immune effectors such as NK or CTL cells (E), and the cytokine IL-2 (L) as the three state variables in the ODE model:

$$\frac{dE}{dt} = cC - u_2 E + \frac{p_1 L}{g_1 + L} E + s_1$$

$$\frac{dC}{dt} = r_2(1 - bC)C - \frac{aC}{g_2 + C} E \qquad (15.2)$$

$$\frac{d(L)}{dt} = \frac{p_2 C}{g_3 + C} E - u_3 L + s_2$$

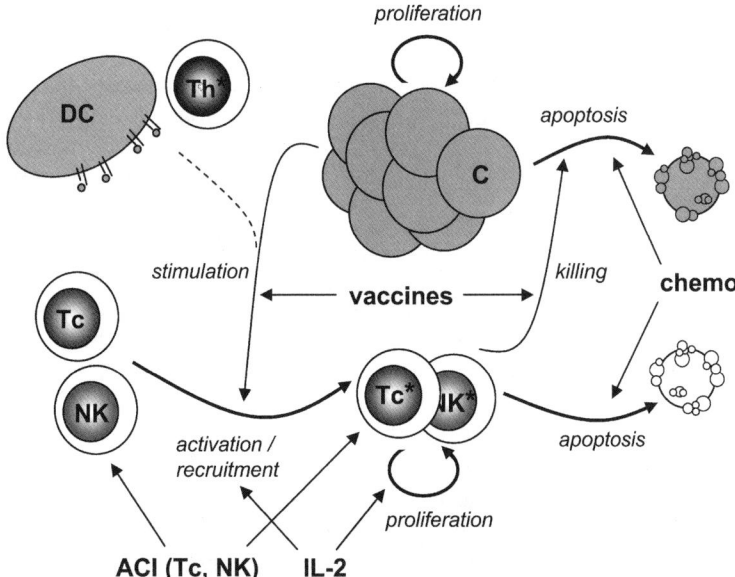

FIGURE 15.2 Biological Components and Mechanisms Represented in Typical Mathematical Models of Tumor–Immune Interactions.
Cytotoxic NK cells and cytotoxic lymphocytes (Tc) are recruited and activated (denoted by *) in response to stimulatory signals from the tumor (C) that can involve the participation of dendritic cells (DC) and CD4[+] helper T cells (Th). Both tumor and cytotoxic cells proliferate and die, with cytotoxic cells actively contributing to killing the tumor cell. Therapies modeled include *chemotherapy* (chemo), which differentially kills both cancer and immune cells, *vaccination* (vaccines), in which antigen (possibly administered using loaded dendritic cells) enhances lymphocyte recruitment/activation and killing potency, *adoptive cellular immunotherapy* (ACI), in which NK and Tc cells are directly administered to the patient, and *interleukin-2 administration* (IL-2), which enhances cytotoxic cell recruitment/activation and proliferation.

Mathematical aspects of this model that are representative of this class of model include:

- Logistic formulation of the tumor growth term, $r_2(1 - bC)C$, describing growth towards an asymptotic tumor size (r_2) known as the "carrying capacity."
- First-order terms for natural death (u_2E) and degradation (u_3L)
- Michaelis–Menten formulation of the cross-regulation terms such as cytokine-stimulated effector cell proliferation: $p_1LE/(g_1 + L)$; tumor-stimulated effector cell killing of cancer cells: $aCE/(g_2 + C)$; tumor-stimulated effector cell secretion of cytokine: $p_2CE/(g_3 + C)$.
- Source terms for cell or cytokine immunotherapy (s_1, s_2)
- Phenomenological representation of complex immunologic functions such as the first-order tumor-induced lymphocyte recruitment, cC, which may actually proceed via a sequence of steps involving several cells and mechanisms.

Even this simple formulation and scope generates complex behaviors. Equation (15.2) results in a cyclic tumor load, with amplitude and periodicity inversely related to tumor antigenicity (c), until, at very high antigenicity, the system sustains a small persistent (i.e., dormant) tumor. Although tumor dormancy is a known phenomenon and periodic recurrence has been observed in certain clinical situations, oscillations may also indicate a need for representing additional mechanisms (immunosuppression or memory, for instance) that influence system dynamics. NK cells, CTLs and IL-2 have received much attention, but $CD4^+$ T lymphocytes and dendritic cells contribute to the antigen-mediated activation and expansion of cytotoxic cells, and additional cytokines and chemokines expressed by these and other cells, including macrophages, stimulate or inhibit the activation and recruitment of cytotoxic cells. Other models have explicitly represented state variables for additional cells and cytokines (De Boer et al., 1985), or have used differential equation models that explicitly address time delays (DeConde et al., 2005; Nani and Oguztoreli, 1994). The solution space of the ODE models has typically been analyzed using stability and bifurcation analyses to characterize outcome regimens that include tumor eradication, dormancy, progression and oscillation. Simulation of immunotherapy is implemented as increased preactivated immune cell populations as a result of adoptive transfer (for cell infusion), increased cytokine concentrations or modification of associated parameters (for cytokine administration), or modifications in efficiency of cell recruitment/activation and immune cell killing of tumor cells (vaccination). Therapeutic protocols can then be investigated or optimized using optimal control approaches in which the magnitude and timing of treatment administration are determined to minimize a cost function, such as the cumulative tumor load during the observation time (Cappuccio et al., 2007; Nanda et al., 2007). For the Kirschner–Panetta model, for example, an investigation of optimal control indicated that combined immunotherapy of IL-2 and CTL was most effective at reducing the tumor burden, and that CTL monotherapy was more effective than IL-2 monotherapy because of the slower loss of administered CTLs compared with that of IL-2. For the oscillatory tumors described by the model, the protocols prescribed dosing at peak tumor mass—although, interestingly, dose itself was not correlated to the magnitude of the tumor peaks. These studies show how combining a mathematical model of immune–tumor interactions with optimal control analysis can be used to evaluate and optimize therapeutic regimens including both the time of administration and the dose of the drug(s).

Two studies have used local ODE models to analyze patient outcomes in clinical trials and to investigate criteria for successful therapy. De Pillis et al. (2006) presented a model of tumor–immune interactions that included CTLs and NK cells and considered cellular and cytokine immunotherapy, vaccine therapy, chemotherapy and combinations thereof (Fig. 15.2). In addition to stability and bifurcation analysis, the authors used specific animal and patient data to generate different parametric solutions, reproduce observed results and make predictions. For one parameterization presented, they showed that the zero-tumor state represents an unstable equilibrium, whereas a high-tumor equilibrium was stable. In such a case, stable elimination of a large tumor would require fundamental changes to system parameters corresponding to, for example, rates of turnover of tumor cells and immune activity. In addition, the authors compared the abilities of chemotherapy, immunotherapy and combined therapy to control tumors of different sizes. After recapitulating successful responses of two patients with metastatic melanoma to combined administration of IL-2 and lymphocyte, they assessed the impact of immune strength and initial tumor size on outcome and predicted (i) the need for combined chemo- plus immunotherapy for larger tumors and (ii) differences between the two patients in threshold tumor size at which combined therapy becomes necessary. The modeling of both chemotherapy and immunotherapy, including complementary (tumor-cytotoxic) and antagonistic (immune-boosting compared with immunotoxic) interactions, is particularly relevant, given that immunotherapy and chemotherapy are frequently combined in clinical trials. The explicit representation of the therapies with some basic associated pharmacokinetics also links the model more closely to the preclinical and clinical settings. Finally, this model was used to investigate individual patient behavior and highlight the fact that outcome is highly dependent on patient-specific parameters, emphasizing the need for customizing treatment protocols on the basis of patient-specific measurements.

Kronik et al. (2008) used a mathematical model to analyze clinical trials of intratumoral delivery of activated CTL for treatment of glioma brain tumors. In addition to cancer cells and CTLs, this model also explicitly considered major histocompatibility complex (MHC) class I and class II molecules used by tumor- and antigen-presenting cells to engage T cells, in addition to the immunogenic and immunosuppressive cytokines interferon (IFN)-γ and transforming growth factor-β (TGFβ) respectively. Specifically, as modeled: MHC class I (MHCI) molecules expressed on the tumor promote CTL activity and thereby killing efficiency; MHC class II (MHCII) levels (on antigen-presenting cells) promote general immune activity and, thereby, CTL recruitment to the tumor; IFN-γ produced by activated CTLs stimulates expression of MHC molecules; TGFβ, present in the central nervous system and augmented by cancer cells, inhibits MHCII production and also suppresses CTL recruitment and activation/killing efficiency. The authors validated their model by recapitulating successful outcomes against grade III malignant gliomas of anaplastic oligodendrioglioma and astrocytoma, and failed outcomes for comparative lower dosing in two patients with glioblastoma multiformae. Subsequently, they used the model to analyze different hypotheses of delayed failure in another patient with malignant glioma and to suggest alternative successful protocols. Finally, they explored the cause for failure and improved protocols for glioblastoma multiformae. Simulation results suggest that the trial failed because of inadequate dosing (20-fold below the concentrations needed). However, successful outcome is predicted for two alternate dose-intensive protocols with more frequent, numerous administrations and/or greater dose per administration, depending on tumor size (Table 15.2). This study is a clear example of how even relatively simple modeling (six coupled ODEs) might guide optimization of trial design and determination of patient-based protocols by offering specific recommendations on treatment

TABLE 15.2 Validation of Glioma Cytotoxic Lymphocyte Immunotherapy Model and Recommendations for Improving Failed Results (Kronik et al. 2007)

Tumor[1]	Dose/Regimen[2]	Clinical Result	Model Assumption[3]	Model Result
Grade III MG	[3 × (3e8 aCTL q5d) + 45d rest] × 5	Successful	1e10 cells	Eradication
Refractory Grade III MG	[3 × (3e8 aCTL q5d) + 45d rest] × 5	Failed	8e10 cells or weaker CTL	Failure
	[3 × (5e8 aCTL q5d) + 45d rest] × 5	(Not tested)	8e10 cells	Eradication
	[3 × (2e9 aCTL q5d) + 45d rest] × 5	(Not tested)	1e10 cells, weaker CTL	Eradication
	[15 × (3e8 aCTL q1d) + 45d rest] × 5			
GBM	[2 × (3e8 aCTL q7d) + 45d rest] × 2	Failed	1e10 cells or 8e10 cells	Failure
	[3 × (3e8 aCTL q5d) + 45d rest] × 5	(Not tested for GBM)	1e10 cells or 8e10 cells	Failure
	[15 × (3e8 aCTL q1d) + 45d rest] × 6	(Not tested)	8e10 cells	Eradication
	[3 × (2e9 aCTL q5d) + 45d rest] × 5			
	[4 × (3e8 aCTL q4d) + 45d rest] × 5	(Not tested)	1e10 cells	Eradication

aCTL, activated cytotoxic lymphocyte; GBM, glioblastoma multiformae; MG, malignant glioma.
[1]Clinical tumor type/grade.
[2]Notation described by Kronik et al. 2008. For example, "[3 × (3e8 aCTL q5d) + 45d rest] × 5" represents: 3 consecutive doses of 3e8 activated CTL given every fifth day, followed by 45 days rest, with this entire sequence repeated 5 times. Multiple protocols may be listed if the outcome was the same.
[3]Assumed tumor cellularity at treatment initiation and any assumptions diverging from baseline parameterization.

dose and timing, and identifying patient characteristics that would necessitate more aggressive protocols.

Lymphocyte Trafficking and Tumor Infiltration: Spatial and Multicompartment Models

The models discussed above treat the interaction of tumor and immune cells as occurring in a well mixed compartment. Thus the spatial effects of the distribution of immune cells compared with that of tumor cells, or issues hampering efficient delivery of adoptively transferred cells, were not addressed. However, infiltration of solid tumors by leukocytes is heterogeneous and, furthermore, the efficient delivery of adoptively transferred leukocytes to the tumor-bearing tissue and into the tumor itself is a considerable challenge in cellular immunotherapy.

Matzavinos and Chaplain (2004) and Matzavinos et al. (2004) developed a PDE model of lymphocyte infiltration into immunogenic preangiogenic tumors and reproduced the phenomenon of dormancy, corresponding to irregular distributions of relatively few cancerous cells amidst immune cell infiltration, and the phenomenon of progression, corresponding to traveling wave solutions of a representative model subsystem in which the tumor cells invade the surrounding host tissue. Mallet and De Pillis (2006) used a hybrid cellular automaton–PDE model to address both spatial heterogeneity and stochastic effects. Distribution of nutrients necessary for proliferation and survival were modeled by classic reaction–diffusion equations under quasi-steady-state assumptions. Tumor and immune cell (CTL and NK) occupancy of a two-dimensional rectangular spatial grid evolved from a single mutated tumor cell according to rules for proliferation, death or migration in response to nutrient and cell profiles. This approach yielded oscillatory behaviors, with T cell recruitment and death determining the stability of oscillations, yielding complete tumor destruction in some cases. Models such as these reiterate the critical role of leukocyte delivery to and penetration of the tumor in tumor control and immunotherapy—mechanisms not addressed in the "well mixed" ODE models.

Focusing upstream on the trafficking of circulating leukocytes to the tumor tissue, Melder et al. (2002) and Zhu et al. (1996) developed a physiologically based kinetic model of the biodistribution of circulating cells, and subsequently used the model to help analyze the distribution of adoptively transferred labeled lymphocytes *in vivo*. Their model considers a physiologically connected and parameterized network of major organs involved in lymphocyte traffic in a tumor-bearing animal, and uses ODEs to model the dynamics of leukocyte distribution among different tissues (including the tumor), on the basis of vascular flow, adhesion, arrest, tissue extravasation and lymphatic drainage of the cells (Fig. 15.3). The model consists of 45 ODEs comprising cellular material balances in the blood and in the vasculature (separate balances for free, adhered and arrested cells) and extravascular space of each tissue, and includes volumetric flow balances on lymph and blood. Data from rodent and human were used in conjunction with scaling approaches, to estimate parameters and to translate them to make predictions in different species, including mouse, rat and human. Results indicated that tumor infiltration was a function of lymphocyte migration rate and tumor site and size. Furthermore, simulations indicated that poor localization reflected entrapment in other tissues, especially the lung (Zhu et al., 1996). Subsequent laboratory experiments, in which lymphocytes were administered to mice with mammary tumors implanted in their legs, were simulated (Melder et al., 2002). The model successfully predicted the kinetics of cell distribution among organs in both splenectomized and non-splenectomized mice. Predictions captured initial lymphocyte partitioning to the lungs and subsequent redistribution to the liver and spleen. Predictions also captured the minimal increase in accumulation in the tumor but increased retention in the liver as a result of splenectomy. Finally, the accuracy of the predictions, which did not include any preferential migration of tumor-specific compared with non-specific cells, supported the accompanying experimental suggestion that both sets of lymphocytes partitioned similarly during the week after administration. The authors thus suggested that non-antigen-specific adhesive interactions between administered lymphocytes and the tumor vasculature pose a limiting step to lymphocyte infiltration of the tumors. Thus model predictions, confirmed by experimental results, identify lymphocyte–vascular interactions as an important area of focus for successful adoptive cellular immunotherapy, with the model allowing rapid evaluation of how interventions (in this case splenectomy) may modulate biodistribution. This finding is particularly interesting, given the continuing interest in immunotherapy of tumors of the brain, where the vascular

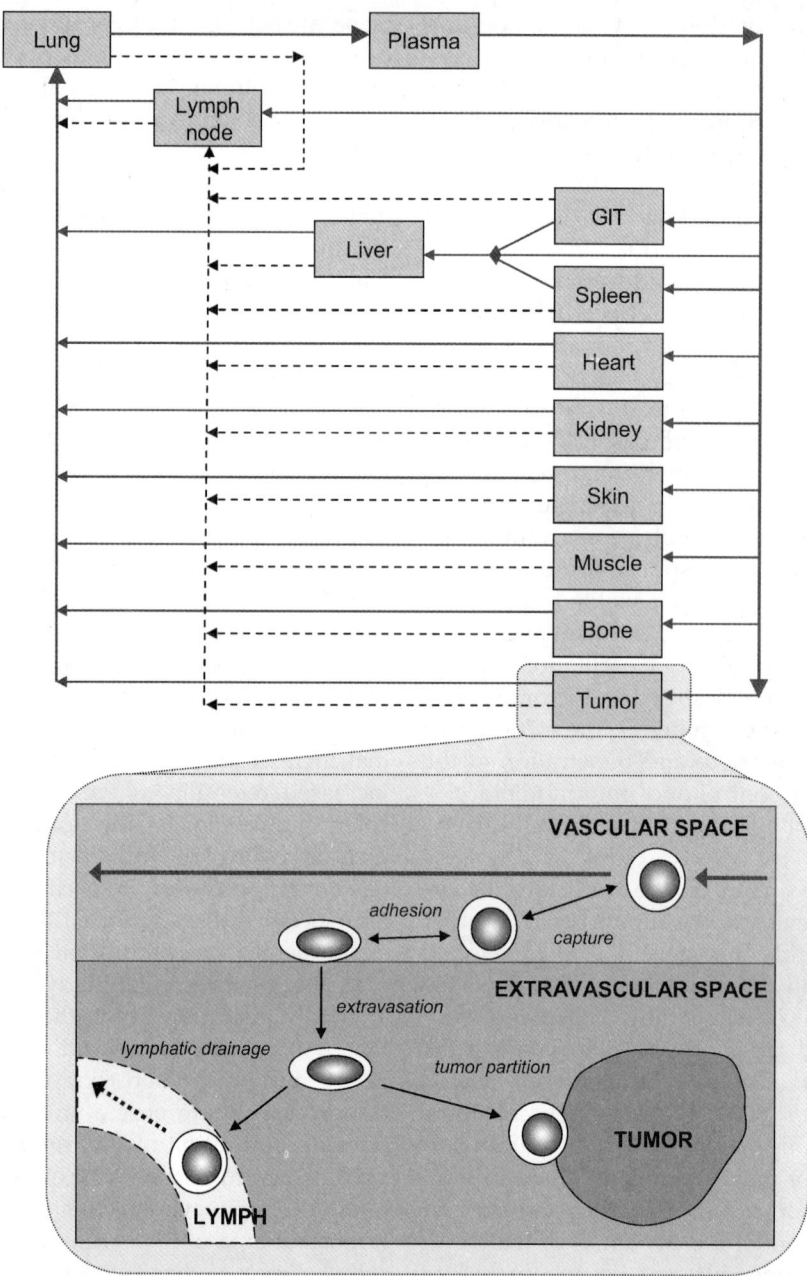

FIGURE 15.3 Schematic Diagram of Pharmacologic Kinetic Model of Lymphocyte Biodistribution in a Tumor-bearing Animal.
Solid red arrows indicate blood flow and dashed blue arrows indicate lymph flow. Within each organ, vascular and extravascular spaces are treated separately, with lymphocyte migration modeled via a cascade of steps involving initial capture by tissue vasculature, firm adhesion to teh endothelium and extravasation into the tissue space. GIT, gastrointestinal tract.
Adapted from Zhu et al. (1996), with permission.

blood–brain barrier poses a major impediment to cellular and molecular infiltration.

Future Work

The specific examples discussed focused on lymphocyte administration or activation via cytokines and vaccines, but other modeling efforts have addressed other approaches, including administration/vaccination of dendritic cells, vaccination with tumor-cytotoxic virus, and macrophages as vehicles for the delivery of anti-tumor drugs (Castiglione and Piccoli, 2006; Owen et al., 2004; Wodarz, 2001). As clinical trials of immunotherapy progress, mathematical models that can reproduce the measurements and results from these trials can shed insight into the reasons for successes and failures, and suggest improved strategies or protocols that increase the likelihood of successful outcomes. As novel immunologic mechanisms are elucidated, these, too, may offer therapeutic opportunities in tumor biology. A recent area receiving growing attention in the field of tumor immunology is the role of regulatory cells in suppression of anti-tumor immune responses. Regulatory-cell-boosting therapies are already under development for autoimmune diseases; in cancer, the role of regulatory cells in permitting tumor development and the impact of reducing this protection may offer new therapeutic strategies. In all, given the complexity of tumor biology and immunology, mathematical modeling offers a unique framework to help clinical and pharmaceutical researchers develop, optimize and test immunotherapeutic strategies in a cost-effective, efficient manner.

ALLERGIC AND AUTOIMMUNE DISEASES

In contrast to infection and cancer, in which the immune system must control a foreign or self-derived threat to maintain health, allergic and autoimmune diseases arise when the immune system responds inappropriately to generally innocuous environmental stimuli or the body's own tissues, respectively. Some of the more common allergic diseases include asthma, allergic rhinitis and food allergy, whereas purported autoimmune diseases include rheumatoid arthritis, multiple sclerosis, type 1(insulin-dependent) diabetes mellitus and inflammatory bowel disease. The etiologies of most allergic and autoimmune diseases are poorly understood and thought to be multifactorial. Because it is believed that every individual harbors lymphocytes with reactivity to environmental and/or self antigens, there is considerable interest in understanding why some individuals develop disease, whereas others do not. In fact, the debate on this fundamental question of how the immune system differentiates antigens that pose a health threat (e.g. those that are virally derived) from antigens that do not, may account for the relatively small number of mechanistic mathematical models addressing these diseases. More specifically, it has been argued that insufficient primary data exist to support mathematical modeling of these immunologic disease processes. However, we maintain that mathematical models, representing the current state of knowledge, can be effectively used to test alternate hypotheses and focus research efforts on those experiments that are most likely to be enlightening. Further, such models present a quantitative summary of known data and disease behaviors that form a foundation on which new data are integrated and understood.

Of the relatively few allergic or autoimmune disease mathematical models that have been reported, several have focused on delineating factors that differentiate normal health from disease and/or account for particular disease manifestations (Freiesleben et al., 1999; Iwami et al., 2007; Louzoun et al., 2001; Wang et al., 2006).

For example, Iwami et al. (2007) have elaborated a basic model of autoimmunity:

$$\frac{dT}{dt} = g(T) - \beta TC$$
$$\frac{dD}{dt} = \beta TC - \alpha D$$
$$\frac{dC}{dt} = f(D) - \gamma C \qquad (15.3)$$

which describes populations of target cells (T), damaged cells releasing self-antigens (D), and immune cells (C). The target cell population is regulated by a growth function $g(T)$; the activation of immune cells by antigen is described by $f(D)$. βTC reflects the damage induced by immune cells, and α and γ reflect death rates for damaged and immune cells, respectively. The authors explored two forms of $g(T)$, one reflecting production and death, the other including target cell proliferation. They further evaluated two forms of $f(D)$, one reflecting linear immune activation in response to antigen, the other sigmoidal. Simulations permitted the researchers to identify the parameter conditions under which tolerance or autoimmunity are generated and conditions that account for mild or severe disease progression, flares and dormancy. Although many of the same elements were included, other authors introduced more immunological detail by representing specific immune cells (e.g. macrophages, T cells) and different activation states, effector activities or regulatory mechanisms (Freiesleben et al., 1999; Louzoun et al., 2001; Nevo et al., 2004; Wang et al., 2006). Interestingly, some mathematical models developed to address a very specific pharmacologic question have included minimal representation of immune system components. For example, Choudat et al. (1999) applied a simple mathematical model including inhaled dose of allergen, allergen concentration, duration of exposure, and deactivation of inhaled allergens and inflammatory mediators to evaluate the bronchial response of asthmatic patients to challenge with flour.

Despite some early efforts (e.g. Waniewski and Prikrylova 1988, 1989), there have been few recent attempts to apply mechanistic modeling to drug discovery and development for allergic or autoimmune diseases. These include small-scale models representing specific aspects of disease developed to research a therapeutic approach, and large-scale models representing the disease more broadly to address multiple therapeutic strategies.

T Cell Vaccination

The importance of autoreactive T and B lymphocytes to the progression of autoimmune disease has been demonstrated through laboratory experiments showing, for example, prevention or amelioration of disease after the removal of autoreactive lymphocytes. Somewhat surprisingly, priming the immune system with autoreactive T cells at subpathogenic doses or in an attenuated form can also invoke protection. This therapeutic strategy, termed T cell vaccination (TCV) has been successfully executed in several animal models of autoimmune disease (Ben-Nun et al., 1981; Holoshitz et al., 1983). Efficacy is attributed, at least in part, to the induction of anti-idiotypic regulatory T cells (i.e., regulatory T cells with specificity for the T cell receptors of autoreactive T cell clones), although the findings of recent studies have also implicated regulatory T cells with other specificities. Clinical trials are currently under way to assess the efficacy of TCV in patients with multiple sclerosis (*see* Internet Resources). Borghans et al. (1998) developed a mathematical model to investigate the mechanisms of TCV. Based on experimental data from experimental autoimmune encephalomyelitis (EAE, a model of multiple sclerosis), the mathematical model includes an autoreactive T cell clone (A), an anti-idiotypic CD4$^+$ regulatory T cell clone (R_4), and an anti-idiotypic

CD8$^+$ regulatory T cell clone (R_8). The cellular dynamics are represented as:

$$\frac{dA}{dt} = m_A + pAS_A - iAR_8 - dA - \varepsilon_A A^2$$

$$\frac{dR_4}{dt} = m_R + pR_4 S_R - dR_4 - \varepsilon_R R_4^2 \quad (15.4)$$

$$\frac{dR_8}{dt} = m_R + pR_8 S_R H - dR_8 - \varepsilon_R R_8^2$$

where S_A is the number of presented self-epitopes and S_R is the number of presented autoreactive TCRs, described as:

$$S_A = \frac{A}{k_A + A} \quad \text{and} \quad S_R = \frac{A}{k_R + A} \quad (15.5)$$

and paramaters m_A and m_R represent influx of newly generated autoreactive and regulatory cells, while p is the maximum proliferation rate for all T cells. The interaction between CD4$^+$ and CD8$^+$ T cells is represented by $H = R_4/(k_h + R_4)$. CD8$^+$ regulatory cells inhibit autoreactive cells at rate i. For small clonal populations, cells die at rate d. For larger clonal populations, an additional term is added in consideration of concentration-dependent cell death ($\varepsilon_N N^2$). Given the activation of autoreactive T cells by self-peptides and the activation of regulatory T cells by TCR peptides of the autoreactive T cells, the model replicates the experimentally observed transient autoimmunity that follows injection of EAE-susceptible animals with the autoantigen, myelin basic protein (MBP). Similarly, stable protection from EAE is induced by vaccinating with autoreactive T cells, provided enough cells are administered to activate feedback loops between the autoreactive T cells and regulatory T cells. Interestingly, the model predicted that vaccination with attenuated autoreactive T cells would provide transient protection while the cells remained in the animal, but would fail to provide long-term protection once the attenuated cells had been cleared. This failure is attributed to the inability of attenuated cells to activate the feedback loop between autoreactive and regulatory T cells. Thus the authors were able to explain the TCV phenomena by hypothesizing that autoreactive T cells are controlled by regulatory T cells. Further, they provided a testable prediction on the efficacy of attenuated autoreactive T cells. The use of mathematical models to understand therapeutic mechanisms of action in animal models could help in the design of key experiments, to improve the likelihood of success in translating therapies from animal models to humans.

Disease-specific Efficacy of Cytokine Blockade

Tumor necrosis factor α is a cytokine that has been implicated as contributing to the pathology of a number of disorders. Interestingly, agents that block its action, including infliximab (Remicade®), etanercept (Enbrel®), and adalimumab (Humira®), have demonstrated clinical benefit in some, but not all, diseases in which TNFα is implicated. Jit et al. (2005) constructed a mathematical model of TNFα dynamics to gain a better understanding of why TNFα blockade successfully treats patients with rheumatoid arthritis but has shown limited efficacy in patients suffering from systemic inflammatory response syndrome (SIRS). The model allows for free TNFα to bind cell surface receptors or antibody within the "receptor compartment," meant to represent the inflamed synovial joint. TNFα production and the possibility of autocrine amplification of TNFα production were explicitly modeled. The authors predicted that inhibitors strongly reduce the concentration of bioactive TNFα, although the total TNFα concentration (free + bound) increases. Interestingly, the long-term effect of the inhibitor is predicted to be dramatically affected by the TNFα dynamics. When production of TNFα is chronically increased, representing a pathological equilibrium that might be consistent with rheumatoid arthritis, the inhibitors are predicted to stably reduce bioactive TNFα concentrations. In contrast, if increased TNFα concentrations are transient, similar to what is observed in SIRS, the inhibitor-bound TNFα is predicted to act as a slow-release reservoir, ultimately leading to a net increase in bioactive TNFα concentrations. This latter scenario would be consistent with the poor results of TNF blockade therapy in SIRS. Through this modeling analysis, the authors were able to evaluate the dynamic interaction between endogenous TNFα concentrations and blocking agents, to predict conditions leading to therapeutic success or failure.

Evaluation and Prioritization of Drug Targets for Rheumatoid Arthritis

In the previous two examples, small-scale models were developed to understand a specific therapeutic modality within the confines of a tightly focused set of biological parameters. These models can clearly provide insight into the problem of interest; however, our group has developed large-scale models representing more broadly the fundamental interacting elements of disease, to make these models applicable to a wider suite of research questions. These mechanistic ODE models have been developed for immune/inflammatory diseases including rheumatoid arthritis, asthma and type 1 diabetes. These models are designed to provide a mechanistic link between clinically observable disease measures and the underlying molecular interactions.

Rheumatoid arthritis is a disease characterized by chronic inflammation and degradation of the joints. More specifically, the synovial tissue that surrounds the joint space becomes inflamed and contributes to structural damage, including loss of articular cartilage and bone erosions. Therapeutic responses in rheumatoid arthritis have been defined by composite scores. For example, the sAmerican College of Rheumatology (ACR) defines the "ACR20 score" as 20% improvement in the number of tender and swollen joints, in addition to 20% improvement in three of the five following core measures: patient and physician global assessments, pain, disability and a laboratory measurement. We developed a platform for rheumatoid arthritis, comprising more than 900 ODEs, to predict the ACR score of "virtual patients" on the basis of specific initial parameters defining a prototypical rheumatoid arthritis joint and the simulated effects of approved and novel therapies on synovial inflammation. Each virtual patient is defined by a particular set of parameters, which may represent known or hypothesized heterogeneity in genetics, environment or lifestyle. Inflammation is explicitly represented by the abnormal increase in the number of cells in the joint, termed synovial hyperplasia, including macrophages, fibroblast-like synoviocytes, T cells, B cells and other inflammatory cells. Specific cellular life cycles (e.g. recruitment, activation, proliferation, apoptosis) and cellular interactions via soluble mediators or cell–cell contact are represented, to provide the molecular network that ultimately drives the predicted ACR score. The model also includes structural biology (e.g. chondrocytes, extracellular matrix, osteoclasts) that predicts measures of joint structural damage, providing the ability to carry out a mechanistic examination of the effects of therapy on cartilage and bone. Virtual patients are validated by simulating published clinical trial protocols for therapies with distinct mechanisms of action and comparing the predicted outcomes (e.g. ACR score, joint space narrowing) with published data from clinical trials (Fig. 15.4).

Rullmann et al. (2005) applied the rheumatoid arthritis platform to investigate and prioritize 31 molecular targets. As these targets were not explicitly represented in the platform, target modulation was simulated by modulating the downstream functional effects of each target.

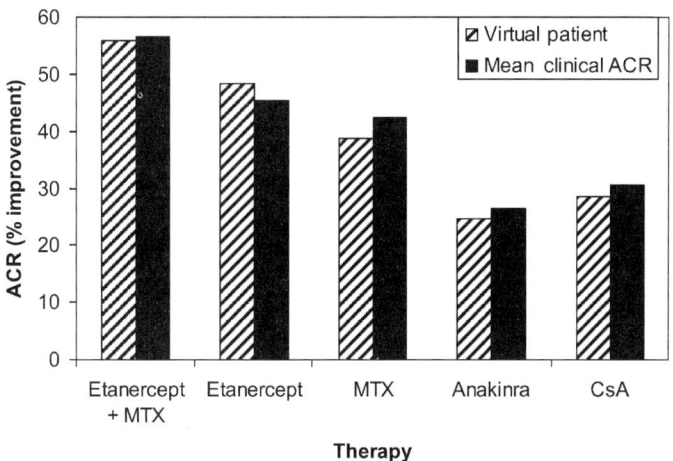

FIGURE 15.4 Example of Virtual Patient Validation.
The ACR score of the virtual patient, reflecting a therapy-induced change in the modeled synovial hyperplasia after 48 weeks of treatment, was compared against the mean ACR score estimated from clinical trial data, reporting the frequency of ACR20, ACR50 and ACR80 responses at 48 weeks. The mean ACR score is calculated as: $ACR_{mean} = (1 - f_{20})r_0 + (f_{20} - f_{50})r_{20} + (f_{50} - f_{70})r_{50} + f_{70}r_{70}$ where f_n is the fraction of patients achieving $\geq n\%$ improvement in ACR score, and r_n is the improvement assumed to characterize the group ($r_{70} = 80\%$, $r_{50} = 60\%$, $r_{20} = 35\%$, and $r_0 = 10\%$). CsA, ?; MTX, methotrexate.
Adapted from Rullmann et al. (2005), with permission.

For example, Lck is a tyrosine kinase found in T lymphocytes and activated after ligation of the T cell receptor. To predict the clinical efficacy of inhibiting Lck, the primary scientific literature was examined to identify effects of pharmacologic or genetic Lck blockade on downstream functions (e.g. T lymphocyte proliferation). To account for functional redundancy with other tyrosine kinases and the reported non-specificity of some pharmacologic inhibitors, a range of potential drug effects was defined and simulated. The result was a range of predicted clinical efficacy for Lck blockade, which could then be compared against the predicted clinical efficacy for other targets, and for methotrexate, a currently approved treatment for rheumatoid arthritis (Fig. 15.5A). This analysis permitted prioritization of the candidate targets on the basis of their relative efficacy, in addition to the predicted degree of target modulation required to achieve competitive efficacy with methotrexate. After the high-priority candidate targets had been identified, additional simulations were conducted to systematically identify the primary mechanism(s) of action responsible for target efficacy. More specifically, simulations were conducted in which only a single mechanism of action for each target was active. Reciprocal simulations were also conducted, to evaluate the effects of activating all but one possible mechanism of action. For Lck antagonism, these analyses predicted that inhibition of the production of IFN-γ by T cells would be a primary mechanism of action (Fig. 15.5B), suggesting that the target could be experimentally validated by confirming a strong effect of Lck inhibition on the production of IFN-γ by T cells. Thus, by identifying likely key mechanisms of action within the model, the authors were able to direct research efforts to confirm only high-priority targets, and improve efficiency by focusing experiments on those target effects predicted to have the greatest impact on clinical efficacy.

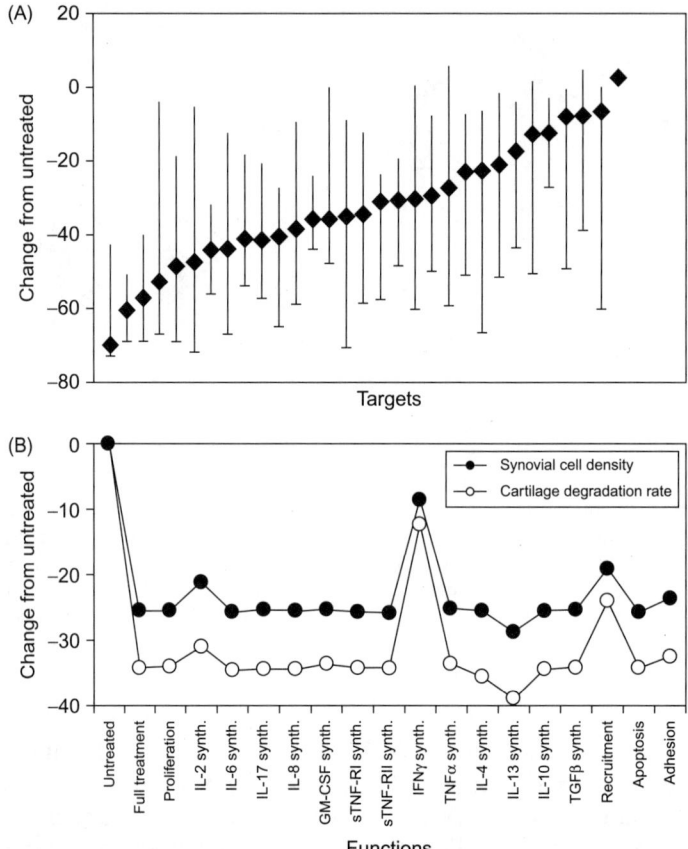

FIGURE 15.5 Investigating and Prioritizing Molecular Targets.
(A) Predicted clinical efficacy of 31 drug targets. Efficacy is the % change relative to the untreated state, averaged over two clinical outputs: ACR score (reflecting synovial cell density) and joint space narrowing (reflecting the cartilage degradation rate). Error bars reflect the upper, lower and most likely (♦) quantifications. The dotted line is the predicted efficacy of methotrexate, a standard treatment for rheumatoid arthritis. (B) Critical mechanisms of action for the tyrosine kinase, Lck. The vertical axis shows the ACR score in a series of simulations in which, in every simulation, a different biological function of Lck antagonism was excluded. The two left-most entries indicate simulations in which there was no simulated Lck antagonism (i.e., untreated) and in which all downstream functions of Lck were antagonized. GM-CSF, granulocyte macrophage-colony stimulating factor; IFN-γ, gamma-interferon; IL, interleukin; sTNF-RI, sTNF-RII, ? tumor necrosis factor receptors I and II; TGFβ, transforming growth factor-β; TNFα, tumor necrosis factor-α.

Adapted from Rullmann et al. (2005), with permission.

CONCLUSION

Effective and safe treatment of immunologic diseases remains a challenging goal because of the complex, context-dependent function of numerous immunologic components. Although experimental investigations continue to elucidate fundamental immunologic principles, key uncertainties remain that slow the discovery and development of new therapeutic agents. In addition, patient data detailing disease characteristics (e.g. early-stage progression) are frequently incomplete, leaving only hypotheses to bridge failures of the immune system and disease. Finally, patient heterogeneity can render treatments effective in some patients, yet ineffective or even unsafe in others.

The techniques of systems biology have been applied to the study of immunologic diseases to integrate disparate datasets, formulate and test new hypotheses, and further scientific understanding of complex biological processes. Such approaches maximize the utilization of data and formulate coherent, testable models. Moreover, models can be used for systemic investigation of areas of the biology in which data are sparse, leading to the identification of critical illuminating experiments.

In this chapter, we reviewed applications of mathematical modeling in the areas of infectious disease, cancer, allergy and autoimmunity. The studies discussed above illustrate how mathematical models can be used to guide drug discovery and development by: (i) identifying "sensitive" parameters corresponding to biological functions the modulation of which can restore healthy outcomes; (ii) evaluating specific targets to determine whether and why modulation can influence disease activity; (iii) evaluating the benefits of specific therapies alone or in combination, and predicting the criteria for success vs. failure; (iv) proposing optimized therapeutic regimens, including timing and dose; (v) determining optimal personalized therapeutic approaches. The quantitative and predictive models reviewed address many of the unique challenges impeding drug discovery and development in each of these disease areas, including drug resistance in HIV, optimal immunotherapy approaches in cancer treatment and the prioritization of promising drug targets in rheumatoid arthritis.

Although modeling and simulation will continue to have increasing roles in immunologic research, drug discovery and development, caution should be used when using model predictions in the absence of supporting *in-vitro* and *in-vivo* data. Systems modeling can be best used to clearly delineate meaningful, testable predictions, which can be used to design more efficient and effective laboratory and clinical studies. Cross-disciplinary collaboration among engineers, mathematicians, researchers and clinicians is essential to sound model development and interpretation of the results of simulations. As systems biology approaches are applied and refined, we anticipate continued advances in our understanding of immunologic disease processes, including associated genomic and environmental risk factors, ultimately leading to the development of more targeted, individualized treatments for human patients.

ACKNOWLEDGEMENTS

We would like to thank Cynthia Stokes, Michael Cole, Gene Napolitano and Jill Fujisaki for their critical reviews.

References

Altfeld, M., Walker, B.D., 2001. Less is more? STI in acute and chronic HIV-1 infection. Nat. Med. 7, 881–884.

Bajaria, S.H., Webb, G., Cloyd, M., Kirschner, D., 2002. Dynamics of naive and memory CD4+ T lymphocytes in HIV-1 disease progression. J. Acquir. Immune Defic. Syndr. 30, 41–58.

Bajaria, S.H., Webb, G., Kirschner, D.E., 2004. Predicting differential responses to structured treatment interruptions during HAART. Bull. Math. Biol. 66, 1093–1118.

Ben-Nun, A., Wekerle, H., Cohen, I.R., 1981. Vaccination against autoimmune encephalomyelitis with T-lymphocyte line cells reactive against myelin basic protein. Nature 292, 60–61.

Borghans, J.A., De Boer, R.J., Sercarz, E., Kumar, V., 1998. T cell vaccination in experimental autoimmune encephalomyelitis: a mathematical model. J. Immunol. 161, 1087–1093.

Cappuccio, A., Castiglione, F., Piccoli, B., 2007. Determination of the optimal therapeutic protocols in cancer immunotherapy. Math. Biosci. 209, 1–13.

Castiglione, F., Piccoli, B., 2006. Optimal control in a model of dendritic cell transfection cancer immunotherapy. Bull. Math. Biol. 68, 255–274.

Choudat, D., Fabries, J.F., Martin, J.C., et al., 1999. Quantification of the dose of inhaled flour: relation with nonspecific bronchial and immunological reactivities. Eur. Respir. J. 14, 328–334.

Chun, T.W., Carruth, L., Finzi, D., et al., 1997. Quantification of latent tissue reservoirs and total body viral load in HIV-1 infection. Nature 387, 183–188.

Coffin, J.M., 1995. HIV population dynamics in vivo: implications for genetic variation, pathogenesis, and therapy. Science 267, 483–489.

De Boer, R.J., Hogeweg, P., Dullens, H.F., De Weger, R.A., Den Otter, W., 1985. Macrophage T lymphocyte interactions in the anti-tumor immune response: a mathematical model. J. Immunol. 134, 2748–2758.

DeConde, R., Kim, P.S., Levy, D., Lee, P.P., 2005. Post-transplantation dynamics of the immune response to chronic myelogenous leukemia. J. Theor. Biol. 236, 39–59.

Deeks, S.G., 2003. Treatment of antiretroviral-drug-resistant HIV-1 infection. Lancet 362, 2002–2011.

De Pillis, L.G., Gu, W., Radunskaya, A.E., 2006. Mixed immunotherapy and chemotherapy of tumors: modeling, applications and biological interpretations. J. Theor. Biol. 238, 841–862.

Flexner, C., 2007. HIV drug development: the next 25 years. Nat. Rev. Drug. Discov. 6, 959–966.

Freiesleben, D.B., Bak, P., Pociot, F., Karlsen, A.E., Nerup, J., 1999. Onset of type 1 diabetes: a dynamical instability. Diabetes 48, 1677–1685.

Friedrich, C.M., Paterson, T.S., 2004. In silico predictions of target clinical efficacy. Drug. Disc. Today 3, 216–222.

Gallant, J.E., DeJesus, E., Arribas, J.R., et al., 2006. Tenofovir DF, emtricitabine, and efavirenz vs. zidovudine, lamivudine, and efavirenz for HIV. N. Engl. J. Med. 354, 251–260.

Holoshitz, J., Naparstek, Y., Ben-Nun, A., Cohen, I.R., 1983. Lines of T lymphocytes induce or vaccinate against autoimmune arthritis. Science 219, 56–58.

Iwami, S., Takeuchi, Y., Miura, Y., Sasaki, T., Kajiwara, T., 2007. Dynamical properties of autoimmune disease models: tolerance, flare-up, dormancy. J. Theor. Biol. 246, 646–659.

Jit, M., Henderson, B., Stevens, M., Seymour, R.M., 2005. TNF-alpha neutralization in cytokine-driven diseases: a mathematical model to account for therapeutic success in rheumatoid arthritis but therapeutic failure in systemic inflammatory response syndrome. Rheumatology (Oxford) 44, 323–331.

Kirschner, D., Panetta, J.C., 1998. Modeling immunotherapy of the tumor-immune interaction. J. Math. Biol. 37, 235–252.

Kronik, N., Kogan, Y., Vainstein, V., Agur, Z., 2008. Improving alloreactive CTL immunotherapy for malignant gliomas using a simulation model of their interactive dynamics. Cancer Immunol. Immunother. 57, 425–439.

Lifson Jr., J.D., Rossio, J.L., Piatak, M., et al., 2001. Role of CD8(+) lymphocytes in control of simian immunodeficiency virus infection and resistance to rechallenge after transient early antiretroviral treatment. J. Virol. 75, 10187–10199.

Lori, F., Lewis, M.G., Xu, J., et al., 2000. Control of SIV rebound through structured treatment interruptions during early infection. Science 290, 1591–1593.

Louzoun, Y., Atlan, H., Cohen, I.R., 2001. Modeling the influence of Th1- and Th2-type cells in autoimmune diseases. J. Autoimmun. 17, 311–321.

Mallet, D.G., De Pillis, L.G., 2006. A cellular automata model of tumor–immune system interactions. J. Theor. Biol. 239, 334–350.

Matzavinos, A., Chaplain, M.A., 2004. Travelling-wave analysis of a model of the immune response to cancer. C. R. Biol. 327, 995–1008.

Matzavinos, A., Chaplain, M.A., Kuznetsov, V.A., 2004. Mathematical modelling of the spatio-temporal response of cytotoxic T-lymphocytes to a solid tumour. Math. Med. Biol. 21, 1–34.

Melder, R.J., Munn, L.L., Stoll, B.R., et al., 2002. Systemic distribution and tumor localization of adoptively transferred lymphocytes in mice: comparison with physiologically based pharmacokinetic model. Neoplasia 4, 3–8.

Nanda, S., Moore, H., Lenhart, S., 2007. Optimal control of treatment in a mathematical model of chronic myelogenous leukemia. Math. Biosci. 210, 143–156.

Nani, F.K., Oguztoreli, M.N., 1994. Modelling and simulation of Rosenberg-type adoptive cellular immunotherapy. IMA J. Math. Appl. Med. Biol. 11, 107–147.

Nevo, U., Golding, I., Neumann, A.U., Schwartz, M., Akselrod, S., 2004. Autoimmunity as an immune defense against degenerative processes: a primary mathematical model illustrating the bright side of autoimmunity. J. Theor. Biol. 227, 583–592.

Nowak, M.A., Bangham, C.R., 1996. Population dynamics of immune responses to persistent viruses. Science 272, 74–79.

Nowak, M.A., May, R.M., 2000. Virus Dynamics: Mathematical Principles of Immunology and Virology. Oxford University Press, Oxford.

Owen, M.R., Byrne, H.M., Lewis, C.E., 2004. Mathematical modelling of the use of macrophages as vehicles for drug delivery to hypoxic tumour sites. J. Theor. Biol. 226, 377–391.

Perelson, A.S., 2002. Modelling viral and immune system dynamics. Nat. Rev. Immunol. 2, 28–36.

Perelson, A.S., Neumann, A.U., Markowitz, M., Leonard, J.M., Ho, D.D., 1996. HIV-1 dynamics in vivo: virion clearance rate, infected cell life-span, and viral generation time. Science 271, 1582–1586.

Roeder, I., Glauche, I., 2007. Pathogenesis, treatment effects, and resistance dynamics in chronic myeloid leukemia—insights from mathematical model analyses. J. Mol. Med. 86, 17–27.

Rong, L., Feng, Z., Perelson, A.S., 2007. Emergence of HIV-1 drug resistance during antiretroviral treatment. Bull. Math. Biol. 69, 2027–2060.

Rosenberg, E.S., Altfeld, M., Poon, S.H., et al., 2000. Immune control of HIV-1 after early treatment of acute infection. Nature 407, 523–526.

Rullmann, J.A., Struemper, H., Defranoux, N.A., Ramanujan, S., Meeuwisse, C.M., van Elsas, A., 2005. Systems biology for battling rheumatoid arthritis: application of the Entelos PhysioLab platform. Syst. Biol. (Stevenage) 152, 256–262.

Smith, R.J., Wahl, L.M., 2005. Drug resistance in an immunological model of HIV-1 infection with impulsive drug effects. Bull. Math. Biol. 67, 783–813.

Struble, K., Murray, J., Cheng, B., Gegeny, T., Miller, V., Gulick, R., 2005. Antiretroviral therapies for treatment-experienced patients: current status and research challenges. AIDS 19, 747–756.

Von Bertalanffy, L., 1976. General Systems Theory: Foundations, Development, Applications. George Braziller, New York.

Wang, X., He, Z., Ghosh, S., 2006. Investigation of the age-at-onset heterogeneity in type 1 diabetes through mathematical modeling. Math. Biosci. 203, 79–99.

Waniewski, J., Prikrylova, D., 1988. Autoimmunity and its therapy: mathematical modelling. Immunol. Lett. 18, 77–80.

Waniewski, J., Prikrylova, D., 1989. A mathematical model of extracorporeal antibody removal in autoimmune disease. Int. J. Artif. Organs. 12, 471–476.

Wiener, N., 1948. Cybernetics: Or Control and Communication in the Animal and the Machine. MIT Press, Cambridge, MA.

Wodarz, D., 2001. Viruses as antitumor weapons: defining conditions for tumor remission. Cancer Res. 61, 3501–3507.

Wodarz, D., Nowak, M.A., 1999. Specific therapy regimes could lead to long-term immunological control of HIV. Proc. Natl. Acad. Sci. USA 96, 14464–14469.

Wu, H., Huang, Y., Acosta, E.P., et al., 2005. Modeling long-term HIV dynamics and antiretroviral response: effects of drug potency, pharmacokinetics, adherence, and drug resistance. J. Acquir. Immune Defic. Syndr. 39, 272–283.

Zhu, H., Melder, R.J., Baxter, L.T., Jain, R.K., 1996. Physiologically based kinetic model of effector cell biodistribution in mammals: implications for adoptive immunotherapy. Cancer Res. 56, 3771–3781.

Internet Resources

Phase I–III clinical trials ongoing in various types of cancer http://www.clinicaltrials.gov/ct2/results?term=immune+therapy+cancer

T cell vaccination clinical trial in multiple sclerosis http://clinicaltrials.gov/ct/show/NCT00245622?order=1; http://clinicaltrials.gov/ct/show/NCT00228228;jsessionid=F1BE92AFEFC0FD40E422EE3211C9F1AF?order=1

CHAPTER 16

Systems Pharmacology in Cancer

Qiang Yu and Edison T. Liu
Genome Institute of Singapore, Singapore

OUTLINE

From Molecule to System	377	Networks, Robustness and Cancer Therapeutic Strategies	388
Complexity of Human Diseases and Drug Action: the Need for a Systems Approach to Pharmacology Highlighted	378	Mining the Regulatory Program in the Cancer Transcriptome for Novel Targets	390
Target-based Therapy and its Limitations	379	Integrating Experimental and Primary Tumor Expression Data for Novel Biomarkers for Therapeutic Efficacy	393
Combination Therapy and Synthetic Lethality	382	Gene Signatures to Reveal the Drug Action–Gene Function Connectivity Map	394
Deconvoluting Mechanisms	385	Concluding Remarks	395
Perturbation Analysis of Constrained Systems to Discover New Anti-cancer Drugs	386		

FROM MOLECULE TO SYSTEM

Proteins rarely function in isolation; rather, they act as part of highly coordinated and interconnected cellular networks. Traditional pharmacology considers the "mechanism" of a drug action at the level of the individual gene product and thus has been focused on developing compounds targeting particular families of "druggable" proteins. In the past 10 years, significant progress has been made in the development of technologies—mainly genomics and proteomics—that enable molecular interrogations at a "systems" level; that is, at the level of interacting networks. These breakthroughs in technology have made possible investigations of the global response of a drug, so that we can begin to understand the action of the drug in the context of cellular and disease networks. Systems-level analysis considers that the human cell and human body are systems of connected gene networks that work together to control the functions of a living organism, and that diseases arise from perturbations of this system. Knowledge of these systems can be used to devise the best therapeutic strategy.

The challenge for system-level investigation of pharmacology is the appropriate integration of the overwhelming datasets that have been generated, so that the data can be interrogated and used to create models that will enable predictions to be made concerning therapeutic interventions. In this chapter, we will focus on how the systems approach can be successfully applied to the processes aimed at developing better anticancer therapeutic agents.

COMPLEXITY OF HUMAN DISEASES AND DRUG ACTION: THE NEED FOR A SYSTEMS APPROACH TO PHARMACOLOGY HIGHLIGHTED

The etiology of many human diseases, such as diabetes, cancer, asthma and depression, are multifactorial, both genetically and environmental. Given the complexity of the human disease and the robust phenotypes of biological systems, it seems unlikely that modulating a single protein will be able to effectively reverse the disease process for every patient. This is particularly true in cancer, as the malignant process involves several aberrant compensatory signaling routes that bypass the inhibition of individual proteins (Hanahan and Weinberg, 2000). A number of factors sustain the malignant state: unlimited growth potential ("stemness" properties), proliferative drive, abrogation of apoptosis, release of growth-inhibitory signals, enhanced invasiveness and angiogenic stimulus. Each one of these cancer-sustaining mechanisms is a rational target for anticancer therapeutics. Each system is controlled by a network of genes and the systems themselves intersect because of the pleiotropic function of oncogenes (Fig. 16.1): for example, *ras*, *myc* and *E2F1* have both growth promoting and apoptotic actions; activation of phosphatidyl inositol 3 kinase induces cellular motility and survival.

An additional challenge in cancer pharmacology is that cancer is a genetic moving target, capable of mutating into resistant or more aggressive forms. Further pharmacokinetic hurdles are presented by tumor physiology that

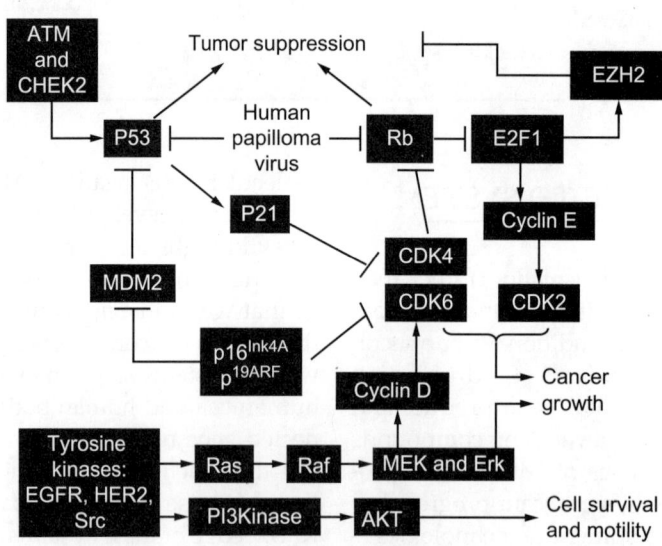

FIGURE 16.1   Interconnecting Network of Cancer-relevant Signaling Molecules Discussed in This Chapter.

limits the penetration of anticancer compounds, making effective cancer treatment a great challenge.

That cellular processes or human diseases are complex has never been in doubt; however, the major advance has been acquisition of the ability for precise measurement of the fundamental units of a complex system in a multiplex fashion, and thereby the ability to measure and to quantify the complexity. Accurate models of such systems provide the potential for predicting cellular outcomes. However, this goal has been elusive and it is more likely that systems approaches in pharmacology will allow investigators to limit their experimental "space," thus conferring on each experiment directed by systems information a greater likelihood of a significant outcome. Systems strategies in cancer pharmacology can therefore be used to:

1. Direct experimental focus.
2. Identify new targets for specific disease states.
3. Uncover mechanisms of action of a compound.
4. Identify likely combination therapies.
5. Generate biomarkers of response.

TARGET-BASED THERAPY AND ITS LIMITATIONS

Since the 1980s, knowledge of the precise molecular etiology of cancer has led to the identification of many cancer-specific abnormalities and the development of targeted treatments tailored to reverse these changes. The most obvious examples are in breast and prostate cancer, for which the nuclear hormone receptor— the estrogen receptor in breast cancer and the androgen receptor in prostate cancer—are among the most effective therapies for these malignancies. Such targeted hormonal strategies have previously been shown to be perhaps more effective than chemotherapy in the treatment of these diseases. The targeting, however, was based on the state of differentiation of these tumors, the expression of receptors associated with the tissue type being exploited. As these pathways are used for normal function, the side-effects of hormonal deprivation were guaranteed. Later, the targeting of specific cancer-associated genetic mutations improved the therapeutic index of these drugs. The first example was in a chronic leukemia. The chromosome translocation t(9;22) occurs in chronic myelogenous leukemia (CML) and creates a chimeric transcript encoding a novel fusion protein known as BCR-ABL, a misregulated Abl kinase that drives aberrant growth of CML cells. The development of the small-molecule compound, imatinib (Gleevec), which specifically targets this aberrant enzyme activity, represents the most notable success in targeted-cancer therapy. Patients with CML treated with imatinib have a response rate up to 80%, although none is cured by this monotherapy. The targeting of mutations specific for cancer is theoretically attractive, because treatments targeting these genetic mutations should improve the therapeutic index of the treatment.

Until recently, identification of such common translocations in solid tumors has been limited because of the complexity of the cytogenetics

---

BOX 16.1

THERAPEUTIC INDEX

Therapeutic index is the ratio of the intended effect over the unintended effect, or the ratio of targeted to off-target effects. It is intended to be a qualitative measure of the specificity of a cancer therapeutic. Therefore, a cancer drug with a high therapeutic index is one that has significant anticancer effect, with low toxicity.

changes in epithelial cancers. However, with the application of increasingly powerful genomic strategies, specific translocations have been detected. Soda et al. (2007) discovered the echinoderm microtubule-associated protein-like 4 (EML4) and the anaplastic lymphoma kinase (ALK) translocation in approximately 7% of non-small-cell lung cancers. Within one year of the description of this finding, an inhibitor of the ALK kinase was shown to inhibit cell growth of lung cancer cell lines (Koivunen et al., 2008), thus providing proof of principle for a small-molecule therapeutic against this subset of lung cancers. In a case potentially of greater clinical impact, Tomlins et al. (2005) identified a recurrent translocation in prostate cancer involving TMPRSS2 and the ETS family of transcription factors (ERG and ETV1), using a bioinformatics strategy called cancer outlier profile analysis (COPA). This translocation generates a fusion transcript linking the first exon of TMPRSS2 to the body of the ETS transcription factors (Tomlins et al., 2005). Intriguingly, this generates a fusion transcription factor that is androgen dependent and inappropriate expression of which transforms prostate epithelia (Tomlins et al., 2007). Importantly, this class of translocation is seen in approximately 60–70% of prostate cancers, making this the most common mutation in the disease.

In solid tumors, such targeted therapeutic strategies have also been used with significant success. The spectrum of activity of imatinib includes inhibiting, not only the ABL kinase, but also the KIT kinase, a gene that is mutated in about 90% of an unusual tumor known as gastrointestinal stromal tumor (GIST). This tumor type is resistant to most forms of chemotherapy, but shows a 50% response rate to single-agent imatinib therapy (Fabian et al., 2005). In non-small-cell lung cancer, activating epidermal growth factor receptor (EGFR) mutations have been seen predominantly in a form of lung cancer, common in Asia, that tends to afflict women who are non-smokers. It was found that therapeutic inhibition of EGFR tyrosine kinase by gefitinib (Iressa) or erlotinib (Tarceva) can result in tumor regression, albeit in only 10–20% of patients (Janne, 2005). This indicates that additional genetic abnormalities also contribute to this disease process. Indeed, the status of PTEN and ErbB family members has been found to influence the clinical efficacy of EGFR inhibition (Engelman et al., 2005; Mellinghoff et al., 2005). This is limitation is also seen in the (12–34%) response rate of breast cancer patients with HER-2 amplification treated with specific anti-HER2 therapy in the form of a humanized monoclonal antibody, trastuzamab. This indicates that, for the more common tumors, the clinical efficacy of targeted therapy is ultimately determined by several contributing pathways that may also need to be targeted.

In all these cases, the efficacy of monotherapy with specific targeted therapeutics either is dramatic in a small number of unique cancers primarily driven by a single pathway (e.g. CML), or is only partially effective in more complex (and also common) cancers. In all cases, relapse with a clone of the cancer resistant to the monotherapy occurs (often as a result of mutation / amplification of the specific molecular target). In many cases, monotherapy is partially effective and requires combination with chemotherapy to optimize clinical outcome (as with trastuzamab anti-HER-2 therapeutics).

In some instances, this resistance to treatment results from the presence of mutations that reduce the affinity of the target kinase for the small-molecule inhibitor. In other cases, resistance appears to be caused by the activation of several receptor tyrosine kinase pathways (Fig. 16.2). It has been observed that EGFR and Met are co-activated in lung tumors. Redundant signaling inputs drive and maintain downstream growth signals, thereby limiting the efficacy of monotherapies targeting single receptor tyrosine kinases (Stommel et al., 2007). Indeed, treatment of with either the EGFR inhibitor, erlotinib, or the MET inhibitor, SU11274, alone had little

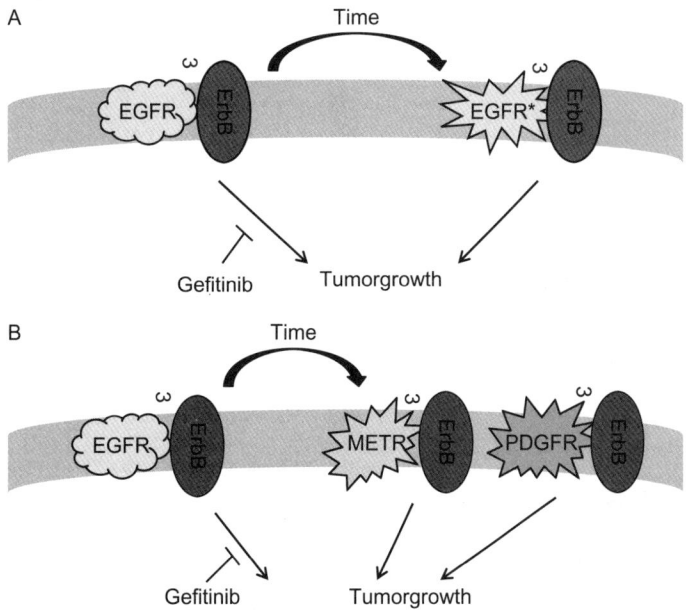

FIGURE 16.2 Evasion of Gefitinib Blockade of EGFR Signaling. Blockade of EGFR signaling by gefitinib is evaded through acquisition of a secondary mutation (A) or activation of receptors METR and PDGFR (B).

effect; however, combination treatment not only reduced the downstream signaling, but also significantly decreased cell viability and growth. Therefore, targeting several molecules contributing to this redundant signaling network may be necessary for effective treatment of these tumors.

In fact, many clinically successful drugs exert their efficacy through multitarget effects. The recent launch of several protein kinase inhibitors illustrated the emerging realization of the importance of polypharmacology. Sorafenib has been recently approved as a multi-kinase inhibitor, affecting both tumor growth (Raf and platelet-derived growth factor receptor [PDGFR]) and tumor angiogenesis (vascular endothelial growth factor receptor [VEGFR]). In addition, sunitinib is another recently launched protein kinase inhibitor with a target footprint similar to that of sorafenib (Fabian et al., 2005). Progressively, the benefits of multi-kinase inhibition for cancer therapy are being recognized, with the development of an even wider spectrum of targets. ABT869, an orally administered, potent and specific inhibitor of all VEGF and PDGF family tyrosine kinases, including FLT-3, and c-kit receptors showed significant clinical effect in a range of tumors in phase I studies (Wong et al., 2007). Drugs acting on several targets with "polypharmacologic" actions are proving to be effective in cancer treatment and, contrary to earlier concerns, with no increase in toxicity. These efforts, however, still rely on empirical, trial-and-error approaches in deciding which target spectrum is the optimal for specific cancers (Fig. 16.3).

To make polypharmacology rationally directed, the global relationships between chemical structure and biological targets need to be better delineated. Paolini et al. (2006) constructed a data warehouse that contains 4.8 million nonredundant chemical structures; among them, 275 000 are classified as biologically active. To date, there are approximately 836 genes in

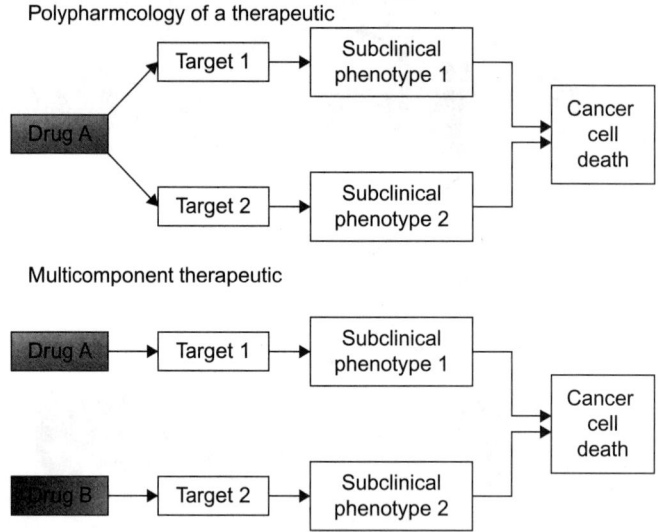

FIGURE 16.3 Polypharmacology and Multicomponent Therapeutics.

the human genome for which small-molecule chemical tools have been discovered. Among them, only 158 human proteins have been identified as the primary nodes of action for clinically approved small-molecule drugs. Thus the remaining genes need to be explored as clinically relevant drug targets. Such catalogues of drugs and targets are the first steps to assembling the "components list" for a systems pharmacology map.

COMBINATION THERAPY AND SYNTHETIC LETHALITY

The use of combination therapies in medicine has a long history, and many successful cases can be found in infectious diseases and human cancers. In the past, the use of combination chemotherapy with cytotoxic agents has been based on optimizing non-overlapping toxicities, rather than on optimizing combinatorial effectiveness. The blunt instrument of cytotoxic chemotherapy does not require precise understanding of mechanisms of action. However, the current availability of targeted therapeutic agents raises the possibility of intelligent combinations for synergistic anticancer effects. This need for a combination approach is pronounced for mammalian cells and tissues, which are composed of complex, networked systems with redundant, convergent and divergent signaling pathways. For example, the *cyclin D1* gene is frequently overexpressed in a broad range of human tumor types. This overexpression is often the result of aberrant genetic events, including chromosomal rearrangement or gene amplification of the *cyclin D1* locus, but it can also be transcriptionally upregulated as a result of oncogenic activation of Ras, Myc and Wnt pathways (Figs 16.1 and 16.4). These pathways interact at several points; they act synergistically or redundantly. Therefore targeting one specific pathway such as Ras might not necessarily result in ultimate abrogation of the expression of *cyclin D1*. In order to treat the cancer patient effectively, one might need to understand all the molecular events that converge to induce *cyclin D* activation, and to exploit multicomponent therapies to achieve optimal blockade of the pathway.

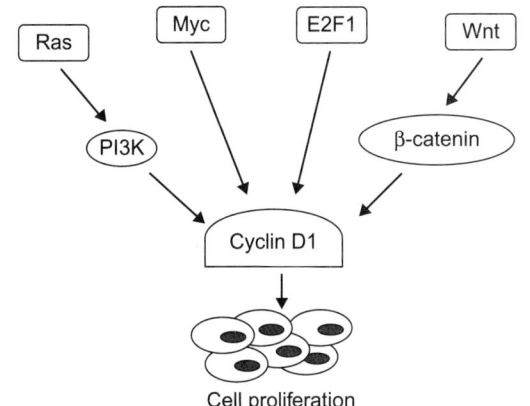

FIGURE 16.4 Convergence of Pathways to *Cyclin D1* and Cell Proliferation.

In genetics, the same strategy is seen in synthetic lethal mutational mapping. Two mutations are termed "synthetic lethal" if the disruption of two genes gives a discernible phenotype when the knockout of either one has no effect. Synthetic lethal phenotypes are indicative of an interaction in function between the products of the two mutant genes in the cell. Such synthetic lethality mapping has been expanded to a genome scale in yeast genetics, and has contributed to the refined understanding of interacting networks in both *Saccharomyces cerevisiae* and *S. pombe*. In fact, the first genome-scale analysis of anticancer drugs in this manner was performed in yeast strains treated with chemotherapeutic agents assessed using high-throughput methodologies (Marton et al., 1998; Simon et al., 2000). The investigators used this strategy to uncover putative cellular pathways that render yeast more sensitive to genotoxic agents. This has now been extended to mammalian systems. Contemporary strategies have revealed that a drug targeting a gene product might be more effective in the presence of a specific mutation in the cancer cell (Kaelin, 2005). For example, gain- or loss-of-function changes in genes that occur specifically in cancer cells might render cells more susceptible to additional therapeutic attacks, but would have no consequence in normal cells.

Small chemical entities can inhibit gene function in a manner analogous to genetic loss-of-function mutation in a synthetic lethal interaction. For example, the DNA repair enzyme, poly (ADP-ribose) polymerase (PARP) has been identified as a synthetic lethal partner of *BRCA1* and *BRCA2*. Inhibiting PARP with small-molecule compounds in cancer cells carrying mutant *BRCA1* results in tumor cell death, whereas cancer cells with normal *BRCA1* are not susceptible to PARP inhibition (Farmer et al., 2005) (Fig. 16.5). These PARP inhibitors (Aladjem et al., 1998) are able to achieve similar results in xenograft models and also in animal models of spontaneous *BRCA2* loss of function (Farmer et al., 2005). The success of this approach in experimental models has led to the initiation of clinical trials using PARP inhibitors as a monotherapy for *BRCA*-deficient tumors. Cells bearing such combinations of PARP inhibition with *BRCA* deficiency would have unique liabilities that might be exploited therapeutically.

The recent advent of functional genomics based on RNA-mediated interference (RNAi) has provided the opportunity to derive unbiased and comprehensive collections of validated gene targets. Taking advantage of this technology, Whitehurst et al. (2007) have performed a genome-wide synthetic screening to identify gene targets that specifically reduce cell viability in the presence of otherwise sublethal concentrations of paclitaxel. Given that the unifying principle governing the molecular pathology of cancer is the co-dependent aberrant regulation of core machinery driving proliferation and suppressing apoptosis, this kind of synthetic lethal screening effort may be able to reveal the optimal intervention targets. Efforts to systematically identify genetic alterations in human cancers will provide new strategy for such therapeutic exploitation, again, by providing a components list for systems pharmacology maps (Sjoblom et al., 2006). For example, genomic detection of gene mutations in breast and colorectal cancers indicates that the large number of somatic mutations

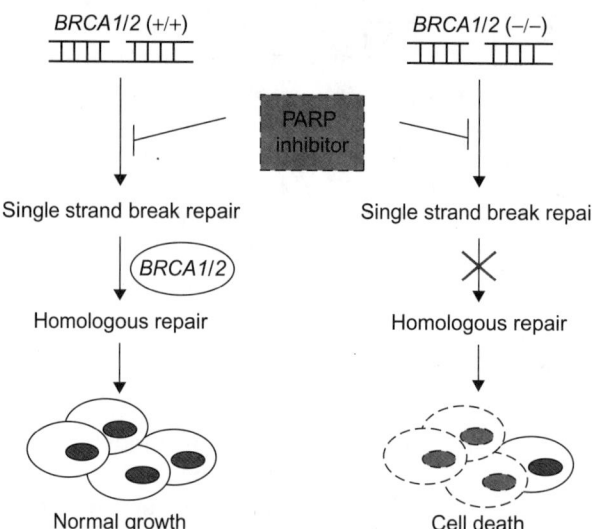

FIGURE 16.5 Exploiting Aberrant DNA Repair. Exploiting the unique liability of *BRCA1*- and *BRCA2*-deficient cancer cells that show aberrant DNA repair. Inhibitors of poly (ADP-ribose) polymerase (PARP) induce cancer cell death only in *BRCA1*- and *BRCA2*-null cells.

actually reflects alterations in a much smaller number of cell signaling pathways (Wood et al., 2007). Many of these pathways have previously been studied in specific cancers: p53, PTEN/AKT, Wnt, RAS/mitogen-activated protein kinase (MAPK), nuclear factor κB (NF-κB). However, the breadth of cancers in which these pathways are perturbed was wider than previously thought. For example, IKBKE and several other components of the NF-κB pathway were found to be frequently mutated in breast cancer, implicating the NF-κB pathway as a therapeutic target in breast cancer. Scientists from the Sanger Institute focused their sequence analysis on the 274 megabases of the coding exons of 518 kinases in 210 diverse human cancers, thus narrowing the specificity of the mutational analysis (Greenman et al., 2007). The mutation rates differed between the cancers, with the highest in lung cancers at 4.2 mutations per megabase, followed by GI cancers at 1.2–2.1 mutations per megabase, and the lowest in breast cancers (0.19 mutations per megabase). The gene spectrum of mutational frequency showed that the BRAF and ATM kinases were among the most commonly mutated. On the basis of pathways analysis, however, the fibroblast growth factor (FGF) signaling network showed the greatest enrichment of non-synonymous mutations in this class of kinases. In addition, the c-Jun N-terminal kinase (JNK) pathway was also generally involved in the cancers represented. These genomic sequencing efforts describe a high level of genetic mutational diversity, but convergence to a manageable number of pathways involved in cancer. Pathway targeting is therefore a rational strategy.

Although it is possible that desired combination effects can be found using specifically targeted therapeutics that attack known pathways, Borisy and colleagues (2003) exploited massively parallel screening technologies for an empiric determination of emergent properties of pharmaceutical compounds. A relatively small number of compounds provided large number of different combinations: a collection of 1000 compounds yielded approximately 500 000 pairwise combinations. By phenotypic screening combinations of compounds with non-relevant uses (e.g. antipsychotic drugs for anticancer effects), Borisy's group identified unique combinations of known drugs for different indications. For example, CRx-026 was discovered in a high-throughput screening of tens of thousands of different combinations of existing drugs for synergistic killing in human tumor cell lines. CRx-026 is a combination of chlorpromazine, a phenothiazine sedative, and pentamidine, an anti-infective agent, and neither has been used as anticancer drugs. CRx-026 effectively inhibited tumor growth in a nude mouse xenograft model in which the individual drugs by themselves had no effect (Borisy et al., 2003). Although the mechanism underlying this effect needs to be explored, it is obvious that what we know about the single compound is insufficient to predict the effect seen in combinations. Instead of "rational" drug design, this might be considered an example of combinatorial screening for emergent properties. This approach is an extension of the multidrug strategy commonly used in infectious diseases and in cancer therapy. Keith et al. (2005) suggested new terminology for drug combinations. The standard strategy commonly used today is to identify drugs known to have an effect on a specific cancer and then to optimize combinations; they call these "congruous" combinations. By contrast, the example of CRx-026 is a multicomponent therapeutic that combines two active ingredients at least one of which is not known to have any effect on the disease as a single agent; this Keith et al. call a "syncretic" combination (defining syncretic as "the fusion of two or more originally different inflectional forms").

DECONVOLUTING MECHANISMS

The use of complex libraries of chemical entities to induce specific cellular phenotypes is also referred to as "chemical genetics" (Strausberg and Schreiber, 2003). The output of such screens requires subsequent deconvolution of the molecular target or mechanism responsible for the observed phenotypic response. A variety of technologies and approaches are being explored for target identification after phenotypic screening (Terstappen et al., 2007). Direct approaches such as affinity chromatography are often used to identify the molecule to which the compound binds. In contrast, genomic approaches based on the genome-wide activity profile in comparison with known drug often provide mechanistic insight into pharmacological activities of combination treatment.

Tan et al. (2005) used this strategy to identify compounds that will improve the outcome of chemotherapy in a p53-dependent fashion. Wild-type p53 can induce cell cycle arrest, which is cytostatic, or apoptosis, which is associated with tumor shrinkage. The HCT116 colon carcinoma cell line shows p53-dependent cell cycle arrest after exposure to one kind of chemotherapeutic agent, doxorubicin, but apoptosis in response to the administration of 5-fluorouracil. These investigators sought to identify compounds that would convert the doxorubicin-induced cell cycle arrest to apoptosis in a p53-dependent manner. Instead of screening genetic mutants, they screened a number of small-molecule kinase inhibitors that would function as inactive mutants of that kinase. They discovered that pharmacological inhibition of glycogen synthase kinase 3 beta (GSK3β) was capable of converting the characteristic G2 arrest to p53-dependent apoptosis. The mechanism appeared to be an augmentation of the p53-dependent conformational activation of the pro-apoptotic protein, Bax, leading to heightened apoptosis through a mitochondrial pathway. This synthetic lethality required the presence of p53, administration of a genotoxic agent such as doxorubicin and inhibition of GSK3β to augment cancer cell death (Tan et al., 2005). Importantly, these experiments broadened the use of GSK3β inhibitors, which were originally developed as antidiabetic agents, to the treatment of cancer. Thus such a systems approach to p53 biology resulted in the expanded use of leads already in clinical development (Fig. 16.6). This is, moreover, another example of a syncretic combination therapy described above.

For such a p53-dependent therapeutic agent to be effective, a precise method of determining the p53 status of a tumor will be necessary. Here again, comprehensive genomic technologies may be better than standard diagnostic approaches. Compared with the conventional methods that assess cancer genotypes through the use of various biochemical assays, such as immunohistochemistry, fluorescent *in-situ* hybridization and mutation analyses, gene profiling has the potential to provide a more precise assessment. For example, in work described by Miller et al. (2005), the status of the p53 pathway in individual breast cancers has been more precisely assessed when based on the expression of p53 signature genes rather than on the presence of the p53 mutational sequence itself. It is clear from this study that many p53 wild-type breast tumors manifest mutant p53-like expression signatures as a result of alternative mechanisms leading to attenuated levels of p53 transcript. This is an example of the coupling of precise diagnostics with precise therapeutics.

PERTURBATION ANALYSIS OF CONSTRAINED SYSTEMS TO DISCOVER NEW ANTI-CANCER DRUGS

It is further recognized that p53 wild-type tumors constitute only 50% of human tumors, and that therapies targeting wild-type p53, such

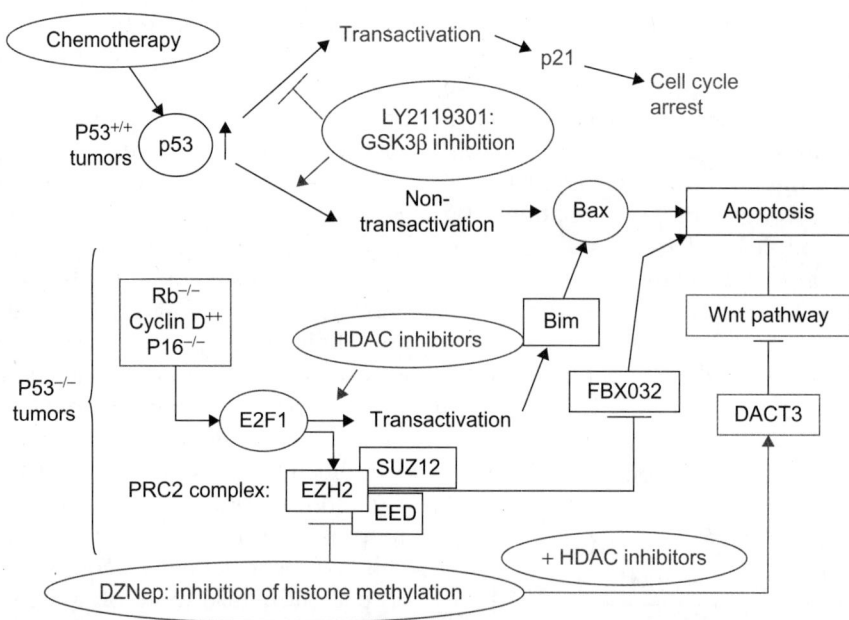

FIGURE 16.6 Therapeutic Nodes in Anticancer Treatment. Small molecules (highlighted in red) have been identified using a systems strategy to uncover compounds that would induce cancer cell apoptosis in a constrained cellular model system. For more detail, see text. DZNep, 3-deazaneplanocin; GSKβ, glycogen synthase kinase 3 beta; HDAC, histone deacetylase; PRC2, polycomb repressive complex 2; Rb, retinoblastoma.

as the GSK3β inhibitors, will not help those individuals with mutant p53-bearing tumors. Zhao et al. (2005) screened for drugs that would be active in cells with a mutant retinoblastoma gene (pRb) in a background that is p53 null. They accomplished this by engineering an inducible transcription factor, E2F1. The E2F1 complex specifically associates with and is inhibited by the active hypophosphorylated retinoblastoma protein, RB1. During late G_1 phase of the cell cycle, as the cell prepares to enter the S phase, RB1 is phosphorylated and is dissociated from the E2F complex, rendering E2F transcriptionally active. Thus overexpression of E2F1 is akin to depletion of pRB and/or p16, both of which are common events in human tumors. This system was used to screen compounds that would induce apoptosis upon activation of E2F1, and identified that histone deacetylase inhibitors (HDACI) induced programmed cell death in cells perturbed in the E2F1/Rb/p16 pathway (Zhao et al., 2005).

Epigenetic control of gene expression is partially modulated through chemical alterations—usually by methylation and acetylation—of DNA binding proteins, the histones. A major enzyme controlling histone acetylation is a family of deacetylases which can be pharmacologically inhibited by HDACIs. It was found that HDAC inhibition augmented E2F1 binding and activation of the *Bim* promoter. *Bim* was subsequently uncovered as the key factor in the induction of apoptosis arising after combined HDAC inhibition and E2F1 activation. These experiments outline the concept of perturbation analysis of "constrained" systems to uncover specific mechanisms for conditional lethality. Instead of screening potential anticancer agents that directly induce cell death, use of the constrained system identified drugs that could conditionally induce death upon E2F1 activation. This systems constraint reduces non-specific cellular toxicity and therefore increases the probability of scoring a true positive (Fig. 16.6).

An advantage of a strategy using systems constraints is that the output is tuned for a more specific set of targets and therefore the range of experimental possibilities can be restricted. For example, cell death can be caused by many factors, but narrowly constraining the operational induction of death to that caused only by available biological factors will uncover tumor necrosis factor (TNF) among the specific inducers of death. Following this principle, the E2F1 system was further used by Tan et al. (2007) to identify chemical entities with HDAC-inhibitor-like effects relative to E2F1. They found one compound, 3-deazaneplanocin A (DZNep), an S-adenosylhomocysteine hydrolase inhibitor, that induced apoptotic cell death in cancer cells but was not an HDAC inhibitor. The constrained system also allows for prioritization of pathways to interrogate. In this case, because DZNep functioned in an HDAC-inhibitor-like manner, the action of DZNep on the epigenetic configuration of the cell was explored and was found to deplete cellular concentrations of components of the epigenetic remodeling complex, the polycomb repressive complex 2 (PRC2, comprising EZH2, SUZ12 and EED) (Kleer et al., 2003; Varambally et al., 2002). This complex is responsible for histone H3-lysine 27 methylation as a mark for gene repression. Intriguingly, EZH2 is often upregulated in human cancers and is associated with blocked expression of key genes associated with tumor suppression. Thus, as a consequence of reversal of de-repression, treatment of cancer cells with DZNep leads to the upregulation of a large number of genes, many involved in the suppression of the cancer phenotype. This has been exploited to discover new cancer-suppressor genes. For example, analysis of gene expression changes induced by DZNep identified one gene, *FBXO32*, encoding the muscle atrophy F-box protein, atrogin-1, as a major mediator of DZNep-induced apoptosis (Fig. 16.6).

Constrained systems can assist in uncovering underlying mechanisms, as the possibilities are more directed and limited. The same team of investigators found empirically that a combination of DZNep and HDAC inhibitors is highly synergistic in triggering cancer cell death, with little apoptotic effect on normal cells. Given that epigenetic changes alter gene transcription, they used expression arrays to identify candidate genes that might be induced by the combined treatment. It was found that the synergy is explained by the dramatic upregulation of a natural Wnt pathway inhibitor, DACT3 (Jiang et al., 2008), which is normally silenced in colon cancer. Thus this combination of DZNep and HDAC inhibitors was pharmacologically able to reverse cancer-associated epigenetic gene repression. Intriguingly, in the course of the analysis, the investigators identified potential biomarkers for pharmacodynamic response to DZNep and HDAC inhibitors.

NETWORKS, ROBUSTNESS AND CANCER THERAPEUTIC STRATEGIES

Phenotypic analysis after specific gene disruption had been the fundamental pursuit of the field of genetics for nearly a century. With genetically tractable experimental organisms, geneticists were able to explore genetic connectivity maps and pursue experimental approaches such as synthetic lethality. Pharmacology had lagged behind because of the limited number of chemical molecules with highly specific biochemical effects, thus a systems approach was not readily applicable until recently. Contemporary systems pharmacology has matured only with the knowledge of the genome, and the availability of pharmacologic agents (small molecules, antibodies, short interfering RNA reagents) that can specifically modify isolated molecular targets within a cell. The output of targeted inhibition by a small molecule is akin to gene disruption, and effective combination therapy with targeted agents is the same as identifying synthetic lethality (Table 16.1). When experimentally tested, the correlation is good between synthetic lethality in yeast identified by either genetic or pharmacologic (small-molecule) strategies (Haggarty et al., 2003). In higher organisms, such detailed synthetic lethal maps are difficult because of the inherent complexity of the control mechanisms. Nevertheless, as will be described in subsequent sections, these connectivity maps and pharmacologic synthetic lethality tables, specific to cancer therapy, are now being drawn.

In cancer treatment, the main goal is to attack the natural robustness of any malignant cell using drugs and radiation therapy. Fundamentally, it is a strategy of inducing catastrophe in robust systems. Alternatively stated, it is targeted disruption to achieve a controlled systems failure. This is different from other pharmacologic strategies used to treat other diseases. For example, replacement therapy seeks to achieve precision in both the singularity and specificity of the replacement and the control of expression. On this point, systems pharmacologic solutions for cancer may be easier to accomplish, because there are many ways to disrupt a system. However, the difficulty lies in the level of redundancy that gives robustness to cancer cells. Therefore, in order to achieve this controlled systems failure, it is useful to be able to quantify robustness. Complex robust systems are usually characterized as having redundant systems. However, redundancy with the amplification of identical components is still subject to a systematic breakdown if a specific inherent weakness of the components is targeted; it is

TABLE 16.1 Terminology of Genetic and Pharmacologic Strategies

Genetic Terminology	Pharmacologic Equivalent
Gene disruption	Targeted inhibition
Synthetic lethality	Combination therapeutic
Phenotypic pleiotropism	Polypharmacology

just that a larger level of a single perturbation is necessary. Redundancy comprising functionally overlapping but non-identical components that are interactive with each other provides the most robust system (Figs. 16.7–16.9). Blockade of one or more nodes can still be bypassed by the many alternative pathways to downstream targets.

Experimentally, most biological systems are structured along the lines of complex systems with redundant and interactive components

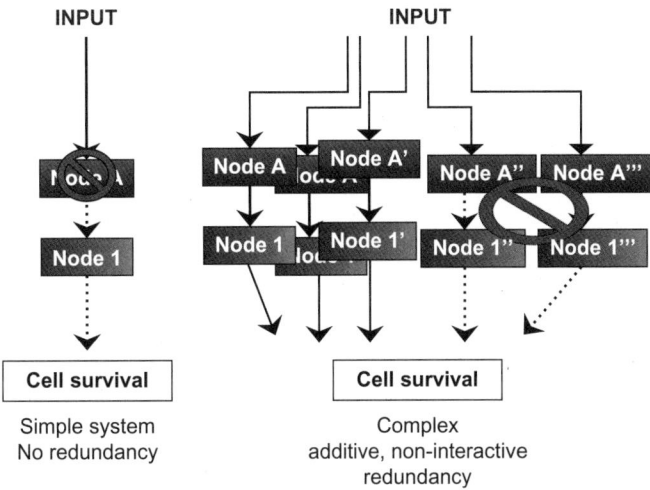

FIGURE 16.7 Robustness and Redundancy. Schematic examples of a simple system without redundant pathways, and a complex system with multiple non-interactive pathways redundant by replication. In the complex system, a single targeted perturbation, if applied with sufficient force, will neutralize all downstream components of a redundant pathway.
After Lehar et al. (2008), under the terms of the Creative Commons Attribution License.

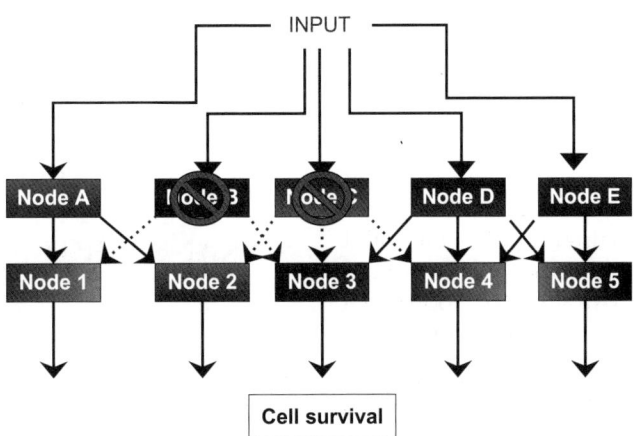

FIGURE 16.8 Robustness and Redundancy. Schematic of a complex system with redundant, non-overlapping and highly interactive redundant pathways. This model allows for alternative routing of signals even if a node is neutralized.
After Lehar et al. (2008), under the terms of the Creative Commons Attribution License.

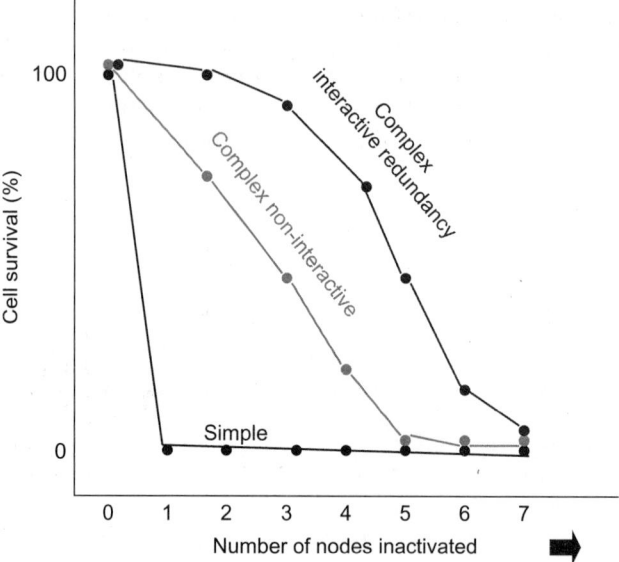

FIGURE 16.9 Robustness and Redundancy. Graphical representation of the robustness of the three systems depicted in Figures 16.7 and 16.8, as measured by cell survival.

After Lehar et al. (2008), under the terms of the Creative Commons Attribution License.

although with varying degrees of redundancy and interactivity between the nodes. In such models of robustness, a system is progressively more fragile and prone to failure as critical nodes are sequentially removed or inactivated. This fragility or robustness can be measured as a "combination order of fragility," which is defined as the point at which successive removal of nodes in a network blocks all possible alternative pathways leading to system failure (Lehar et al., 2008). Systems strategies for cancer pharmacology would seek to identify the critical nodes maintaining tumor viability, understand their connectivity and, through perturbation analysis, assess which nodes have greater influence on the system than others. The goal would be to model the robustness of a cancer and potentially to predict those combinations of targeted interventions that will lead to cancer cell death. Because each cancer is likely to represent a different system with idiosyncratic components and connectivity, it is probable that no general connectivity map can be created for all malignancies. Therefore, a truly predictive model for discovering therapeutic champions common to all cancers will not be forthcoming with current knowledge. However, it is within the horizon to be able to project possible combinations of targeted therapies that will reduce the robustness of a specific cancer cell once its component parts have been identified.

MINING THE REGULATORY PROGRAM IN THE CANCER TRANSCRIPTOME FOR NOVEL TARGETS

Towards this goal of a systems map of cancer, several strategies are now available for the comprehensive and precise identification of the regulatory components that form the critical control nodes of a cancer.

One approach to identify such regulators is through the integration of transcription factor binding sites analysis with gene expression data to define directional pathways activated in cancer signatures. Rhodes and Chinnaiyan (2005) have utilized the computational approach to identify the highly enriched putative transcription factor binding sites in the promoter sequence of the human genes. By comparing them with the gene expression signatures in cancer, transcription factors that are responsible for the observed gene expression might be identified. In this study, up to 232 regulatory programs have been identified through analysis of a large dataset from 65 independent studies that included 6732 microarray experiments. Strikingly, more than 50% of these were found to be linked to the transcription factor, E2F1, in many cancer types. These results reaffirm the importance of E2F1 in human cancer. They also provide a rationale for developing therapeutic strategies for targeting the E2F1 pathway for more cancer-selective killing. As described before, HDACIs can activate E2F1-induced apoptosis through transcriptional activation of the pro-apoptotic gene, *Bim* (Zhao et al., 2005). NF-Y is a CCAAT-box binding transcription factor that plays a part in tissue-specific major histocompatibility complex class II gene transcription. Sites of NF-Y binding to genes involved in cancer signatures were also found to be common, and usually coincided with the E2F1 regulatory program. Given that NF-Y binding to certain gene promoters is necessary for E2F1 activity, and that NF-Y transactivation is dependent on phosphorylation by the cyclin-dependent kinase 2 (CDK2), it is therefore possible to target CDK2 for repressing the NF-Y and E2F1 regulatory program in cancer.

Obviously, the computation-based identification of putative transcription factor-binding sites has its limitations and might generate false predictions. Recently developed new technologies such as chromatin immunoprecipitation coupled with genomic tiling arrays (ChIP-on-chip) or a sequencing-based approach such as paired-end ditag (ChIP–PET) allow experimental genome-wide identification of genome-wide transcription factor binding sites (Wei et al., 2006a). Using these technologies, genomic binding sites have been mapped out for increasing numbers of oncogenic transcriptional factors that are important in cancer, such as p53, Myc, E2F1, NF-κB and ER (Bieda et al., 2006; Lim et al., 2007; Lin et al., 2007; Wei et al., 2006a; Zeller et al., 2006). The data generated from these studies, when integrated into a comprehensive transcriptional network, will provide precision in identifying direct targets of key transcription factors.

Transcriptional signatures of physiologic responses can uncover fundamental control networks in cancer, which can triangulate to new therapeutic targets. Genes coordinately induced in fibroblasts in response to serum stimulation has been used as surrogates for a tissue "wound response" (Iyer et al., 1999), which has been

---

BOX 16.2

TARGETING TRANSCRIPTION FACTORS

Targeting transcription factors has historically been difficult, because their functional domains are not as structurally amenable to tight docking as are those of enzymes. This limits the specificity of chemical disruptors to the individual transcription factor targets. Also, the amount of drug required to inhibit the action of a transcription factor is usually much greater than is required of those that inhibit enzymatic functions. For these reasons, pharmaceutical development of anti-transcription factor therapeutics has not been pursued. Nevertheless, the recent development of small-molecule disruptors of p53–MDM2 interaction, such as nutlin-3, appears to be countering this bias (Vassilev, 2007).

correlated with poor prognosis in breast cancer, even when proliferative genes are removed from the gene list (Chang et al., 2005). As gene amplification is a mechanism for "hard wiring" overexpression of genes in cancer, Adler and colleagues (2006) sought to explain the transcriptional origin of the wound signature in aggressive breast cancer by correlating the wound response signature (defined by expression microarrays) to gene copy number changes (defined by array-comparative genomic hybridization (CGH) assessing chromosomal amplification). Using the wound response expression cassette in tumors as the dependent variable, they asked which regions of gene amplification appeared to be correlated with this expression profile. The purpose was to identify those genes within genomic amplicons that might transcriptionally affect the wound response cassette. In this study, several genes on chromosome 8q, specifically 8q24 and 8q13, were found to be amplified in those tumors with the activated wound signature. Within these linked amplicons, the oncogene, *MYC*, and *CSN5*, a general activator of the cullen ubiquitin ligase complexes, were both found to be amplified in tumors with the activated wound expression signature, and Adler et al. hypothesized that they may functionally interact to regulate the transcription of the wound response cassette. In the validation experiments, these two genes, *MYC* and *CSN5*, were overexpressed in MCF10A cells (derived from non-cancerous human breast epithelial cells). Whereas overexpression of *MYC* and *CSN5*, individually, yielded only partial modulation of the wound signature genes, the simultaneous overexpression of both genes induced the synergistic transcriptional response indicative of the wound signature (Adler et al., 2006). This is an example of transcriptional epistasis, in that the interaction of two genes was necessary to fully regulate the prognostic wound signature phenotype, and it underscores the need for simultaneous interruption of several targets for full anticancer effects to be seen.

Pujana et al. (2007) used a similar network modeling strategy to uncover novel genes potentially associated with the risk for breast cancer. Using gene expression profiling from primary tumors, cross-referenced with functional genomic and protein association data from various species, they generated a network of 118 genes connected through 866 potential functional associations that arose from exploring relationships with four known genes encoding tumor suppressors in breast cancer. The higher-order signaling network map implicated a new candidate cancer susceptibility gene, HMMR, from this network analysis. HMMR encodes a centrosome subunit and is linked in function with the breast-cancer-associated gene, *BRCA1*, and in a case–control association study of breast cancer susceptibility the HMMR locus appeared to be associated with greater risk of breast cancer. Thus computational network analysis uncovered a potential new target for cancer therapeutics.

The above pathways were constructed using two-hybrid systems, and data/text mining associations. Although the analysis can infer hierarchy and directionality, the data are not truly quantitative, and therefore not subject to certain statistical approaches. Sachs et al. (2005) approached this problem by using single-cell analysis and labeled phospho-specific antibodies to assess differences in phospho-signaling configurations in primary human $CD4^+$ T cells. Using multicolor flow cytometry, they assessed the simultaneous measurement of 11 phosphorylated protein and phospholipid components in individual hematopoietic cells, following 10 antibody or targeted small-molecule challenges that either activate or inhibit specific signaling nodes. The uniqueness of their approach is that tens of thousands of cells could be analyzed for each condition for the 11 parameters, and therefore could be subjected to Bayesian network modeling of signaling pathways. With this approach, statistically meaningful relationships and dependencies between the molecular components of a signaling network were inferred, allowed for the *de-novo* ordering of connections between network components, and predicted new pathway interactions. This map correlated very well to others drawn from several decades of biochemical and genetic experimentation. The same group of investigators also subjected primary acute myelogenous leukemia cells to similar perturbations, and found that a limited phosphoprotein profile could segregate patients into clinically meaningful subsets (Irish et al., 2004). This represents a dynamic diagnostic derived from perturbation-generated systems maps.

INTEGRATING EXPERIMENTAL AND PRIMARY TUMOR EXPRESSION DATA FOR NOVEL BIOMARKERS FOR THERAPEUTIC EFFICACY

The rapidly expanding repositories of primary tumor gene expression data contain a vast amount of information about the process of human cancer. However, this information currently is largely static, in that there is sparse perturbation analysis and it is not possible easily to define the mechanisms underlying a disease process. However, as described above, expression profiling using established cancer cell lines can be analyzed dynamically by following temporal changes in expression after chemical perturbations. As cancer cell lines have been shown, to a certain degree, to retain the majority of the gene deregulation present in primary tumors, integrating results from *in-vitro* experiments with *in-vivo* cancer signatures might make it possible to infer the activity of a specific oncogenic pathway *in vivo*. Bild et al. (2006) explored this approach and generated gene signatures that represent the state of activation of individual oncogenic pathways.

They used recombinant retroviruses to express various oncogenic signals in quiescent human mammary epithelial cells (HMECs) so that the generated gene expression profiles could be used to predict the status of a particular oncogenic event. The experimentally derived gene signatures have been successfully used to predict Myc and Ras status in mammary tumors in transgenic mice expressing *Myc* or *Ras*. Furthermore, combining of pathway signatures shows a real predictive power. Analysis of lung tumors showed that adenocarcinomas predicted to have low-level *Ras* activity generally also have increased *Myc, E2F3, β-catenin* and *Src* activity. This information is particularly important in guiding target-based therapeutics. Indeed, growth inhibition measured in cell lines exposed to Ras or Src inhibitors correlated well with the predicted status of the corresponding pathway (Bieda et al., 2006). In the past 20 years, a substantial number of therapeutic drugs targeting specific oncogenic pathways have been developed. Thus the real power of genomic profiling technology is its capability of developing a sufficient complexity of data, thereby providing a comprehensive view of the underlying deregulation of many pathways simultaneously and helping in the development of an effective therapeutic strategy.

In addition to the success of using biomarkers to select individuals for targeted therapeutics, the same approach can also be applied to chemotherapeutic agents that affect several pathways and are thus more complex in action. The US National Cancer Institute has screened more than 100000 anticancer compounds, using a panel of 60 diverse human cancer cell lines (NCI-60). Microarray analysis of the expression levels has been used to identify a set of genes that are most associated with drug sensitivity. The findings have provided a rich database of the *in-vitro* effects of these compounds, which can be used to predict the clinical response of patients (Lee et al., 2007; Potti et al., 2006; Staunton et al., 2001). This integrated approach seems to be valid, because the *in-vitro*-developed expression profiles can accurately predict clinical response in individuals treated with these drugs (Potti et al., 2006). For example, a set of 50 genes with expression levels most likely to correlate with drug sensitivity in cancer cell lines has been successfully used to identify individuals who respond to docetaxel in the clinic. Using this approach, a panel of gene signatures that predict chemotherapeutic sensitivity has been identified. Strikingly, these individual signatures can also predict responses to combinations of drugs. Furthermore, by integrating with the oncogenic pathway signature, tumors predicted to be resistant to chemotherapy can be rendered sensitive using specific pathway-targeted agents. For example, cancer cells predicted to be topotecan resistant were found to have a greater likelihood of Src pathway deregulation, and thus can be treated in combination with an Src inhibitor. Thus these studies demonstrated the power of using systems approaches to guide the use of anticancer drugs and to identify the optimal therapeutic options in cancer (Potti et al., 2006).

In another application of expression signatures, Antipova et al. (2008) used a gene expression signature as a surrogate of a biological state associated with a specific signaling pathway. Perturbations of this gene expression signature were then used as the readout in small-molecule screens for inhibitors of a specific pathway, PDGFR/ERK. How they extracted this signature is informative. First, a neuroblastoma cell line was treated with the BB homodimer of PDGF (PDGF-BB), resulting in PDGFRβ and downstream ERK activation. The temporal activation of constituents of the PDGFβ pathway was monitored for changes in their levels of phosphorylation after administration of the growth factor. The investigators then performed gene expression profiling at the peak time for PDGF stimulation. In order to devolve the component of the gene expression signature attributable to ERK activation by PDGFR (as opposed to other pathways downstream of PDGFR), gene expression profiles were obtained from cells pretreated with either an MAPK kinase (MEK) inhibitor or an ERK inhibitor. Genes not affected by the MEK inhibitor, but reversed by the ERK inhibitor after PDGF stimulation, were deemed markers that reflect the PDGF-stimulated state. Using the top three genes strongly upregulated by activation of ERK through PDGFR (c-fos, early growth response 1 [EGR1], and activity-regulated cytoskeleton-associated protein [ARC]), they then screened 1739 compounds in active use for their inability to inhibit the induction of the three-gene cassette after PDGF induction. Three compounds were identified from this screen. Upon detailed studies, one, aurintricarboxylic acid (ATA), showed a unique mechanism of action. ATA appeared to inhibit PDGFR signaling by potentially inhibiting PDGF binding to the extracellular domain of PDGFR, and/or disrupting ligand-induced activation of the receptor. Thus expression signatures can be used simply to identify new leads for targeted therapeutics in cancer.

GENE SIGNATURES TO REVEAL THE DRUG ACTION–GENE FUNCTION CONNECTIVITY MAP

Some agents are known to target specific cellular targets but selectively induce the death of cancer cells by as yet unknown mechanism. Examples include HDACIs and heat-shock protein 90 (HSP90) inhibitors such as geldanamycin. These agents might induce the therapeutic effect in cancer cells through a collection of cancer-specific changes not seen in normal cells (Nebbioso et al., 2005; Zhao et al., 2005). A great challenge in current pharmacology research is to develop a systematic approach that connects gene function and drug action using one analytic system with high-throughput capability for quantitative and digital measurements. This concept has been recently illustrated by scientists at Broad Institute, who have successfully developed a solution to the problem of identifying functional connections between drugs and genes and diseases (Lamb et al., 2006). In this study, a "connectivity map" was generated in which a large reference collection of gene-expression data from cultured human cells treated with many bioactive small-molecule chemicals has been used to find connections among small molecules sharing a mechanism of action and to uncover the target pathways of poorly characterized small molecules.

This new approach was further applied to solve the real-world problems in cancer research as demonstrated in two recent studies. In the first case, the generated gene activity map derived from cell lines treated with 167 compounds was used to predict the action of poorly characterized compounds. This chemical genomics approach classified HSP90 inhibitors as having activity similar to that of androgen-receptor activation inhibitors, and found gedunin, an HSP90 inhibitor, to be active in inhibiting androgen-receptor signaling. This work identified new modes of HSP90 modulation through the use of a strategy based on gene expression, which can be applied as a general approach to discovery and target prediction of modulators of cancer phenotypes (Hieronymus et al., 2006). In the second case, the same gene expression database was screened for molecules having profiles that overlapped with a gene expression signature of glucocorticoid sensitivity/resistance in acute lymphoblastic leukemia cells. The screen found that the mammalian target of rapamycin (mTOR) inhibitor, rapamycin, induced a gene expression signature that matches glucocorticoid sensitivity, immediately suggesting the possibility for rapamycin to induce glucocorticoid sensitivity in lymphoid malignancy cells. This hypothesis was further experimentally confirmed by showing that rapamycin sensitizes to glucocorticoid-induced apoptosis via modulation of antiapoptotic myeloid cell leukemia-1 (MCL1) and identified a drug that is capable of reversing glucocorticoid resistance in acute lymphoblastic leukemia (ALL) cell (Wei et al., 2006b). The study represents an example of a strategy for the identification of promising combination therapies for cancer, based on predictions from the expression signatures that are linked to specific functions.

Together, these two studies demonstrate that the connectivity map can be used to generate testable hypotheses about the target pathways of poorly characterized small molecules. In each case, the database mining predicted an anticancer activity that was subsequently demonstrated in model systems.

CONCLUDING REMARKS

The complexity of cellular network control in cancer requires a systems approaches to dissect and exploit several nodes for perturbation. Systems strategies in human cell biology and in therapeutics are limited by the sheer complexity of higher organisms. However, with the knowledge of the genome sequences, genetic tools to interrupt the function of specific genes and the availability of large libraries of small molecules targeting specific protein products, such systems approaches are now productive. Although the future is bright, applications of systems approaches in cancer pharmacology remain nascent and incomplete. There are, however, special characteristics of cancer that both challenge and accelerate discovery in this field. The greatest challenge is the genetic plasticity and resulting complexity of the cancer genome; because of the unique mutations, rearrangements and epigenetic changes, every cancer is a special genome in itself. Thus knowledge of these individual cancer genomes will need to be included in the systems modeling. Fortunately, new sequencing technologies will permit the precise identification of all mutations in a cancer genome in a cost-effective and timely manner. The advantage of systems pharmacology in cancer treatment is that dismantling protective redundancies to induce a state of relative fragility can be accomplished by many means, as compared with reconstructing perfectly controlled normal systems.

Going forward, we will need to re-examine the cellular systems that cancer pharmacology has frequently used as model systems utilizing all the comprehensive tools in genomics and proteomics. These component maps will be the first step in building the true cartography of the cancer cell that ultimately can be used as a roadmap for targeted therapeutics.

References

Adler, A.S., Lin, M., Horlings, H., Nuyten, D.S., van de Vijver, M.J., Chang, H.Y., 2006. Genetic regulators of large-scale transcriptional signatures in cancer. Nat. Genet. 38, 421–430.

Aladjem, M.I., Spike, B.T., Rodewald, L.W., et al., 1998. ES cells do not activate p53-dependent stress responses and undergo p53-independent apoptosis in response to DNA damage. Curr. Biol. 8, 145–155.

Antipova, A.A., Stockwell, B.R., Golub, T.R., 2008. Gene expression-based screening for inhibitors of PDGFR signaling. Genome. Biol. 9, R47.

Bieda, M., Xu, X., Singer, M.A., Green, R., Farnham, P.J., 2006. Unbiased location analysis of E2F1-binding sites suggests a widespread role for E2F1 in the human genome. Genome. Res. 16, 595–605.

Bild, A.H., Yao, G., Chang, J.T., Wang, Q., et al., 2006. Oncogenic pathway signatures in human cancers as a guide to targeted therapies. Nature 439, 353–357.

Borisy, A.A., Elliott, P.J., Hurst, N.W., et al., 2003. Systematic discovery of multicomponent therapeutics. Proc. Natl. Acad. Sci. USA 100, 7977–7982.

Chang, H.Y., Nuyten, D.S., Sneddon, J.B., et al., 2005. Robustness, scalability, and integration of a wound-response gene expression signature in predicting breast cancer survival. Proc. Natl. Acad. Sci. USA 102, 3738–3743.

Engelman, J.A., Janne, P.A., Mermel, C., et al., 2005. ErbB-3 mediates phosphoinositide 3-kinase activity in gefitinib-sensitive non-small cell lung cancer cell lines. Proc. Natl. Acad. Sci. USA 102, 3788–3793.

Fabian 3rd, M.A., Biggs, W.H., Treiber, D.K., et al., 2005. A small molecule-kinase interaction map for clinical kinase inhibitors. Nat. Biotechnol. 23, 329–336.

Farmer, H., McCabe, N., Lord, C.J., et al., 2005. Targeting the DNA repair defect in BRCA mutant cells as a therapeutic strategy. Nature 434, 917–921.

Greenman, C., Stephens, P., Smith, R., et al., 2007. Patterns of somatic mutation in human cancer genomes. Nature 446, 153–158.

Haggarty, S.J., Koeller, K.M., Wong, J.C., Butcher, R.A., Schreiber, S.L., 2003. Multidimensional chemical genetic analysis of diversity-oriented synthesis-derived deacetylase inhibitors using cell-based assays. Chem. Biol. 10, 383–396.

Hanahan, D., Weinberg, R.A., 2000. The hallmarks of cancer. Cell 100, 57–70.

Hieronymus, H., Lamb, J., Ross, K.N., et al., 2006. Gene expression signature-based chemical genomic prediction identifies a novel class of HSP90 pathway modulators. Cancer Cell 10, 321–330.

Irish, J.M., Hovland, R., Krutzik, P.O., et al., 2004. Single cell profiling of potentiated phospho-protein networks in cancer cells. Cell 118, 217–228.

Iyer, V.R., Eisen, M.B., Ross, D.T., et al., 1999. The transcriptional program in the response of human fibroblasts to serum. Science 283, 83–87.

Janne, P.A., 2005. Ongoing first-line studies of epidermal growth factor receptor tyrosine kinase inhibitors in select patient populations. Semin. Oncol. 32, S9–S15.

Jiang, X., Tan, J., Li, J., et al., 2008. DACT3 is an epigenetic regulator of Wnt/beta-catenin signaling in colorectal cancer and is a therapeutic target of histone modifications. Cancer Cell 13, 529–541.

Kaelin Jr., W.G., 2005. The concept of synthetic lethality in the context of anticancer therapy. Nat. Rev. Cancer 5, 689–698.

Keith, C.T., Borisy, A.A., Stockwell, B.R., 2005. Multicomponent therapeutics for networked systems. Nat. Rev. Drug Discov. 4, 71–78.

Kleer, C.G., Cao, Q., Varambally, S., et al., 2003. EZH2 is a marker of aggressive breast cancer and promotes neoplastic transformation of breast epithelial cells. Proc. Natl. Acad. Sci. USA 100, 11606–11611.

Koivunen, J.P., Mermel, C., Zejnullahu, K., et al., 2008. EML4-ALK fusion gene and efficacy of an ALK kinase inhibitor in lung cancer. Clin. Cancer Res. 14, 4275–4283.

Lamb, J., Crawford, E.D., Peck, D., et al., 2006. The Connectivity Map: using gene-expression signatures to connect small molecules, genes, and disease. Science 313, 1929–1935.

Lee, J.K., Havaleshko, D.M., Cho, H., et al., 2007. A strategy for predicting the chemosensitivity of human cancers and its application to drug discovery. Proc. Natl. Acad. Sci. USA 104, 13086–13091.

Lehar, J., Krueger, A., Zimmermann, G., Borisy, A., 2008. High-order combination effects and biological robustness. Mol. Syst. Biol. 4, 215.

Lim, C.A., Yao, F., Wong, J.J., et al., 2007. Genome-wide mapping of RELA(p65) binding identifies E2F1 as a transcriptional activator recruited by NF-kappaB upon TLR4 activation. Mol. Cell 27, 622–635.

Lin, C.Y., Vega, V.B., Thomsen, J.S., et al., 2007. Whole-genome cartography of estrogen receptor alpha binding sites. PLoS Genet. 3, e87.

Marton, M.J., DeRisi, J.L., Bennett, H.A., et al., 1998. Drug target validation and identification of secondary drug target effects using DNA microarrays. Nat. Med. 4, 1293–1301.

Mellinghoff, I.K., Wang, M.Y., Vivanco, I., et al., 2005. Molecular determinants of the response of glioblastomas to EGFR kinase inhibitors. N. Engl. J. Med. 353, 2012–2024.

Miller, L.D., Smeds, J., George, J., et al., 2005. An expression signature for p53 status in human breast cancer predicts mutation status, transcriptional effects, and patient survival. Proc. Natl. Acad. Sci. USA 102, 13550–13555.

Nebbioso, A., Clarke, N., Voltz, E., et al., 2005. Tumor-selective action of HDAC inhibitors involves TRAIL induction in acute myeloid leukemia cells. Nat. Med. 11, 77–84.

Paolini, G.V., Shapland, R.H., van Hoorn, W.P., Mason, J.S., Hopkins, A.L., 2006. Global mapping of pharmacological space. Nat. Biotechnol. 24, 805–815.

Potti, A., Dressman, H.K., Bild, A., et al., 2006. Genomic signatures to guide the use of chemotherapeutics. Nat. Med. 12, 1294–1300.

Pujana, M.A., Han, J.D., Starita, L.M., et al., 2007. Network modeling links breast cancer susceptibility and centrosome dysfunction. Nat. Genet. 39, 1338–1349.

Rhodes, D.R., Chinnaiyan, A.M., 2005. Integrative analysis of the cancer transcriptome. Nat. Genet. 37 (suppl), S31–S37.

Sachs, K., Perez, O., Pe'er, D., Lauffenburger, D.A., Nolan, G.P., 2005. Causal protein-signaling networks derived from multiparameter single-cell data. Science 308, 523–529.

Simon, J.A., Szankasi, P., Nguyen, D.K., et al., 2000. Differential toxicities of anticancer agents among DNA repair and checkpoint mutants of Saccharomyces cerevisiae. Cancer Res. 60, 328–333.

Sjoblom, T., Jones, S., Wood, L.D., et al., 2006. The consensus coding sequences of human breast and colorectal cancers. Science 314, 268–274.

Soda, M., Choi, Y.L., Enomoto, M., et al., 2007. Identification of the transforming EML4-ALK fusion gene in non-small-cell lung cancer. Nature 448, 561–566.

Staunton, J.E., Slonim, D.K., Coller, H.A., et al., 2001. Chemosensitivity prediction by transcriptional profiling. Proc. Natl. Acad. Sci. USA 98, 10787–10792.

Stommel, J.M., Kimmelman, A.C., Ying, H., et al., 2007. Coactivation of receptor tyrosine kinases affects the response of tumor cells to targeted therapies. Science 318, 287–290.

Strausberg, R.L., Schreiber, S.L., 2003. From knowing to controlling: a path from genomics to drugs using small molecule probes. Science 300, 294–295.

Tan, J., Zhuang, L., Leong, H.S., Iyer, N.G., Liu, E.T., Yu, Q., 2005. Pharmacologic modulation of glycogen synthase kinase-3beta promotes p53-dependent apoptosis through a direct Bax-mediated mitochondrial pathway in colorectal cancer cells. Cancer Res. 65, 9012–9020.

Tan, J., Yang, X., Zhuang, L., et al., 2007. Pharmacologic disruption of Polycomb-repressive complex 2-mediated gene repression selectively induces apoptosis in cancer cells. Genes. Dev. 21, 1050–1063.

Terstappen, G.C., Schlupen, C., Raggiaschi, R., Gaviraghi, G., 2007. Target deconvolution strategies in drug discovery. Nat. Rev. Drug Discov. 6, 891–903.

Tomlins, S.A., Rhodes, D.R., Perner, S., et al., 2005. Recurrent fusion of TMPRSS2 and ETS transcription factor genes in prostate cancer. Science 310, 644–648.

Tomlins, S.A., Laxman, B., Dhanasekaran, S.M., et al., 2007. Distinct classes of chromosomal rearrangements create oncogenic ETS gene fusions in prostate cancer. Nature 448, 595–599.

Varambally, S., Dhanasekaran, S.M., Zhou, M., et al., 2002. The polycomb group protein EZH2 is involved in progression of prostate cancer. Nature 419, 624–629.

Vassilev, L.T., 2007. MDM2 inhibitors for cancer therapy. Trends Mol. Med. 13, 23–31.

Wei, C.L., Wu, Q., Vega, V.B., et al., 2006a. A global map of p53 transcription-factor binding sites in the human genome. Cell 124, 207–219.

Wei, G., Twomey, D., Lamb, J., et al., 2006b. Gene expression-based chemical genomics identifies rapamycin as a modulator of MCL1 and glucocorticoid resistance. Cancer Cell 10, 331–342.

Whitehurst, A.W., Bodemann, B.O., Cardenas, J., et al., 2007. Synthetic lethal screen identification of chemosensitizer loci in cancer cells. Nature 446, 815–819.

Wood, L.D., Parsons, D.W., Jones, S., et al., 2007. The genomic landscapes of human breast and colorectal cancers. Science 318, 1108–1113.

Wong, C.I., Thng, C.H., Soo, R., et al., 2007. Phase I and biomarker study of ABT869, a multiple receptor tyrosine kinase inhibitor, in patients with refractory solid malignancies. Journal of Clinical Oncology, 2007 ASCO Annual Meeting Proceedings Part I. Vol 25, No. 18S (June 20 Supplement), 3519.

Zeller, K.I., Zhao, X., Lee, C.W., et al., 2006. Global mapping of c-Myc binding sites and target gene networks in human B cells. Proc. Natl. Acad. Sci. USA 103, 17834–17839.

Zhao, Y., Tan, J., Zhuang, L., Jiang, X., Liu, E.T., Yu, Q., 2005. Inhibitors of histone deacetylases target the Rb-E2F1 pathway for apoptosis induction through activation of proapoptotic protein Bim. Proc. Natl. Acad. Sci. USA 102, 16090–16095.

CHAPTER 17

Systems Biology in Drug Discovery: Using Predictive Biomedicine to Guide Development Choices for Novel Agents in Cancer

Greg Tucker-Kellogg[1,2], Amit Aggarwal[1], Kerry Blanchard[2] and Richard Gaynor[3]

[1]Lilly Singapore Centre For Drug Discovery, Singapore
[2]National University of Singapore, Singapore
[3]Lilly Research Laboratories, Indianapolis

OUTLINE

Summary	399	Integrating and Extending Cancer Cell Model Data	404
Introduction	400	Systems-oriented Target Identification	405
Systems Biology in Drug Discovery	401	Translating from Discovery to the Clinic	407
From Clinical Genomics to Model Systems	403	Concluding Remarks	412

Summary

Whole-systems approaches have radically integrated the use of computational analysis with high-throughput experimentation in discovery biology. In clinical practice, such approaches have also changed the clinical description of disease, using molecular signatures to identify new subtypes of disease and new standards of prognosis. These data-driven approaches are useful well before, or in the absence of, obtaining an understanding of the molecular disease etiology. A similar strategy is being used, not only to characterize disease and prognosis, but also to predict clinical response, with the aim of guiding the use of chemotherapeutic and targeted agents in cancer. We describe how systems approaches for predictive biomedicine—integrating discovery and clinical data—can be applied to identify novel targets, predictive biomarkers of response to agents in development and targeted use of drug combinations. Our aim in these approaches is for new agents, the development of which is guided by predictive biomedicine to improve outcomes for individual cancer patients.

INTRODUCTION

In the past 25 years, we have seen the beginnings of what promises to be a dramatic change in approaches to therapeutic treatment of cancer (Di Cosimo and Baselga, 2008; Jordan 2003). This clinical prospect stems from the advancing science of cancer biology, especially the broad recognition that, as cancers are highly heterogeneous diseases acquired over a lifetime through accumulation of somatic genetic and epigenetic aberrations, new pharmacologic interventions should target the molecular basis of disease in each patient, rather than just the proliferative nature of cancer cells. However, the initial optimism of targeted agents in cancer has been tempered with the increasing understanding of the complexity of disease, the pleiotropic role of genes in disease etiology and the multitargeted actions of many drugs, leading to the realization that both diseases and disease interventions need to be seen as dynamic systems instead of highly specific drugs attacking a well characterized target.

The first molecularly targeted agent approved for use in cancer with an accompanying *in-vitro* diagnostic assay was trastuzumab (Hall and Cameron, 2009), a monoclonal antibody targeting the oncogene ErbB2 (HER-2/neu) receptor involved in epidermal growth factor receptor (EGFR) signaling in HER2-positive breast cancers.

Following the approval of trastuzumab, other agents were develpoed that also targeted known somatic genetic defects: cetuximab and erlotinib for EGFR activation (Mendelsohn and Baselga, 2006) and gefitinib targeting the Bcr–Abl fusion protein in chronic myelogenous leukemia (CML). Even agents designed to target a specific genetic defect can have benefit in other tumor types, through inhibiting secondary target; this is exemplified by the action of gefitnib in gastrointestinal stromal tumors, in which it targets activated c-Kit instead of Bcr–Abl. Some more recently approved agents, such as sorafenib, intentionally target several members of signaling cascades dysregulated in tumors, taking advantage of the multitargeted nature of many kinase inhibitors (Petrelli and Giordano, 2008).

During the same period, we have seen a phenomenal explosion in the generation of experimental data in the wake of the human genome project, making possible a wide range of whole-genome measurements unimaginable just a few years before. Gene expression microarrays, proteomics, metabalomics, next-generation sequencing, epigenomics and RNA interference (RNAi) studies have each increased the complexity and volume of data beyond what might otherwise be simple biological experiments, and have pushed biologists to lift their eyes from any single target to focus instead on networks, pathways and systems at several levels of regulation.

Finally, rapid advances in computational processing power, data storage, modeling and analysis have become available to make such data interpretable. It is now increasingly the case that biologists turn to computer scientists for help dealing with the mountains of complex data, as computer scientists turn to biologists for inspiration and interesting challenges. Indeed, significant advances in computational biology are now frequently made in collaboration with experimental biologists, and even small experimental laboratories are now hiring computational professionals to help manage and analyze increasingly complex data. The complexity of modern biological studies is such that it is possible to see a time in the near future when studying biology will be virtually impossible without informatics and computational biology specialists.

The convergence of these three trends—targeted therapies in cancer, post-genomic system-wide experimentation platforms and unprecedented advances in information technology—lays the foundation for the application of systems biology to drug discovery in cancer. This convergence has already begun to affect the clinical practice of medicine; the challenge is to apply this approach to developing the next generation of drugs to improve outcome in individual patients.

SYSTEMS BIOLOGY IN DRUG DISCOVERY

When Systems Biology was first conceived, the potential for accurate modeling of dynamic multi-scale biological processes was seen by many as the ultimate toolbox, integrating large-scale experimental data with accurate modeling and simulation (Kitano, 2002). It is indeed true that systems-level approaches to biology have generated increasingly sophisticated models of pathways and gene regulatory networks. The integration of computational analysis with systems-level experimental data to affect clinical practice has, however, more often advanced using predictive models without any such representation. The first use of systems-level data from clinical cancer samples was a data-driven predictive model (Golub et al., 1999), and that has been followed by a flood of studies taking a data-driven approach instead of the dynamic modeling approach.

Does the success of data-driven models mean that the systems biology vision of dynamic multi-scale biological modeling has less opportunity in a drug discovery environment? Not at all, but the axiom "all models are wrong, but some are useful" is especially pertinent here. Systems biology provides an integrative means of approaching drug discovery that enables better decisions to be made: choosing the right targets, alone and in combination, choosing the right models to study those targets, understanding more completely the role of those targets and pathways in disease, and making better choices when taking programs into clinical development. Applying systems biology in drug discovery requires integrating the processes of systems biology studies with the processes—the systems—governing research and development in a large organization. Dynamic systems models of biology also have a role in drug discovery (Fitzgerald et al., 2006; Kumar et al., 2006), and may play an essential bridging function with the increasing importance of quantitative pharmacology and model-based approaches to drug development (Zhang et al., 2006, 2008).

Several authors have written extensively about applying systems biology approaches to problems of drug discovery. Zhu and co-workers (2008) have taken a rigorous network-based approach to the problem of the identification of metabolic and cardiovascular targets, constructing probabilistic causal networks from integration of gene expression data, genetic variation data and clinical or model system covariates. This integrative approach allows systematic identification of pathways underlying the causal factors of genetically associated diseases in cases in which more conventional approaches would have failed. In parallel to advances in rigorous *in-silico* target identification, some systems biologists have chosen explicitly to set aside the problem of target identification, and instead take an approach driven by experimental biology, screening compounds using complex cellular systems that are believed to be more relevant to disease (Butcher et al., 2004). This latter approach coincides with a general increase in interest in phenotypic screening, an acknowledgment of the challenges of target validation and the recognition of the value of multitargeted agents.

When applied to cancer, systems-based approaches to drug discovery present a unique opportunity to take advantage of the growing compendium of clinical cancer genomic data and to integrate these data with available model systems through informatics. We see systems biology as having a number of currently important roles in our drug discovery and development needs, most centrally (Fig. 17.1):

1. Identifying and validating targets in discovery, utilizing clinical genomic data and genome-wide perturbation.
2. Identifying and implementing clinically relevant biomarkers from preclinical studies.
3. Implementing quantitative and testable models to test hypotheses on dosing, combination and patient-stratification.

These are, ultimately, choices enabling translational decisions, made possible in cancer drug development by the increasing availability of genomic data from diseased tissue. They are also urgent decisions: it is not sufficient to use early clinical response data as the first pieces of evidence to decide which patients are likely to respond to a novel agent, when translational approaches promoting model systems may provide an opportunity to gather reliable evidence for such choices before the first patient response is observed.

It should not go without mention that systems-based approaches to small-molecule design and characterization have also been used productively in drug discovery (Vieth et al., 2004, 2005), but those approaches are not the focus here.

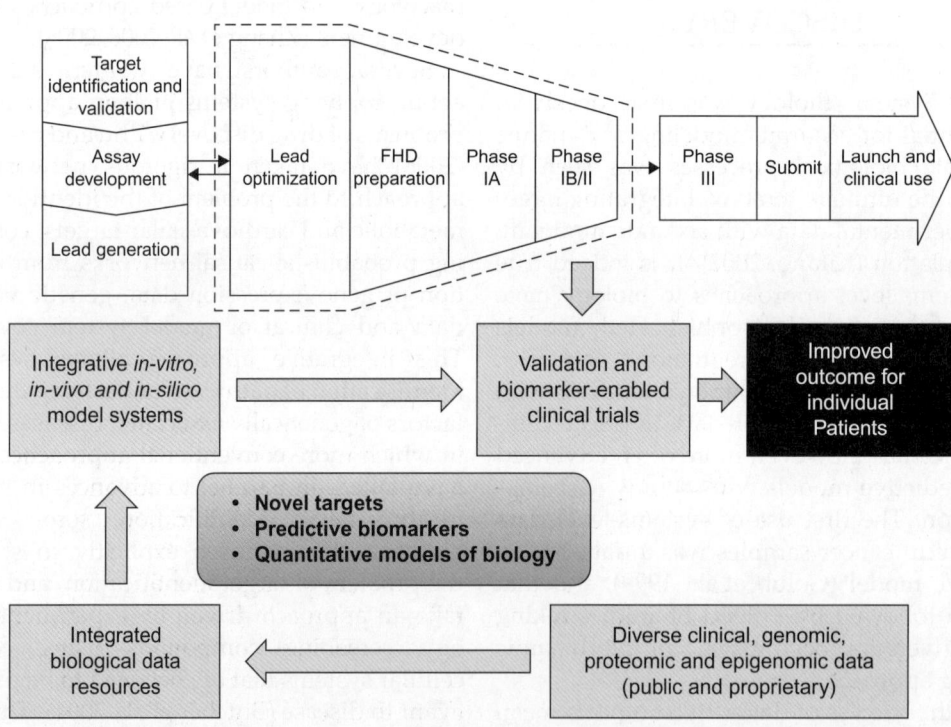

FIGURE 17.1   Leveraging Integrative Systems Approaches in Drug Discovery.

From Clinical Genomics to Model Systems

Applying systems approaches translationally to drug discovery presents a two-way challenge. The common objective of translational research is to apply basic research to clinical practice, in the form of improved diagnostics, decision support systems, imaging technology, patient monitoring and countless other areas that can improve patient care. However, the translational challenge in drug discovery also runs the other direction: experiments in cell lines and preclinical models need to be performed before a drug is administered to a patient. A standing challenge is choosing and using these models in such a way that they improve successful prosecution of the drug discovery pipeline and provide translational utility in the clinic.

Fortunately, the increased availability of integrative clinical genomic data has provided an opportunity to assess the ultimate translational utility of models used in discovery, and to provide evidence to connect the models used in experimentation to clinical practice. An illustration of the cycle from integrative clinical data to essential model systems to decision-making with clinical impact is shown in Figure 17.1, with the essential process of generating integrated "omics" data resources from clinical disease tissue data shown in the arrow on the bottom. The vast majority of these clinical genomic data studies come from patient studies initiated by universities, clinical centers and research institutes around the world. For our purposes in the business of drug discovery, we do not expect to compete with these efforts, but to (i) underpin them and (ii) supplement them as needed.

Cancer is a diverse family of acquired genetic diseases, diversity of disease being defined, not by the diversity among cell lines—many of which may be far removed from their deceased tissue of origin—but by the molecular diversity observed in disease tissue itself. A central theme when choosing models along the lines described above is that clinical samples, not model systems, determine the clinical relevance of targets. As the first challenge of target identification is to develop evidence that a target is causally related to cancer, integrative clinical genomic studies provide an essential path forward towards later confirmation in model systems. Using model systems experimentally to try to address clinically relevant questions is always an imperfect and uncertain process, but the observation of sustained genomic pathway dysregulation conserved from tumor sample to cell line gives some hope that it is not irrelevant.

A key advance in the use of cancer cell lines as models with some translational utility was the observation that gene expression in cancer cell lines such as the NCI 60 panel changed to resemble the patterns of gene expression observed in the lineage and tumor tissue type from which the cell line was derived (Ross et al., 2000). This observation both allows the broad characterization of cell lines from tumor tissues of different patient origin and also, when seen as lineage dependence, provides a way of structuring pathway-specific hypotheses for therapeutic intervention.

An excellent example of the utility of this approach can be seen in the case of breast cancer systems. As before, clinical molecular data are the driving force: many clinical genomic breast-cancer datasets have become available over the past several years, from patient samples acquired at the time of diagnosis or during the course of treatment (Miller and Liu, 2007; Perou et al., 2000; Ross et al., 2000; Sørlie et al., 2001; West et al., 2001). These datasets have been used for the finer assessment of clinically relevant subtypes of disease not apparent from pathology at presentation, and have been integrated into meta-analysis studies to identify both new targets and the importance of functional signatures for key tumor suppressor pathways such as p53 (Miller et al., 2005). Importantly, collections of breast cell lines have been assessed on the same platforms (Neve et al., 2006) in order to provide a collection of model systems that can be associated back to the functionally distinct subtypes as they are understood at any time. The clinical genomic data on breast cancer serve as a growing reference dataset for translation, and the cell lines serve as an advancing experimental resource for testing (Stemke-Hale et al., 2008). The opportunity to derive clinical relevance of experimental tests performed with this system grows over time, as new platforms are added to the existing datasets and testing of the cell-line panel becomes sufficiently sophisticated to identify clinically relevant subgroups of models sensitive to targeted agents (Mirzoeva et al., 2009).

Integrating and Extending Cancer Cell Model Data

The focus on integrative omics for systems biology described here relies on data resources drawn from several sources, both public and private. Because the proven value of integrative and meta-analyses is to align genomic data from disparate sources for more powerful inference, and as new clinical genomic datasets continue to become available, we take a systematic informatics approach to support the data resourcing process (Fig. 17.1, bottom). Lilly, like other organizations, has made a substantial commitment to the informatics integration of these data, and has developed a systematic service-oriented architecture for data and application integration—Lilly's Life Sciences Grid (LSG) framework—a version of which has been released to the public domain, and will be described ("Integrating scientific data for drug discovery and development using the Life Sciences Grid (LSG)" elsewhere. A semantic data integration architecture to support oncology discovery platforms is also described elsewhere (Manning et al., 2009).

Using such integrative informatics platforms, we can start a systematic integration of corresponding data types between model systems and clinical patient samples (Fig. 17.2) and extend them to new tumor and data types. The genetic, genomic and proteomic data common to clinical and model system samples provide a bridge, as illustrated below via signatures, via which to associate clinically heterogeneous disease with differential sensitivity and response in model systems. The breast-cancer model system approach described above has been applied to

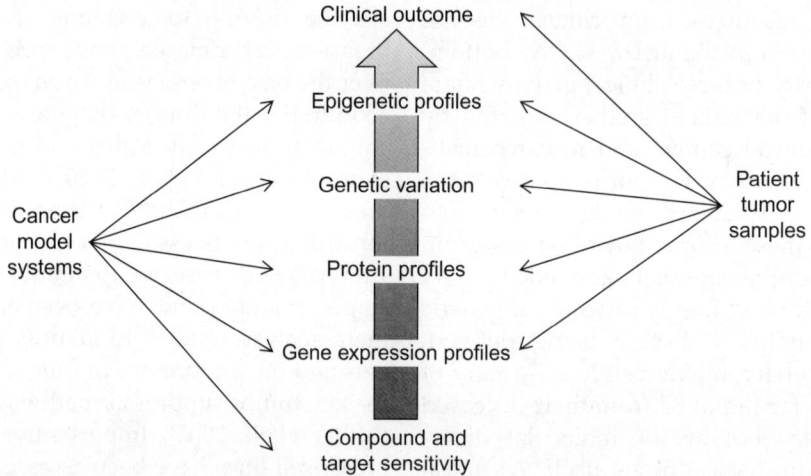

FIGURE 17.2   Integration Between Model Systems and Clinical Cancer "Omics" Data.

many other cancer types with high prevalence in Europe and North America, to provide panels of models that can be used in rational testing of hypotheses about genetic and lineage dependencies of targets and pathways. We are developing similar model system panels to support other tumor types, integrating clinical and model systems data for tumors of high incidence and prevalence in east Asian populations, such as gastric and hepatocellular carcinomas.

The integration of genomic data from both model systems and clinical samples provides an important translational bridge, but cancer cell lines are still not highly predictive of clinical response. Human cancer xenografts in the nude mouse derived from conventional cell lines, while providing a useful *in-vivo* model, have also shown limited ability to predict human clinical responses to therapeutic intervention (Sausville and Burger, 2006). As an alternative to immortalized settings, some groups (Garber, 2009; Smith et al., 2008) are developing primary tumor xenograft models, transplanting patient tumors directly into a xenograft setting for experimental use. A fraction of tumors implanted grow as xenografts and can be used for efficacy studies. Fiebig and his colleagues at Oncotest GmbH have developed a large panel of such models that appear to show more promising predictive value when studied *in vivo* and from which an *in-vitro* tumor clonogenic assay can be used to choose among models for *in-vivo* studies. When combined with integrated genomic data such as described above for cell lines, this model collection provides an attractive platform for translation from discovery to the clinic (Fiebig et al., 2004, 2007).

Systems-oriented Target Identification

With cancer cell and *in-vivo* models associated ever more precisely with clinical disease based on molecular systems data, the challenge is to use these models effectively to modulate and understand the role of cancer targets, often by the use of RNAi. In mammalian cell culture, RNAi has long been seen as an attractive platform for systematic measurement of the biological effects of loss of gene function with minimal genetic manipulation (Chi et al., 2003; Czauderna et al., 2003; Elbashir et al., 2001).

Concerns have been raised about RNAi as a large-scale target-screening approach, because of its lack of target specificity, prevalence of false positives, transfection effects in short interfering (si)RNA screens requiring automation, and many other issues. RNAi remains, however, the workhorse for screening target modulation in cellular systems. After a series of studies to establish the viability of RNAi in mammalian cell culture and the ability of the RNAi phenomenon to recapitulate biological effects from known causes of pathway interference, focused target studies were followed by pathway-level and, eventually, whole-genome loss-of-function screens. In an early proof-of-concept and platform validation, Hsieh and co-workers (2004) demonstrated that carefully designed short siRNA duplexes could be used in a pathway-based cellular genetic screen to identify genetic regulators of activation of the phosphatidyl inositol 3-kinase (PI3K) pathway. At around the same time, Berns and colleagues (2004) constructed a lentiviral short hairpin (sh)RNA library to confirm known and identify new modulators of p53-dependent arrest of proliferation. The methods used by these authors and others have been extended to a range of pathway screens, target-by-class screens and whole-genome screens, to identify phenotypic changes induced by loss of gene function.

As the technology for systems-level RNAi studies has advanced, a variety of strategies have been developed for utilizing knockdown libraries in a screening context (Table 17.1). Using pools of reagents against a single target has been particularly valuable for minimizing the off-target effects of any single siRNA oligonucleotide. When extended to shRNA vectors,

TABLE 17.1 Alternative RNA Interference Formats for Target Identification Screens

Format	Advantages	Drawbacks
siRNA Oligonucleotides		
Single well	Known and available reagents; target specifity inferred by multiple hits	Replicates are resource consuming; need to validate target specificity
Pooled	Higher target specificity	Have to test individual siRNAs for hits anyway
shRNA in Lentivirus		
Single well	Each well can be scaled	Low knockdown efficiency; automation requirements
Pooled	Can be done on the benchtop; identify shRNA by microarray or sequencing	Reagents generally unavailable; need to generate normalized validated collections

shRNA, short hairpon RNA; siRNA, short interfering RNA.

the pooled approach can be further extended to run large RNAi screens without automation, identifying the reagents conferring phenotype either by hybridization to a specialized microarray (Ngo et al., 2006) or by polymerase chain reaction (PCR) followed by insert sequencing.

RNA Interference Synthetic Lethality to Identify Targets, Biomarkers and Combinations

RNA interference loss-of-function screens can rapidly identify targets of interest in a cell line, but such screens can also be seen as a form of synthetic genetic screening. In a conventional synthetic lethal setting, knockout of either one of two genes does not lead to a lethal phenotype, but knockout of both genes in the same setting is lethal. RNAi knockdown can be substituted for one of the genes in a synthetic lethal experiment, and when performed in a screening context becomes a form of RNAi synthetic lethality screening (Fig. 17.3). However, RNAi screens in cancer cells are *always* performed on a background of genetic aberrations, known or unknown, so each RNAi screen in such models is dependent on its genetic context. This fact can be a complication or a tool. This observation has been used as a feature to identify targets the knockdown of which is lethal in the context of models derived from activated B-cell-like diffuse large B-cell lymphoma (ABC-DLBCL), but not of those derived from germinal centre B-cell-like tumors; these are two subtypes of disease originally defined by their molecular genomic patterns (Ngo et al., 2006). The resultant ABC-DLBCL-specific target, CARD11, was later shown to be oncogenically activated in ABC-DLBCL tumors (Lenz et al., 2008), providing an exquisite example of the path from clinical samples to clinically relevant model systems to the identification of a molecular target for a devastating clinically unmet need.

This can also lead to unexpected results, as in the case of the study by Shaffer et al. (2008), who used RNAi to study synthetic lethal effects over the heterogeneous genetic background of multiple myeloma. Amazingly, they found that the transcription factor, IRF4, is required in myeloma cells, regardless of the underlying genetic background, and is at the center of regulatory networks commonly dysregulated by the diverse genetic aberrations that lead to disease.

The concept of synthetic lethality can be further extended to substitute inhibition of a drug target for gene knockdown (Fig. 17.3, bottom),

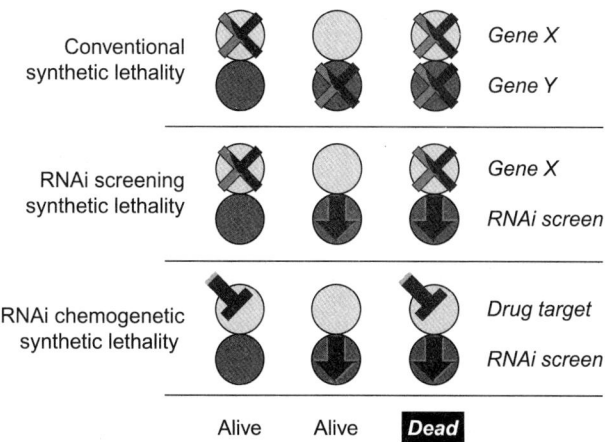

FIGURE 17.3 RNA Interference (RNAi) as a Form of Synthetic Lethality.

in a form of RNAi chemogenetic synthetic lethality. Chemogenetic synthetic interaction studies provide a systematic means of identifying genes associated with drug sensitivity. Whitehurst and co-workers (2007) used such an approach to identify 87 genes that sensitized the NCI-H1155 NSCLC cell line to low doses of paclitaxel. When the genes so identified are integrated with knowledge of genomic aberrations in clinical samples, they can point the way for patient populations with a higher probability of predicted response; when integrated in the context of the mechanisms of other drugs, they can explain or point the way to combinations with a higher likelihood of clinical efficacy. This was the case in the paclitaxel study, in which several pathways and complexes stood out in the sensitizer gene list, including seven subunits of the proteasome, consistent with the observed clinical synergy between the proteasome inhibitor, bortezomib, and paclitaxel.

Although the study described above is one of synthetic lethality, the idea can be generalized to synthetic rescue experiments, in which knockdown of the gene rescues the phenotypic effect of drug action, and marker rescue experiments, in which overexpression of the gene product reverses the drug effect.

The clinically relevant diversity of these experiments is daunting (Fig. 17.4), with at least three obvious dimensions to consider: genetic diversity, target perturbation and compound effects. Furthermore, whereas some of the existing data on compound profiling, such as the NCI 60 panel, provide a window into chemosensitivity, most RNAi screens are heavily reliant on automation. Happily, advances in technology may solve this problem. As vector-based platforms such as shRNA and overexpression libraries can be amplified by PCR, it is possible rapidly to expand the range of available screens by running studies in pooled experiments, amplifying the inserts and quantifying the hits using next-generation sequencing of the amplicons.

Translating from Discovery to the Clinic

With advances in both informatics and experimental platforms, promoting integrative genomics data from the clinic for discovery, we and others are looking to utilize systems biology approaches for predictive biomedicine: to maximize the opportunity for patient benefit before going to the clinic. Not surprisingly, gene

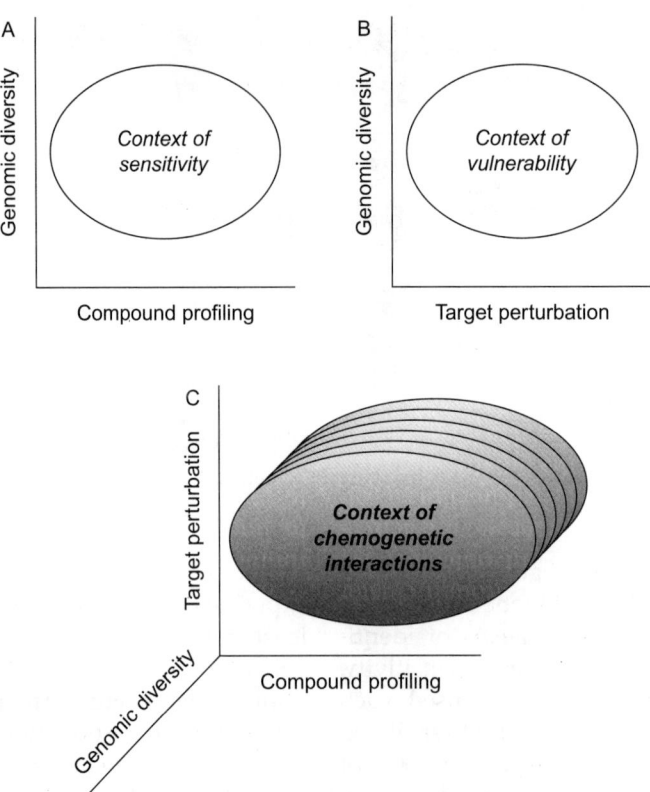

FIGURE 17.4   Integrating Compound, Target and Genetic Profiles.

expression studies have been at the forefront of this effort. Since the first studies on class discovery and class prediction by microarray profiling in 1999 (Golub et al., 1999), systems-based approaches have steadily advanced towards the goal of using genomic data to direct the administration of clinical agents (Potti and Nevins, 2008). Some of the results have already influenced clinical practice, such as the acceptance of genomics-defined subtypes of clinical disease, and the use of a limited number of microarray-based tests for clinical decision-making (Dowsett and Dunbier, 2008).

From the identification of molecular subtypes (Alizadeh et al., 2000; Golub et al., 1999; Ivshina et al., 2006), to the identification of gene signatures that substitute for clinical phenomena in model sytems (Chang et al., 2004), to association with and prediction of chemosensitivity (Staunton et al., 2001) and patient outcome (Huang et al., 2003; Sørlie et al., 2001; West et al., 2001), gene expression signatures have proven their worth. It is notable, however, that in a high number of cases in which integrative studies have been carried out, gene expression signatures have also been predictive of the underlying known genetic lesions in tumors (de Tayrac et al., 2009; Miller et al., 2005). This opens up a further potential for the use of gene signatures: it is clear from the growing compendia of cancer genome sequencing data that the genetic events underlying cancer progression are even more diverse and widespread than was earlier believed (Greenman et al., 2007; McLendon et al., 2008; Parsons et al., 2008), with implications for dynamics models of genetic progression towards cancer (Beerenwinkel et al., 2007). With individually powerful genetic drivers of disease sparsely populated, gene expression signatures may prove to be, not just a surrogate for genetic etiology, but a point of convergence between diverse genetic etiologies. In other words, genomic surrogates such as expression signatures may be both retrospective and prospective tools for understanding cancer at a molecular level.

Bild et al. (2006) have used gene expression signatures as a tool to deconvolute the events of pathway activation. In a series of experiments, they introduced controlled oncogenic activators, such as Myc, Ras and E2F3, into human mammary epithelial cells and measured the resultant levels of gene expression to define signatures of activation. They showed, not only that gene expression signatures induced in such a controlled setting could accurately predict the oncogenic activation status in a set of independent samples, but also that the pathway activation signatures generated could be observed in clinical tumor samples and, through cluster analysis, associated with patient outcome. We ourselves have assessed whether *in-vitro* activation signatures could be detected in clinical settings of varying relation to the *in-vitro* signature derivation (Fig. 17.5). When tested in a clinical lung cancer setting, the *in-vitro* Ras activation signature of Bild et al. (2006) was clearly distinct from expectations of a random gene set (Fig. 17.5A). Similarly, an *in-vitro* signature of estrogen response was clearly detectable in a breast cancer setting (Fig. 17.5B). However, as expected, the estrogen response signature was not detected in lung cancer clinical settings (Fig. 17.5C). This shows that the strength of signature-like behavior can be detected in unrelated clinical genomic datasets and has the potential to optimize the use of prediction tools for signatures in individual patients.

Related work from another laboratory has resulted in the development of an integrated strategy using model systems and clinical genomic data to predict the chemotherapeutic response in patients with several types of cancer, and its application to a range of existing treatment options (Dressman et al., 2007; Potti et al., 2006; Salter et al., 2008). The investigators approached the problem by developing signatures predictive of sensitivity to chemotherapeutic agents, and validated those signatures in separate *in-vitro* studies. They associated these signatures with clinical response in both ovarian and breast cancers, and used the signatures of individual treatment response to associate patient responses with the pathway activation signatures developed by Bild et al. (2006). This approach, and other work, have been sufficiently promising to enable the proposal a general framework to test the use of genomically guided chemotherapy for primary agents in current use (Potti and Nevins, 2008).

Predicting Patient Benefit from Preclinical Data for Novel Agents

In a drug discovery and development environment, we cannot wait until clinical practice to understand which patients are most likely to respond to agents in development. Instead, we are continually faced with the challenge of interpreting data for decisions on the fate of novel compounds, perhaps with unprecedented mechanisms of action. With the success of predictive, systems-based approaches to identify patients responsive to chemotherapeutic agents in the clinic, can we take an analogous, predictive approach to predict patient benefit for agents entering clinical development?

We believe the answer to this question is "yes," provided sufficiently reliable biomarkers are available to guide successive decision stages in the development process. Integrative systems biology is used at several stages of this process: (i) identification of pharmacodynamic and pathway modulation biomarkers that can be used to determine a biologically efficacious dose; (ii) identification and use of model systems that

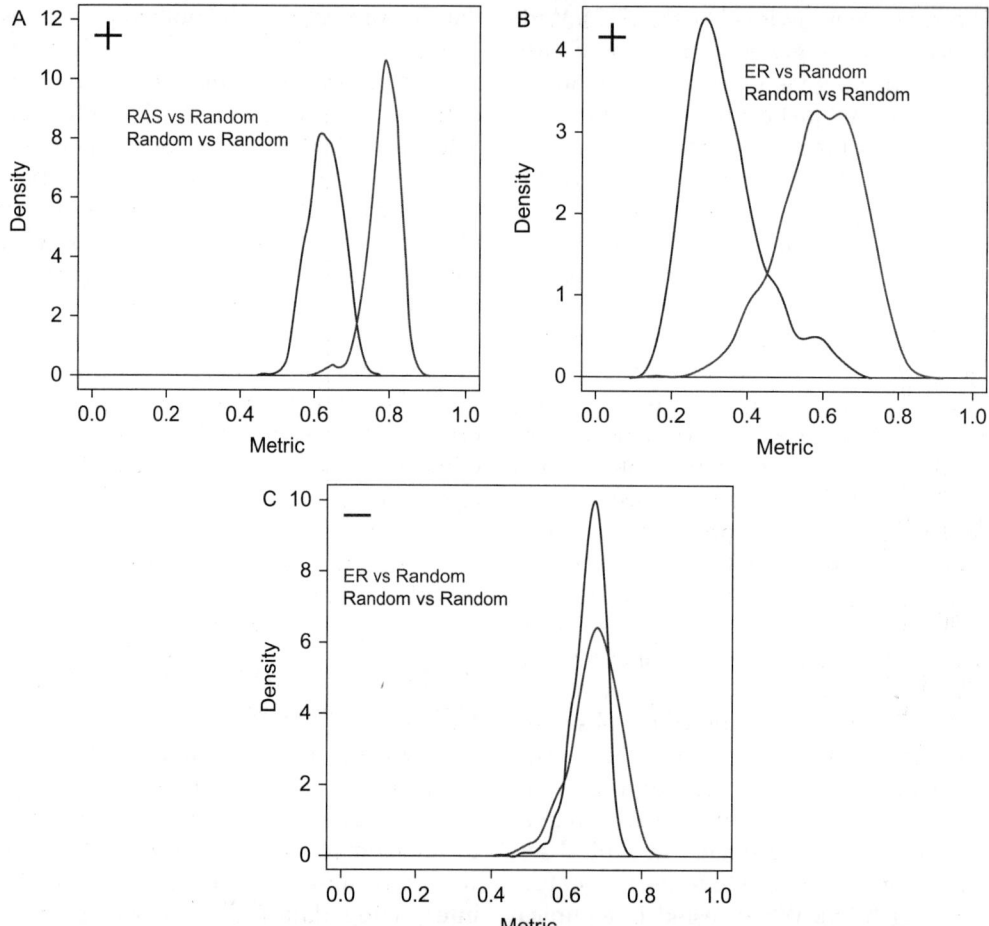

FIGURE 17.5 Assessment of Signatures in Disparate Clinical Settings.
Positive detection of a signature is detected by the separation of peaks from expectations of a random signature. (A) A distinct Ras activation signature in a clinical cancer setting. (B) A clearly detectable estrogen response signature in a breast cancer setting. (C) No estrogen response signature detectable in a clinical lung cancer setting. (A. Aggarwal et al., unpublished observations).

are associated, by clinical genomic data, with target dependence in patient samples; (iii) identification of patient groups, or individual patients, most likely to respond to treatment. Finally, in favorable cases, dynamic models of cancer biology—signaling pathways (Ventura et al., 2009), cell cycle, angiogenesis and other critical cancer-associated processes—can add mechanistic insight and predictability to indirect pharmacodynamic models (Sharma and Jusko, 1998).

To use signatures for clinical prediction, we apply all of the systems biology resources described above in the framework outlined in Figure 17.5. The strategy as outlined uses signatures at several stages, *in vitro* to *in vitro*, *in vitro* to *in vivo*, and from both to predicted clinic response. Although the use of *in-vitro* signatures to predict clinical response to current chemotherapeutic regimens has shown considerable promise, in our experience, patient-derived tumor models tested *in vivo* and in tumor clonogenic assays can show a greater variation in sensitivity than conventional cell lines, and this presents an opportunity to understand chemosensitivity profiles in more clinically relevant samples. In addition, many somatic genetic aberrations commonly seen in tumors are infrequent or absent in cell lines (Li et al., 2008; Nupponen et al., 1998), and primary tumor models represent the most attractive opportunity to bridge the gap in experimentation.

It should be noted that not all successful predictions of patient response in the clinic should require the use of a genomic test in clinical practice. A common challenge faced in oncology clinical development is to decide which indications to focus on in a Phase II clinical trial. A large range of indications may be attractive for a particular development program, but only a few may be practical for initial Phase II studies. The choice of which indications to prioritize is based on the best possible understanding of the target, accumulated results of studies from discovery through to preclinical models, and whatever limited patient response has been observed in Phase I clinical studies. With broad systems-based approaches to translation, predictive patient stratification signatures can be used to rank potential indications on the basis of the likelihood of observing a significant clinical response, thus enabling better options for a decision that has to be made in any case. We expect that this sort of prediction, identified as a clinically responsive group setting in Figure 17.6, will be used more commonly in advance of the need to predict response in individual patients.

In the same vein, low-frequency somatic events characterized by systems-based approaches can provide strong evidence to drive proof-of-concept decisions about a target or compound, even when the patient population is not practical to stratify in clinical trials. For example, the activating AKT1 mutation, AKT1(E17K), was discovered and characterized in an integrative study of colon and breast tumors, and shown to provide a novel route to activation of the

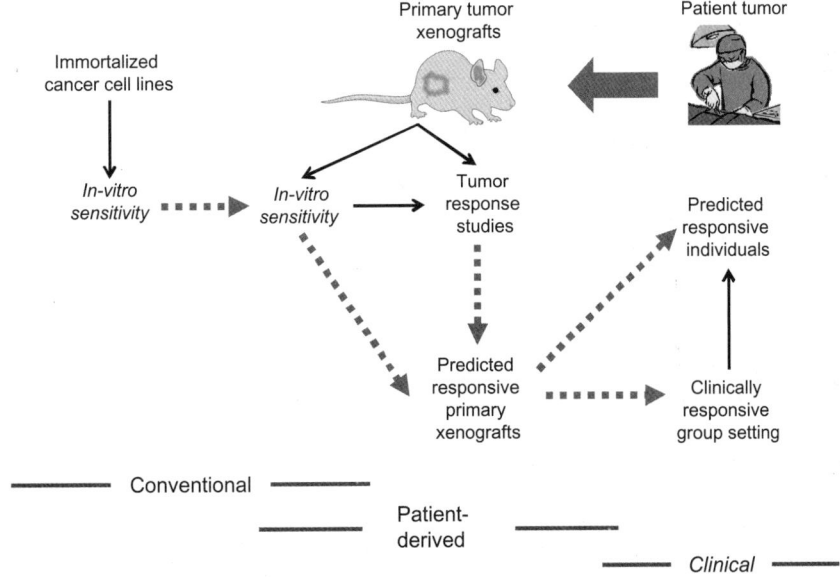

FIGURE 17.6 Use of Signatures to Make Clinical Predictions from Model Systems. Dashed arrows represent application of signatures for prediction.

PI3K/AKT pathway (Carpten et al., 2007). Other mutations along the same pathway, particularly the upstream activating mutations at PIK3CA and loss at PTEN (Stemke-Hale et al., 2008), are well characterized in many tumor types. The frequency of the AKT1(E17K) mutation in most tumor types is low (Kim et al., 2008), but the consequences for activation of the pathway are clear. Activation thus provides an opportunity for clinical proof-of-concept: a competitive AKT1 inhibitor administered using appropriate pharmacodynamic markers and pharmacokinetic/pharmacodynamic models to define a biologically efficacious dose in tumors should be expected to show some evidence of response in patients harboring a somatic AKT1(E17K) variant. This type of approach can build the case for the likely observation of response before clinical trials in broader populations of patients.

CONCLUDING REMARKS

Systems-based approaches to translational medicine are being made possible by the convergent acceleration of several disciplines—computational, post-genomic platform and biomedical sciences—working together to offer a more complete picture of the complexities of disease and disease treatment. Molecular targeting of tumorigenic aberrations in cancer has become the standard by which modern treatment is defined, but single molecular targets do not tell the whole story of disease, which must be understood, within cancer cells, in terms of dsyregulated pathways, aberrant molecular networks and selective pressures in response to treatment, and, in whole tumors, by the complex interactions between the cancer cell, the tumor microenvironment, and developmental lineage. Systems-based approaches offer an increasingly less biased set of platforms with which to observe the phenomenal diversity of cancers and conduct experiments in a wider range of more clinically relevant models. The opportunity in cancer is driven by the rapid growth of integrated clinical cancer genomic data to determine the clinical relevance of targets and pathways in these models.

The complexity of disease is a fact of life, but systems-based approaches allow us to accept this complexity and even recognize what opportunities it affords (Gund et al., 2007; West et al., 2006). Because pathways and networks dysregulated in disease can function as points of convergence for diverse molecular etiologies (Shaffer et al., 2008), understanding disease and intervention at the level of pathways and networks sustains the promise using predictive models to individualize treatment for cancer patients, even when the molecular basis of disease is incompletely understood.

Data-driven predictive models from whole-systems studies have already begun to affect the clinical understanding of disease, and will increasingly be used to guide treatment of agents in the clinic (Potti and Nevins, 2008). In discovering and developing novel treatments, the challenge is not only to identify new targets, but to capitalize upon the growing wealth of integrative clinical genomic data to drive clinically relevant decisions before clinical trials begin. Data-driven models and dynamic multi-scale models of biological systems—intracellular, multicellular and physiological—can together optimize these data to provide more accurate and useful model-based tools for representing biology (Kumar et al., 2006), transforming drug discovery to a more holistic, model-based approach that accelerates innovation and improves outcome in individual patients.

References

Alizadeh, A.A., Eisen, M.B., Davis, R.E., et al., 2000. Distinct types of diffuse large B-cell lymphoma identified by gene expression profiling. Nature 403, 503–511.

Beerenwinkel, N., Antal, T., Dingli, D., et al., 2007. Genetic progression and the waiting time to cancer. PLoS Comput. Biol. 3, e225.

Berns, K., Hijmans, E.M., Mullenders, J., et al., 2004. A large-scale RNAi screen in human cells identifies new components of the p53 pathway. Nature 428, 431–437.

Bild, A.H., Yao, G., Chang, J.T., et al., 2006. Oncogenic pathway signatures in human cancers as a guide to targeted therapies. Nature 439, 353–357.

Butcher, E.C., Berg, E.L., Kunkel, E.J., 2004. Systems biology in drug discovery. Nat. Biotech. 22, 1253–1259.

Carpten, J.D., Faber, A.L., Horn, C., et al., 2007. A transforming mutation in the pleckstrin homology domain of AKT1 in cancer. Nature 448, 439–444.

Chang, H.Y., Sneddon, J.B., Alizadeh, A.A., et al., 2004. Gene expression signature of fibroblast serum response predicts human cancer progression: similarities between tumors and wounds. PLoS. Biol. 2, E7.

Chi, J.T., Chang, H.Y., Wang, N.N., Chang, D.S., Dunphy, N., Brown, P.O., 2003. Genomewide view of gene silencing by small interfering RNAs. Proc. Natl. Acad. Sci. USA 100, 6343–6346.

Czauderna, F., Fechtner, M., Aygün, H., et al., 2003. Functional studies of the PI-kinase signalling pathway employing synthetic and expressed siRNA. Nucleic. Acids. Res. 31, 670–682.

de Tayrac, M., Etcheverry, A., Aubry, M., et al., 2009. Integrative genome-wide analysis reveals a robust genomic glioblastoma signature associated with copy number driving changes in gene expression. Genes Chromosomes Cancer 48, 55–68.

Di Cosimo, S., Baselga, J., 2008. Targeted therapies in breast cancer: where are we now? Eur. J. Cancer 44, 2781–2790.

Dowsett, M., Dunbier, A.K., 2008. Emerging biomarkers and new understanding of traditional markers in personalized therapy for breast cancer. Clin. Cancer Res. 14, 8019–8026.

Dressman, H.K., Berchuck, A., Chan, G., et al., 2007. An integrated genomic-based approach to individualized treatment of patients with advanced-stage ovarian cancer. J. Clin. Oncol. 25, 517–525.

Elbashir, S.M., Harborth, J., Lendeckel, W., Yalcin, A., Weber, K., Tuschl, T., 2001. Duplexes of 21-nucleotide RNAs mediate RNA interference in cultured mammalian cells. Nature 411, 494–498.

Fiebig, H.H., Maier, A., Burger, A.M., 2004. Clonogenic assay with established human tumour xenografts: correlation of in vitro to in vivo activity as a basis for anticancer drug discovery. Eur. J. Cancer 40, 802–820.

Fiebig, H.H., Schuler, J., Bausch, N., Hofmann, M., Metz, T., Korrat, A., 2007. Gene signatures developed from patient tumor explants grown in nude mice to predict tumor response to 11 cytotoxic drugs. Cancer Genomics Proteomics 4, 197–209.

Fitzgerald, J.B., Schoeberl, B., Nielsen, U.B., Sørger, P.K., 2006. Systems biology and combination therapy in the quest for clinical efficacy. Nat. Chem. Biol. 2, 458–466.

Garber, K., 2009. From human to mouse and back: "tumorgraft" models surge in popularity. J. Natl. Cancer Inst. 101, 6–8.

Golub, T.R., Slonim, D.K., Tamayo, P., et al., 1999. Molecular classification of cancer: class discovery and class prediction by gene expression monitoring. Science 286, 531–537.

Greenman, C., Stephens, P., Smith, R., et al., 2007. Patterns of somatic mutation in human cancer genomes. Nature 446, 153–158.

Gund, P., Maliski, E., Brown, F., 2007. Embracing complexity in drug discovery. Curr. Opin. Drug Discov. Devel. 10, 252–253.

Hall, P.S., Cameron, D.A., 2009. Current perspective-trastuzumab. Eur. J. Cancer 45, 12–18.

Hsieh, A.C., Bo, R., Manola, J., et al., 2004. A library of siRNA duplexes targeting the phosphoinositide 3-kinase pathway: determinants of gene silencing for use in cell-based screens. Nucleic. Acids Res. 32, 893–901.

Huang, E., West, M., Nevins, J.R., 2003. Gene expression profiling for prediction of clinical characteristics of breast cancer. Recent Prog. Horm. Res. 58, 55–73.

Ivshina, A.V., George, J., Senko, O., et al., 2006. Genetic reclassification of histologic grade delineates new clinical subtypes of breast cancer. Cancer Res. 66, 10292–10301.

Jordan, V.C., 2003. Tamoxifen: a most unlikely pioneering medicine. Nat. Rev. Drug. Discov. 2, 205–213.

Kim, M.S., Jeong, E.G., Yoo, N.J., Lee, S.H., 2008. Mutational analysis of oncogenic AKT E17K mutation in common solid cancers and acute leukaemias. Br. J. Cancer 98, 1533–1535.

Kumar, N., Hendriks, B.S., Janes, K.A., de Graaf, D., Lauffenburger, D.A., 2006. Applying computational modeling to drug discovery and development. Drug. Discov. Today 11, 806–811.

Lenz, G., Davis, R.E., Ngo, V.N., et al., 2008. Oncogenic CARD11 mutations in human diffuse large B cell lymphoma. Science 319, 1676–1679.

Li, A., Walling, J., Kotliarov, Y., et al., 2008. Genomic changes and gene expression profiles reveal that established glioma cell lines are poorly representative of primary human gliomas. Mol. Cancer Res. 6, 21–30.

Manning, M., Aggarwal, A., Gao, K., Tucker-Kellogg, G., 2009. Scaling the walls of discovery: using semantic metadata for integrative problem solving. Brief. Bioinform. 10, 164–176.

McLendon, R., Friedman, A., Bigner, D., et al., 2008. Comprehensive genomic characterization defines human glioblastoma genes and core pathways. Nature.

Mendelsohn, J., Baselga, J., 2006. Epidermal growth factor receptor targeting in cancer. Semin. Oncol. 33, 369–385.

Miller, L.D., Liu, E.T., 2007. Expression genomics in breast cancer research: microarrays at the crossroads of biology and medicine. Breast Cancer Res. 9, 206.

Miller, L.D., Smeds, J., George, J., et al., 2005. An expression signature for p53 status in human breast cancer predicts mutation status, transcriptional effects, and patient survival. Proc. Natl. Acad. Sci. USA 102, 13550–13555.

Mirzoeva, O.K., Das, D., Heiser, L.M., et al., 2009. Basal subtype and MAPK/ERK kinase (MEK)-phosphoinositide 3-kinase feedback signaling determine susceptibility of breast cancer cells to MEK inhibition. Cancer Res. 69, 565–572.

Neve, R.M., Chin, K., Fridlyand, J., et al., 2006. A collection of breast cancer cell lines for the study of functionally distinct cancer subtypes. Cancer Cell 10, 515–527.

Ngo, V.N., Davis, R.E., Lamy, L., et al., 2006. A loss-of-function RNA interference screen for molecular targets in cancer. Nature 441, 106–110.

Nupponen, N., Hyytinen, E.R., Kallioniemi, A.H., Visakorpi, T., 1998. Genetic alterations in prostate cancer cell lines detected by comparative genomic hybridization. Cancer Genet. Cytogenet. 101, 53–57.

Parsons, D.W., Jones, S., Zhang, X., et al., 2008. An integrated genomic analysis of human glioblastoma multiforme. Science 321, 1807–1812.

Perou, C.M., Sørlie, T., Eisen, M.B., et al., 2000. Molecular portraits of human breast tumours. Nature 406, 747–752.

Petrelli, A., Giordano, S., 2008. From single- to multi-target drugs in cancer therapy: when aspecificity becomes an advantage. Curr. Med. Chem. 15, 422–432.

Potti, A., Nevins, J.R., 2008. Utilization of genomic signatures to direct use of primary chemotherapy. Curr. Opin. Genet. Devel. 18, 62–67.

Potti, A., Dressman, H.K., Bild, A., et al., 2006. Genomic signatures to guide the use of chemotherapeutics. Nat. Med. 12, 1294–1300.

Ross, D.T., Scherf, U., Eisen, M.B., et al., 2000. Systematic variation in gene expression patterns in human cancer cell lines. Nat. Genet. 24, 227–235.

Salter, K.H., Acharya, C.R., Walters, K.S., et al., 2008. An integrated approach to the prediction of chemotherapeutic response in patients with breast cancer. PLoS ONE 3, e1908.

Sausville, E.A., Burger, A.M., 2006. Contributions of human tumor xenografts to anticancer drug development. Cancer Res. 66, 3351–3354.

Shaffer, A.L., Emre, N.C., Lamy, L., et al., 2008. IRF4 addiction in multiple myeloma. Nature 454, 226–231.

Sharma, A., Jusko, W.J., 1998. Characteristics of indirect pharmacodynamic models and applications to clinical drug responses. Br. J. Clin. Pharmacol. 45, 229–239.

Smith, V., Wirth, G.J., Fiebig, H.H., Burger, A.M., 2008. Tissue microarrays of human tumor xenografts: characterization of proteins involved in migration and angiogenesis for applications in the development of targeted anticancer agents. Cancer Genomics Proteomics 5, 263–273.

Sørlie, T., Perou, C.M., Tibshirani, R., et al., 2001. Gene expression patterns of breast carcinomas distinguish tumor subclasses with clinical implications. Proc. Natl. Acad. Sci. USA 98, 10869–10874.

Staunton, J.E., Slonim, D.K., Coller, H.A., et al., 2001. Chemosensitivity prediction by transcriptional profiling. Proc. Natl. Acad. Sci. USA 98, 10787–10792.

Stemke-Hale, K., Gonzalez-Angulo, A.M., Lluch, A., et al., 2008. An integrative genomic and proteomic analysis of PIK3CA, PTEN, and AKT mutations in breast cancer. Cancer Res. 68, 6084–6091.

Ventura, A.C., Jackson, T.L., Merajver, S.D., 2009. On the role of cell signaling models in cancer research. Cancer Res. 69, 400–402.

Vieth, M., Higgs, R.E., Robertson, D.H., Shapiro, M., Gragg, E.A., Hemmerle, H., 2004. Kinomics-structural biology and chemogenomics of kinase inhibitors and targets. Biochim. Biophys. Acta 1697, 243–257.

Vieth, M., Sutherland, J.J., Robertson, D.H., Campbell, R.M., 2005. Kinomics: characterizing the therapeutically validated kinase space. Drug. Discov. Today 10, 839–846.

West, M., Blanchette, C., Dressman, H., et al., 2001. Predicting the clinical status of human breast cancer by using gene expression profiles. Proc. Natl. Acad. Sci. USA 98, 11462–11467.

West, M., Ginsburg, G.S., Huang, A.T., Nevins, J.R., 2006. Embracing the complexity of genomic data for personalized medicine. Genome. Res. 16, 559–566.

Whitehurst, A.W., Bodemann, B.O., Cardenas, J., et al., 2007. Synthetic lethal screen identification of chemosensitizer loci in cancer cells. Nature 446, 815–819.

Zhang, L., Sinha, V., Forgue, S.T., et al., 2006. Model-based drug development: the road to quantitative pharmacology. J. Pharmacokinet. Pharmacodyn. 33, 369–393.

Zhang, L., Pfister, M., Meibohm, B., 2008. Concepts and challenges in quantitative pharmacology and model-based drug development. AAPS J. 10, 552–559.

Zhu, J., Zhang, B., Schadt, E.E., 2008. A systems biology approach to drug discovery. Adv. Genet. 60, 603–635.

CHAPTER 18

Quantitative Biology and Clinical Trials: a Perspective

Robert A. Harrington[1] and Edison T. Liu[2]

[1]Duke University Medical Center, Durham
[2]Genome Institute of Singapore, Singapore

OUTLINE

The Role of Clinical Trials in Modern Medicine	415
Clinical Trials of Therapeutics	417
Understanding the Problem	419
Another View of "Systems" Biomedicine	421
Conclusion and Summary	422

THE ROLE OF CLINICAL TRIALS IN MODERN MEDICINE

Clinicians depend on a variety of sources of evidence to guide decision making and the care of patients. Traditionally, patient management decisions were based on an understanding of pathophysiological reasoning and knowledge of the basic biology of a disease or condition. During their training, physicians are initially taught a reductionist approach to disease as they learn the basics of molecular and cell biology, biochemistry, anatomy and organ physiology. Following this grounding in "normal" human biology, students next learn to recognize diseases as being pathological perturbations of normal physiological function. Many students sense that, if they understand the pathway to a disease, knowing how to treat it must emerge logically (and almost linearly) from that understanding.

The concept of evidence-based medicine emerged from a recognition that treating human diseases required more than an understanding of basic science; that, while it was clear that basic discovery science could provide great insights into the biology of the human organism, thinking must shift towards quantitative experimentation and measurement in order to discover effective therapeutic strategies (Straus and Sackett, 1998). Medical care should be driven by the best quantitative evidence that can be used to achieve optimal outcomes, and then applied to the care of patients in the context of their individual values and preferences. Although clinical trials have always required quantification of endpoints such as death or occurrence of disease, a proliferation of biomarkers has caused the field to develop quantitative analytical approaches that take into account the analog nature of the data (as opposed to the binary, yes/no, outcomes of survival and death) that are assessed in a multiplex fashion. The shift in thinking initiated by the evidence-based medicine movement has moved medical decision making from relying on the judgment of experts to algorithmic representations of decision branch-points, such that evidence can be weighed objectively and quantitatively. Medical history is deeply steeped in the tradition of expert opinion; decision-tree analysis is relatively new in medical practice.

The fundamental basis of systems biology is to render descriptive biological observations into quantitative forms such that systems models can be constructed and used to predict outcome. Moreover, systems biology seeks to quantify and to embrace component complexity, in order to build more accurate models. In clinical medicine and clinical trials, we have not achieved the predictive power of a true systems biological model, but we have come a long way in the form of quantitative medicine; enough so that decision analyses using quantitative data to project optimal processes in medical care are increasingly common. The importance of quantitative evidence arising from clinical trials has become ever more obvious. For this reason, our focus in this chapter will be on quantitative strategies in clinical research that will, one day, form the framework for systems biology in clinical trials.

In the pantheon of evidence, there is a distinct, quality-based hierarchy that guides clinical decision making (Alonso-Coello et al., 2008). Although all knowledge and information might be considered "evidence," data on medical therapeutics that are derived from well performed (and typically large) randomized clinical trials are considered to be the highest-quality evidence, whereas evidence based on limited observation might be considered of low quality. Increasingly, society has demanded that clinicians make healthcare decisions that are based on the best available data/evidence. For example, health regulatory authorities demand a high level of evidence regarding benefits and risks of a therapy before granting market approval and, increasingly in the United States, healthcare payers are targeting reimbursement to the practice of evidence-based prescribing. Professional societies such as the American College of Cardiology, the European Society of Cardiology (http://www.escardio.org/guidelines-surveys/esc-guidelines/about/Pages/rules-writing.aspx) and the American Heart Association (http://circ.ahajournals.org/manual/) now produce numerous practice guidelines that provide recommendations for clinical care that are based on varying strengths of evidence.

The concept of perturbation analysis, common in systems biology, fits nicely into the construct of the modern randomized clinical trial, as a trial typically is developed when a scientific idea (frequently one that addresses a single disease pathway) is ready to be tested in the intact human through a therapeutic intervention (i.e., "perturbation"). In the early phases of therapeutic development, the information to be gained in a clinical trial is largely centered on understanding an individual's biological response to an intervention (typically a drug, or a biological therapeutic) such as abciximab or low molecular weight heparin. In these types of investigation, the linkage between the concentrations of a drug or a biological therapeutic agent (pharmacokinetics) and the measurement of physiological responses (pharmacodynamics) is critical. These pharmacokinetic–pharmacodynamic experiments are often the first movement from reductionist science that focused on a basic pathway into a more systems-based approach of seeing how the intact organism responds as a particular pathway is perturbed. Often, such detailed quantitative studies are carried out in the context of early-phase (I or II) clinical trials in which small numbers of patients are studied intensely. Phase I studies, which focus on drug tolerance and effective dosing, are ideal experimental situations for systems perturbation analysis. Commonly, it is in phase I studies that the most intensive pharmacokinetic investigations are conducted. Pharmacokinetic modeling is perhaps one of the best examples of the application of quantitative methods in clinical trials, and is a mainstay of drug development. In pharmacokinetics, a drug is administered and, most commonly, the serum concentrations of that drug are followed over time. Here, compartment models and decay curves can be partially predicted by *in-vitro* knowledge of the solubility of a drug and its lipid partition coefficients, metabolic pathways and protein binding affinities, but the final model, which takes into account entire physiologic effects, must be empirical. On the basis of pharmacokinetic models constructed from experimental data, the dosing of a new therapeutic agent is decided.

Later-phase clinical trials (phase III, comparing the efficacy of treatments against each other or against a placebo) take the systems approach one step further, progressing from measuring the effects of an intervention on an individual to quantifying its effects (the good and the bad) on a population. Here, the goals of systems biomedicine are to have a positive effect on populations and to optimize practice processes. This approach provides investigators with insight into the trade-offs of risks and benefits that form the central core of an evidence base. In a similar way, the conduct of a large clinical trial that is designed to *quantify* population effects also is consistent with a systems biology approach. Large clinical trials conducted around a single question such as adjuvant chemotherapy for breast cancer can be aggregated in meta-analyses to estimate the effect of an intervention on the larger population. In this manner, therapeutic effect is sought under conditions that take into account the complexity of medical practice. This generalizes the concept of systems biomedicine even further. Additionally, with the integration of biomarker studies into large clinical trials, basic hypotheses can be raised from analyses of such investigations, which can then be moved back into the basic laboratory for further exploration and study. Califf and colleagues (2007) have described this as a therapeutic development cycle (Fig. 18.1).

CLINICAL TRIALS OF THERAPEUTICS

Earlier in history, clinical studies were often based on testing an empirical therapeutic agent (one for which there was no firm knowledge of the mechanism of action) to seek optimal outcomes. However, knowledge of biology and biochemical pathways inspires the creation of a new therapeutic. Currently, this not only means a focus on an individual molecule, but the exploitation of an understanding of an entire pathway or physiologic system. One can consider this as a progressive movement towards a systems biomedical approach.

A useful example with which to understand the movement from empirical observation to systems and mechanistic strategies in clinical trials is the development of the platelet glycoprotein IIb/IIIa inhibitors (Katz and Harrington, 2009). The first clinical observation was that there were a group of patients with a bleeding diathesis known as Glanzmann's thrombasthenia in whom the platelets did not normally aggregate in response to various stimuli such as thrombin or ADP (Charo et al., 1986, 1987; Eldor et al., 1985). Basic laboratory investigation revealed that these patients had a hereditary disorder in which their platelets did not bind fibrinogen between adjacent platelets. Eventually, a series of investigations showed

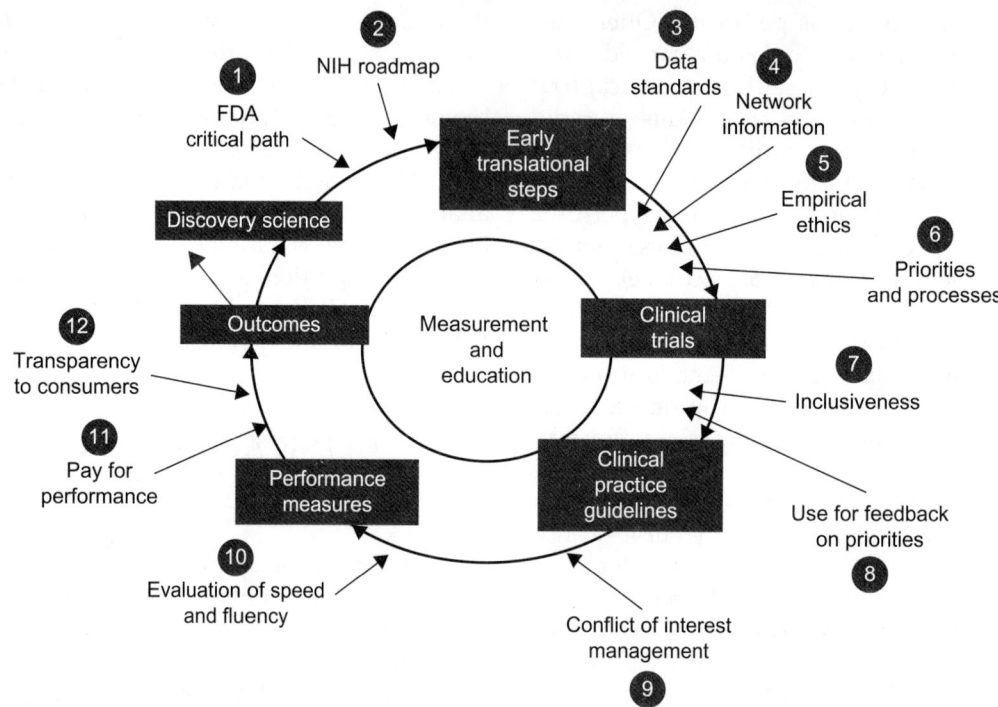

FIGURE 18.1 The Cycle of Quality: Generating Evidence to Inform Policy.
FDA, Food and Drug Administration; NIH, National Institutes of Health. Modified from Califf et al. (2007), with permission.

that fibrinogen could bind adjacent platelets (the process known as platelet aggregation) through an activated surface glycoprotein (GP) receptor complex that became known as the GP IIb/IIIa receptor complex (Charo et al., 1986, 1987; Eldor et al., 1985; Phillips et al., 1987). Patients with Glanzmann's thrombasthenia have a defect in this GP IIb/IIIa receptor complex.

As this work in basic science was progressing in the laboratory, observational studies in patients were demonstrating the importance of platelets and thrombosis in the etiology of the acute ischemic syndromes such as acute myocardial infarction (Charo et al., 1991; Genton and Turpie, 1983). In addition, large randomized clinical trials such as the Second International Study of Infarct Survival (ISIS-2) proved that aspirin, an anti-inflammatory drug with antiplatelet properties, could reduce mortality when administered acutely to patients with myocardial infarction (ISIS-2 Collaborative Group, 1988). Given that aspirin is a weak antiplatelet agent, basic investigators believed that more potent platelet inhibitors could be valuable therapeutics.

On the basis of their knowledge of the role of GP IIb/IIIa in platelet physiology, Coller and colleagues first postulated that blocking the ability of fibrinogen to bind to the GP IIb/IIIa receptor might be a useful way to treat patients who had or were at risk for platelet-mediated thrombotic diseases such as myocardial infarction. This group developed a monoclonal antibody fragment (and eventually a chimeric antibody fragment) that could prevent *ex-vivo* platelet aggregation in response to a variety of stimuli such as ADP and thrombin (Coller et al., 1983, 1986). Others developed small-molecule inhibitors of the GP IIb/IIIa receptor (Charo et al., 1991; Scarborough et al., 1991, 1993).

Early *ex-vivo* studies showed that these agents were very potent inhibitors of platelet aggregation. There was an intuitive appeal to pursue the development of these drugs for use as therapeutic agents in humans. On the basis of the observation that the patients with Glanzmann's thrombasthenia had a lack of GP IIb/IIIa that accounted for their platelet dysfunction, but they did not suffer from serious spontaneous bleeding (Phillips and Agin, 1977), it was hypothesized that inhibition of GP IIb/IIIa could be safely achieved without serious bleeding complications. However, moving from the bench to the intact human organism is always fraught with danger, so these investigators tested their hypothesis in a highly controlled manner.

How does one deliver a potentially dangerous drug to the clinic on the basis, largely, of no more than the knowledge that it blocks a single specific pathway that might play a part in human disease? Testing in intact human beings under clinical trials conditions is essential so that measures of physiological functions can be performed. Because this GP IIb/IIIa blocking drug has potential for inducing dangerous bleeding, regardless of the experience with Glanzmann's thrombasthenia, the first human experience with this class of drugs involved the administration of the monoclonal antibody fragment to a patient who had been declared brain dead and whose next of kin agreed to allow this critical next scientific step to occur (Coller et al., 1988). This experience showed that these drugs could be given to a human being without inducing major spontaneous bleeding, and it was used to usher in a major new class of therapeutic agents for use in humans.

Subsequently, dose-finding studies were performed (Harrington et al., 1995; Tcheng et al., 1994), establishing pharmacokinetic–pharmacodynamic relationships that provided the preliminary evidence necessary to move into larger, definitive, population-based studies that would document that administration of these drugs to patients with a variety of acute ischemic syndromes was associated with improved clinical outcomes and acceptable bleeding risks (Boersma and Westerhout, 2004; EPIC Investigators, 1994; EPILOG Investigators, 1997; ESPRIT Investigators, 2000; Kong et al., 2003; PURSUIT Investigators, 1998; Tcheng et al., 1995). These agents are now included in professional society practice guidelines that inform the care of patients with acute coronary syndromes and those undergoing percutaneous coronary intervention (Anderson et al., 2007; Harrington et al., 2008a; Smith et al., 2006).

Over the course of more than 20 years, discovery science centered on the GP IIb/IIIa receptor moved from the bench into intact human beings into individual patients and, finally, into large population-based studies. Collectively, these studies represent the different "systems" approaches in clinical research: the interrogation of a molecular system, of a physiologic system within a single individual and then of a delivery-of-care system.

UNDERSTANDING THE PROBLEM

The complexity of human disease necessitates that a systems experimental approach be taken in the ultimate study of any new therapeutic agent, especially those that represent a new class of drugs with a unique mechanism of action. Over-reliance on systems models is hazardous, however, and rigorous experimental validation remains essential.

Cardiovascular medicine has many examples in which a biological hypothesis, based on reasonable discovery science and laboratory investigation, completely fails and experimentation reveals the opposite to be true when the hypothesis is subjected to the rigors of whole-system testing in large clinical trials. It is clearly insufficient to claim a positive (or harmful) health effect on the basis of an understanding

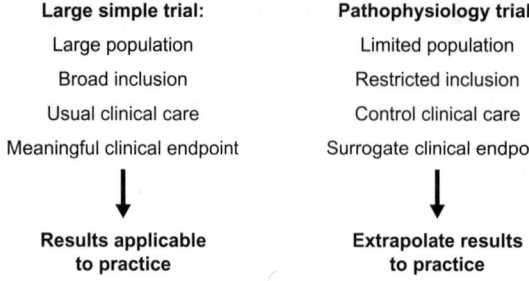

FIGURE 18.2 Comparison of Trial Models. Modified from Topol and Califf (1992), with permission.

of a disease pathway and knowledge that some drug or biological interferes with that pathway.

One might describe two types of clinical trials, one exploratory or mechanistic and the other pragmatic or evaluative. Mechanistic trials seek to uncover some underlying biology in the study, whereas evaluative studies focus on best-of-practice outcomes (e.g. treatment A is better than treatment B). Each has its uses, but their intentions and goals are different and therefore their optimal designs will also differ. Topol and Califf (1992) have previously articulated these differences (Fig. 18.2). For mechanism-inspired studies, an advantage is also that new biomarkers can be inferred that can be used as surrogates for drug effectiveness. Often, these surrogates or substitutes function as intermediate endpoints. Clearly, the more accurate the mechanistic model, the better the biomarker will perform clinically. Normally in a clinical trial, the medical endpoint is an important clinical outcome such as death, or a disease event such as diabetes, disease relapse or stroke. An intermediate endpoint is a related measurable outcome that can be used as a surrogate for the final outcome. The advantage of this approach is that biomarkers can be used as such surrogate endpoints for these clinical outcomes if the mechanistic understanding links a particular marker to a specific clinical outcome. Blood pressure, for example, has been considered a surrogate endpoint for heart attacks, stroke and kidney failure because there is a known association between blood pressure and cardiovascular death. Drugs are then tested to lower abnormal blood pressure, on the assumption that normalizing hypertension will result in fewer deaths.

Such intermediate outcomes are attractive, because they tend to be readily measured and occur sufficiently frequently in the populations under study that sample sizes can be markedly reduced. Examples of relevant biomarkers are the low-density lipoproteins (LDL). Decreasing the serum concentrations of LDL functions as an intermediate endpoint for targeted therapeutics in place of the clinical outcomes of death, myocardial infarction or stroke. It has been long observed that LDL concentrations are predictive of risk for heart attack, so some clinical trials are directed at decreasing LDL levels rather than seeking a primary reduction of cardiovascular deaths. Among others, however, Fleming and DeMets (1996) have cautioned that it can be misleading to draw therapeutic implications on the basis of measuring intermediate outcomes instead of meaningful clinical outcomes (Figs. 18.3 and 18.4). Granger and McMurray (2006) specifically pointed out examples from myocardial infarction and heart failure trials in which such intermediate outcomes were unreliable as true surrogates for the clinical events of interest. This especially is true when the surrogate biomarker is simply associated with, rather than causative of, the clinical outcome. (An example of this difference between associative and causal relationships might be the association between African descent and sickle-cell anemia: these two factors are simply linked by statistical association, but it is incorrect to say that being African causes sickle-cell anemia.) It is quite a challenge to raise a biomarker or intermediate outcome to the level of a true surrogate that reliably does indeed predict the clinical event of interest (Harrington et al., 2008b; Prentice, 1989). Definitive, practice-changing evidence predominantly comes from large, population-based randomized clinical trials that enroll large numbers of patients with the disease of interest and demonstrate an effect on meaningful clinical

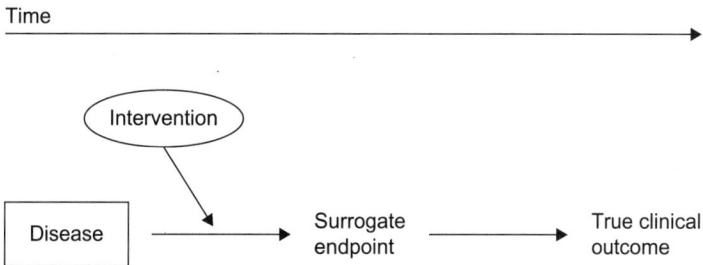

FIGURE 18.3 The Use of Surrogate Endpoints.
The setting that provides the greatest potential for the surrogate endpoint to be valid. Modified from Fleming and DeMets (1996), with permission.

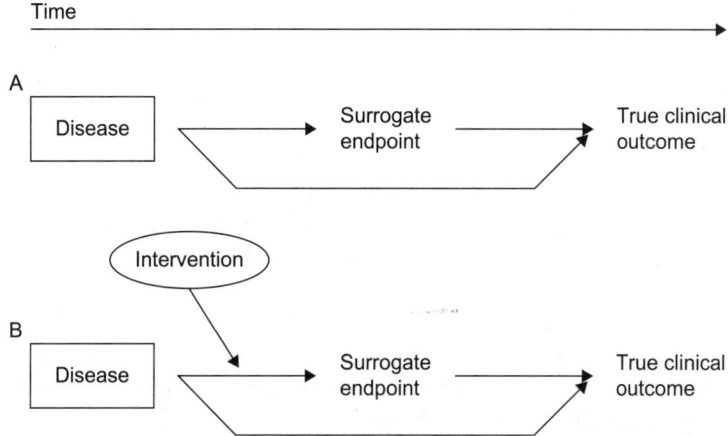

FIGURE 18.4 Drawbacks of Using Surrogate Endpoints.
Reasons for failure of surrogate endpoints. A. The surrogate is not in the causal pathway of the disease process. B. Of several causal pathways of disease, the intervention affects only the pathway mediated through the surrogate. Modified from Fleming and DeMets (1996), with permission.

outcomes, especially death (Table 18.1) (Califf and DeMets, 2002). Nevertheless, unexpected results in which the performance of a biomarker deviates from an expected mechanistic model may lead to insights that will refine the original model. This is another form of iterative improvement of biological modeling through perturbation analysis.

ANOTHER VIEW OF "SYSTEMS" BIOMEDICINE

From a biologist's point of view, systems biology is molecular, mechanistic and explanatory at the level of a cell or a biochemical pathway. Clinical trialists also consider systems biomedicine to include effects on larger population systems such as an entire healthcare system. Clinical trials, especially pragmatic or evaluative ones, represent a systems approach to answering questions that inform clinical practice and decision making. The World Health Organization Global Burden of Disease Project (WHO, 2004) indicated that the major global public health problems are vascular diseases, mental health disorders and cancer. This is true in both developed countries and economically emerging ones. With global disease come both the opportunity and the obligation to understand therapeutic approaches within the societal context

TABLE 18.1 Medical Therapies Proven to Reduce Death

Therapy	Indication	No. Patients	Reduction in Deaths (%)		C/E
			Relative	Absolute	
Aspirin	MI	18 773	23	2.4	+++++
Fibrinolytics	MI	58 000	18	1.8	++++
β-Blocker	MI	28 970	13	1.3	++++
ACE inhibitor	MI	101 000	6.5	0.6	+
Aspirin	2nd prev	54 360	15	1.2	+++++
β-Blocker	2nd prev	20 312	21	2.1	++++
Statins	2nd prev	17 617	23	2.7	++++
ACE inhibitor	2nd prev	9297	17	1.9	++++
ACE inhibitor	CHF	7105	23	6.1	+++++
β-Blocker	CHF	12 385	26	4	+++++
Spironolactone	CHF	1663	30	11	+++++

ACE, angiotensin-converting enzyme; C/E, cost-effectiveness; CHF, chronic heart failure; MI, myocardial infarction; 2nd prev, secondary prevention. Adapted from Califf and DeMets (2002), with permission.

in which the patient lives, works and receives care (the healthcare systems environment). If one views clinical trials of therapeutics in a "system" of information discovery and dissemination, there is much to be learned that can address questions relevant to global health. For example, information technology tools allow collaboration to take place at any time using the internet; the emphasis on establishing widely available electronic health records should allow better integration of clinical research into daily clinical care. The conduct of a clinical trial that involves hundreds of medical centers has immediate impact on the subsequent adoption of new treatments, should the trial show benefit. The mobilization of manpower for a clinical trial that has parallel functions in the standard delivery of care is a systems logistical problem. Data management and data analysis have the same challenges as those seen in systems biological investigations in cellular models. To many in the field, this will be the ultimate in systems biomedicine: when clinical research questions are being asked, addressed and answered continuously and seamlessly within regular care.

CONCLUSION AND SUMMARY

In the other chapters of this book, the concept of systems biology and biomedicine was highly focused on the cell as the unit of study. In clinical investigations, however, the entire human is the unit of systems study. We believe that the first requirement of such a systems approach is to quantify all parameters, so that mathematical models can be constructed. Such an approach is not new; for example, in cardiology, given the mechanical nature of the heart, quantitative medicine has been standard practice. To date, cardiac physiology has modeled the heart as a cylindrical pump with parameters that can be reduced to measurable values: cardiac output, stroke volume, ejection fraction, etc. The intriguing new approach in cardiological systems biology is to refine this pump model to take into account the dynamics of billions of contracting muscle cells (*see* Chapter 13). Such contemporary approaches seek to integrate cell biology with physiologic models. This then is the second tenet of systems biomedicine: the focus on characterizing complexity with mathematical formalism. In contrast to basic scientists, clinical investigators practice systems approaches at the community and population level, in many ways like social and organizational scientists. Surprisingly, the same mathematical principles, such as the power law, hold true across these scales of difference.

The challenge is to bring these new concepts to clinical practice, which is steeped in the tradition of expert opinion and expert judgment. As formal decision analysis becomes mandated by funding bodies in the guise of practice guidelines, one must always keep in mind that no model today can describe all contingencies of human physiology; models must allow for "override" from individual judgments of expert clinicians. Here, we can learn from our basic colleagues in systems biology and systems engineering, who routinely warn us of overfitting models and overengineeing solutions.

References

Alonso-Coello, P., Garcia-Franco, A.L., Guyatt, G., Moynihan, R., 2008. Drugs for pre-osteoporosis: prevention or disease mongering?. BMJ 336, 126–129.

Anderson, J.L., Adams, C.D., Antman, E.M., et al., 2007. ACC/AHA 2007 guidelines for the management of patients with unstable angina/non–ST-elevation myocardial infarction—executive summary. J. Am. Coll. Cardiol. 50, 652–726.

Boersma, E., Westerhout, C.M., 2004. Intravenous glycoprotein IIb/IIIa inhibitors in acute coronary syndromes: lessons from recently conducted randomized clinical trials. Curr. Opin. Invest. Drugs 5, 313–319.

Califf, R.M., DeMets, D.L., 2002. Principles from clinical trials relevant to clinical practice: Part I. Circulation 106, 1015–1021.

Califf, R.M., Harrington, R.A., Madre, L.K., Peterson, E.D., Roth, D., Schulman, K.A., 2007. Curbing the cardiovascular disease epidemic: aligning industry, government, payers, and academics. Health Affairs 26, 62–74.

Charo, I.F., Fitzgerald, L.A., Steiner, B., Rall, Jr. S.C., Bekeart, L.S., Phillips, D.R., 1986. Platelet glycoproteins IIb and IIIa: evidence for a family of immunologically and structurally related glycoproteins in mammalian cells. Proc. Natl. Acad. Sci. USA 83, 8351–8355.

Charo, I.F., Bekeart, L.S., Phillips, D.R., 1987. Platelet glycoprotein IIb-IIIa-like proteins mediate endothelial cell attachment to adhesive proteins and the extracellular matrix. J. Biol. Chem. 262, 9935–9938.

Charo, I.F., Nannizzi, L., Phillips, D.R., Hsu, M.A., Scarborough, R.M., 1991. Inhibition of fibrinogen binding to GP IIb-IIIa by a GP IIIa peptide. J. Biol. Chem. 266, 1415–1421.

Coller, B.S., Peerschke, E.I., Scudder, L.E., Sullivan, C.A., 1983. A murine monoclonal antibody that completely blocks the binding of fibrinogen to platelets produces a thrombasthenic-like state in normal platelets and binds to glycoproteins IIb and/or IIIa. J. Clin. Invest. 72, 325–338.

Coller, B.S., Peerschke, E.I., Seligsohn, U., Scudder, L.E., Nurden, A.T., Rosa, J.P., 1986. Studies on the binding of an alloimmune and two murine monoclonal antibodies to the platelet glycoprotein IIb-IIIa complex receptor. J. Lab. Clin. Med. 107, 384–392.

Coller, B.S., Scudder, L.E., Berger, H.J., Iuliucci, J.D., 1988. Inhibition of human platelet function in vivo with a monoclonal antibody. With observations on the newly dead as experimental subjects. Ann. Intern. Med. 109, 635–638.

Eldor, A., Vlodavsky, I., Martinowicz, U., Fuks, Z., Coller, B.S., 1985. Platelet interaction with subendothelial extracellular matrix: platelet-fibrinogen interactions are essential for platelet aggregation but not for the matrix-induced release reaction. Blood 65, 1477–1483.

EPIC Investigators, 1994. Use of a monoclonal antibody directed against the platelet glycoprotein IIb/IIIa receptor in high-risk coronary angioplasty. The EPIC Investigation. N. Engl. J. Med. 330, 956–961.

EPILOG Investigators, 1997. Platelet glycoprotein IIb/IIIa receptor blockade and low-dose heparin during percutaneous coronary revascularization. N. Engl. J. Med. 336, 1689–1696.

ESPRIT Investigators. Novel dosing regimen of eptifibatide in planned coronary stent implantation (ESPRIT): a randomised, placebo-controlled trial. Lancet 356:2037–2044.

Fleming, T.R., DeMets, D.L., 1996. Surrogate end points in clinical trials: are we being misled? Ann. Intern. Med. 125, 605–613.

Genton, E., Turpie, A.G., 1983. Anticoagulant therapy following acute myocardial infarction. Part I. Incidence of and factors predisposing to thromboembolism associated with acute myocardial infarction. Mod. Concepts Cardiovasc. Dis. 52, 45–48.

Granger, C.B., McMurray, J.J., 2006. Using measures of disease progression to determine therapeutic effect: a siren's song. J. Am. Coll. Cardiol. 48, 434–437.

Harrington, R.A., Kleiman, N.S., Kottke-Marchant, K., et al., 1995. Immediate and reversible platelet inhibition after intravenous administration of a peptide glycoprotein IIb/IIIa inhibitor during percutaneous coronary intervention. Am. J. Cardiol. 76, 1222–1227.

Harrington, R.A., Becker, R.C., Cannon, C.P., et al., 2008a. Antithrombotic therapy for non-ST-segment elevation acute coronary syndromes. Chest 133, 670S–707S.

Harrington, R.A., Hasselblad, V., Califf, R.M., 2008b. Defining and utilizing surrogates in the evaluation of coronary stents: what do we really want and need to know? J. Am. Coll. Cardiol. 51, 33–36.

ISIS-2 (Second International Study of Infarct Survival) Collaborative Group, 1988. Randomised trial of intravenous streptokinase, oral aspirin, both, or neither among 17,187 cases of suspected acute myocardial infarction: ISIS-2. Lancet 2, 349–360.

Katz, J.N., Harrington, R.A., 2009. Intravenous glycoprotein IIb/IIIa antagonists. In: Freedman, J. E., Loscalzo, J. (Eds.), New Therapeutic Agents in Thrombosis and Thrombolysis. 3rd ed. Informa Healthcare USA, Inc., New York (2009), pp. 00–00.

Kong, D.F., Hasselblad, V., Harrington, R.A., et al., 2003. Meta-analysis of survival with platelet glycoprotein IIb/IIIa antagonists for percutaneous coronary interventions. Am. J. Cardiol. 92, 651–655.

Phillips, D.R., Agin, P.P., 1977. Platelet membrane defects in Glanzmann's thrombasthenia. Evidence for decreased amounts of two major glycoproteins. J. Clin. Invest. 60, 535–545.

Phillips, D.R., Fitzgerald, L.A., Charo, I.F., Parise, L.V., 1987. The platelet membrane glycoprotein IIb/IIIa complex. Structure, function, and relationship to adhesive protein receptors in nucleated cells. Ann. NY Acad. Sci. 509, 177–187.

Prentice, R.L., 1989. Surrogate endpoints in clinical trials: definition and operational criteria. Stat. Med. 8, 431–440.

PURSUIT Investigators, 1998. Inhibition of platelet glycoprotein IIb/IIIa with eptifibatide in patients with acute coronary syndromes. N. Engl. J. Med. 339, 436–443.

Scarborough, R.M., Rose, J.W., Hsu, M.A., et al., 1991. A GPIIb-IIIa-specific integrin antagonist from the venom of Sistrurus m. barbouri. J. Biol. Chem. 266, 9359–9362.

Scarborough, R.M., Naughton, M.A., Teng, W., et al., 1993. Design of potent and specific integrin antagonists. Peptide antagonists with high specificity for glycoprotein IIb-IIIa. J. Biol. Chem. 268, 1066–1073.

Smith Jr., S.C., Feldman Jr., T.E., Hirshfeld, J.W., et al., 2006. ACC/AHA/SCAI 2005 guideline update for percutaneous coronary intervention – summary article. J. Am. Coll. Cardiol. 47, 216–235.

Straus, S.E., Sackett, D.L., 1998. Using research findings in clinical practice. BMJ 317, 339–342.

Tcheng, J.E., Ellis, S.G., George, B.S., et al., 1994. Pharmacodynamics of chimeric glycoprotein IIb/IIIa integrin antiplatelet antibody Fab 7E3 in high-risk coronary angioplasty. Circulation 90, 1757–1764.

Tcheng, J.E., Lincoff, A.M., Sigmon, K.N.for the IMPACT II Investigators, , et al., 1994. Platelet glycoprotein IIb/IIIA inhibition with Integrilin during percutaneous coronary intervention: the IMPACT II Trial [Abstract]. Circulation 92 (suppl I), I–I543.

Topol, E.J., Califf, R.M., 1992. Answers to complex questions cannot be derived from "simple" trials. Br. Heart J. 68, 348–351.

WHO, 2004. http://www.who.int/healthinfo/global_burden_disease/GBD_report_2004update_full.pdf. Global Burden of Disease Project.

Index

Note: Page numbers followed by *f* indicate figure; page numbers followed by *t* indicate table.

A

ABC-DLBCL. *See* Activated B-cell-like diffuse large B-cell lymphoma (ABC-DLBCL)
ABM, of cellular networks. *See* Agent-based modeling (ABM), of cellular networks
Accounting cycle, 317
   for receptors, 319, 320*f*
Acetylation, 127
Acquired immunodeficiency syndrome (AIDS), 355
ACR. *See* American College of Rheumatology (ACR)
Activated B-cell-like diffuse large B-cell lymphoma (ABC-DLBCL), 406
Activator
   binding sites for, 60
   and enhanceosome, 60–61
   sequence-specific DNA binding transcription factors, 60
Active proteins, production of, 124
Acute lymphoblastic leukemia (ALL) cell, 395
Adalimumab, 369
Adhesome
   classification of components, 144
   constructing network, 141–142
   domains associated, with components of, 149
   functional families of, 142–143
   holistic view, 141
   protein domains and switchable links for, 147, 149, 150
Affymetrix arrays, 27, 28
Agent-based modeling (ABM), of cellular networks, 239–245
   agents, 240
   initial conditions and scaling, 241–242
   of neural tube domain patterning, 242*f*–243*f*
   rules sets, 240–241
   simulation space, 241
   validation of, 242, 244
Agents, of ABM, 240
AIDS. *See* Acquired immunodeficiency syndrome (AIDS)
ALK. *See* Anaplastic lymphoma kinase (ALK)
ALL. *See* Acute lymphoblastic leukemia (ALL) cell
Allergic, 367
American College of Rheumatology (ACR), 370
Analytical models, statistical/probabilistic information into, 191
Anaplastic lymphoma kinase (ALK), 380
Andre's CellML tools, 299
Androgen-receptor, 395
API. *See* Application Programming Interface (API)
Apple QuickTime, 281
Application Programming Interface (API), 302
Arabidopsis thaliana
   circadian rhythm in, 263
Array datasets, variation in, 27
Arrestin, 204
ATA. *See* Aurintricarboxylic acid (ATA)
ATF5 in neural development, 123
Aurintricarboxylic acid (ATA), 394
Autocrine signaling, 179
Autoimmune diseases, 367
   cytokine blockade, 369–370
   mathematical model for, 367–368
   overview, 367
   TCV in, 368
Autoregulation, 124–126
   in ESCs, 124
   Lin28 and *let-7*, 126
   mir-21, to target gene, 125
   Nanog and REST, role of, 124–125
Average sensitivity rank, of parameters, 267*f*

B

bantam, regulating apoptosis in *Drosophila*, 112
Batch correction method, 74
Bayesian networks, 8, 235, 392
   discretization, 237
   dynamic, 236
   goal of, 236–237
   modeling of Hedgehog target genes, 237–239, 238*f*
   scoring metric and, 237
Bayes' rule, 236
B cells, 204
Bcl2, anti-apoptotic gene, 113
Bim promoter, 387
Binary variables (u_i), 197
Biochemical descriptive language, 295
Biochemical kinetics calculation, 4
Biochemical models, 181–182
   challenges in building
      integration of diverse data, 186–188
      proteomic states and interactions, 184–186
   temporal state of, 188
      correlation networks, 188–189
      dynamic and temporally causal networks, 189–190
      static pseudocausal directional networks, 189
Biochemical systems
   Bayesian networks, 183
   biochemical model. *See* Biochemical model
   biomolecular network database, 182
   cell-specific constraining of parameters, 184
   computational model, 182

425

Biochemical systems (*Continued*)
  mathematical model, 182
  SBML format, 183
  simple input–output models, 183
  systems biology software, 183
  three-level modeling strategy, 181
Biochemiluminescence-based assay, 18
Biological fluids, proteomics of
  biomarkers for, 48
  in cancer, 48, 50
  isobaric tag labeling method for, 50
  plasma proteins for disease-related changes, 48–49
  strategies for, 48
Biological Pathway Exchange (BioPAX), 307
Biological processes, genome-wide systems analyses of, 16
Biological systems, importance of control theory in, 5
Biomarkers, for therapeutic efficacy in cancer, 393–394
BioModels database, 308–309
BioNetGen, 297, 299
Biopathways Workbench tool, 185
BioPAX. *See* Biological Pathway Exchange (BioPAX)
BioSens, 268–269
BioTapestry, 297
Black boxes, 318
B lymphocyte, 113, 368
Bmal1 knockout mice
  fibroblasts from, 10
  sensitivity to cyclophosphamide, 11
BMP. *See* Bone morphogenic protein (BMP)
Bone morphogenic protein (BMP), 244
Boolean variables, 240
Branched DNA technology, 32–33
Breast cancer
  target-based therapy, 379
  translational impact in
    biological heterogeneity of, 66
    expression cassettes, 67
    molecular markers, 67
    p53 mutations and gene expression, association between, 68
    transcriptional signatures, 66–67
Breast-cancer model system, 404
Browsers, database, 275

C

Cable theory, equations of, 284
Ca^{2+} concentration, 206
CADLive, 297

Caenorhabditis elegans, 112, 330
  endogenous RNAs in, 35–36
  lin-4 in, 127
  RNAi tools in, 36–37
Calcium
  binding proteins, 208
  influx, 204
  modeling, 209
  signaling, 199–200, 204
Calcium dynamics in RAW 264.7 cells, regulation of, 204
  mathematical representation, 207–208
  mechanisms, 204–206
    calmodulin and PKC, feedback effects from, 207
    GTPase cycle module, 206–207
    IP3 module, 207
    receptor module, 206
  simulation and parameter estimation, 208–209
    dose response, 209–210, 212
    knockdown response, 210, 211
    receptor recovery system, analysis of, 210–211
    sensitivity analysis, 210
Calcium-induced calcium release (CICR) mechanism, 208
Calponin homology, 147
Cancer, 360–367 specific entries
  biomarkers for therapeutic efficacy, 393–394
  cell model data, integrating and extending, 404–405
  hard wiring mechanism, 392
  homogenous single-compartment models, 361–364
  natural robustness of malignant cells, 388–389
  systems-based approaches to drug discovery, 402
  therapeutic strategies, 388–390
  transcriptome for novel targets, 390–393
Cancer outlier profile analysis (COPA), 380
Cancer patient prognosis, transcriptional regulation
  cis-regulatory motifs binding, 70–71
  E2F binding motifs, 71
  embryonic stem cell expression, 69–70
  ESC-specific binding of transcription factors, 71
  exogenous c-myc, 70
  five-gene genetic grade signature, 69
  gene expression "signatures", 68
  stem cell phenotype, 69
Cancer signatures, in vivo, 393

Cardiovascular medicine, 419
Casein kinase 1 and oscillator, 9
Caspase, 260, 261
CCA1. *See* Circadian clock associated 1 (CCA1)
CCAAT-box binding transcription factor, 391
CDK2. *See* Cyclindependent kinase 2 (CDK2)
cDNA fragments, 26
cDNA library, primed, 33
Cell adhesion, 157
Cell-based proteomics
  discovery workflow, 47
  enzyme activities, 47–48
  glycoproteins, 47
  isotopic labeling for, 46
  of ovarian adenocarcinoma cell lines, 46–47
  of ovarian cancer cell lines, 47
  post-translational modifications, 47
Cell culture, mammalian, RNAi and, 405
Cell culture systems, in-situ PCR technology in, 33
CellDesigner, 298
Cellerator / xCellerator, 299
Cell Illustrator, 298
Cell isotopic labeling, 46
Cell lines, cancer, 403
Cell Markup Language (CellML). *See* CellML
CellML, 305
  Andre's tools, 299
  applications based on, 298–299
  component based implementation, 321–324
  incorporate models into tissue and organ models, 325–327
  schematic file of IP3, 322, 323*f*
  VCell and, 276
Cell motility, 202
Cell signaling, enzyme–substrate interactions, 57
Cellular complexity, 120
Cellular processes, 253–254
Cellular signaling, 179
Cellular systems, transcription network in
  acting as activators/repressors in, 111
  transcription factors, defining roles in, 111
  unspliced mRNA molecules, production of, 110–111
Cellware, 297
CH. *See* Calponin homology
Channel flux (J_{ch}), 210
Chemical master equation (CME), 254–255

Chemotherapy, *vs.* immunotherapy, 363
ChIP. *See* Chromatin immunoprecipitation
ChIP analyses for OCT4, SOX2 and NANOG, 160
ChIP-enriched DNA, 157, 158
ChIP-on-chip arrays
   advantages of, 29–30
   and DNA microarrays, 29
   labeled using fluorescent dyes, 29
   probe design challenges, 30
ChIP-on-chip/ChIP–PET data, 161
ChIP–PET analysis, 158
ChIP–PET cluster, 159
ChIP–PET method, of mapping, 159
ChIP-sequencing technologies, 157, 159
Chromatin-associated proteins, 167
Chromatin immunoprecipitation, 157
Chromatin structure, 167
Chromatography, 385
Chromosome conformation capture (3C), 64
Chromosome translocation
   in CML, 379
Chronic lymphocytic leukemia, 113
Chronic myelogenous leukemia (CML), 379
Circadian clock, components of, 9
Circadian clock associated 1 (CCA1), 263
Circadian cycles
   and metabolism, link between, 10
   as model for systems biomedicine
     in animal models, 10
     molecular mechanism, 9
     schematic representation, 10
Circadian entrainment, flies and, 265–268
Circadian rhythm, 262
   of arabidopsis thaliana, 263
   of fly, 264–265
   mouse, 268–270
Cis-regulatory modules, 343
   role of, in Dorsal–ventral patterning of *Drosophila* Embryo, 345f
   spatial and temporal regulation of *endo-16*, 344f
cis-regulatory motif role, 66
cis-regulatory region, of gene, 128
c-Jun N-terminal kinase (JNK) pathway, 384
Classical genetics and systems biology, 5
Classifier, 74
Client-server architecture, of VCell, 285
Clinical genomic data, 403
Clinical trials
   comparison of, models, 420
   role of, in modern medicine, 415–417
   of therapeutics, 417–419

Clock genes and metabolic phenotypes, associations between, 10
Clustering strategies for gene, 72–73
CME. *See* Chemical master equation (CME)
CML. *See* Chronic myelogenous leukemia (CML)
Co-activators, 60
Coarse-grained model, 194
Coarse-graining
   advanced research in, 213
   mixed-integer non-linear programming approach to
     basic concept, 197
     graph-theoretic approach, 198–199
     MINLP, formulation of, 197–198
     network structure and estimation of parameters, 197
   modularity of networks, an additional advantage of, 193
   steps for, 195
Co-inertia analysis (CIA), 187
COMBAT algorithm, 74
Combination therapy, 382–385
   DNA repair, 383
   in human cancers, 382
Combinatorial interaction, 126
Complex robust systems, 388
CompMoby, 161
Component, 317
   functional, 317
   messenger, 317
Computational modeling of cell signaling networks
   activation of ERK, 96
   Boolean logic description, 96
   differential equation models, 95–96
   Fuzzy logic extension, 96
   PCA and PLSR algorithms, 96–97
   software tools for, 97
Computational models, challenges in building
   cell-specific and subpopulational variability, 204
   distance and time, variation in, 201–202
   multiple scales, 203
   stochastic simulation, 202–203
   unknown parameters, 199–200
   parameter estimation, approaches to, 200–201
Computational Proteomics Analysis System, 52
Computational systems biology, 190, 211
   paradigms in, 178
Computational tools for network construction and modeling, 160

Bayesian network, 162
network dynamics, 162–163
network mapping, 161–162
regulatory module, 161
Conditional probability, 235–236
Conrad, Emery, 300
Coordinated target genes, regulation of burst-like manner, in eukaryotic cell, 122
   coherent circuits, 120–121
   coherent motif, 120
   ESCs, Oct4 expression, 122
   incoherent circuits, 121, 122
   incoherent motif, 120
   regulation, of common target genes, 120
   repression, of RESTtargeted protein-coding genes and, 122
   silencing effects, 121
   synergism of upstream factors, 120
   Tcf3 role of, 122
   temporal gap, 122
   transcription factor–miRNA pairing, 120
   transcriptions of *miR-29* and *miR-135b*, 122
COPA. *See* Cancer outlier profile analysis (COPA)
COPASI, 294–295
COR, CellML-based tool, 299
Co-regulators, 60
Co-repressors, 60
Core promoter, 61
Corrected phase trajectories, 257, 258f
Correlation, diagrams
   comparison of sensitivity measures using, 266f
CPAS. *See* Computational Proteomics Analysis System
Crk protein, 147
   protein domains and switchable links of, 150
CRx-026, 385
CTCF in regulating gene expression, 64
CTL. *See* Cytotoxic lymphocyte (CTL)
Cullen ubiquitin ligase complexes, 392
Cyclindependent kinase 2 (CDK2), 391
Cyclin D1 gene, 382
   convergence of pathways, 383f
Cytokine blockade, disease-specific efficacy of, 369–370
Cytokine-induced differentiation, 114
Cytokines, 186
Cytoscape, 187, 297
CytoSim, 304

Cytotoxic chemotherapy, 382
Cytotoxic lymphocyte (CTL), 355

D

DAG. *See* Directed acyclic graph (DAG)
Data acquisition in biology, 4
Database
  BioModels, 308–309
  VCell, 275–278
DCC in neural development, 123
DCL. *See* Diagrammatic Cell Language (DCL)
Death, medical therapies to reduce, 421, 422t
3-deazaneplanocin A (DZNep), 387
Decapentaplegic (dpp), 336
Deconvoluting mechanisms, 385–386
Delaunay triangulation, 283
Delta/Notch signaling pathway, 330, 331f
Dendritic cells, 354, 355
Deterministic simulation, 201
DGCR8, RNA-binding domain protein, 112
Diagrammatic Cell Language (DCL), 298
Dicer, 36, 112, 113
Differential equations, problems with, 291
Directed acyclic graph (DAG), 236
Discretization, in Bayesian networks, 237
Distal promoter elements, 61
Distance weighted discrimination method, 74
Dizzy, 304
DNA binding factors, 157
DNA interactions, mapping, 157–160
DNA library
  immobilization of, 19
  preparation. *See* DNA library preparation
DNA library preparation, 20–21
  bridge amplification, 21
  DNA fragments for, 20–21
  in Roche/454 sequencing platform
    DNA fractionation, 18
    dsDNA fragments separation, 19
    ligation of short adapters, 19
  in SOLiD platform, 23
DNA methylation, 167
  for epigenetic control of transcription, 63
DNA microarray, generation of, 29
DNA probes
  double-stranded cDNAs, 26
  matched and mismatched, 27
DNA promoters, 124
DNA sequencing
  parallel, 19
  using DNA polymerase and nucleotide terminators, 17
  using reverse transcriptase, 24
  using SOLiD platform
    fluorescence tag, 24
    primer hybridization, 23–24
D-optimal design, 253
  in Fas apoptosis model, 262, 262f
Dorsal-ventral (DV) axis, 244
Dorsal–ventral patterning, of *Drosophila* Embryo, 345f
Dose-response curve, 240
dpp. See Decapentaplegic (dpp)
Drosophila Embryo, 332
  Dorsal–ventral patterning of, role of *Cis*-regulatory sequences in, 345f
Drosophila melanogaster
  endogenous RNAs in, 35–36
  RNAi tools in, 36–37
Drosophila melanogaster, circadian rhythm of, 264–265
Drug discovery
  cancer and. *See* Cancer
  challanges in treating HIV. *See* Human immunodeficiency virus (HIV)
  challanges to, in immune-related disease, 352–353
  immunology, 354–355
  leveraging integrative systems approaches in, 402f
  system biology for, 353–354, 354t
  systems biology in, 401
    cancer cell model data, integrating and extending, 404–405
    from clinical genomics to model systems, 403–404
    systems-oriented target identification, 405–407
Druggable proteins, 377
Drug resistance, viral, 358
DV axis. *See* Dorsal-ventral (DV) axis
Dynamic Bayesian networks, 236
Dynamic causal networks, 189–190
DZNep. *See* 3-deazaneplanocin A (DZNep)
DZNep-induced apoptosis, 387

E

EAE. *See* Experimental autoimmune encephalomyelitis (EAE) model
E-Cell, 299–300
Echinoderm microtubule-associated protein-like 4 (EML4), 380
EC_{50} value, 210
Edinburgh Pathway Editor, 297

Editors, visual, 297
  CellDesigner, 298
  commercial visual design tools, 298
  JDesigner, 298
EGFR. *See* Epidermal growth factor receptor; Epidermal growth factor receptor (EGFR)
Ehox transcription factor, 161
E3 ligase, 145
Embryoid body formation, 114
Embryonic stem cells, 111
  associated transcription factors, 114
  depletion of, 115
  differentiation, 123, 161, 167, 171
  genetic perturbation strategies, for regulators of, 164
  proliferation, 161
  properties of, 158
  specific genes, 156
  specific motifs, 161
  specific transcripts, 156
  transcriptional regulation, of microRNAs in, 171–172
  transcriptome of, 156
EML4. *See* Echinoderm microtubule-associated protein-like 4 (EML4)
Emulsion polymerase chain reaction process, 19
endo-16, spatial and temporal regulation of, 344f
Endocrine system, 179
Endoplasmic reticulum (ER), 204, 207
Engineering miRNA networks, 119–120
Enhanceosomes, 60–61
Enhancers
  functionality, 61
  location, 62
ENU. *See* N-ethyl-N-nitrosourea (ENU)
Enzyme (E)-catalyzed reaction, 280, 280f
Enzyme–substrate (ES), 280
  databases, 57–58
Epidermal growth factor receptor, 46
  activation, 180
Epidermal growth factor receptor (EGFR), 380
  gefitinib blockade of, 381f
Epigenetic control of transcription
  DNA methylation for, 63
  histone modification, 63–64
Epigenetics, 167
Epistasis, mathematical representation of, 5
ER. *See* Estrogen receptor
Eras-deficient cells, 166
Eras gene, 166
ErbB receptor phosphorylation, 180
Erlotinib, 380

ES. *See* Enzyme-substrate (ES)
ESC. *See* Embryonic stem cells (ESC)
Estrogen receptor
  activatation, 82
  binding sites
    and ERE motif, 83
    genome-wide positioning and
      characteristics of, 83–84
    for transcription factors, 84
  dimerization, 82
  genome-wide positioning and
    characteristics of, 83–84
  interaction of modulators of
    transcriptional regulation with, 83
  in-vivo studies of, 83
Etanercept, 369
Eukaryotes, 254
Eukaryotic kinases, 84–85
Euler method, 282
Evidence-based medicine, 415
Evolvable systems, 5
Exact stochastic simulators, 284
Experimental autoimmune
  encephalomyelitis (EAE) model,
  368
Expressed Sequence Tag (EST), 156
Expression arrays, 26
  Affymetrix arrays, 27, 28
  complexity in, 28
  datasets, variation in, 27
  oligonucleotide probes, 58
  performance analysis of, 27
Expression for $J_{PM,IP3dep}$, 208
Expression quantitative trait loci (eQTL)
  in humans, 8
Extracellular-signal-regulated kinase
  (ERK) phosphorylation, 162

F

Factorization, of matrix, 229
False discovery rate (FDR), 73
Familial advanced sleep-phase syndrome
  (FASPS), 9
Fas apoptosis model, 260–262, 260f
  D-optimal design, 262, 262f
  hypothesis discrimination, 260–262,
    261f
FasL. *See* Fas ligand (FasL)
Fas ligand (FasL), 260
F-box protein, 387
Feed-forward loops, 77–78, 123
FERM domains, 147
FFL. *See* Feed-forward loops (FFL)
FGF. *See* Fibroblast growth factor (FGF)
Fibroblast growth factor (FGF), 244, 333,
  384
Fick's second law, 240

FieldML, 327
Filamin, 149
FIM. *See* Fisher information matrix (FIM)
Firegoose, 187
Fisher information matrix (FIM), 251
  optimization of data quality and,
    253
  stochastic system and, 255
Five-gene genetic grade signature, 69
Flies
  circadian entrainment and, 265–268
  circadian rhythm of, 264–265
Fluidigm Biomark, 32
Fluorescence-based competition assay,
  165
Forger and Peskin model, 269–270
Forward genetics
  ENU mutagenesis, 35
  phenotypic assays, 34
FoxD3 transcription factor, 161
Frameworks, in SBW, 296
Funahashi, Akira, 298
Functional biological network map, for
  Halobacterium salinarum, 6
Functional component, 317
Functional protein families, 144–145
Functional subnets, 145–146

G

GA–DE–PSO algorithm, 201
Gastrointestinal stromal tumor (GIST),
  380
Gaussian noise, FIM and, 251
Gefitinib, 380
Gene, transcriptional regulatory region
  of, 59
Gene-based technologies for systems
  studies, 16
Gene clustering strategies, 72–73
Gene disruption by homologous
  recombination, 35
Gene expression data, Shh pathway and,
  237–238
Gene identification signature pair-end
  ditag (GIS-PET), 26
Gene profiling experiments, circadian
  periodicity, 10
Generalized minimal residuals method
  (GMRES), 283
General transcription factors, 59–60
  binding to core promoter, 61
Gene regulatory networks, 120, 190
Gene signature
  assessment of, in disparate clinical
    settings, 410, 410f
  for clinical predictions, from model
    systems, 411f

  for drug action–gene function
    connectivity map, 394–395
Genetic perturbation strategies, 164
Genome Analyzer, 20
Genome Sequencer 20 (GS20), 17
  sequencing process in, 22
Genome-to-systems, 16
  technologies for, 17
Genome-wide mutagenesis, strategies for
  forward genetics
    ENU mutagenesis, 35
    phenotypic assays, 34
    reverse genetics, 35
Genome-wide transcription factor
  location analysis, 114
Genomic data, integration of, 405
Genomic medical approaches, advantage
  of, 73
GEPASI, 294
GFP. *See* Green fluorescent protein (GFP)
Gibson – Bruck Next Reaction method,
  284
Gillespie algorithms, 284
Gillespie method, 303
GIST. *See* Gastrointestinal stromal tumor
  (GIST)
Glanzmann's thrombasthenia, 417
Glioma cytotoxic lymphocyte
  immunotherapy model,
    validations of, 364t
Gli transcription factor, 227
Glycogen synthase kinase 3 beta (GSK3
  β), 385
Glycoprotein (GP), 418
Glycoproteins, 47
GMRES. *See* Generalized minimal
  residuals method (GMRES)
GoSurfer, software tool, 157
GP. *See* Glycoprotein (GP)
GPCR module, 319, 320f
GP IIb/IIIa receptor complex, 418
G-protein, 184, 206, 283
  activation, 206–207
G-protein-coupled receptor (GPCR)
  kinase (GRK), 204
Granulocyte-colony stimulating factor
  (G-CSF), 187
Graphical modeling applications, 306
green fluorescent protein (GFP), 337
  expression cassettes, 165
GS 20. *See* Genome Sequencer 20 (GS20)
GSK3 β. *See* Glycogen synthase kinase 3
  beta (GSK3 β)
GTF. *See* General transcription factors
  (GTF)
GTPase cycle, 206
Gurken gradient, 337

H

HAART. *See* Highly active antiretroviral therapy (HAART)
Halobacterium salinarum, functional biological network map for, 6
HBV. *See* Hepatitis B virus (HBV)
HCT116 colon carcinoma cell, 385
HCV. *See* Hepatitis C virus (HCV)
HDACI. *See* Histone deacetylase inhibitors (HDACI)
HDAC inhibitor, 387
Heart, multi-scale modeling for, 325, 326f
Hedgehog (Hh), 333
Hedgehog target genes, Bayesian-network modeling of, 236–239, 238f
Heparan sulfate proteoglycan (HSPG), 336
Hepatitis B virus (HBV), 355
Hepatitis C virus (HCV), 355
Hh. *See* Hedgehog (Hh)
Hierarchical clustering, 73
High-level modeling, 226–245
  partial least squares. *See* Partial least squares modeling
Highly active antiretroviral therapy (HAART), 356
Highly Optimized Theory (HOT), 5
High-sensitivity fluorescence detection, 22
Hill coefficient, 208
Hill kinetics, 263
Hill-type equation, 208
Histone deacetylase inhibitors (HDACI), 387
Histone modification, epigenetic control of transcription, 63–64
Histone modifications, 167
H3K4 methylation, 167, 168
H3K27 methylation, 167
HMEC. *See* Human mammary epithelial cells (HMEC)
Homogenous single-compartment models, 361–364
Homologous recombination, 165
  strategies, gene disruption by, 35
Homozygous *Clock*-mutant mice, 10
HSPG. *See* Heparan sulfate proteoglycan (HSPG)
HSP90 inhibitor, 395
Human Genome Project, 17
Human immunodeficiency virus (HIV)
  challenges in treating, 355–356
  mathematical models of, 356–358, 357f
  STI and, 358–360
  viral drug resistance, 358
Human mammary epithelial cells (HMEC), 393
Human medicine, 5

Human Protein Reference Database (HPRD), 85

I

Illumina Genome Analyzer, sequencing process in, 22
IL-4-specific pathways, 187
Imatinib, 379
Immune cells, 364
  distribution of, 364
  lymphocyte trafficking, 364–367
Immune-related diseases, and drug discovery and development, 352–353
Immunology, 354–355
Immunotherapy, *vs.* chemotherapy, 363
Infliximab, 369
Ingenuity Pathways Analysis (IPA), 94
Inositol triphosphate (IP3), 319
  CellML schematic file of, 322, 323f
  reaction scheme of, 319, 320f
Inositol 1,4,5-trisphosphate (IP3), 184
Insulators/boundary elements
  importance of, 62–63
  transcription regulation by, 63
Intact Protein Analysis System (IPAS), 50
Integrin, 147
Interconnecting network of cancer-relevant signaling molecules, 378f
interfering RNAs (siRNAs), 111
Interferon (IFN)α, 187
Interleukin-2 (IL-2) pathway, 180
Interleukins (IL)-1α, -6 and -10, 187
IP3. *See* Inositol triphosphate (IP3)
IP3R channels, 205
IP3 receptor (IP3R) proteins, 184
ISIS-2. *See* Second International Study of Infarct Survival (ISIS-2)
Isobaric tag labeling method (iTRAQ), 50

J

Jacobian matrix, 291
Jarnac, 295
JDesigner, 298
JigCell, 300
JNK. *See* C-Jun N-terminal kinase (JNK) pathway
JSIM, 295
JWS, online database, 308

K

KEGG compound database
  searching for species in, 276, 277f
Kinases, 142
KineCyte, 297

Kinetic Algorithm Ontology (KiSAO), 307
Kirchoff's equations, current and voltage, 283
KiSAO. *See* Kinetic Algorithm Ontology (KiSAO)
K-means clustering, 73
Knockdown responses, 210
Knockout mice, reverse genetics in, 35

L

Langevin equation, 292
Laplace-Beltrami operator, 283
Late elongated hypocotyl (LHY), 263
Layilin, 147
LDL. *See* Low-density lipoproteins (LDL)
Lectin arrays, 51
Lentiviruses, 165
Leukemia cells, 393
Leukocytes, 365
LHY. *See* Late elongated hypocotyl (LHY)
Libraries, software, 301
  libSBML, 302, 306
  libStructural, 303
  re-usable, 310
  SOSLib, 302
LibSBML, 302, 306
LibStructural, 303
Ligand binding, to receptors, 341
Lilly's Life Sciences Grid (LSG), 404
LIM domains, 147
Limit cycle behavior, of oscillatory system, 256f
Lin28, blocking processing, 130
Linear dynamic Bayesian network, 190
lin-14 mRNA, 127
Lipid subnet, 146
Llipidomics, 178
Loadings vectors, 229–230
Locus control regions (LCRs), 62
Long-range chromosomal looping, 64
Low-density lipoproteins (LDL), 420
LRH1 gene, 115
LSG. *See* Lilly's Life Sciences Grid (LSG)
Luminex assays, RNA detection using, 33
Lumped parameter, 318
Lumping reactions, 199
Lymphocyte trafficking, 364–367
  in vivo, 365
Lymphocytic leukemia, 113

M

Macrophage-colony stimulating factor (M-CSF) -specific pathway, 187
Macrophage inflammatory protein (MIP)-1α, 187

INDEX

Macrophages, 204
Major histocompatibility complex (MHC), 363
Mammals, circadian rhythms of, 268–270
MAPK. See Mitogen-activated protein kinases (MAPK)
Markov stochastic process, 284
Mass action, 263, 278
Mathematical model
  challenges in building. See Mathematical model, challenges in building
  of HIV, 356–358, 357f
  hypothesis generation and discrimination, 253
  optimization of data quality, 253
  refinement of, sensitivity analysis and, 251–252
  of tumor–immune interaction, 361f
Mathematical model, challenges in building, 190
  incomplete knowledge and coarse graining, 193–195
    implementation and case study, 196
    multiparametric variability analysis, 195–196
    reduced-order models, generation of, 196
  incorporating statistical/probabilistic information, 191
  utilizing qualitative constraints, 191–192
    additional simulations, for validation, 193
    semi-quantitative constraints, 192–193
    temporal responses, qualitative trend of, 192
Mathematics and biological problems, 5
MathSBML, 295–296
Matlab®, 196
Matrix
  dependent blocks, 230–231
  factorization of, 229
  independent blocks, 230–231
  Jacobian, 291
  for sensitivity analysis, 255–258
Mature miRNA, 112, 130
MCA. See Metabolic control analysis (MCA)
MCF10A cells, 392
MCL1. See Myeloid cell leukemia-1 (MCL1)
Mechanism-derived biomarker discovery, 68
Membrane transport kinetics, 278–279

Mendes, Pedro, 294
Messenger component, 317
Meta-analysis procedures, 74
Metabolic control analysis (MCA), 292
Metabolic engineering, 180
Metabolomics, 178
Methylation, 127
Methyl-CpG binding proteins, 167
MHC. See Major histocompatibility complex (MHC)
MHC class I (MHCI), 363
MHCI. See MHC class I (MHCI)
MIASE. See Minimum Information About a Simulation Experiment (MIASE)
Michaelis-Menten flux expression, 197
Michaelis-Menten formulation, 362
Michaelis-Menten rate, 278
Microarray-based approaches
  protein microarrays
    classes of, 51
    concept of, 50–51
    detection of binding in, 51
    for glycomic analysis, 51–52
    lectin arrays, 51–52
    uses of, 50
Microarray data analysis
  and clustering of similarly regulated genes, 28
  complexity in, 28
Minimum Information About a Simulation Experiment (MIASE), 307
Minimum information requested in the annotation of biochemical models (MIRIAM), 276, 306–307
MINLP approach, 197
miR-1, inducing differentiation, 113
mir-14, regulating apoptosis in *Drosophila*, 112
mir-16-1, of chromosome, 13, 113
mir-17-92, for animal development, 114
mir-134
  induced differentiation, 113
  induced translation, 115
  and mRNA, 115
mir-181, modulating hemopoietic stem cells in mice, 112
miR-203, repressing transcription factor, 113
mir-273, controling neuronal cell, 112
mir-15a, of chromosome, 13, 113
mir-372 and *mir-373*, for testicular germ cell tumors, 113
mir-371/2/3 family, in human, 113

MIRIAM. See Minimum information requested in the annotation of biochemical models (MIRIAM)
miR-296 in mouse ESCs, overexpression, 171
miRNA, 35, 111
  act as translational activators, 124
  activation/repression in ESCs, 115
  alterations in expression patterns, 115
  altering expression of genes in mammalian cell types, 113
  binding sites, 129
  binding to 5′ UTR binding sites, and, 129
  biogenesis and function, 111–113
  and cloning of cDNA libraries, 130
  combinatorial interaction among, 126
  concentration in primary tumors, 113
  downregulation, 114
  in embryonic stem cells, 169–170
  ESCs deficient in components of, 113
  extensive roles in, 112
  features for swift response to differentiation signals, 124
  forward feedback loop, to suppress a transcriptional factor, 171
  founding members, in nematode, 112
  functions, 127
    inhibitory function, 169
    models for, 169
  hubs, 114
  identification of targets, 117
  inducing ESC differentiation, 115
  intersection of targeting networks, 118
  in metazoans, 112, 115, 126–127
  microarray techniques, 170, 171
  miRNA–TF networks, 116
  network and interface with transcriptional factors, 115
  in plants, 112
  post-transcriptional control by, 64–65
  post-transcriptional processing, 124
  production of, 124
  recycling of, 124
  rheostat model, 127
  rules for switch, deciphering, 128
    blockade of translation, 128
    degree of complementarity of, 128
    elongation, 128
    iron-responsive element, 129
    length of 3′ UTR and binding sites, 128, 129
    miRNA-mediated gene regulation, 128
    net repressive effect, 128
    RNP complexes, 128

miRNA (Continued)
    sequestration of Argonaute-bound mRNA into P-body, 128
    translational inhibition, 128
    translational repression/mRNA degradation, 128
    in silico prediction models, 115
    and siRNAs, 36
    spatial and temporal control, interaction on, 129–130
    stem cell factors, at promoters of, 114
    target gene regulation by, 117
    target hubs, 126
    targeting of pluripotency factors, 115
    and target mRNAs, 168
    target prediction, 118
        Bayesian-based data analysis algorithm, 119
        GenMiR++, improving accuracy of, 119
        miRanda program, 118
        PicTar program, 118
        programs, major publicly available, 119
        rna22 program, 118, 119
        TargetScan program, 118
        TargetScanS program, 118
    tissue-specific, 119
    titer, levels of mRNAs and proteins, 126
    transcription factor interactions, 113
    transcription units, 114
    3′ untranslated region (UTR), 115, 117
    upregulation, 115
miRNA-mRNA interactions, 115
miRNA-mRNA pairing, 127
miRNA-UTR duplex, 36
Mitogen-activated protein kinases (MAPK), 342, 384
Mixed-integer non-linear program (MINLP), 195, 197–198
Model Comparator Tool, 275
Model control language, 295
Model systems, 403
    integration between, and clinical cancer omics data, 404f
Modern medicine, role of clinical trials in, 415–417
Modularization
    conceptual, 319–321
    implicatioons of, 324–325
Modules
    defined, 318
    in SBW, 296
Molecular entourages, identification of, 147
Molecular switches, 126–128

Monte Carlo multidimensional analysis sensitivity rankings of, 263, 264f
Morphogens, 226, 332–341
    multicell, application to, 244–245
    Shh, 336
    spatial patterning by, 333f
    transport
        role of receptor–ligand trafficking in, 334, 335f
Mouse, circadian rhythm of, 268–270
Mouse *mir-290-295* family, 113
Mouse sperm treatment with ENU, 34
MPVA. See MultiParametric Variability Analysis
MPVA-based approach, 195
mRNA
    decay activities, 124
    gene-specific, estimation in PCR, 31
    susceptibility to siRNA-mediated knockdown, 36
mTOR inhibitor, 395
Mtpn, myotrophin mRNA, 117
Multicolor/multiparameter flow cytometry, 8
Multicompartment models, 364–367
Multidimensional analysis, Monte Carlo sensitivity rankings of, 263, 264f
MultiParametric Variability Analysis, 195
Multiplexing strategies, 50
Muscle contraction, 157
Mutant mouse
    reverse genetics in, 35
    sperm treatment with ENU, 34–35
Myc pathways, 382
Myeloid cell leukemia-1 (MCL1), 395
MyoD, myogenic differentiation factor, 111

N

Na^+–Ca^{2+} exchanger (NCX), 206
N-acetylglucosaminyltransferase III (GnT-III) expression, 47
Nanog gene, 115
Nanog mRNA coding region, 129
Nanog transcription factors, 157
Natural killer (NK) cells, 354
ncRNAs, subclasses of, 65
N-ethyl-*N*-nitrosourea (ENU), 34–35
NetPhorest, 88
Network analyses, 7
Network Analysis Tools (NeAT), 94
NetworKIN, 88
Network model
    input information to construct, 7
    of subsystems, 8

Network motifs
    B-cell lymphomas, 79–80
    dysregulated interactions, 80
    ERK1, 79
    examples, 76
    feed-forward loops, 77–78
    gene co-expression, 79
    miR-17-92–E2F–Myc interaction, 78
    NF-κB localization, 76
    P53 and MDM2 (proteins), 76
    promoter motifs data, 78
    single-edge reactions, 75
    single-input module, 76–77
    transcription modules, 78–79
Networks
    cellular, agent-based modeling of. See Agent-based modeling (ABM)
    high-level modeling of. See High-level modeling
    transcriptional, Bayesian modeling of. See Bayesian networks
Neural tube, domain patterning ABM of, 242f–243f
New Species dialog box, 277f
NF-κ B. See Nuclear factor κB (NF-κ B)
N-fold cross-validation procedure, 75
NK cells. See Natural killer (NK) cells
Noise in gene expression, 122
Non-parametric procedures, 74
Non-TLR ligands, 186
Novel biomarkers
    predicting patient benefit from preclinical data for, 409–412
Nuclear factor κ B (NF-κ B), 384
Nuclear hormone receptors
    of oscillator loop, 10
    REV-ERB and ROR, 11
Nuclear receptor co-repressor (N-CoR), 60
Nucleocytoplasmic transport, 3D spatial simulation of, 281, 281f
Nucleosomes, 127

O

OCT4 and NANOG circuitries, 160
Oct4 binding site, mapping of, 159
ODE. See Ordinary differential equation (ODE)
Off-target effects, 41
Oligo expression array platforms, 27
Omics data, 404f
Oncogenic pathway, 393
Ontologies, 307
Oocyte maturation, 113
Optimization, of data quality, 253
Ordinary differential equation (ODE), 360
    JSIM models and, 295

Organ-level models, 4
  incorporate CellML into, 325–327
Orthogonal data
  definition, 6
Oscill8, 300
Oscillators, 9
Oscillatory system
  angular phase of, 256
  limit cycle behavior of, 256f
  period sensitivity and, 256–257
Overfitting problem, 74–75

P

p63, for stratified epithelial stem cells, 113
Paired-end ditag (PET), 157
Paracrine signaling, 179
PARP inhibitors, for *BRCA* -deficient tumors, 383
Partial differential equation (PDE)
  JSIM models and, 295
  spatial discretization of, in VCell, 282
Partial least squares modeling, 230–231
  implementation of, 231
  overview of, 228
  principal components analysis. *See* Principal components analysis
  Shh signaling networks. *See* Shh signaling networks, application to of Shh simulations, 232–234
Patched (Ptch1), 227, 227f
Pathway Studio, 94
Pattern recognition receptor (PRR), 354
P-bodies, 124
PCEnv, 299
PCR. *See* Polymerase chain reaction; Polymerase chain reaction (PCR)
p^{53}-dependent cell cycle, 385
PDGFR. *See* Platelet- derived growth factor receptor (PDGFR)
PER – CRY repressor complex degradation, 9
Perturbation analysis, 386–388, 416
PET sequencing technology, 157–158
Pharmacokinetic/pharmacodynamic experiments, 416
Pharmacologic kinetic model of lymphocyte biodistribution, 365, 366f
Phenotypic assays, 34
Phenotypic interactions, between genes/alleles, 5
PHOSIDA, 86
Phosphatases, 142, 146, 147, 149
Phosphatidylinositol bisphosphate, 143, 146, 184, 206

Phosphatidylinositol-4,5-bisphosphate (PIP2), 276, 277, 278f
Phosphatidyl inositol 3-kinase (PI3K), 405
Phosphatidylinositol (PtdIns) kinase family, 143, 145
Phosphatidylinositol triphosphate (PIP3), 143, 146
Phospho.ELM, 85
Phospholipase C beta (PLCβ), 184
Phosphopeptide binding domain
  binding site for, 89–90
  HPRD and ELM, 91
  Polo-box domain and BRCT domain, 90–91
  substrates identification, 90
Phosphopeptide binding domains, 89
Phosphopeptide databases
  HPRD, 85
  PHOSIDA, 86
  Phospho.ELM, 85
  PhosphoSitePlus, 85–86
  UniProtKB/Swiss-Prot, 85
Phosphoproteins, 84
Phosphorylation, 127, 140, 162, 167, 206, 207
Phosphorylation-mediated disruption of sequence-specific effects, 91
PhosphoSitePlus, 85–86
Phosphotyrosine phosphatase (PTP)-1B, 147
Physiome project, 325
Picotiter plate (PTP)
  DNA beads and enzyme beads deposition on, 20
  fiberoptic faceplate, 19
  in fixed order during sequencing run, 19
PI3K. *See* Phosphatidyl inositol 3-kinase (PI3K)
PIP2. *See* Phosphatidylinositol bisphosphate; Phosphatidylinositol-4,5-bisphosphate (PIP2)
PIP2 binding, 147
piwi-interacting RNAs (piRNAs), 111
PKC.DAG.Ca$_i$ complex, 207
Plasma membrane calcium ATPase (PMCA) pump, 206
Platelet aggregation, 418
Platelet-derived growth factor (PDGF), 199
Platelet- derived growth factor receptor (PDGFR), 381
Pleckstrin homology (PH), 147
Pluripotency, 111, 113
Pluripotent embryonic stem cells, 155

epigenetic and chromatin features, 166–168
POINTILLIST software, 187
Poisson stochastic processes, 284
Polycomb group proteins, 114
Polymerase chain reaction (PCR), 406
  and laser scanning technology integration, 31
  probe primer, 32
  microarray analysis, 31
  primer sets evaluation by, 31
  products, radio-labeling of, 30
  real-time quantitative, 31
  SyBr green dye incorporation during, 31
  TaqMan, 32
Polypharmacology, 381, 382f
Position × weight matrices (PWM), 161
Post-transcriptional control by miRNAs, 64–65
Post-transcriptional regulation, 111, 126, 129
PottersWheel, 300
pRb. *See* Retinoblastoma gene (pRb)
Preclinical data, predicting patient benefit from, for novel agents, 409–412
Predicting MicroRNA Targets, 117–119
Prey proteins, 33
pri-miRNA, 112
Principal components analysis, 228–229
  implementation of, 229–230
  vs. partial least squares, 231
Probability, conditional, 235–236
Probe primer, 32
Process modeling tool, 300
Prokaryotes, 254
ProMoT, 300
Prostate cancer, target-based therapy, 379
Protease inhibitor, pretreatment condition and, 357
Proteases, 142, 146
Protein-coding genes, 111, 113
Protein–DNA interaction, 158
Protein entourages, of Actin and PKC, 148
Protein kinase C (PKC), 147
Protein kinases
  catalytic activity, 84, 85
  domains, diversity among, 85
  downstream products of, techniques for identifying, 87
  protein phosphorylation by, 85
  in-vivo functions of, 89–91
  requirements for, 86

Protein kinases (*Continued*)
  putative substrates, database tools for identifying
    ELM, 88
    HPRD, 87–88
    NetworKIN, 88
  substrate specificities of, 87
Protein microarrays
  classes of, 51
  concept of, 50–51
  detection of binding in, 51
  for glycomic analysis, 51–52
  lectin arrays, 51–52
  uses of, 50
Protein networks
  analysis of
    computational modeling, 95–97
    pathway visualization, 93
    tools for, 94
    topological, 94–95
  knowledge integration for, 93
  protein interaction networks, 92
  signaling networks, 91, 92–93
Protein output, fine-tuning of, 123
Protein phosphatases, 91
Protein phosphorylation, in-vivo functions of
  conformational change induction, 89
  phosphopeptide binding domain
    binding site for, 89–90
    HPRD and ELM, 91
    Polo-box domain and BRCT domain, 90–91
  substrates identification, 90
  protein phosphatases, 91
  sequence-specific effects, 91
Protein–protein interaction (PPI) networks, 147, 161–162
Protein signaling networks, 91
  epidermal growth factor receptor as model for
    EGFR–EGFR homodimers, 98
    ErbB family, 97
    HER2-overexpressing cells, 99
    Kholodenko framework, 98
    PLSR modeling, 99
    Ras/Raf/MEK/ERK and PI3K/Akt pathways, 98
  proteomic and phosphoproteomic datasets, 92–93
Proteomics, 45
  of biological fluids
    biomarkers, 48
    in cancer, 48, 50
    isobaric tag labeling method, 50
  plasma proteins for disease-related changes, 48–49
  strategies, 48
  cell-based
    discovery workflow, 47
    enzyme activities, 47–48
    glycoproteins, 47
    isotopic labeling for, 46
    of ovarian adenocarcinoma cell lines, 46–47
    of ovarian cancer cell lines, 47
    post-translational modifications, 47
  computational aspects
    CPAS, 52
    datasets integration, 52–53
    transcriptomic data, 52
Proteomic states, complexity, 184–186
PRR. *See* Pattern recognition receptor (PRR)
Ptch1. *See* Patched (Ptch1)
Pyrosequencing, 17–18
PySCeS, 296
Python-based
  simulator, 296
  tool, 301

Q

Quantigene assays, 33
Quantitative model of I kappa B, 194
Quasi-one-dimensional case, 284

R

RA. *See* Retinoic acid (RA)
Radiation therapy, natural robustness of malignant cells, 388–389
Radio-labeling of polymerase chain reaction products, 30
Radivoyevitch, Tomas, 300
Ramsey, Stephen, 304
Rapamycin, 395
Ras-like gene, 166
Ras-mediated arrest, 113
RAS/mitogen-activated protein kinase (MAPK). *See* Mitogen-activated protein kinases (MAPK)
Ras pathways, 382
RAW 264.7 cells, 204, 208
Raw phase trajectories, 257, 257*f*
Reaction– diffusion equations, 282
Real-time PCR-based assays, 28
Real-time quantitative polymerase chain reaction, 31
Receptors
  accounting cycle for, 319, 320*f*
  conservation cycle for, 319, 321*t*

Receptor tyrosine kinases, signaling hubs for, 8
Reduced-order models
  for linear systems, 194
  re-estimated within constraints, 196
  using Matlab®, 196
Regulated on activation normal T cells expressed and secreted (RANTES), 187
Regulatory-cell-boosting therapies, for autoimmune diseases, 367
Regulatory proteins, 156
Reproducibility probability score, 156
REST, transcription repressor, 122
Retinoblastoma gene (pRb), 387
Retinoic-acid-induced differentiation, 165
  in mouse ESCs, 171
Retinoic acid (RA), 244
Retinoic treatment, 114
REV-ERBα induction by BMAL1/CLOCK, 9
Reverse-engineering algorithm, 163
Reverse transcriptase inhibitor, pretreatment condition and, 357
Reverse transcriptase-polymerase chain reaction, 30
Rheostat, 126
Rheumatoid arthritis, drug targets for, 370–372
  therapeutic responses in, 370
Rho-family GTPases, 142
Ribonucleoprotein RNA-induced silencing complex (RISC), 112
RISC components, 124
RISC–miRNA complex, 112
RNA detection using Luminex assays, 33
RNAi. *See* RNA interference (RNAi)
RNAi-mediated depletion approach, 166
RNA-induced silencing complex (RISC), 112
RNA interference (RNAi), 110, 160, 184
  alternative formats for target identification, 405, 406*t*
  as biological mechanism, 35
  delivery methods, 36–37
  intelligent design of, 39
  libraries, 39
  machinery, 112
  in mammalian cells
    dsRNA, 37
    siRNA selection process, 37–38
  as synthetic lethality, 406–407, 407*t*
  in systems biology, 40
  use of, 39
RNAi screening, factors influencing experimental design of

duration of inhibition, 40
off-target effects, 41–42
routes of RNAi administration, 40
shRNA vectors, 41
target mRNA reduction, 42
using pools of vectors, 40–41
RNA-mediated interference (RNAi), 383
RNA pol II promoters, 61
RNA polymerase II, 112
RNA polymerase (RNAP) binding, 163
RNA processing, 157
RNase III enzyme, 112
RNA transport, 157
Robustness, representation of, 5–6
Roche/454 sequencing platform
  DNA library preparation process in, 18
  pyrosequencing in, 17–18
  titanium, 20
ROM. *See* Reduced-order models (ROM)
R Packages, 300
R statistics package, 187
RTK. *See* Receptor tyrosine kinases (RTK)

S

Saccharomyces cerevisiae, 258, 383
Saccharomyces pombe, 383
SAM analysis, 156
Sandwich assays, 51
Sanger sequencing, 17
SBGN. *See* Systems Biology Graphical Notation (SBGN)
SBML. *See* Systems Biology Markup Language (SBML)
SBML-based Parameter Estimation Tool (SBMLPET), 300–301
SBMLPET. *See* SBML-based Parameter Estimation Tool (SBMLPET)
SBML (Systems Biology Markup Language), 305–306
  VCell and, 276
SBMLToolbox, 301
SBML-to-XPP translator, 300
SBO. *See* Systems Biology Ontology (SBO)
SBToolbox², 296
SBW. *See* Systems Biology Workbench (SBW)
SCAMP, 295
Scheduled treatment interruption (STI), 358–360
Scores vectors, 229–230
Second-generation sequencing technologies
  platform in, 17
  vs. Sanger-based capillary electrophoresis, 17

Second International Study of Infarct Survival (ISIS-2), 418
Sensitivity Analysis
  circadian rhythms and. *See* Circadian rhythms
  classical, review of, 251
  Fas apoptosis model and, 260–262, 260f
  hypothesis generation and discrimination, 253
  low-level model, of Shh network, 233–234, 234f
  for mathematical model refinement, 251–252
  matrices for, 255–258
  optimization of data quality, 253
  stochastic systems and, 253–255
  UPR and, 258–259
Sensitivity measures, 266f
Sequencer
  flow cell, 19
  genome analyzer, 20
  Roche/454 sequencing platform. *See* Roche/454 sequencing platform
Sequence-specific DNA binding transcription factors/activators, 60
Sequencing technologies
  second-generation, 17
  for templates, 22
SERCA pump, 207
Serial analysis of gene expression (SAGE), 26, 156
S662G mutation, 9
SH2 domains, 149
Shh. *See* Sonic hedgehog (Shh)
Shh signaling networks, application to gene expression data and, 237–238
  low-level model of, 231–232
  sensitivity analysis of, 233–234, 234f
  parameters of, 232
short gastrulation (*sog*), 336
Short hairpin RNAs
  specificity validation, 165
  vectors encoding, 38
shRNA. *See* Short hairpin RNAs (shRNAs)
Sigmoid, 309
Signal transduction, 324
SILAC-based quantitative mass spectrometry, 46
Silencers, 62
Silencing short interfering RNAs (siRNA)
  knockdown efficiency, 36–37, 38
  and miRNAs, 36
SimWiz, 297

Single nucleotide polymorphisms (SNP), 8
siRNA. *See* Silencing short interfering RNAs (siRNA)
SIRS. *See* Systemic inflammatory response syndrome (SIRS)
Skin miRNA, 113
Sleep disorders, 9
sloppyCell, 301
Smo. *See* Smoothened (Smo)
Smoothened (Smo), 227
Soft tissue tumors, molecular characterization of, 74
Software
  libraries. *See* Libraries, software
  in modeling biochemical networks, 292–293
  need for, 292
  test suites, 309
  tools, for modeling, 293
    BioNetGen, 299
    cellerator/xcellerator, 299
    commercial, 301
    COPASI, 294–295
    E-Cell, 299–300
    Jarnac, 295
    JigCell, 300
    JSIM, 295
    MathSBML, 295–296
    Oscill8, 300
    PottersWheel, 300
    ProMoT, 300
    PySCeS, 296
    R Packages, 300
    SBMLPET, 300–301
    SBMLToolbox, 301
    SBToolbox², 296
    SBW, 296–297
    sloppyCell, 301
    VCell, 297
  visual editors. *See* Editors, visual
  XPPAUT, 301
sog. *See* Short gastrulation (*sog*)
SOLiD platform, 22
  DNA library preparation using, 23
  sequencing chemistry, 25
Soluble cues. *See* Morphogens
Sonic hedgehog (Shh), 226. *See also* Shh signaling networks, application to morphogens, 336
  signaling pathway, 227f
  stimulation, partial least squares modeling of, 232–234
SOSLib, 302
Sox family of transcription factors, 157
Sox2 gene, 115

Spatial discretization, of PDE, in VCell, 282
Spatial modeling, VCell, 283
Spatial models, 364–367
Spatial patterning, 333f
Spatial simulation, 3D, 281, 281f
Specification cues
  long-range, 332–341
  morphogens, 332–341
  short-range, 330–332
    Delta/Notch signaling pathway in, 330, 331f
  signals downstream of
    processing, refining, and integrating, 341–346
specific short interfering RNA (siRNA), 146
Splenectomy, 365
Src homology 2 (SH2) domain, 147
Src homology 3 (SH3) domain, 147
SRES. See Stochastic ranking evolution strategy (SRES)
SSA. See Stochastic simulation algorithm (SSA)
Standards, for modeling
  CellML. See CellML
  graphical layout, 306
  MIRIAM, 306–307
  SBML. See SBML (Systems Biology Markup Language)
  SBO, 307
Static pseudocausal directional networks, 189
Stem cells, 154–155
  factors, 114
  model, 113, 115
  for systems biology, 155–156
STI. See Scheduled treatment interruption (STI)
S/T kinases, 146, 149
Stochastic ranking evolution strategy (SRES), 300
Stochastic simulation, 202–203. See also Computational models, challenges in building
  methods for, 202
  in parameter estimation studies, 202–203
  tools for, 303–304
Stochastic simulation algorithm (SSA), 254–255, 291
Stochastic switching mechanism, 82
Stochastic systems, 253–255
StochKit, 304
StochSim, 304
STRING (protein–protein interaction database), 88
Su(H). See Suppressor of Hairless (Su(H))

Suppressor of Hairless (Su(H)), 330
Suprachiasmatic nucleus (SCN), 9
Swiss-Prot. See UniProtKB
SwissProt database, 276
SyBr green dye, incorporation during polymerase chain reaction, 31
Synthetic lethality, 382–385
  DNA repair, 383
  loss-of-function mutation in, 383
  RNAi as, 406–407, 407t
  RNAi in, 383
Systemic inflammatory response syndrome (SIRS), 210, 369
Systems analysis, prerequisite for, 7
Systems biology
  characteristics, 4
  critical enabling factors for, 16
  definition, 4
  epistatic relationships, 5
  experimental strategies in, 6–7
  RNA interference approaches in
    Caenorhabditis elegans, 36–37
    Drosophila melanogaster, 36–37
    mammalian cells, 37–38
Systems Biology Graphical Notation, 298
Systems Biology Graphical Notation (SBGN), 306
Systems Biology Markup Language (SBML), 292
Systems biology markup language (SBML), 183
Systems Biology Ontology (SBO), 307
Systems Biology Workbench (SBW), 296–297
Systems biomedicine
  definition, 4, 7
  vs. systems studies, 11
Systems-level analysis
  in living organisms, 377
Systems-level modeling, 180–181
Systems models
  biochemical kinetics, 16
  oscillators, 9
Systems pharmacology, cancer
  cancer therapeutic strategies, 388–390
  combination therapy, 382–385
  deconvoluting mechanisms, 385–386
  gene signatures, 394–395
  human diseases and drug action, 378–379
  molecule to system, 377–378
  novel biomarkers, 393–394
  perturbation analysis, 386–388
  systemic lethality, 382–385
  target-based therapy, 379–382
  transcriptome for novel targets, 390–393

T

Talin protein, 147
  domains and switchable links of, 150
TaqMan quantitative polymerase chain reaction assay, schematic of, 32
Target-based therapy, 379–382
  in breast cancer, 379
  in prostrate cancer, 379
  for solid tumour, 380
TATA box, 61
T cell receptor (TCR), 355
T cells, 113
  anti-idiotypic regulatory, 368
  CD8 $^+$regulatory, 369
T cell vaccination (TCV), 368–369
TCR. See T cell receptor (TCR)
TCV. See T cell vaccination (TCV)
TEDDY. See Terminology for the Description of Dynamics (TEDDY)
Temporally causal networks, 189–190
Terminology for the Description of Dynamics (TEDDY), 307
Test suites, software, 309
Tetracycline-regulated Oct4 transgene, 165
TGF β. See Transforming growth factor-(TGF β)
Therapeutic development cycle, 417, 418f
Therapeutic nodes in anticancer treatment, 386f
Therapeutics, clinical trials of, 417–419
Thermodynamic limit, 254
Thickveins (Tkv), 336
Threshold cycle (C_T), 31
Time discretization, 282
Timing of cab (TOC1), 263
Tissue-level models, CellML and, 325–327
Tkv. See Thickveins (Tkv)
tld. See Tolloid (tld)
T lymphocyte, 354, 355, 368
TOC1. See Timing of cab (TOC1)
Toll-like receptor (TLR) ligands, 186
Tolloid (tld), 336
Topological analysis
  of protein interaction networks
    disease-related genes, 94–95
    disease-relevant subnetwork, 95
    signal transfer, 95
  of transcriptional network
    genetic buffers, 81
    HSP90, 81
    mice with mutations in miRNAs, 81–82
    power-law relationships, 80

scale-free networks, 81
transcription factor hubs, 80–81
Topology. *See* Networks, biological
Transcriptional machinery
  components of, 59
  co-regulators, 60
  enhanceosomes, 60–61
  general transcription factors, 59–60
  sequence-specific DNA binding
    transcription factors/activators,
    60
Transcriptional network analysis
  network motifs
    B-cell lymphomas, 79–80
    dysregulated interactions, 80
    ERK1, 79
    examples, 76
    feed-forward loops, 77–78
    gene co-expression, 79
    miR-17-92–E2F–Myc interaction, 78
    NF-κB localization, 76
    P53 and MDM2 (proteins), 76
    promoter motifs data, 78
    single-edge reactions, 75
    single-input module, 76–77
    transcription modules, 78–79
  statistical approaches
    association with disease outcome,
      73–74
    batch correction method, 74
    classifier, 74
    COMBAT algorithm, 74
    expression profiles of tumors,
      72–73
    hierarchical clustering, 73
    meta-analysis procedures, 74
    N-fold cross-validation procedure,
      75
    non-parametric procedures, 74
    overfitting problem, 74–75
  stochasticity in cellular systems, 82
  topological analysis, biological
    interactions
      genetic buffers, 81
      HSP90, 81
      mice with mutations in miRNAs,
        81–82
      power-law relationships, 80
      scale-free networks, 81
      transcription factor hubs, 80–81
Transcriptional regulation on genomic
  scale
  in breast cancer
    expression cassettes, 67
    molecular markers, 67
    p53 mutations and gene expression,
      association between, 68

transcriptional signatures, 66–67
to cancer patient prognosis
  cis-regulatory motifs binding, 70–71
  E2F binding motifs, 71
  embryonic stem cell expression,
    69–70
  ESC-specific binding of transcription
    factors, 71
  exogenous c-myc, 70
  five-gene genetic grade signature, 69
  gene expression "signatures", 68
  stem cell phenotype, 69
cis-regulatory motif role in, 66
mechanism-based approaches in
  DLBCLs
  gene expression, germinal center B
    cells, 71
  NF-κB activity, 72
organizational principles for, 65
in wound healing, 69
Transcriptional regulatory elements
  core promoter, 61
  enhancers
    functionality, 61
    location, 62
  insulators/boundary elements
    importance of, 62–63
    transcription regulation by, 63
  locus control regions (LCRs), 62
  silencers, 62
  upstream promoter elements, 61
Transcriptional regulatory networks
  gene expression regulation, 58
  and protein, mapping of, 58
  regulating self-renewal in ESCs, 166
Transcriptional regulatory region of
  gene, 59
Transcription factor binding sites, 28–29
Transcription factors, 111, 114
  Gli, 227
  mapping, 157–160
Transcription-factor-specific antibodies,
  28
Transcription networks, 156–157
Transcript loading of ribosomes, 123
Transcriptome
  assessment, 24, 58
  cloning strategies, 26
  complexity of, 65
  genomic representation of, 24, 26
  for novel targets, 390–393
Transcytosis, 334, 335*f*
TRANSFAC database, on 5 K upstream
  regions, 161
Transforming growth factor-β (TGFβ),
  333
Transient cues, 342*f*

Translationally repressed mRNAs, 129
Trimethylation, of histone 3 lysine 4
  (H3K4me3), 124
tsg. See Twisted gastrulation (tsg)
Tumor-cytotoxic virus, 367
Tumorigenesis, 113
Tumor–immune interaction
  mathematical models of, 361*f*
Tumor necrosis factor α, 369
Tumor necrosis factor (TNF) β, 187
Twisted gastrulation (tsg), 336
Two-hybrid screens
  bait of, 33
  molecular basis of, 33
  transcription initiation, reporter
    gene(s), 34
  yeast. *See* Yeast two-hybrid screens
Tyrosine kinases, 145, 149

U

Ubiquitination, 127
Unfolded Protein Response (UPR),
  258–259
  mean, sensitivity, 259*t*
UniProtKB, 85
UPR. *See* Unfolded Protein Response
  (UPR)
Upstream promoter elements (UPEs), 61
3' UTR silencing, 129

V

van der Pol oscillator, limit cycle
  behavior of, 256*f*
Vascular endothelial growth factor
  receptor (VEGFR), 381
VCell. *See* Virtual Cell (VCell)
VCML. *See* Virtual Cell Markup
  Language (VCML)
Vectors, 229–230
  encoding short hairpin RNAs, 38
VEGFR. *See* Vascular endothelial growth
  factor receptor (VEGFR)
VIC reporter probe, fluorescence of, 32
Vinculin, 149
Viral clearance, 357
Virtual Cell Markup Language (VCML),
  276
Virtual Cell (VCell), 297
  binding new species in, 276, 277*f*
  biomodel interface, modeling process
    in, 278–281, 279*f*
  CellML and, 276
  client–server architecture, 285
  database, 275–278
    import of reactions from, in Virtual
      Cell Reaction Editor, 278*f*

Virtual Cell (VCell) (*Continued*)
  defining new species in, 276, 277f
  framework of, 285, 286f
  impact of, 286t
  MIRIAM and, 276
  numerical algorithm in, 282–284
  overview of, 274–275
  SBML and, 276
  simulation process, 280, 280f
  spatial discretization of PDEs in, 282
  spatial modeling, 283
  web based deployment of, 285, 286f
  XML and, 275–276
Virtual patient validation, 371f
Visual editors, 297

CellDesigner, 298
commercial visual design tools, 298
JDesigner, 298
von Neumann, John Louis, 239

W

Web based deployment, of VCell, 285, 286f
Wg/Wnt. *See* Wingless (Wg/Wnt)
Whole-heart cardiac model, 325, 326t
Wiener, Norbert, 353
Wingless (Wg/Wnt), 333
Wnt pathways, 382

X

Xenopus oocyte, 342
XML (Extensible Markup Language)
  VCell and, 275–276
XPPAUT, 301

Y

Yeast two-hybrid screens, molecular components of, 34

Z

Zeitgeber, 267
Zfx-deficient ESCs, 166
Zfx gene, 166

有奖征集反馈意见

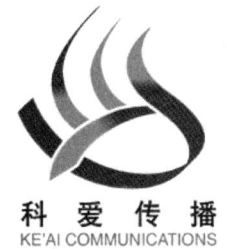

尊敬的读者：

科学出版社科爱森蓝文化传播有限公司（简称"科爱传播"）立足国际合作，致力于为科技专业人士提供优质的信息服务。我们很想通过自己的努力最大限度地满足您的需求，您的哪怕是一点点的建议和意见，都将成为我们改进工作的重要依据。

我们将在每年的 6 月份、12 月份各一次从半年的参与者中抽取幸运者 10 名，幸运者可以从"科爱传播"的出版物中任选价值 1000 元的图书（10 册以内）作为奖品（全部出版物信息可在我们的网站上查到）。

1. 您所购买的图书书名：《＿＿＿＿＿＿＿＿＿＿＿＿＿＿＿＿＿＿＿＿＿＿＿》

    您于＿＿＿年＿＿月＿＿日在（通过）＿＿＿＿＿＿＿＿＿＿＿购买到此书。

    你认为本书的定价：□偏高　　□合适　　□偏低
    你认为本书的内容有约＿＿％对您有用。

2. 你认为我们出版物的质量：

    内容质量（学术水平、写作水平）：□很好　□较好　□一般　□较差
    译介质量（翻译水平、文字水平）：□很好　□较好　□一般　□较差
    印制质量（印制、包装）：□很好　□较好　□一般　□较差

3. 您所在的专业领域：＿＿＿＿＿＿＿＿＿＿＿

4. 在你获取专业知识和专业信息的主要渠道中，排在前三位的是：

    1.＿＿＿＿　2.＿＿＿＿　3.＿＿＿＿
    A.网络　B.期刊　C.图书　D.报纸　E.电视　F.会议　G.内部交流　H.其他：＿＿＿

5. 你还需要哪些类型的图书？

    □专著　□教材　□实验手册　□辞典工具书　□文集　□其他：＿＿＿
    □书摘（原版书摘编）　□刊摘（国外学术期刊重要文献摘编）

6. 您还希望我们从国外引进哪些专业方向的图书（或期刊）？

7. 您建议采用何种引进形式？
   □翻译　□影印　□摘编（只从原书中选部分内容引进）
   □导读（原文影印加少量中文介绍）　□注解（原文影印加大量中文介绍）

8. 您是否愿意与我们合作，参与编写、编译、翻译图书或其他科技信息？

9. 请列举您近两年看过的，您认为最有参考价值、对您帮助最大的 1~2 本书：

书名	著作者	出版社	出版日期	定价

10. 您还有什么别的意见、建议？（可另附纸）

● 请告诉我们您准确的地址和联系办法：

   姓名：_____　性别：_____　生日：_____年__月__日
   单位：_____职务/职称：_____
   地址：_____
   E-mail：_____电话：_____
   传真：_____手机：_____

回邮地址（也可以通过 E-mail 反馈）：
北京东黄城根北街 16 号　科学出版社 科爱传播中心 杨 琴（收）　邮编：100717
联系电话：010-64006871；传真：010-64034056

编辑部电话：010-64034507
投稿及读者反馈：editor@kbooks.cn, keai@mail.sciencep.com
（注：本反馈单复印有效，也可以在线下载：http://www.kbooks.cn）